Register Now for Online Access to Your Book!

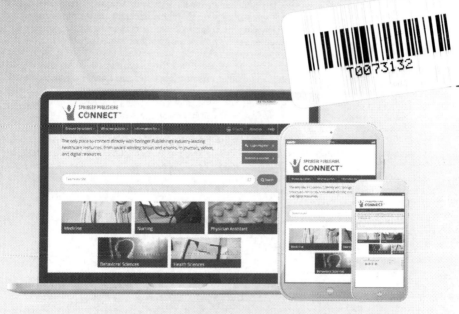

Your print purchase of *Legal and Ethical Issues in Nursing Education: An Essential Guide* **includes online access to the contents of your book**—increasing accessibility, portability, and searchability!

Access today at:
http://connect.springerpub.com/content/book/978-0-8261-6193-2
or scan the QR code at the right with your smartphone
and enter the access code below.

5EBE9M0U

Scan here for quick access.

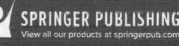

SPRINGER PUBLISHING
View all our products at springerpub.com

MARY ELLEN SMITH GLASGOW, PhD, RN, ACNS-BC, ANEF, FAAN, is Dean and Professor at Duquesne University School of Nursing. She completed a fellowship at Bryn Mawr College and HERS, Mid-America Summer Institute for Women in Higher Education Administration. Dr. Glasgow was selected as a 2009 Robert Wood Johnson Foundation Executive Nurse Fellow. As dean, under her leadership, enrollment and NCLEX-RN® scores increased, and research and scholarship have significantly expanded. The school is recognized as a national leader in nursing education, emphasizing social justice, digital technologies, and graduates with strong ethical reasoning skills. Recently, she led the development of the first dual undergraduate Biomedical Engineering and Nursing Program in the country, and a PhD in Nursing Ethics. Dr. Glasgow is an innovator in nursing and health professions, both nationally and internationally. Dr. Glasgow previously served as Associate Dean for Nursing, Undergraduate Health Professions, and Continuing Education and Chair of Undergraduate Programs at Drexel University. At Drexel, she created a BSN Co-op Program, BSN Accelerated Career Entry Program, Pathway to Health Professions Program, and other forward-thinking educational programs. She also advanced online pedagogy developing one of the largest online nursing programs in the country.

She previously served as Associate Editor for *Oncology Nursing Forum,* responsible for the Leadership and Professional Development feature. She is the coauthor of three books, two of which have won the *American Journal of Nursing* Book-of-the-Year Award, first place. She was inducted as a Fellow in the American Academy of Nursing and as an NLN Academy of Nursing Education Fellow. She has been honored with the Villanova University College of Nursing Alumni Medallion for Distinguished Contribution to Nursing Education, Gwynedd-Mercy University Distinguished Alumni Award, and the Nightingale Award of Pennsylvania. Recently, she served on the Health Service Executive and National Nursing and Midwifery Quality-Care Metrics Project Team to develop quality metrics for the country of Ireland. Dr. Glasgow brings years of academic administrative experience on the undergraduate and graduate levels as a co-author of this text, *Legal and Ethical Issues in Nursing Education: An Essential Guide.*

H. MICHAEL DREHER, PhD, RN, FAAN, ANEF, is currently the Associate Vice Provost at Medgar Evers College, City University of New York in Brooklyn, NY, and Professor in the Department of Nursing. Previously, he served as Associate Vice President for Healthcare Innovation and Special Projects, 2017 to 2019 at The College of New Rochelle (CNR). Previously he served as Dean of the School of Nursing and Healthcare Professions at CNR, 2014 to 2017. Dr. Dreher has long been an innovator in healthcare professions in and outside nursing education, both nationally and internationally. At Drexel, he co-created a BS in Nursing, which became the largest provider of nurses in Pennsylvania. He developed an MS in Nursing Innovation, and as Chair of the Doctoral Nursing Department, he also founded one of the first Doctor of Nursing Practice programs in the United States. He has served as Associate Editor of *Holistic Nursing Practice,* writing a column on "Innovation, Health, and Healing." In 2010, he was appointed as the only non-UK citizen to the UK Council on Graduate Education's *2011 Report on Professional Doctorates Review Panel.* He is the coauthor of five books, three of which have won the *American Journal of Nursing* Book-of-the-Year Award. He has been funded by the John A. Hartford Foundation, the Center for American Nurses, Health Resources and Services Administration, and various other agencies. He was inducted as a Fellow in the American Academy of Nursing in 2012 and an Academy of Nursing Education Fellow in 2017. He is a graduate of the University of South Carolina, Widener University, and the University of Pennsylvania.

MICHAEL D. DAHNKE, PhD, is a philosopher and bioethicist who has designed and taught courses in philosophy, ethics, bioethics, and medical humanities, currently teaching nursing ethics at the Mercy College and ethics and philosophy at the College of Staten Island. Prior to Mercy College, he was Clinical Associate Professor at the College of Nursing and Health Professions at Drexel University.

He is author of *Film, Art, and Filmart: An Introduction to Aesthetics through Film* (2007) and coauthor (with H. Michael Dreher, PhD, RN, FAAN, ANEF) of *Philosophy of Science for Nursing Practice* (2011, 2016 [second ed.]), awarded *American Journal of Nursing* Book-of the-Year Award second place, research division. His research interests include end-of-life ethics, ethics education for health professions students, and ethics and family caregiving. His recent publications include "Devotion, Diversity, and Reasoning: Religion and Medical Ethics" (*Journal of Bioethical Inquiry*), "What We Learn (and Don't Learn) from the Terri Schiavo Autopsy" (*Functional Neurology, Rehabilitation, and Ergonomics*), and "Utilizing Codes of Ethics in Health Professions Education" (*Advances in Health Sciences Education*).

JOHN GYLLENHAMMER, JD, joined the Drexel University Office of the General Counsel in 1997. Mr. Gyllenhammer is the chief attorney responsible for all legal matters affecting the College of Medicine, College of Nursing and Health Professions, and the School of Public Health, and serves as the Office's managing attorney for all administrative, financial, and personnel matters. He provides legal counsel and support to senior management, department chairs, faculty, and staff in a wide variety of areas including contracts and business transactions, healthcare law, litigation prevention and management, faculty and student affairs, sponsored research, patient safety, regulatory compliance, real estate, and employment law matters. John has worked in higher education law since 1992. Prior to joining the Office of the General Counsel, John spent 5 years in the Legal Affairs Office at George Mason University in Virginia, from which he received his Juris Doctor. He received his Bachelor of Arts from the State University of New York at Binghamton.

Legal and Ethical Issues in Nursing Education

AN ESSENTIAL GUIDE

Mary Ellen Smith Glasgow, PhD, RN, ACNS-BC, ANEF, FAAN
H. Michael Dreher, PhD, RN, FAAN, ANEF
Michael D. Dahnke, PhD
John Gyllenhammer, JD

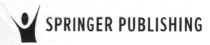

Springer Publishing Company, LLC
11 West 42nd Street, New York, NY 10036
www.springerpub.com
connect.springerpub.com/

Acquisitions Editor: Joseph Morita
Compositor: S4Carlisle Publishing Services

ISBN: 978-0-8261-6192-5
ebook ISBN: 978-0-8261-6193-2
DOI: 10.1891/9780826161932

Qualified instructors may request supplements by emailing textbook@springerpub.com

Instructor's Manual ISBN: 978-0-8261-5608-2

20 21 22 23 / 5 4 3 2 1

The author and the publisher of this Work have made every effort to use sources believed to be reliable to provide information that is accurate and compatible with the standards generally accepted at the time of publication. The author and publisher shall not be liable for any special, consequential, or exemplary damages resulting, in whole or in part, from the readers' use of, or reliance on, the information contained in this book. The publisher has no responsibility for the persistence or accuracy of URLs for external or third-party Internet websites referred to in this publication and does not guarantee that any content on such websites is, or will remain, accurate or appropriate.

Library of Congress Cataloging-in-Publication Data
Names: Glasgow, Mary Ellen Smith, editor. | Dreher, Heyward Michael,
  editor. | Dahnke, Michael D., editor. | Gyllenhammer, John, editor.
Title: Legal and ethical issues in nursing education : an essential guide /
  Mary Ellen Smith Glasgow, Heyward Michael Dreher, Michael Dahnke, John Gyllenhammer, editors.
Description: First Springer Publishing edition. | New York : Springer
  Publishing Company, [2021] | Includes bibliographical references and index.
Identifiers: LCCN 2020018440 (print) | LCCN 2020018441 (ebook) | ISBN
  9780826161925 (paperback) | ISBN 978-0-8261-5608-2 (instructor's manual) | ISBN 9780826161932 (ebook)
Subjects: MESH: Education, Nursing--legislation & jurisprudence |
  Education, Nursing–ethics | Civil Rights | Liability, Legal | United States
Classification: LCC RT71 (print) | LCC RT71 (ebook) | NLM WY 33 AA1 | DDC 610.73071–dc23
LC record available at https://lccn.loc.gov/2020018440
LC ebook record available at https://lccn.loc.gov/2020018441

Printed in the United States of America.

To my husband Tom, my strongest supporter. What can I say about a man who is intelligent, kind, and a great cook; I am so glad we found each other.

MEG

To my partner in life and husband, Michael D. Dahnke, who I count on 24/7 and to Freud, Drucilla, Eudora, Reggie, Buddy, Wayne, and Mandy, you gave us a lot and a couple of you still do.

HMD

To H. Michael Dreher, my loving husband and personal expert on all matters of nursing education.

MDD

I dedicate this book to the three most important persons who have touched my life. My wife Renee, and my parents Elaine and Roland. Words can never adequately express what I owe to each of you for the love, understanding, support, and encouragement you have given to me. You will always be in my thoughts and heart.

JG

Contents

Section I REVISITING THE LEGAL PROCESS

Section II THE ETHICS DIMENSION OF LEGAL AND ETHICAL ISSUES IN NURSING EDUCATION

Section III LEGAL AND ETHICAL CASES WITH NURSING STUDENTS, FACULTY, AND ADMINISTRATORS

Section IV SPECIFIC CLINICAL EDUCATION ISSUES

Section V SPECIFIC ISSUES CONFRONTING ADJUNCT FACULTY IN THE CLINICAL AGENCY AND CLASSROOM

Contributors

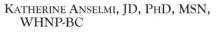

KATHERINE ANSELMI, JD, PhD, MSN,
WHNP-BC
Clinical Professor
Drexel University College of Nursing and
Health Professions
Philadelphia, Pennsylvania

SETH BECKMAN, DA
Dean of the College of Fine Arts
Ball State University
Muncie, Indiana

STEPHEN F. GAMBESCIA, PhD, MEd, MBA,
MHum, MCHES
Clinical Professor
Drexel University College of Nursing and
Health Professions
Philadelphia, Pennsylvania

MARCIA R. GARDNER, PhD, RN,
CPNP, CPN
Dean and Professor
Barbara H. Hagan School of Nursing
Molloy College
Rockville Centre, New York

ANDREW LOGAN-GRAF, MA, PC
Associate Director, Disability Services
Duquesne University
Pittsburgh, Pennsylvania

WILLIAM LORMAN, JD, PhD, PMHNP-BC,
CARN-AP, FIAAN, FAAN
Clinical Assistant Professor
Drexel University College of Nursing and
Health Professions
Philadelphia, Pennsylvania

FAYE A. MELOY, PhD, RN, MSN, MBA
Dean, Allied Health, Emergency Services
and Nursing
Delaware County Community College
Media, Pennsylvania

CARL "TOBEY" OXHOLM III, JD
Senior Vice President and General Counsel
(Retired)
Drexel University College of Medicine
Philadelphia, Pennsylvania

ENEST RICHARDS, MPH, MS, RN
Assistant Professor
Department of Nursing
Medgar Evers College
City University of New York
Brooklyn, New York

JAMES SCHREIBER, PhD
Professor
Advanced Role Department
Duquesne University School of Nursing
Pittsburgh, Pennsylvania

CYNTHIA STERLING-FOX, FNP, MS, RN
Assistant Professor
Department of Nursing
Medgar Evers College of the City University
of New York
Brooklyn, New York

ADAM WASILKO, ED. D.
Assistant Vice President, Student Involvement
Director, Disability Services
Duquesne University
Pittsburgh, Pennsylvania

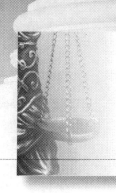

Note From the Authors

The case studies in this book are drawn principally from the experiences of the two nurse educator coauthors of this book. The judgments about the facts, the conduct, and the better practices are theirs alone, not that of Drexel University, nor of the lawyer coauthor, John Gyllenhammer. He has participated in the editing of each chapter, and we thank him for his contributions, but we hasten to note that, as in legal practice, the lawyer does not have to share his client's opinions, and "for the record," we do have our differences—but the clients get to decide. As Drexel's chief attorney responsible for all legal matters affecting the College of Medicine, College of Nursing and Health Professions, and School of Public Health, for close to a decade, John Gyllenhammer is charged with the primary responsibility for counseling and representing the College of Nursing and Health Professions, and was our "go-to" attorney for many years whenever the College faced a "hot issue." His experience and expertise are broad; quick to recognize when more in-depth legal knowledge is appropriate, he has called on several colleagues with whom he works in Drexel's Office of the General Counsel to take the lead in editing chapters related to their respective legal expertise. We wish to acknowledge and thank them here:

DANA AUGUSTE, JD, MS
Associate General Counsel
Office of the General Counsel
Drexel University
Philadelphia, Pennsylvania
Chapters 22 and 23

PAUL FLANAGAN, JD, MS
Assistant Professor of Law
Director of Privacy, Cybersecurity and Compliance
   Program
Thomas R. Kline School of Law
Philadelphia, Pennsylvania
Chapters 7 and 8

JARED MILLER, JD 2021
Candidate
Thomas R. Kline School of Law
Drexel University
Philadelphia, Pennsylvania
Chapters 7 and 8

TIMOTHY RAYNOR, JD, MS
Associate General Counsel
Office of the General Counsel
Drexel University
Philadelphia, Pennsylvania
Chapter 11

Foreword

Nursing education situates within two of the most highly regulated and compliance-driven industries in modern times: higher education and healthcare. Practitioners in this important field confront on a daily basis clinical and educational questions that stem from an overriding concern for doing the right thing for the individual. From state laws, to federal regulations, to institutional policies, to common sense, a dizzying array of considerations come into play for nurse educators seeking to teach ethical practitioners. Perhaps in no other field of education do hypothetical problems for the student so quickly become "real-world" problems in practice.

Like talented nurses everywhere, this book fills a void and meets a need. Students and educators alike will benefit from its straightforward, accessible treatment of complex topics, such as addressing students with mental health issues and managing student complaints of discrimination. In addition to perpetually problematic issues like academic freedom, conflicts of interest, and substance misuse, the book also addresses topics of more recent vintage, such as medical marijuana and nursing students, and managing professional boundaries with students in the age of social media. Chapters are replete with real-life scenarios, case studies, and prevention tips that will allow readers to prepare for confronting complex decisions with confidence grounded in knowledge. Ample case references in each chapter provide opportunity for further exploration of topics of interest.

Nurse educators and students with no background in law or ethics will not be put off by this book's topical approach to practice-based problems. Drawing on the diverse expertise of its authors, the book should become a go-to reference for anyone looking to make sound decisions in the modern nursing landscape that is so often marked with peril for the uninitiated or uninformed.

JACOB H. ROOKSBY, JD, PhD

Dean and Professor
Gonzaga University School of Law
Spokane, Washington

Preface

"You'll be hearing from my lawyer!"

Unfortunately, this is a phrase that all too many of us get to hear in our lives. In many sectors, including academia, it has become the "trump card" in how students and faculty think they can get a dispute resolved their way: threaten to get "the lawyers" involved, and people cave.

If you practice the healing arts and teach others who will do the same, your objective is to care for patients and teach students to do so; but you will not always be able to help individuals as much as you (or they) will like, and sometimes there will be an adverse result. In academia, there will be disputes—about agreements allegedly made, quality of services rendered, costs incurred, attitudes expressed. With our society becoming increasingly diverse, the opportunities for misunderstanding—and causing offense—are expanding rapidly.

The law is the framework that allows each of us to deal with others in a predictable way.[1] For centuries, the courts have been where disputes were resolved. Our modern legal practices date back over eight centuries to England in 1215 and the Magna Carta—a reform imposed upon the king by the populace, which, among many other things, guaranteed that disputes between the people would be decided by the people themselves in their own community, in public. This system of justice—trial by jury—remains the dominant feature of American law, but it is no longer the primary way that disputes are resolved. In most cases and for most people, lawyers and courts are too formal, too slow, and too expensive. But they are always there, waiting for when other methods fail.

The first chapter discusses rights and claims, the different ways they get resolved, and the process that dispute resolution typically takes. The next chapters provide a quick overview of the legal principles and specific laws that all nursing faculty need to know and provide some instruction on how to read "a case." Then the role of university counsel is addressed. The remaining chapters analyze academic nursing cases in order to provide the reader with legal background, prevention tips, and resources to navigate common and not-so-common legal issues in nursing education. Society has become increasingly litigious. This book will serve as a resource to aspiring nursing faculty, current faculty, and academic administrators on how to manage legal issues encountered in their daily professional lives.

This book, *Legal and Ethical Issues in Nursing Education: An Essential Guide* was conceptualized based on a previous book which bears a similar name, *Legal Issues Confronting Today's Nursing Faculty: A Case-Study Approach*. This text provides aspiring nursing faculty, current faculty, and academic administrators with practical advice on how to deal with the vast array of legal issues that arise in nursing education. These issues are *rarely addressed* in the literature, and faculty often struggle with how to solve some of the legal issues they confront daily in the classroom

---

[1] Everybody knows the famous quote from Shakespeare's *Hamlet*: "The first thing we do, we kill all the lawyers." While this is commonly thought to be a slam against attorneys, it is in fact an accolade. The persons discussing this strategy were intent on causing social chaos. They knew that, in the absence of law and those who "guarded" it, they could better achieve their ends.

and clinical environment. This book assists faculty in making real-life decisions about academic issues such as harassment, discrimination, academic dishonesty, and conflict of interest, with the legal bases in mind. The two nursing faculty authors, Drs. Mary Ellen Smith Glasgow and H. Michael Dreher, have extensive backgrounds in academic nursing administration (as Chair, Associate Dean, Dean, and Associate Provost); management of large, complex nursing programs; and expertise in the faculty role. The university attorney author, John Gyllenhammer, has served as chief attorney responsible for all legal matters affecting a College of Medicine, College of Nursing and Health Professions, and a School of Public Health at a large, private university for 20 years. The authors offer their knowledgeable perspectives on how to address simple and complex nursing academic legal issues based on their collective experience. A unique feature of this book is Section II: The Ethics Dimension of Legal and Ethical Issues in Nursing Education, written by philosopher and ethicist, Michael D. Dahnke. Dr. Dahnke provides an ethical perspective to each legal case study presented throughout the book.

Whether you are a new or seasoned nursing professor/academic, nursing administrator, or graduate student taking a master's or doctoral nursing program in legal issues in nursing education course, we believe this text can serve as an important guide for your career. The nursing education environment today is complex and challenging. Navigating the legal issues that every faculty member will at some point face (regardless of role) requires, at minimum, some familiarity with critical higher education legal issues and their management, in addition to attention to the ethical considerations.

MEG
HMD
MDD
JRG

Acknowledgments

To Carl "Tobey" Oxholm III, attorney author on our first legal book, *Legal Issues Confronting Today's Nursing Faculty: A Case-Study Approach*, who has a brilliant legal mind and tons of energy. We appreciate your expertise and contributions. Many thanks! MEG, HMD, MDD, and JG

To Susan Pickup, my niece, and Pittsburgh girlfriend, I am glad you decided to stay in Pittsburgh after Law School; it is great to have your friendship and support. MEG

To Karen Robson, a Duquesne University School of Nursing PhD student and my graduate assistant; thanks for your exemplary research for this book. MEG

Authors' Disclaimer

We have a combined 58 years of university nursing education experience and 27 years of university legal experience. The case studies utilized in this book are not "fact," but composites drawn from that experience, as well as from the decided case law so that we can discuss the specific points at issue in the chapter. All the names of the characters in the case studies are fictional.

We have included copies of policies and procedures in use at Drexel University at the time this book was being written. We are happy to share these as examples, but they are only examples. Drexel University is a private university—in corporate form, a private not-for-profit corporation. It is governed by a charter, articles of incorporation, and bylaws. Its faculty members are not unionized, and there are no collective bargaining agreements with faculty. It has not adopted, officially or unofficially, the policies or procedures of the American Association of University Professors (AAUP), whose policies and procedures we have also referenced. Finally, Drexel is located in Philadelphia, Pennsylvania, which has a fairly well-developed body of judicial case law applicable to higher education. As a result, the Drexel policies and procedures have been developed to fit Drexel's situation and should only be considered as an example. And our lawyer-authors are quick to add that they are offered entirely without any warranties or representations. You really should check with your university counsel before using these examples at your institution.

As this book will make clear, "the law" is not a "one-size-fits-all" menu, nor is it a list of rules and regulations that you can consult and get specific answers in every situation. Lawyers are famous for giving "two-handed advice"—"on the one hand, this; on the other, that"—for good reason: Judges have issued opinions that are diametrically opposed in virtually identical situations, and legislators have not been comprehensive (or even thoughtful) when they add the "next" piece of legislation to an already complicated area.

What this means is that judgment on your part is always involved; and what the lawyer does is provide advice on how to increase the likelihood that one answer will be the final answer in a particular situation. What this also means is that this book provides examples, but not specific legal advice, on ways to address situations that we face regularly, if not every day. How we interact with students is driven by the same legal principles that apply to how we interact with colleagues (employees), so there is overlap in the discussion; and you ought to read pairs of chapters (for students/for faculty) to more fully understand what is going on in the legal realm.

In many ways, the point of this book is to get you to the point of appreciating the legal framework that provides the structure of our business. Sometimes—even most of the time—the principles will be easy to apply, and the way to resolve a situation will be clear. The higher the "price" of a wrong decision, the more the bottom line becomes clear: Consult your own university counsel.

I

REVISITING THE LEGAL PROCESS

1

An Introduction to the Legal Process: A Primer

THE ORIGIN OF RIGHTS

"You cannot do this to me. I know my rights!"

In fact, virtually none of us knows our rights. What we have is a sense of entitlement that results from living in one of the world's richest countries, having the privilege of attending a college or university, and enjoying the luxury of reading and thinking. Add to this situation an excess of lawyer advertising[1] and the publicity given to some seemingly outrageous jury awards.[2]

In a legal sense, rights come from a number of sources that can be identified and consulted.[3] These include the following:

- Contracts: Agreements both oral and written in which one party obligates itself to do something for another
- Common law: Rules and principles arising from the judgments of juries and judges and the way that they articulate the bases for their decisions
- Statutory law: Rules that legislatures of all levels have enacted
- Administrative law: Rules and procedures that have been developed by government agencies charged with the interpretation and enforcement of statutes
- Constitutional law: Pronouncements made in a federal or state government's highest charter
- International law: Treaties among nations and the laws of other nations

A variety of rights can be involved in a particular event. For example, it is a crime to hit someone. That means the conduct violates a written law that is part of the criminal code (perhaps of both the state and federal government). It is also a violation of the common law (battery), because that law protects the "right to bodily integrity" even if the state had not also stepped in. These rules have different consequences if they are broken. Break a criminal statute, and one can be put in jail and made to pay a fine, which goes to the state; violate the common law, and one will pay money (damages or restitution) to the victim.

There are also two systems of justice at work: state and federal. In most cases, it is only the law of the state in which the dispute arose that will matter. In some instances, however, there is an overlay of

---

[1] It is virtually impossible to complete a round-trip to campus from home without seeing or hearing an advertisement for a lawyer, making it clear that a (bad) situation is someone else's fault, and that the lawyer will fight "to the death" to vindicate your rights. They have toll-free numbers and promise that there will not be a fee "unless we win for you." What's not to like?

[2] How many tens of millions of dollars did that woman win from McDonald's, after she sued because the fresh cup of coffee she had purchased from the drive-through and placed between her legs spilled and scalded her?

[3] This is to distinguish the discussion of rights as lawyers and judges argue about them from the kinds of inherent rights that flow from religious or political philosophies. The latter typically inform the former, but only the former can be cited to a court or a judge as justification for a particular position.

federal rights and obligations stemming from the Constitution of the United States, the laws enacted by Congress and the president, and the rules and regulations promulgated by federal agencies. When a federal contract or right is involved in a dispute, federal law is triggered and the federal courts can become involved. If the person one has punched has rights that are protected by federal law (e.g., the right to be free of discrimination on the basis of age, sex, race, disability, or national origin), one's conduct may be subject to investigation in two proceedings at the same time.

In academia, rights under the law can acquire new and added dimensions. It is likely, for example, that a university prohibits faculty members from punching a colleague or a student—it's far enough removed from academic freedom to be punishable as a violation of the university's code of conduct. Faculty could be suspended or even lose a job. That's a matter of contract law: When faculty members took the job (or when students accepted the offer of admission), they agreed to live by the rules of the university. Not knowing that was a possible consequence of their actions is not a defense.[4]

Another example worth considering is academic dishonesty. Suppose a junior member of the faculty, intent on tenure, is "creative" in their research, borrowing data from another source and claiming it as their own, and entirely making up other data. The original author had her work stolen, so there is a violation of the common law. The university has its most fundamental precept of integrity dashed, so the employment contract was broken. The researcher may also have violated the terms of a grant that was funding the research, threatening adverse consequences to the university (possibly disqualification from future grants, not to mention damage to its reputation). It may have violated federal or state regulatory requirements, for which there might be fines or penalties. And what about those who read the fraudulent results and relied on them—perhaps using a therapy that really was not proved and that ended up causing harm? All of a sudden, satisfying tenure requirements seems inconsequential.

DECIDING WHO'S RIGHT

We all decide dozens of disputes every day—conflicts in our calendars, disagreements in an approach to a problem, competition for a parking spot, and confrontations with aggressive drivers. We don't spend much time or effort on them because they are so small. The bigger the issue—the more important to our future, our family, or our wallet—the more time and effort we'll spend. And when it's really important, that's when most of us head for a lawyer.

Because of the way that our country was founded, we strive to make our courts open to those who have complaints. Not only are the filing fees relatively low, but in the United States, plaintiffs can engage their attorneys on a contingency fee basis, meaning that the attorney will be paid only out of money won for the plaintiff; and the attorney is even allowed to pay the out-of-pocket costs for the plaintiff on the same basis.

Going to court can be incredibly expensive for defendants—costs can easily rise to six figures to defend hotly disputed claims such as employment discrimination or medical malpractice. Oftentimes defendants won't get the opportunity to testify or to defend themselves at trial because they signed away that right to their insurance company in the policy they bought: For the insurance company, it's only money, and the company is not obligated to worry about the defendant's reputation. Insurance companies also know that juries (and judges) make mistakes, and sure-win claims can be lost. Even a "win" at trial won't mean it's over (or that the meter has stopped running), because decisions can be easily taken to an appellate court.

The expense, the time, and the publicity involved in litigation are all reasons that people have decided to take their disputes to other places to have them resolved. "Alternative dispute resolution" is a phrase that encompasses many different methods, each of which one may experience as a member of a college or university faculty.

---

[4] This is where the phrase "ignorance of the law is no excuse" comes from. Because the law is what sets the boundaries of behavior, all of us have the right to expect that those boundaries will be observed—whatever they are. If one crosses a line unknowingly, this violates someone else's rights; and the fact that it was not intended, and the offender didn't realize it, does not reduce that other person's right. Where ignorance does come into play is often in considering the remedy for the misconduct: Intentional bad acts get punished far more severely than do innocent ones. In most instances, the amount of the punishment is left to the discretion of the decision-maker (judge, juror, arbitrator, or other decider).

OMBUDSMAN

Often a university has a standing position called the *ombudsman*. This is not a process but a person who is available to help resolve certain kinds of complaints or issues. This person has no power, cannot order anyone to do anything, and cannot punish anyone for not participating. The university cannot force anyone to use ombudsmen. They don't decide anything. All they can do is ask questions, make suggestions, and help the disputants work through their issues. Typically, the ombudsman is someone whom everyone respects and holds in high regard; typically, the ombudsman is sworn to secrecy, keeps no notes, and cannot be forced to divulge what anyone said. But "typically" means not always: The role of the ombudsman is defined by university policy or procedure, which must be read carefully.

MEDIATION

Like the ombudsman, a *mediator* helps disputants reach an agreed-on solution, but the mediator's role is more formal than that of the ombudsman: There is a process to be followed and the expectations for each are better defined. The disputants often get to choose the person who will serve as the mediator. The mediator is subject to a code of ethics. The mediation process is typically described in a written document to which the disputants are required to agree, but in all respects it is a voluntary process that requires agreement of both sides every step along the way.

Before actually tackling the problem at hand, the mediator will typically require the different sides to discuss and agree on the way the mediation will be handled, dates, what issues will be discussed, whether they will submit written materials (e.g., their statements of claims and defenses), ground rules for behavior (complete confidentiality being the most important), and when and how the process might end. The role of the mediator then becomes that of "shuttle diplomat," operating in the zone between the two sides and working to bring them closer together.[5] Sometimes mediation will resolve the whole dispute, sometimes just part; it can clear away collateral issues and forge agreements on how the remaining parts of the dispute can be handled. It is important that it ends with an agreement between the parties—an enforceable contract—if it results in anything at all.

INTERNAL ADMINISTRATIVE HEARINGS BY THE COLLEGE OR UNIVERSITY

Codes of conduct, student and faculty handbooks, and collective bargaining agreements routinely specify ways of resolving certain kinds of disputes in a way that is more formal than mediation but less formal than going to court. Objections about how a member of the faculty has been treated (grievances) or behaved (disciplinary problems) are typically required by the university to be submitted to this kind of process. Universities do this because the courts will enforce that kind of requirement and not allow lawsuits to be filed until the process is over.

The governing document (code, handbook, policy, or contract) will specify both what the process is and who will sit as the hearing officer(s); the disputants typically are given very little say in either matter. The hearing officers are members of the university community—faculty, staff, or students as appropriate given the nature of the panel and dispute. They are given certain stated powers—for example, they can require university employees to appear and give evidence. They also have certain specified duties, including performing their duties in fairness to all and rendering a decision within a set period of time. Lawyers may or may not be allowed to participate. The time for presenting each side may be limited. Witnesses may or may not be allowed to be called to testify. The decision-makers may be allowed to render only certain kinds of decisions or dispense only certain kinds of remedies. All of these issues are typically specified in the governing documents, but never with enough specificity to answer every question; in those cases, the panel members make the decisions.

The disputants may or may not have rights to appeal the decision to another university official (e.g., dean of students in the case of student disciplinary matters, provost in the case of faculty

---

[5] The word *mediate* comes from the Latin word for "middle," *medias*. The mediator is the one in the middle.

grievances, president in case of tenure denial), but the "scope of review" (what issues can be considered) is typically very small. Once this step is over (or if no appeal is taken), the decision is called final and it must then be implemented. Sometimes one side or the other will take a further appeal to the courts, but the appeal will not postpone (or stay) the duty to comply with the decision. The law strictly limits the issues that a judge can consider. On the merits of the dispute, the law requires judges to defer to the expertise of the university in certain key areas, promotion and tenure being prime examples, unless there is a clear and convincing reason that the university is wrong. In the end, it is only in the rarest of circumstances that the law gives judges the authority to undo a decision made during a grievance or disciplinary proceeding, either about who should win or what the remedy should be.[6] In virtually no case is one party or another ever given the chance to start over.[7]

ARBITRATIONS

Arbitrations are like administrative proceedings, but have broader applicability. The parties to a contract may have agreed (at the start of the contract) that they would submit to arbitration all disagreements arising out of or relating to the contract. They can agree to arbitration after a contract is in place and a dispute has arisen. A judge can force them to take their claims to arbitration before they go to trial before a jury. Employers often insert mandatory arbitration clauses in their employment contracts with employees. Although not without controversy, some colleges and universities have included mandatory arbitration provisions in their enrollment contracts with students.

There are several ways that the arbitrators can be selected: They can be assigned by a judge, chosen from a list of qualified individuals from which unacceptable candidates have been "stricken" by the parties, or selected by agreement. Once selected, the process that is followed will either be set by the document signed by the parties or governed by court rules.

In general terms, arbitrations may follow court procedures but will be less formal. There will be lawyers, and the lawyers will give opening statements. Witnesses will be called, examined, and cross-examined. Documents will be formally marked as exhibits and offered to the arbitrator. Legal memoranda will be submitted. The arbitrator will then issue a decision, rendering an award to one side or the other and specifying the remedy to be provided. In most cases, the award is for damages—money—but where the rules or agreement allows, the arbitrator can specify equitable relief—orders that certain actions must be done (e.g., return to work) or must stop and not happen again (called *injunctions*; e.g., ending a policy).

Whether there can be appeals from arbitration awards depends on the agreement or the rules under which it was conducted. Arbitrations can be binding—that is, the decision rendered by the arbitrator(s) can be final like those in an administrative hearing—or not.[8]

AGENCY PROCEEDINGS

Many federal, state and local laws and regulations are enforced by governmental administrative agencies or bodies designated by the law or regulation. More commonly known administrative agencies include the U.S. Equal Employment Opportunity Commission ("EEOC"), the U.S. Department of Education's Office for Civil Rights, or the U.S. Department of Labor. Although this can depend on the law, often aggrieved parties must first file their allegations with the administrative agency before

---

[6] Appeals from administrative hearings are typically limited to claims that there was a fundamental problem with the hearing (e.g., it did not follow the process that the handbook or agreement specified) or with a hearing officer (the officer had a fundamental conflict of interest that was not disclosed). Under some states' laws, decisions of administrative panels can be modified if the judge finds that there was "capricious disregard of the evidence" or "gross abuse of discretion" but as the words themselves show, the bar is set very high for these kinds of rulings.

[7] A de novo hearing is one that starts "from the beginning." It is awarded extremely rarely, as when a judge determines that one side or another was completely deprived of a fair hearing the first time.

[8] Because so many lawsuits are filed each year and there is only a set number of judges, courts in most jurisdictions have adopted rules of procedure that require disputes of a certain kind and amount to be tried in arbitration before they are allowed to be listed for a trial before a judge or jury. The parties to the dispute have no choice about this—it is a rule—but although the process is mandatory, the decision of the arbitrator(s) is not final. The loser has the right to appeal and receives a de novo hearing. Although this may seem a waste of time, the vast majority of cases referred to arbitration are resolved either by the arbitrators or shortly after an appeal is filed. The principal reasons for this are that the lawyers use the arbitrators to get a fair evaluation of the case and the filing of an appeal is often used as a last step to provoke a negotiated settlement rather than incur the substantial costs associated with formal trials. Judges receiving cases on appeal from arbitrations also see them as ripe for settlement, and use their power to encourage the parties to settle.

they can seek legal redress before a court of law. For example, a claim of employment discrimination under Title VII of the Civil Rights Act of 1964 must first be made to the EEOC or its corresponding state or local agency. Before employees claiming illegal discrimination, harassment, or retaliation can sue in court under Title VII, they must either wait for the agency to complete its investigation or obtain a "right to sue" letter from the EEOC.

The nature of the proceedings required by the administrative agency can vary, but often they will require the aggrieved party to file a complaint or charge with the agency to which the defending party must respond. The agency, through its employees, will investigate the allegations. This investigation may include a fact-finding hearing or conference conducted by an employee of the agency or by the agency employee interviewing parties or witnesses and requiring the parties to produce records and information to the agency. Parties can be represented by attorneys during these proceedings. The agency will issue a written determination as to whether it found the allegations to be proven or not. The agency may also offer to host a voluntary mediation session between the parties to see if it is possible to resolve the matter before the agency investigates the allegations further.

TRIALS

Disputes can go to trial and be resolved by jury verdicts or judicial awards. That happens in a very small percentage of the disputes that find their way to court. There are many reasons for this: Trials are very expensive (costs plus time that people must spend preparing for them and sitting through them), it takes a long time to get to trial (during which time emotions tend to lessen and financial reasons tend to dominate), the process reveals information that makes right and wrong less clear (making settlements possible), and judges regularly use their power to force settlements. Few people actually make it through the entire process, and only a small subset of them think the experience was worth it.

The following section outlines the process that leads from the filing of a complaint to the issuance of a decision ending the case. Virtually every lawsuit will go through each of these steps (unless it is settled earlier).

PARTIES

The person who believes they have been wronged and who starts the lawsuit is called the plaintiff. The plaintiff chooses who must respond to the charges of misconduct, and those persons are called defendants because the law obligates them to defend themselves (if they don't, a judgment by default will be entered against them almost automatically). Being named a defendant, and being served with legal papers, often catches people by complete surprise. Sometimes the plaintiff names people who had nothing to do with the claim; more often, the people had something to do with the events that had something to do with the claim. The defendant(s) and the plaintiff(s) are together termed the parties.[9]

Lawsuits are begun when the facts are least clear; the facts get clearer as the lawsuit progresses, and that often allows innocent defendants to get out of the case before it goes to trial. But at the beginning, an attorney representing a plaintiff will err on the side of including as a defendant anyone who may have played a role in causing the injury to the client. This is because the law puts a very hard deadline on when people can file lawsuits (or, in an administrative setting, assert claims). These limiting rules are called statutes of limitation because they are usually enacted by the legislature (statute) and limit access to the court. If a lawyer learns after the time period has expired that someone else really did have something to do with causing the injury, even the guiltiest person can escape liability. Therefore, it is often out of an abundance of caution that people who are not really responsible—including nurses and nursing students—can find themselves named in medical malpractice cases.

---

[9] The term comes from contract law, as in "the party of the first part" and "the party of the second part" who are on opposite sides of the transaction, as they are in court.

Individuals can be served with legal process by anyone anywhere at any time—at home, in the office, even in the middle of teaching a class.[10] Written in rather stilted English, presented in numbered paragraphs, and referring to long-ago events in which one has no real or current interest, a legal document from the court is exactly the kind of thing that one will be inclined to put to one side to read later. Don't. Process servers and the piece of paper they deliver are the modern-day equivalent of a person being physically arrested by a sheriff and there are penalties (which can include arrest) if the instructions contained in the paper are not followed within the (usually short) period of time allowed. If the claim has anything whatsoever to do with a faculty member's or administrator's service to the university, it is in that person's best interest (and probably required by university policy) to deliver that paper to a university administrator or the university's legal counsel immediately. Never ignore a legal process you receive because a "default" judgment can be entered against you or your institution if you fail to file a proper response to the complaint within the allowed time period.

PLEADINGS

A long time ago, those who were aggrieved submitted pleas to the judiciary to help them. Today, the pleadings are the written statement of what the claims and defenses are. In some jurisdictions (including many state courts), the claim must be stated with specificity, providing a detailed account of what happened and why the grievant (called a *plaintiff*, who starts the process by filing a com*plaint*) should be given some help (called relief), such as money damages, return of property, orders forcing the other party to do something, and so on. In other jurisdictions (such as the federal courts), all the plaintiff needs to do is give a short-form notice that they have a complaint of a certain type against the defendant.

The defendant then has a short amount of time to respond, and is given a choice: They can file a motion that challenges the legal sufficiency of the complaint, or file an answer to it. In most cases, a motion is filed because the defendant's lawyer thinks it might actually succeed in removing some of the claims, or will get the judge involved in the case faster, or just buys time. Few cases are actually dismissed at this point because even if the defendant is right, judges will usually allow the plaintiff a second (and often a third) time to plead a claim properly.

Once the motion practice is concluded and the judge has issued any preliminary orders, the defendant has to file an answer to all of the claims that remain—a response that not only challenges the facts (and defendants are often required to state their own contrary view of what happened, so the court knows where the factual disputes actually lie) but also asserts legal principles that either excuse the conduct or prove that the conduct was not wrong in the first place (defenses). The plaintiff then has the opportunity to test the legal sufficiency of the defenses through motion practice.

DISCOVERY

When the motion practice has ended and the pleadings are closed, the parties engage in what is called *discovery*. This is the period of time in which each party gets the chance to ask questions to discover the truth. They can ask questions of any of the other parties, of independent witnesses,[11] and of experts who have been hired to testify in the trial. The questions can be about the facts, the claims, the defenses, the opinions of the experts and the reasons for them, and anything else that might be important—including the mental abilities and capacities of the people who are witnesses. Great care must be taken in answering questions, because false answers suggest that someone is not a truth teller, and that opens up the questioning to other instances and events in which the person

---

[10] Many universities have policies that require all legal processes addressed to any employee to be served on a specific administrator. This includes lawsuits that have nothing to do with the university, suits in divorce being an easy example. This is not to pry, but to avoid disruption to the class and embarrassment to the faculty member. The process server is not required by law to obey the policy. Process servers are not required to be considerate; they are hired to get the job done.

[11] If a person is not a party to the lawsuit, they will receive these questions by way of a subpoena commanding their presence at a deposition and requiring them to bring various documents with them. The word *subpoena* comes from the Latin words for "under punishment," and the document is as powerful as a complaint in terms of the force of the law that stands ready to enforce it. As with a complaint, this document should also be taken to a university administrator as quickly as possible.

may not have told the truth. But everyone who has ever been involved with litigation will say that the questions are endless, require enormous effort to answer, and are terribly intrusive.

The manner in which the questions get asked are up to the attorneys. They can be in the form of written questions (interrogatories), oral questions (depositions), and requests to produce anything tangible for their inspection and copying. Virtually everything arising out of or relating in any way to the facts that are at issue is fair game for the questioning. The law also permits the attorneys to review any document (graphic, electronic, or other form of recording) and all files—even those marked personal, because they get to prove for themselves that one of the parties has been accurate in filing the information away and is not hiding something.

Electronic records are the greatest source of dispute because of how much we use email and e-documents. Once served with legal process, one's personal obligation is to provide access to every device that might have been used to store or communicate information relevant to the dispute.[12] In addition, there are also federal and state laws that require that any and all records that might be related to a case be preserved, and the lawyers are allowed to check the parties' hard drives (and everyone else's, it seems) for deleted items. Discovery that one has destroyed documents or other kinds of evidence not only leads to the inference that it would have proved bad things against that party, but it can, under certain laws, subject one to criminal penalties, such as fines and even jail.[13]

For everyone involved, discovery represents the largest investment of time and the biggest intrusion into privacy, and the right of the parties (and their lawyers) to look almost everywhere explains why universities have policies that state nothing on an employee's office computer, laptop, or cell phone is exempt from inspection review by the university, at least in certain situations. Collecting and imaging hard drives not only costs quite a lot of money but substantially interferes with everyone's work; and because the law imposes a continuing obligation to disclose, collecting information may have to occur more than once. For those who have undergone this process, it is easy to understand why the university (typically in the role of the defendant) settles cases more often, or more quickly, than the merits of the cases suggest it should: As a purely economic matter, it is often far less expensive to pay early to get out fast.

MOTION PRACTICE AND PRETRIAL PROCEEDINGS

For those subject to it, the process of discovery seems endless, but a date does arrive when the questioning is required to end. At that point, the parties and their lawyers spend enormous amounts of time organizing all of the evidence, presenting it in motions to the court, arguing about the legal sufficiency of the claims and defenses, and getting ready for the actual trial. This can take months or even years. It is also during this period that the parties—by their own decision, or directed by the judge—may try to settle the case through mediation, or agree to have it resolved by arbitration instead of trial.

After the discover period has ended but before the trial begins, parties will often file what is called a motion for summary judgment to try to get all or some of the counts or claims of the lawsuit decided by the judge without the need for a trial. The party filing a motion for summary judgment is asking the judge to agree that there is no genuine issue of material fact on that claim and that if all of the allegations of the claim are accepted as true, the opposing party must lose on the claim as a matter of law. If the judge rules in favor of the moving party, then that specific claim will not be argued during the trial. Should the moving party succeed in getting all of the claims or counts decided in their favor, then there will be no trial at all. However, the losing party may appeal the summary judgment ruling to a higher court.

---

[12] If the parties cannot agree, it's the judge who ultimately decides what is relevant, but the party asking will ask for as much as possible and the party responding will try to limit the request as much as possible.
[13] Federal law, for example, prohibits the alteration or destruction of documents, or interference with witnesses, in any matter that is the subject of an investigation or could become so. For that reason, complaints about sexual harassment or misconduct, or wage and hour violations, or safety in the workplace, all of which involve federal laws, all involve the potential federal penalties.

TRIALS

Real-life trials are nothing like those on television crime dramas. They can span weeks at a time. The lawyers often meet with the judge behind closed doors, while everyone else sits in the courtroom, waiting without explanation. One is not allowed to have cell phones on in the courtroom or to talk above a whisper. If a person has been subpoenaed to testify, they may even be required to sit out in the hallway (so they don't hear what other witnesses are saying), and they will have to remain there until the judge releases them. If a person is a party, the university will most likely require them to be in court every day, from the moment the jury is picked to the minute the judge gavels that the proceeding has ended. Depending on legal rulings made by the judge and tactical decisions made by the lawyers, the person might not even testify. It is a huge imposition on everyone's time and the university's funds.

Almost no one finds the experience satisfying. Witnesses are not allowed to give their stories; instead, they are confined to answering the lawyers' questions, even if that means the full story is not given. The lawyers interrupt each other and the witnesses with objections that are very distracting (and sometimes intended to be). The lawyers will know the facts even better than the witnesses (that's their job), and they will be ready to impeach anyone's testimony with facts they have learned during the discovery process. Their objective is to prove that their client's side of the story is the right one, the one that the judge and jury should believe, and that anyone who speaks against that version is wrong, or lying about it. It may not even seem fair—but it is, in the larger sense that everyone is playing by the same rules.

After all of the evidence has been presented, the lawyers will give their closing arguments in which they marshal all of the facts they have brought out in the trial into the story that they want the jury to accept, and argue why the other party's story is inconsistent with the facts and not worthy of belief. The judge then charges the jury on what the law is and the jury's obligation to interpret those laws to the facts of the case and decide who is right. This charge is not written: As in the rest of the trial, the members of the jury must try to remember what they have been told, as they are not allowed even to take notes in most jurisdictions. They retire to the jury room to discuss the facts and make their decision, and are allowed to be finished only when they have reached and announced their verdict in open court. Unlike criminal cases, the jury does not need to be unanimous: Each jurisdiction decides for itself the number of juror votes required to make the decision.

POSTTRIAL PROCEEDINGS AND APPEALS

After a verdict has been entered, the parties will try to persuade the trial judge that the jury was wrong, and the judge does have the ability to reject the whole of the jury's verdict or to modify it. When the judge is finished with that process, the parties have the right to appeal whatever part of the decision they don't like to a higher court called a court of appeals. At that level, the judges (typically a panel of them) will hear the argument and make what is in most instances the final decisions in the case.[14]

It is in this posttrial process that the law changes from oral (the jury's decisions) to written form. Before the decisions are submitted to an appeals court, the trial court is required to confirm the reasons for its decisions in a written opinion. The appellate court, in turn, reviews that decision and issues its own, which is also written. These are public, recorded in the courthouse, published, and, at the appellate level, reported in both hard copy and electronic journals. It is these decisions to which the lawyers and judges look for guidance in presenting and arguing their next cases, and where most of the law is found.

---

[14] These courts are called intermediate appellate courts because there is usually one higher court, called (in most states and in the federal system) the supreme court. In most cases, however, the supreme court gets to decide whether it will hear the appeal, and the vast majority of requests are denied.

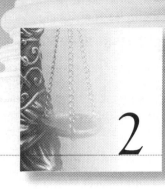

2

Legal Issues Commonly Encountered by Faculty and Academic Administrators

INTRODUCTION

As noted in Chapter 1, An Introduction to the Legal Process: A Primer, the law comes from a wide variety of sources, including the interpretations of hundreds of thousands of judges. There is nothing close to unanimity or consistency across all of these decisions, the main reason lawyers can find precedent (a judge's decision) to support virtually any argument and claim. Therefore, it can be difficult at times to know what the law is or what your rights are.[1]

This chapter provides a broad overview of the law in areas that faculty administrators commonly encounter. The decisions that are most important to faculty administrators are those that have been rendered by judges in the state where they work, because those decisions are binding on the judges who will hear the claims in which they are involved. (The decisions rendered by judges in other states or system are "advisory only" and do not have to be followed.) Familiarity with major legal causes of action that arise in the educational setting can help the faculty administrator to avoid stepping on legal landmines while running a program or department.

BREACH OF CONTRACT

Whether one works at a state or private institution of higher education, the most common legal claim raised in a lawsuit is a breach of contract claim. It is often alleged in the plaintiff's complaint that the institution breached its contract, meaning that it failed to abide by or violated some provision of the contract. A contract can be oral, written, or a combination of both; it can be created formally (e.g., in a legal-looking document with signatures at the bottom) or informally (e.g., through a letter or a telephone call); and it can be formed by action and conduct as well as by words. Both state and private institutions can be held liable for breach of contract to a student, faculty member, or employee because each of these relationships is of a contractual nature. Courts have upheld breach of contract claims under both express and implied theories.

---

[1] This is also why "it depends" is the answer your questions will most likely receive from a lawyer.

EXPRESS THEORY

Under the express theory of liability, the court finds that the school has violated the terms of a written agreement or document, such as an employment, housing, dining or scholarship agreement which the student or faculty member has signed. The court may rely on some other institutional document to establish the terms of the contract, such as an appointment letter, a handbook, a catalog, a brochure, or a course-offering bulletin. As the intermediate appeal court in Pennsylvania[2] held:

> [T]he relationship between a private educational institution and an enrolled student is contractual in nature; therefore, a student can bring a cause of action against said institution for breach of contract where the institution ignores or violates the portions of a written contract…. The contract between a private institution and a student is comprised of the written guidelines, policies and procedures as contained in the written materials distributed to students over the course of their enrollment in the institution.

Therefore, in order to succeed in a breach of an express contractual provision, the plaintiff must be able to point to some provision in the written contract that the institution has not followed. This is frequently difficult for a plaintiff to do. In many cases, the judge dismisses the breach of contract claim because the plaintiff cannot point to a commitment specific enough to hold the institution liable.

IMPLIED THEORY

Because courts have been reluctant to rigidly apply commercial contractual principles on the student–college relationship, several state courts have also recognized an implied contractual relationship between students and their school. The exact terms of this contract are more nebulous and not as easy to find. The implied theory has its modern origin in a 1962 decision of New York's highest appellate court, the New York Court of Appeals,[3] which wrote:

> When a student is duly admitted by a private university, secular or religious, there is an implied contract between the student and the university that, if he complies with the terms prescribed by the university, he will obtain the degree sought.

Under either theory, the prudent faculty administrator will always consult the applicable policies, procedures, regulations, and other institutional documents and seek to apply them in a consistent manner. Institutional counsel should be consulted before deviating from established policies or in situations where such policies are vague, ambiguous, inconsistent, or nonexistent.

DISCRIMINATION, HARASSMENT, OR RETALIATION CLAIMS

Federal, state, and local laws prohibit discrimination on the basis of race, national origin, sex, disability or handicap, religion, and age. Some state or local statutes also prohibit discrimination based on other protected categories such as sexual orientation. Academic institutions will also have established policies and procedures on this subject that the faculty administrator should become familiar with. It is very common for educational institutions to designate a specific office, department, or officer to ensure institutional compliance. This designated official will often have responsibility for the internal investigation and resolution of complaints. To protect the institution, the faculty administrator who becomes aware of discrimination or harassment allegations should immediately consult with the institution's designated official.

RACE AND NATIONAL ORIGIN

Discrimination on the grounds of race, color, or national origin is prohibited under Title VI of the Civil Rights Act of 1964 (42 U.S.C. § 2000d) for an institution that receives federal funds. The statute simply says the following:

[2] Swartley v. Hoffner 734 A.2d 915, 919 (Pa. Super. Ct. 1999)
[3] Carr v. St. John's University of New York, 187 N.E.2d 18 (N.Y. 1962)

No person in the United States shall, on the grounds of race, color, or national origin be excluded from participation in, be denied the benefits of, or be subject to discrimination in any program receiving Federal Financial assistance.

And in the context of employment, discrimination on the basis of race, color, or national origin in any employment decisions is illegal under Title VII of the Civil Rights Act of 1964 (Title VII) (42 U.S.C. § 2000e *et seq.*). This includes employment decisions concerning hiring; firing; promotions; demotions; discipline; compensation; and any other terms, conditions, or privileges of employment.

SEX OR GENDER

Discrimination on the basis of sex is prohibited under Title IX of the Education Amendments of 1972 (Title IX) (20 U.S.C. § 1681 *et seq.*) for those institutions receiving federal funds and, in the employment context, is also prohibited under Title VII. The "Me Too" movement and growing awareness of sexual violence on college and university campuses has focused attention on the protections afforded under these statutes.

In situations in which a student claims sexual harassment by a teacher, in order for an institution to be held liable under Title IX, the student-plaintiff must prove that an appropriate person at the educational institution had actual knowledge of the alleged discrimination and responded with deliberate indifference to the allegation. Actual notice must be given to a person at the institution who has authority to address the alleged discrimination and implement corrective actions. In order to establish institutional liability for student-on-student sexual harassment, the plaintiff must also prove that the offending behavior is so severe, pervasive, and objectively offensive that it denies its victims the equal access to education that Title IX is designed to protect.

Courts recognize two types of sexual harassment claims under Title VII. The first, quid pro quo, occurs when a supervisor requires a subordinate to submit or perform sexual favors or advances as a condition of receiving some tangible job benefit. The second, hostile environment, involves unwelcome, offensive conduct that becomes sufficiently severe and pervasive that it alters the victim's conditions of employment. A hostile environment can be created by supervisors or nonsupervisors such as other employees or third parties. The employer will be held strictly liable if the harassment resulted in some type of tangible or adverse employment action. If there is no tangible or adverse employment action, the employer will not be held liable if it shows (a) that it exercised reasonable care to prevent and promptly correct any harassing behavior; and (b) that the employee unreasonably failed to take advantage of any preventive or corrective opportunities provided by the employer.

One of the key disputes in many discrimination and retaliation cases is whether the plaintiff experienced an adverse employment action. It is clear that courts will consider major actions such as a termination, reduction in pay, demotion, failure to promote, suspension, reassignment, removal, or diminishment of duties and responsibilities to be tangible or adverse. Other minor types of action may not rise to the legal standard of tangible or adverse action. In situations in which an employee or student has raised allegations of discrimination or harassment, is it always a good idea to consult with institutional legal or human resource offices before any type of negative or adverse action is taken.

Federal regulations implementing both Title IX (34 C.F.R. § 106.40) and the Pregnancy Discrimination Act of 1978 (29 C.F.R. § 1604.10) prohibit discrimination on the basis of pregnancy, childbirth, or related illnesses. These laws need to be considered when a nursing program wishes to impose limitations on pregnant students and employees out of concerns that during their work or educational program they could be exposed to substances or diseases that might cause birth defects.

DISABILITY DISCRIMINATION AND REASONABLE ACCOMMODATIONS

State and private schools are prohibited from discriminating against individuals (including employees and students) with disabilities. Although both federal and state laws address disability discrimination, the two leading federal statutes on this subject matter are section 504 of the Rehabilitation

Act of 1973 (29 U.S.C. § 794) and the Americans With Disabilities Act of 1990 (ADA) (42 U.S.C. § 12101 *et seq.*). In most jurisdictions, courts analyzing claims under state disability discrimination law will follow or adopt decisions interpreting the ADA and section 504 federal laws.

The ADA protects qualified individuals with a disability. Under the law, a person is considered disabled if he or she (a) has a physical or mental impairment that substantially limits one or more major life activities, (b) has a record of such impairment, or (c) is regarded as having such an impairment. Major life activities include: caring for oneself, performing manual tasks, seeing, hearing, eating, sleeping, walking, standing, lifting, bending, speaking, breathing, learning, reading, concentrating, thinking, communicating, and working. While temporary impairments of short duration, such as a broken leg, will usually not be considered a protected disability absent long-term or permanent complications, impairments that are episodic in nature or in remission will be protected. Mitigating measures such as medication are also not considered when making disability determinations. The individual must also be "otherwise qualified," meaning she or he must meet the education, experience, expertise, or other qualifications for a program or position. Courts typically defer to an educational institution's determination of its own qualification standards for applicants, students, and academic programs. The deference is far greater when the university has specified the essential functions of the position through a job description or established technical standards stating the key requirements for admission to, participation in, and graduation from the academic program.

The law imposes a duty to provide reasonable accommodations. This duty arises once a disabled individual indicates that they have a disability and need accommodations. The law does not require that the employee or student use any specific words to invoke the law's protection. There is also no duty if the institution is not aware of the disability and the need for an accommodation. Most colleges and universities will have policies that designate a specific office or administrator to handle all aspects of accommodation requests, from evaluating whether the impairment meets the legal definition of disability to considering and approving specific reasonable accommodations. One of the most important roles that the faculty administrator has is recognizing when a student or employee is making a request for accommodations and then referring the individual to the appropriate office for consideration of the accommodation request.

Once the institution becomes aware that there is a disability and a need for accommodation for an individual, the law requires an interactive process to occur between the institution and that person to determine what reasonable accommodations should be provided. Both sides are required to participate in this interactive process. The institution need not provide the specific accommodations requested by the individual. Reasonable accommodations can include almost anything. However, the institution does not need to make an accommodation that would cause it undue hardship. Courts have found an undue hardship occurs when an accommodation would substantially modify the academic program or if there is a direct threat to the health and safety of the disabled individual or to others.

RELIGIOUS DISCRIMINATION AND ACCOMMODATIONS

Title VII also prohibits employers from discriminating against or harassing employees and applicants because of their religious beliefs. It also requires employers to provide employees with reasonable accommodations based on religious beliefs unless the accommodation would cause an undue hardship to the employer. Although the accommodation request process is similar to that followed in disability accommodations, the undue hardship standard is easier for the employer to meet in religious accommodation cases in that they need to show that the accommodation would incur more than a *de minimum* cost.

AGE DISCRIMINATION

It is illegal for any employer, public or private, to discriminate against persons who are 40 years or older under the Age Discrimination in Employment Act (ADEA) (29 U.S.C. § 621 *et seq.*).

RETALIATION CLAIMS

Most federal and state law prohibiting illegal discrimination and harassment also contains provisions that prohibit retaliation by the institution against individuals who bring complaints or participate in the investigation of such allegations. It is not unusual in employment or student discrimination litigation for the institution to prevail on the underlying discrimination complaint but have the court find it liable for retaliating against the plaintiff. In order to state a claim for retaliation, the plaintiff will need to show that they engaged in a protected activity and suffered an adverse employment or academic action, and that there is a causal connection between the protected activity and the adverse action. Many faculty administrators find managing a student or employee who has previously raised an allegation of discrimination or harassment to be particularly challenging.

SARBANES–OXLEY PROTECTIONS

The Sarbanes–Oxley Act of 2002 (15 U.S.C. § 7201) is commonly understood as applying only to publicly traded corporations. In fact, it has two parts that apply to all entities. The first, the Corporate and Criminal Fraud Accountability Act of 2002 (Title VIII), which makes it a crime to "knowingly" alter documents "in relation to or contemplation of" the investigation of "any matter within the jurisdiction of any department or agency" and establishes penalties for retaliating against whistleblowers. The Corporate Fraud Accountability Act of 2002 (Title XI) makes it a violation of the criminal laws to "tamper" with documents involved in, or "otherwise impede," an "official proceeding." The law imposes both civil and criminal penalties for violations.

There are any number of federal laws that apply to universities that go beyond employment and access to education: research, financial aid, housing, occupational and workplace safety, and environmental, just to name a few obvious ones. Any violation of these laws leads to the possibility (or possibility of contemplation) of a federal investigation; the involvement by the U.S. Equal Employment Opportunity Commission (EEOC) in a claim of employment discrimination is almost commonplace at many large universities. What Sarbanes–Oxley does is add a level of prohibitions to what can be said and done once there is the possibility or existence of an official proceeding; and the charge of retaliation or destruction of evidence is often easier to allege and prove than the underlying misconduct.

JUDICIAL DEFERENCE TO ACADEMIC DECISIONS

Be it a student challenging an academic dismissal or a faculty member challenging a decision to deny tenure, both federal and state courts will defer to legitimate academic decisions of the faculty and institution. There are many reasons courts give this deference. The two seminal U.S. Supreme Court cases on this question, involved the dismissal of two medical students. The principles enunciated in these two decisions establish the broad deference granted by courts in academic decision-making and are frequently cited by subordinate federal and state courts.

The Supreme Court's 1978 decision in the *Horowitz* case involved a student's dismissal from medical school.[4] During Horowitz's first year of clinical rotations, faculty noted dissatisfaction with her clinical performance, attendance at clinical sessions, and personal hygiene. Although the student was advanced to the next year on probation, faculty dissatisfaction with Horowitz's clinical performance continued and, when her performance was again reviewed by a faculty committee, it was recommended that she not be permitted to graduate at the end of the year and that she be dismissed unless she showed "radical improvement." Horowitz was permitted to appeal the decision by taking a set of oral and practical examinations given by seven practicing physicians who were to recommend whether Horowitz should be dropped immediately or remain in the program on probation. Two of the evaluating physicians recommended graduation, two of the evaluating physicians recommended immediate dismissal, and three recommended delaying graduation and continuing probation. After receiving the physician evaluations, the committee reconfirmed its decision to withhold graduation, and after receiving poor evaluations in two more clinical rotations, the committee unanimously

---

[4] *Board of Curators of the University of Missouri v. Horowitz*, 435 U.S. 78, 98 S.Ct. 948 (1978)

voted to dismiss Horowitz from medical school. Students were not typically allowed to appear before either of the evaluating committees when the student's academic performance was being reviewed.

In her lawsuit against the medical school, Horowitz claimed that she had not been given procedural due process prior to her dismissal. Assuming that Horowitz had a constitutionally protected interest requiring procedural due process, the Supreme Court held that during her dismissal, Horowitz had been provided with as much due process as the Fourteenth Amendment required:

> The school fully informed respondent of the faculty's dissatisfaction with her clinical progress and the danger that this posed to timely graduation and continued enrollment. The ultimate decision to dismiss respondent was careful and deliberate. (474 U.S. at 85, 98 S.Ct. at 953)

In its opinion, the Court distinguished between decisions to suspend or dismiss a student for academic versus disciplinary reasons:

> Academic evaluations of a student, in contrast to disciplinary determinations, bear little resemblance to the judicial and administrative fact-finding proceedings to which we have traditionally attached a full-hearing requirement.... The decision to dismiss [Horowitz], by comparison, rested on the academic judgment of school officials that she did not have the necessary clinical ability to perform adequately as a medical doctor and was making insufficient progress towards that goal. Such a judgment is by its nature more substantive and evaluative than the typical factual questions presented in the average disciplinary decision. Like the decision of an individual professor as to the proper grade for a student in his course, the determination whether to dismiss a student for academic reasons requires an expert evaluation of cumulative information and is not readily adapted to the procedural tools of judicial or administrative decision-making. (435 U. S. at 89–90; 98 S.Ct. at 955)

The Court found that the committee's consideration of Horowitz's clinical attendance and personal hygiene did not convert the dismissal into one for disciplinary reasons. The Court noted that personal hygiene and timeliness may be factors that are as important in a school's determination of whether a student will make a good medical doctor as is the student's ability to take a case history or diagnose an illness.

After finding that Horowitz had no procedural due process right to a formal hearing prior to her dismissal on academic performance grounds, the Supreme Court considered whether the dismissal had violated her rights to substantive due process. On this question, the majority opinion stated,

> Courts are particularly ill-equipped to evaluate academic performance. University faculties must have the widest range of discretion in making judgments as to the academic performance of students and their entitlement to promotion or graduation. (435 US 78, 96, n. 6., 98 S.Ct. 948, 958, n. 6)

The U.S. Supreme Court provided additional guidance on the substantive due process requirements in its 1985 decision in *Ewing*. In the fall of 1975, Ewing had enrolled in a 6-year program at the University of Michigan, known as the Inteflex program,[5] which offered both an undergraduate and medical degree upon completion of the program. Although encountering academic difficulties, including marginal passing grades, a number of incompletes, and makeup examinations while on a reduced course load, Ewing had by the spring of 1981 completed all of the courses required for the first 4 years of the Inteflex program. One of the requirements of the Inteflex program was for a student to pass the National Board of Medical Examiners (NBME) Part I examination. In his first attempt at the Part I examination, Ewing failed with the lowest score ever received by an Inteflex student in the program.

The school's Promotion and Review Board reviewed the status of several Inteflex program students, including Ewing, and voted to drop him from the program. At Ewing's written request, the board met a week later to reconsider its decision. Ewing personally appeared before the board to explain why he believed his score did not reflect his academic progress or potential. However, the Promotion and Review Board members unanimously reaffirmed their decision to drop him from the program. He then appealed the board's decision to the Executive Committee of the medical school. After giving Ewing an opportunity to be heard in person, the Executive Committee denied his appeal for a leave of absence and another attempt at the Part I examination.

---

[5] *Regents of the University of Michigan v. Ewing*, 474 U.S. 214, 106 S.Ct. 507 (1985)

After exhausting internal appeals within the school, Ewing sued the university, claiming that the school's refusal to allow him to retake the examination was an arbitrary departure from the school's past practice. He claimed the other medical students at the school who had failed the NBME Part I examination had routinely been allowed to take the test a second time.

Ewing pointed to the fact that all 32 medical students who had previously failed the NBME Part I had been permitted to retake the test. He also pointed to a promotional pamphlet issued by the school that stated that a student who failed the examination would be provided an opportunity to retake it. After losing at the trial level, Ewing succeeded before the court of appeals, which held that the failure to permit him to retake the test although all other students who failed had been allowed to do so resulted in Ewing being deprived of his Fourteenth Amendment property right to continued enrollment in the state's medical school program free from arbitrary state action. The Supreme Court reversed, holding that the court of appeals had misapplied the doctrine of "substantive due process." Writing for a unanimous court, Justice Stevens characterized Ewing's claim to be that the university misjudged the student's fitness to remain in the medical school program. Justice Stevens's opinion strongly counsels judges from second-guessing the judgment of faculty:

> The record unmistakably demonstrates, however, that the faculty's decision was made conscientiously and with careful deliberation, based on an evaluation of the entirety of Ewing's academic career. When judges are asked to review the substance of a genuinely academic decision, such as this one, they should show great respect for the faculty's professional judgment. Plainly, they may not override it unless it is such a substantial departure from accepted academic norms as to demonstrate that the person or committee did not actually exercise professional judgment. (474 U.S. at 225; 106 S.Ct at 513)

The *Ewing* Court believed that restrained judicial review of the substance of academic decisions is appropriate because of the lack of standards to guide judicial review, a reluctance to interfere in the prerogatives of state and local educational institutions, and the school's right under the First Amendment to academic freedom and institutional autonomy (474 U.S. at 225–226; 106 S.Ct. at 513–514).

The rationale for judicial deference articulated in the *Horowitz* and *Ewing* opinions are frequently cited by lower federal and state courts. It provides powerful arguments that a nursing program can rely on to defend itself in litigation and makes it extremely difficult for a student to successfully challenge an adverse academic decision in a court of law.

DISTINCTION BETWEEN ACADEMIC AND DISCIPLINARY MATTERS

As noted, courts distinguish between academic dismissals and disciplinary dismissals. They require more due process in disciplinary matters than in academic ones. Although the line is not always clear, it is important to properly classify whether the issue at question is an academic or a disciplinary one. Courts have found the following matters to be academic in nature:

- Matters of personal hygiene, interpersonal skills, and attendance
- Inability to handle stress, make sound judgments, and set priorities
- Repeated failure to produce thesis data when requested
- Incompetent clinical performance because of absence from class and unethical conduct by missing patient appointments
- Sleeping in class, turning in assignments late, and exhibiting behavior that causes concerns about students' commitment to a profession
- Failure to follow supervising faculty's directions or the delivery of unsupervised healthcare

In contrast, courts have required that institutions provide more due process in situations involving academic misconduct or academic dishonesty issues such as cheating or plagiarism. Generally, courts require that the accused student be given adequate notice of the charges and opportunity for a hearing appropriate to the nature of the case.

THE UNIVERSITY–FACULTY RELATIONSHIP

In addition to teaching and supervising students, the nursing administrator may also have responsibility for the management and supervision of faculty members within the department, program, or, as is becoming more common in nursing programs, the delivery of a single course taught by a team of faculty members.

Much of the university–faculty relationship will be governed by the provisions of the individual employment contract or faculty appointment letter as supplemented by any written faculty handbook and applicable policies, rules, regulations, and procedures (hereafter referred to as "institutional policies" of the institution, the nursing college or school, and the faculty member's department or program). Such matters can also be governed by unwritten practices that have been routinely applied or followed in the past to address the same type of matter.

It is critical for the nursing administrator to be familiar with these institutional documents and common conduct because they will govern critical faculty matters such as promotion, nonreappointment, dismissal, tenure, discipline, ownership of intellectual property created or invented by the faculty member, assignment of duties and responsibilities, performance evaluation, and grievance rights, to name just a few. Failure to follow or to consistently apply institutional policies can expose the institution to liability on breach of contract or discrimination grounds.

Of course, it is inevitable that situations will arise in which no written institutional policy or unwritten practice exists to guide decision-making. In those circumstances, consultation with the nursing administrator's supervisors is advisable before any action is taken.

At those educational institutions where faculty are part of a union or collective bargaining unit, the terms of the collective bargaining agreement between the institution and the union will also govern the relationship.

ACADEMIC FREEDOM ISSUES

As an administrator, you will encounter faculty members who may claim an institutional policy or a decision you have made violates the faculty member's right to academic freedom. Despite its importance as a fundamental principle in academia, it is a bit strange to learn that there is no real consensus about the precise meaning of academic freedom and that as a legal principle guiding courts it remains "poorly understood and ill-defined". Your response to this assertion of academic freedom will depend, in part, on whether you work at a state or governmental institution (i.e., public) or at a private one.

Faculty members employed by a public college or university are protected by the First Amendment of the U.S. Constitution. Therefore, they can sue for violation of their constitutional rights when their employer improperly punishes them for engaging in protected speech or expression. A public institution cannot limit or punish faculty members for speech expressed on a matter of public concern or in his or her role as a private citizen, as opposed to being a public employee. However, this does not mean the faculty member can do or say whatever they want in the classroom. The faculty member can be subject to discipline if their speech or conduct in the classroom is unrelated to the course or at variance with the established curriculum. Therefore, the faculty member will not be protected by the courts under either First Amendment or academic freedom principles.

First Amendment constitutional claims cannot be brought against a private institution. However, a private institution (as well as a state institution) may promise academic freedom to faculty members through the faculty contract or an institutional policy. For example, many private and public institutions of higher education have adopted the American Association of University Professors (AAUP) 1940 Statement of Principles on Academic Freedom and Tenure. The AAUP statement defines academic freedoms as including the "full freedom in research and in the publication of the results," "freedom in the classroom in discussing their subject," and freedom from institutional censorship or discipline when the faculty member speaks or writes as a citizen.[6] At institutions that have adopted the AAUP statement or some other definition of academic freedom, a faculty member may assert that this is part of the employment contract.

---

[6] Lawrence White, Fifty Years of Academic Freedom, 36 Journal of College and University Law 791 (2010)

TORT CLAIMS

Negligence

Institutions and individuals can be held liable for deaths or injuries to person or property that are caused by the negligent acts or omission of the school, its employees, or agents. Although negligence is determined by state law, in general, liability can occur if (a) the institution owes a legal duty of care toward the injured party; (b) the institution has failed to meet the requisite standard of care; and (c) the institution's breach of duty was a proximate cause of the plaintiff's injury. However, liability may not be imposed if the defendant can show that the plaintiff was contributorily negligent or assumed the risk. State institutions may have additional defenses or immunity depending on the state's tort claims act. Consultation with your institution's risk management department or legal office is recommended.

Medical Malpractice

Medical malpractice (professional negligence) liability is usually based on tort law. Malpractice occurs when the healthcare provider breaches their duty to exercise reasonable skill and care in the treatment of the patient.

Malpractice claims may be brought against both nursing faculty and students who are involved in patient care activities because of educational and training requirements of the nursing school program. The operation of the clinical training program will usually be governed by the terms of the contract (often referred to as an affiliation agreement) between the nursing school or program and the hospital or healthcare facility where the clinical training occurs. These contracts almost always contain requirements that the faculty and students assigned to the clinical site have appropriate levels of professional liability and other types of insurance coverage. Usually this insurance coverage is provided for both the employed faculty and students by the school under its own insurance policies. However, in some instances, schools do not provide this insurance coverage for their students and require that the students purchase their own personal, professional liability policy. In either event, it is important for the nursing administrator responsible for the affiliation agreement to make sure that all participants have the required coverage or the institution may be in breach of its contract with the training site, as well as exposed to uninsured financial loss.

Defamation

A claim of defamation can be brought in instances in which the faculty administrator communicates negative information about a student or employee to a third party. This could occur in any number of contexts, such as providing a reference for a student or employee, giving an assessment of a tenure candidate, or responding to a questionnaire from a state board or healthcare facility. A defamatory statement is a written or verbal publication of a statement or information that is false and has a tendency to injure a person's reputation. Because defamation is a matter of state law, the elements of a defamatory claim can vary slightly from state to state. In general, to succeed in a defamation case, the plaintiff must prove that a false statement of fact was made that is defamatory in nature and was published to a third party who is not the defendant or plaintiff. Although truth is always a defense to a defamation claim, it may not be easy to prove in court. Because the defamatory statement must be one of fact, an opinion will not be actionable. Another defense to a claim of defamation is that the defamatory statement is protected by an absolute or a qualified privilege. Absolute privileges are available when the plaintiff gives consent or in a legal proceeding. A qualified privilege can be raised when there is a shared legitimate common right, duty, or interest between the defendant publishing the information and the third party receiving it.

Educational Malpractice

Courts have generally not recognized claims of educational malpractice, whether framed in terms of tort or breach of contract, made by students or third parties where the allegation is simply that the educational institution failed to provide a quality education or its pedagogical methods were questionable. Courts are reluctant to recognize educational malpractice as a cause of action because of the difficulty in determining an appropriate standard of care to measure a teacher's conduct, the uncertainty in determining if poor teaching is the reason for the student's failure to learn, the potential burden that permitting such claims might impose on schools and courts, and recognition that courts are not equipped to oversee the daily operations of an educational institution. The Iowa Supreme Court in 1986 relied on these reasons in rejecting an educational malpractice claim brought by a patient against a school, alleging that the patient's injuries were caused by the school's inadequate training of the chiropractor who treated him.[7]

SUMMARY

This chapter provides only a very basic and introductory explanation of the more common types of legal issues that faculty administrators are likely to encounter in their job. Later chapters in this book build on this summary of basic legal issues with more specific situational examples and discussion.

Our objective here is to help you "spot the legal issues" so you can be sensitive to the fact that there are legal ramifications that can form relationships, breach obligations, and expose your institution (and even yourself) to potential financial liability. When you *start* feeling you are out of your depth, *that* is the time you should go to your supervisor and consider contacting university counsel.

---

[7] *Moore v. Vanderloo* (386 N.W.2d 108) (Iowa 1986)

3

How to Read a Judicial Decision

INTRODUCTION

Thanks to LexisNexis®, Westlaw®, and other online research tools, it is easy to research the law and find decisions that have been reported.[1] One has to know what one is reading, though, before one can decide it is meaningful. This chapter explains how judicial decisions are written and reported, to give a sense about how to read and use them.

Cases are always referred to by their citations, an example of which follows:

Wilson v. El-Daief, 600 Pa. 161, 964 A.2d 354 (2009).

What this tells the reader is that those involved in the lawsuit was a person named Wilson, and he was opposed by a person named El-Daief. Their dispute was so seriously contested that they took it all the way to the Supreme Court of Pennsylvania (Pa.), which decided the case in 2009. The court's opinion can be found in two different books (Pa. and A.2d), through the online legal research services mentioned above and other internet search engines (go ahead and try it).

Readers will see that the opinion is divided into the parts described in the following.

CAPTION

At the very top of the decision will be the names of the people or entities that were having the dispute. The title of the case is called its *caption*. At the trial level, the person or organization (called a *party*) who started the lawsuit is called the *plaintiff* (sometimes the *petitioner*). Their names come first. The person who was sued is called the *defendant* (or the *respondent*). At higher levels (i.e., once the case goes up on appeal), the first-named party is typically the one who lost and who is called the *appellant* (the one who is calling on the appellate court for justice). The party that won is called the *appellee*. The v. that separates the plaintiff/appellant from the defendant/appellee stands for *versus*. The abbreviation et al. is sometimes included on one or both sides of the v., which stands for et alia, meaning "and others."

COURT

The next segment of the judicial decision will indicate the name of the court from which the decision was reported, and the name of the judge(s) who wrote it. In the federal system, the trial court is called the United States District Court, the appellate court is called the United States Circuit Court of Appeals, and the highest appellate court is the United States Supreme Court. The states have named

---

[1] Whether one uses LexisNexis® or Westlaw® is really just a matter of personal preference. Each offers different ways of researching the law. Both are excellent.

their courts in inconsistent ways, so be careful. New York State's supreme court is actually its lowest-level court, and its appeals courts have divisions. The *Bluebook* has a list for each state of the state courts from the highest down to the lowest trial court.[2]

KEY NUMBERS

The commercial companies that publish legal decisions have done their best to break down every decision into the specific points that the judge(s) made. They have then organized all of those legal issues into an outline of the law that is astonishing in its scope and complexity (because of how inter-related the law is). The company has assigned each small legal issue its own place in the outline by giving it a unique identifying code (library and number). By doing so, they are collecting in the same location every decision rendered by any judge in any jurisdiction (trial or appellate, state or federal) in any decision that the company has reported. It's a service the company offers, but is neither fool-proof nor official.

This organization of the law does not make any effort to distinguish between the actual holding in the case (the bottom line of the decision) and the legal principles that were specifically required to reach that decision, and the more general discussion about the law that the judges typically employ to frame the issues or describe the process they used to get to their decision. This latter is called *dictum* and, although interesting, instructive, or even persuasive, it is not of precedential value, authoritative, or binding in any way.

SUMMARY AND HOLDING

In a short paragraph, the company then summarizes the parties, claims, and disposition. This is provided as a service by the company; it is not official but usually very instructive concerning the larger points.

THE COURT'S OPINION

The court's opinion is actually the text of the judge's decision. It is typically written in parts: (a) who the parties are, (b) at what point in the process the decision is being rendered, (c) the questions to be addressed in the opinion, (d) a description of facts regarding the lawsuit the court considers important to mention, (e) the answers the judge gives to them, and, often, (f) what happens next. The commercial reporters typically reproduce the full text of the decisions.

Judges are empowered to make their own decisions, but they are required to follow the law. Some decisions are binding on them, namely, decisions rendered by the appellate courts that are higher than theirs in the same system and decisions made in courts that have primary jurisdiction over the issues. This means, for example, that federal courts have primary jurisdiction over federal laws and the U.S. Constitution, and the courts in Pennsylvania have primary jurisdiction over disputes in Pennsylvania.

To show that they are following the law, judges will specifically refer to other decisions that have been rendered on the point they are discussing. These are called *precedents,* and the opinion will therefore cite the decision by the names of the parties (all underlined) and give the address in the libraries of the commercial reporters where those decisions can be found.

REPORTERS AND CITATIONS

When a decision is first issued by the court, it is a separate opinion, by itself, not yet collected for publication with others. At this stage, it is called a *slip opinion*. Most written decisions by judges are then collected and published in sets of books called *reporters* that can be either official or unofficial.[3]

---

[2] The *Bluebook* began in 1926 as *A Uniform System of Citation: Abbreviations and Form of Citations.* In 1939, the paperback was published with blue covers. It formally took the name the *Bluebook* in 1991. As it accurately says of itself, it is "the definitive style guide for legal citation in the United States. For generations, law students, lawyers, scholars, judges, and other legal professionals have relied on *The Bluebook*'s unique system of citation" (www.legalbluebook.com). It is the legal profession's equivalent to Strunk and White's *Elements of Style* or *Publication Manual of the American Psychological Association* style guide for scholarly papers.

There will often be two different publishing companies that have taken the official opinions and reproduced them, in hard volumes and/or over the Internet, adding additions to them that they hope will make people want to buy and use their specific services. The text of the decisions should not be different, but the ways of searching for useful or applicable decisions will be.

Each decision (called a *case*) has its own unique identifier, called a *citation*—usually the name of the reporter, the volume, and the page number on which the case begins. Reporters are generally organized by the kind of court and its location. For state court decisions, the official reporter will usually have a state abbreviation as its name, such as *Pennsylvania Reports* (abbreviated as Pa.). The major commercial publisher has grouped the states into regions and publishes regional reporters containing decisions from that group of state courts. Pennsylvania cases are published in the Atlantic regional reporter (abbreviated as A.), which covers the mid-Atlantic states (Delaware, Maryland, New Jersey, and Pennsylvania). There are so many decisions that there will be a second, third, fourth, and fifth series of the reporters (abbreviated as 2d, 3d, etc.).

When a decision is published in more than one place, the citations are called *parallel citations,* usually referencing the official journal as well as the commercial one (or two) where it can be found. Recall the example from the beginning of this chapter:

Wilson v. El-Daief, 600 Pa. 161, 964 A.2d 354 (2009).

In this example, the same written decision of the Pennsylvania Supreme Court can be found in volume 600 of the *Pennsylvania Reports* (Pa.) beginning on page 161, and also in volume 964 of the *Atlantic Reporter, Second Series* (A.2d), beginning on page 354. One could retrieve the decision either by using books in a law library or by typing one of the citations into a commercial database.

The following are examples of citations of federal court cases:

Miranda v. Arizona, 384 U.S. 436, 16 L.Ed. 2d 694, 86 S.Ct. 1602 (1966).

This Supreme Court decision would be found in volume 384 of the *United States Reports* beginning on page 436. That is the official reporter. The decision is also published in two other unofficial reporters: the *Lawyers Edition* (L.Ed.), and the *Supreme Court Reporter* (S.Ct.). They are parallel citations.

Enron Oil Corp. v. Diakuhara, 10 F.3d 90 (2d Cir. 1993).

This decision from the Second Circuit Court of Appeals, which is an intermediate federal appellate court, would be found in volume 10 of the *Federal Reporter, Third Series,* beginning on page 90.

When there is a published reporter that contains an opinion, the proper citation is to cite the reporter. Before a reporter citation is available, cases may be cited in a more complicated way, typically at Westlaw or LexiasAdvance, that identifies the case by name and the commercial database identifier:

Ji v. Bose Corp., 2010 WL 4722276 (1st Cir. 2010).

Once the case receives a citation to the *Federal Reporter* (it will be included in the F.3d series), that would become its proper citation. There are also some opinions that are never officially published, often because the court has made the judgment that the case does not add to the law and is not significant to persons other than the parties involved. Because a court's decisions are public, the commercial databases will often obtain these opinions from the clerk and publish them anyway. There are rules set by each court about using their so-called unpublished opinions, so caution is needed before relying on one of these.

Remember, just because a case has a citation, don't assume that it is good law or even law at all. The citation just tells someone where to find it. What's inside the decision is what lawyers get paid to fight about!

---

[3] Official reporters are those the state or federal court designates as its own. There are also unofficial reporters containing the same decisions that are published in print by commercial publishers. The same written decisions can also be retrieved on the Internet from commercial databases such as Westlaw and LexisNexis®, or on other sites, including sites the particular court runs. For example, the Supreme Court of the United States posts its decisions on its website as they are issued each term.

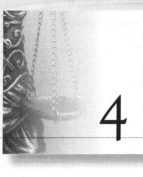

The Role of the University Attorney: When the Academic Nursing Administrator Comes Calling

INTRODUCTION

Society has become very litigious. Everyone seems to want to fight for their rights instead of compromising to find some mutual accord. That's one of the reasons that the law fills so many volumes, is so complicated, and hardly ever provides one definitive, single answer to a question. Academia might once have been protected from these pressures, but the day of the ivory tower is long gone. Today, the law is a constant visitor to the campus. It audits every class and faculty meeting and personal interaction. Its millions of pages are accessible over cell phones to those who believe they have been wronged, and a carefully worded search will produce a decision right on point to support their positions.

A multitude of legal issues confronts the contemporary nursing faculty members in the classroom, in clinical settings, and in their professional role as members of the faculty. Academic nursing administrators not only see these issues directly but also must help guide others through them and manage them as business matters, adding new dimensions (and new exposures to liability) to situations that are already complicated. But although all this may appear overwhelming and poised to swamp the academic enterprise at every possible turn, the fact is that the world is largely no different on campus than it is off. The major difference is that everyone on campus is accustomed to inquiry and argument, and to being rewarded for persistence.

This book was written to help nursing faculty and administrators identify, address, and resolve some of the legal issues that they are likely to confront in the classroom and clinical environment during their tenure as a faculty member and/or academic administrator. It should help you in making real-life decisions with legal and ethical bases in mind about academic issues that range from interpersonal incivility to unconstitutional discrimination. But it cannot address every issue you will face, nor can it provide the specific guidance that you might need in any particular instance. That's why universities have lawyers.

WHEN TO CALL

The old medical saying "An ounce of prevention is worth a pound of cure" also rings true in the legal setting. When you become aware of an issue that could have legal implications, or can see a situation that might get out of control, you should get someone else involved in helping you think it through—a more senior member of the faculty, your department head, or your dean. In the majority of universities and colleges across the country, that's about as far as you will be able to go, because there is no one else to consult.[1] But more and more universities are hiring attorneys as part of the staff, and larger universities may have several in the Office of General Counsel. As its name suggests, it is there to provide advice and counsel on a wide variety of matters to members of the university. It is also the gateway to attorneys who specialize in particular fields such as intellectual property, tax, employment discrimination, federal regulations, and litigation.

If a university has one or more attorneys on staff, be sure that they are busy helping the university's administrators conduct university business: reviewing and negotiating contracts, helping the director of human relations with specific employment-based issues, dealing with insurance companies and municipal authorities, and assisting the president and chief financial officer. Although all these tasks are important and will fill any attorney's day, if you are served with legal process and the time to respond is running out, then dealing with your problem takes precedence over them all. If and when you receive a summons, complaint, or lawyer's letter, do not put it aside: Call the university counsel and deliver that document to them immediately.

The best time to involve the university counsel, however, is before that lawyer comes looking for you, or when you have to seek your own lawyer. At the core, the university attorney's role is managing risks. In almost every context, their objective is to be predictive about all of the things that might go wrong, and build into the situation steps that will reduce the university's exposure to disruption and loss. In contracts, these are the written terms of the deal being negotiated; in ongoing relationships, this is practical advice that will help the attorney's clients avoid issues or solve them before they grow much larger.

THE RULES OF ENGAGEMENT

When you call university counsel, you are making an official call, from one university employee/official to another. Under the legal profession's Code of Ethics, lawyers owe the duty of undivided loyalty to their clients. That means that everything a lawyer does must be done in the client's best interests (or at least, what the lawyer thinks them to be). In conducting their client's affairs with others, lawyers must conduct themselves with honesty and integrity as well as be zealous advocates for their client, using their best efforts at all times. Lawyers must keep their clients well advised about what they are doing and about any developments that are material to the client's interests. Finally, lawyers are duty bound to keep confidential everything that their client tells them in confidence. Therefore, clients may be totally honest and in return receive the best possible legal advice, based on the circumstances having been presented factually.

These ground rules may seem pretty straightforward, and when the client is an individual, they are. But what happens when the client is a corporation, as is a university? To whom is the duty of undivided loyalty owed? The president? The dean? The board of trustees? Whose lawyer are they really? If you tell the lawyer something, from whom must it be held in confidence? When the issue is a lawsuit filed against you, alleging that you caused harm to a student or a third party, the answers to these questions are clear: Your interests are the same as the university's, and you want everyone to know what is going on because you are all working together. But what happens if your dispute is with your department head or dean? Does it matter if your interest is personal (you think you have been unfairly treated) or organizational (you think your superior is breaking university policy)?

---

[1] But do not give up if legal counsel is not directly available to you. Other institutional resources may be available at your college or university to help you manage matters that have legal issues associated with them such as the human resources department, risk management, student and employee disability services office, campus security or police department, campus counseling center, or an equality/equity office. Each of these offices will be staffed by administrators who, although not attorneys, have a wealth of professional experience and training.

These are some of the toughest issues that university counsel have to decide, and there can be significant legal consequences if the attorney makes the wrong decision. For example, the former General Counsel for Penn State University (and former member of the Pennsylvania Supreme Court) faced disciplinary action in 2019 before the Pennsylvania Supreme Court because of her duel representation of Penn State and three individual administrators, the University President, Vice President, and Athletic Director, during 2011 criminal grand jury proceedings in the Jerry Sandusky child sex abuse scandal. It is claimed that the General Counsel violated her professional ethics duty by failing to warn the three administrators of a potential conflict of interest when she represented them during the grand jury testimony. This conflict also later resulted in an intermediate state appeals court dismissing obstruction and perjury charges against the three administrators in 2016. But they are the attorney's issue, not yours.

When you seek the advice of university counsel, begin by telling them the nature of the issue and the dispute and ask them if they will keep in confidence what you are about to tell them. They should respond by telling you that they will do so until such time as they recognize a conflict of interest. At that time, they should tell you that they can no longer help you on a confidential basis and you will have to decide whether to proceed further. Until then, though, you have been the attorney's client and they must not tell anyone else what you have told them unless you give them authorization (consent) to do so.[2]

UNIVERSITY COUNSEL AS ADVISOR

From the discussion of the law in Chapter 2, Legal Issues Commonly Encountered by Faculty and Academic Administrators, you can tell that there is a wide variety of laws that apply to universities that are, in many respects, like small cities. No lawyer can claim to be a master of all legal issues, and it is unlikely that university counsel will be a specialist in any. Instead, university counsel are typically generalists, equipped to handle most matters presenting themselves in the university context because they can do the legal research that is required to produce a reasonably reliable result. In most circumstances, that is enough.

Although it may be the first time that you have ever faced the issue that is troubling you, it is likely that the university's legal counsel has faced it before—you may just not have heard of it because it was handled confidentially. When you call the attorney, you may get the answer right then; however, it is more likely your question will itself be met with lots of questions. You won't find this frustrating after reading the preceding chapters, because you will recognize at once what is going on: The attorney knows the outline of the law and is using these questions to discover the facts and learn where the issue best fits in that outline, so the attorney can give you the most precise answer to your question.

That answer may not be what you expected or wanted. Instead of being a final decision, the answer may be a recommendation that you perform some action or take some step. This is because lawyers know that most disputes are actually resolved not on the merits of a decision, but through procedures that lead to agreements. The advice may include suggestions about things to say as well as steps to take, and will almost always include documenting and making a record of what you are doing. Thinking down the line, the lawyer knows that juries feel more confident in finding the facts if there is a document that was created at the time that proves what the facts were. Take, for example, employment disputes: Saying that you met with someone who reported to you and discussed the problems you had with that person's performance several times before you terminated the employee is far more credible if you kept notes from those meetings at the time and placed them in the personnel file. When the attorney receives a copy of a client's file (as the attorney quickly will) and sees your notes, the employee's attorney will feel very differently about whether to take the case and how zealously the employee's attorney can advocate for the client than if those notes were not there.

A major benefit of university counsel is their ability to help you think of alternatives.[3] If they do their job well, they will be more broadly versed in the university as a whole, and be able to identify

---

[2] There are exceptions to this general rule, but they are extreme. For example, a lawyer may disclose to others a client's intention to break the law or to do someone else bodily harm. You can be sure that university counsel would quickly do so.

resources within the university community unknown to you that may help resolve the situation. You will know more about the subject matter and context in which the problem arises. Working together, you have a better opportunity to figure it out.

The other major role of university counsel is to advise you regarding the obligations you owe—and the rights you have—as a representative of the university. This may be in interpreting the regulations of a government agency or the terms of a grant you have been awarded; analyzing the conflicting duties you may owe to funder, patient, or student; or defining what *due process* means in the context of a grievance hearing or what *academic freedom* means in the context of classroom behavior or academic research. What you think is fair really is not important (or material, as a lawyer would say), and the answers to your questions will not always (or even predictably) be rational. The best course of action is to ask. You won't be faulted if you followed the advice of university counsel or were not provided it when you asked for it.

UNIVERSITY COUNSEL AS MEDIATOR

Because the primary role of university counsel is that of risk manager, they will be ever on guard to reduce the likelihood that disputes within the university community will rise to the level of formal complaints requiring adjudication by grievance officers or courts. The university has many levels of employees and officers, from the most recently hired secretary to the chairperson of the board of trustees, all of whom form the client. On a day-to-day basis, they may have the same interests, or they may not. Because everyone is different, perceives things differently, and communicates imperfectly, conflict can easily arise within the group. In an era of economic shortage and increasing demands, opportunities abound for personnel issues to arise.

In the formal construct, an attorney must choose a client and take a side. In fact, university counsel often acts more as a mediator than an attorney. This can take two different forms: shuttling between disputing colleagues and being an active participant in helping them work out a problem, or advising both sides behind the scenes on how each might approach the other. In this case, the lawyer owes the same obligations to each side. A lawyers can only reveal confidential facts to the extent permitted by the one who gave the facts to them, which requires the lawyer to create an internal barrier to separate the confidences and instructions of one from another. A lawyer cannot help one more than the other. If the dispute is not resolved, the lawyer cannot represent either and must recuse (remove) themselves from further involvement.

These are the ground rules that the lawyer should explain to the university employee whenever advice regarding an intra-university issue is sought. You need to know that the university attorney is providing this service to you because the attorney's client is the university and, in performance of the ethical and professional obligations the attorney owes to that client, the attorney is going to do their very best to resolve the issue at the lowest possible level, thereby reducing the risks and costs to the client. There is a conflict of interest in performing these two very different roles at the same time. You waive that conflict when you seek the attorney's advice on the personal matter because you accept the fact that the attorney is trying to do her best for the university. If you are out for your own purposes, then you need to hire (and pay for) your own attorney.

UNIVERSITY COUNSEL AS ADVOCATE

In dealings with third parties, university counsel has an undivided loyalty to zealously advocate for the university. Within the university, the university counsel's job is to enforce the university's rules and procedures and advance its (corporate) interests. In both realms, there is a hierarchy of authority that begins at the top, above the university president, with the chairperson of the board, and is constrained by published university bylaws, codes, policies, and procedures.

---

[3] This is not a skill that all attorneys have. Unfortunately there are counsel who view their role as simply that of being able to reject requests. The more experienced and valuable counsel are those who say, "You cannot do it the way you propose, but there are other ways to reach the same objective."

In these circumstances, there is a right answer, and the university counsel can be relied on to give it and enforce it. If you have been sued because of something you did within the scope of your duties for the university, you can be confident that university counsel will advocate zealously in your defense—subject to the university making the final decisions about whether to defend the claim and when to settle it.[4]

The role of advocate is different from that of decision-maker. Lawyers do not make substantive decisions. They can advise you about the consequences of certain actions, but the client always has the right to decide which action to take, even if the lawyer thinks it is a bad idea and recommends against it. If the lawyer believes the course of conduct you have decided on is not in the university's best interests, lawyers will tell you that you (and they) cannot proceed with it without getting the approval of someone at a higher level of authority.

There is one part of the university that university counsel does not represent, and that is the student. University counsel will always defend and advocate for the university and any of its employees against a student. The duty that the attorney owes the student derives solely from the promises the university has made to the student, and even here the duty is indirect: The lawyer will advocate to university personnel on behalf of students, but once an issue is decided, the lawyer's duty to the university takes over, and the lawyer will advocate to the student whatever that decision is.

UNIVERSITY COUNSEL AS A TRAINER

Consider utilizing the university's attorney in your faculty and professional staff development program. Attorneys can present on the wide variety of legal issues confronting your faculty and staff, such as federal privacy law applicable to student education records, or can complement larger panels or programs on general topics such as best practices in student evaluations or new faculty orientation by bringing their legal perspective to the subject matter. This is a great way for the institutional counsel and faculty to meet and get to know one another. All general counsel offices will welcome the opportunity to engage with your faculty and answer the questions and concerns they have. Good training programs are a prophylactic and aim at preventing trouble before it starts.

UNIVERSITY COUNSEL AND YOU

University counsel adds an important dimension and can play a valuable role in the academic community. You will find that attorneys will ask you questions (because of their training) that will help you get a clearer picture of the situation you are confronting. If the matter involves something inside the university, the help you get may be more practical than truly legal in nature, because (as every lawyer will tell you) the facts are key. Change the facts just a bit, and the legal implications can be substantial. That's why it is smarter to involve the university counsel earlier in the process rather than later, so that they can help you create and develop options for resolution. It will also give you confidence that you are doing the best you can and that you will be defended by the university if the issue cannot be resolved and develops into a claim.

---

[4] Indeed, virtually every university will carry a variety of insurance policies (such as general liability, errors and omissions, professional liability, etc.) that cover employees and agents when they are alleged to be legally responsible (liable) for actions committed while acting within the scope of the employee's or agent's scope of duties for the university. Often these universities will have an institutional policy that describes the circumstances and conditions under which their employee or agent will be eligible for indemnification and defense from the institution; and that policy will also indicate, directly or by inference, when the university will not protect the employee. Many universities require their employees to disclose potential conflicts of interest. One of the reasons that it is important for the employee to do so thoroughly is to make sure that the university knows what the employee is doing, so that there won't be any question about whether the insurance later covers the employee in case a claim is asserted.

THE ETHICS DIMENSION OF LEGAL AND ETHICAL ISSUES IN NURSING EDUCATION

Basic Primer on Applied Ethics

WHAT IS ETHICS? DESCRIPTIVE, NORMATIVE, PROFESSIONAL

Ethics, in the academic sense of the term, refers to a discipline (or collection of disciplines) the subject of which is moral action, where "moral action" is understood as human activity in relation to fundamental values of right and wrong. This description, however, already oversimplifies. First, under this description, the discipline(s) of ethics is far more complex with various, simultaneous instantiations across various disciplines. Most fundamentally, ethics is a philosophical discipline. But philosophy has no monopoly on ethical thought and inquiry. Certainly, *every* human is capable of such thought (not just philosophers), and, more formally, most disciplines (not just philosophy) engage in ethical inquiry as it relates to the actions and goals of the specific discipline. Further, "ethics" is not only a discipline (or disciplines), but the manner in which the word is commonly used often refers to the actions that are studied as part of the discipline and the actual standards and values that underlie those actions. That is, "ethics" can simply refer to the actions regarding the lives people lead and the moral value of those actions. Thus, before developing the specific questions of ethics relevant here, it will help to tease out and clarify these various meanings and uses, in relation to a variety of conceptual distinctions.

The first important distinction to note is between descriptive ethics and normative ethics. Descriptive ethics, as the name suggests, is a discipline that merely attempts to nonnormatively and nonprescriptively *describe* actions within the moral realm. Descriptive ethics is typically studied within the social sciences: psychology, sociology, anthropology, and so on. A moral psychologist, for example, may want to understand the cognitive processes people employ at different points of their lives to understand the difference between right and wrong. A sociologist might study the moral beliefs and actions of a particular subpopulation: millennials or those with a college degree or women versus men. What makes these studies *descriptive* is that neither the psychologist nor the sociologist is concerned with determining what is actually right or wrong in a moral sense. They merely *describe* the moral thinking, beliefs, and actions that they observe and perhaps infer general factual truths from those observations. The descriptive ethicist does not make moral judgments but observations and factual inferences pertaining to those observations. Moral truths or judgments are beyond and outside the scope of their studies. In contrast, the study of normative ethics focuses on prescription and determining which actions are morally right or wrong. From the perspective of normative ethics, it is not enough to merely describe what people think, feel, or believe about morality—or even their concrete actions—but what the truth is about right and wrong, and often a systematic process for determining such truths, is the goal.

As noted, (normative) ethics is most fundamentally a subdiscipline of philosophy and, along with metaphysics, epistemology, logic, and aesthetics, is commonly included as one of the five basic and traditional branches of philosophy. Yet even in the narrower study of normative ethics, the discipline of philosophy still has no monopoly. For example, most professions express and manifest the value of their profession through an exploration of normative ethics in relation to their practices. Most obvious and ancient is the area of medical ethics. The Hippocratic Oath is well known as an expression of the ethical values and standards of physicians that dates to between the third and fifth centuries BCE (Askitopoulou & Vgontzas, 2018; Catto, 2014). Despite the historical importance of this document, it may not compare well to many modern formal expressions of professional ethics. Arguably, the Hippocratic Oath is more assertion and pronouncement than inquiry, analysis, or argumentation (Dahnke, 2015, Pellegrino & Thomasma, 1996, 1997). Yet, it still represents an acknowledgment of the moral underpinnings of practice and a concern for proper action. In the time since the introduction of the Hippocratic Oath, the medical establishment has engaged in critical reflection on the standards and assumptions found therein and extended the analysis and evaluation of this initial expression (Askitopoulou & Vgontzas, 2018; Catto, 2014). Similar ethical inquiry can be found in most, if not all, other professions: law, engineering, nursing, and so forth. Attention to ethical conduct and inquiry into proper ethical conduct within a profession expresses an acknowledgment of the social value of the profession, the impact of the profession on society, and a definition of proper professional action (Dahnke, 2009). The discourse and inquiry various professions engage in regarding their respective ethical duties and values may or may not be contributed to directly by trained philosophers. However, without question, all these discussions are at least indirectly influenced or informed by the centuries of philosophical study of normative ethics. Thus, despite the various areas of discourse and study in which normative ethics is examined beyond the discipline of philosophy, that fundamental discipline retains a transdisciplinary influence.

Within normative ethics another important distinction to highlight is that between theoretical ethics and applied (or practical) ethics. Theoretical ethics refers to the disciplinary enterprise in which one attempts to understand what ethics truly means, what the foundation of ethical values is, and ultimately to create a systematic, rationally justified process for determining which actions are morally right and morally wrong, or alternatively to distinguish a morally good person from a morally evil person. This systematic process is referred to as an ethical theory. Most ethical theories have been proposed to provide the last word on ethics, a process and the answers that any sufficiently rational person would agree with. However, no theory has in fact achieved such absolute consensus. Some theories have turned out to be stronger than others. Some have endured the test of time better than others. Although none is perfect, that is, a universally accepted expression of what ethics is and how to answer practical moral questions, most have their strengths and their weaknesses. Because of the weaknesses, none by itself may be able to provide all the final answers for what is morally right and wrong. Because of the strengths, some (or most) can provide valuable insight into morality and the moral life or contribute positively to moral discourse. Thus, it becomes important to adopt a nuanced and informed perspective regarding the value of the various ethical theories in particular and of ethical theory in general.

Applied ethics refers to the study in which real-world problems are subjected to analysis and evaluation based on the insights and formulae of theoretical ethics. These problems can be categorized as general social issues such as the death penalty, abortion, or the legalization of illicit drugs. Or, they can be categorized within more specified areas of life such as various professions: legal ethics, medical ethics, nursing ethics, and so on. These distinct studies of professional ethics will then apply the theoretical insights from philosophical ethics toward a deeper understanding of the goals, values, virtues, and duties of members of the profession, as well as duties of the profession as a whole. Within some professions, more particularized approaches to understanding ethics and making decisions may be developed, drawing on general strategies and reasoning from philosophical ethics, and aimed toward constructing a process of analysis and evaluation designed to fit the needs and challenges of the specific profession. For example, Beauchamp and Childress's (2013) *Principles of Biomedical Ethics* lays out a theoretical/practical rubric, which came to be called "principlism," that draws upon the long history of theoretical ethics in Western philosophy for analyzing and evaluating moral issues from within the practice of modern biomedicine. The system they devise is not perfect, nor is it universally assented (similar to ethical theories as noted previously), but it is a widely circulated and recognized attempt to create an ethical system to fit the specific needs of a particular professional area. So, applied ethics, particularly of the professional sort, works discursively with the insights of the broader study of theoretical ethics, sometimes with direct contributions of trained philosophers but sometimes separate from such direct contributions, though with indirect influence nonetheless.

Despite the variety of theories, areas of application, and specific needs of different areas of life, the language and general concepts of ethics (theoretical and applied) are largely uniform—though the relative importance of different central concepts can vary widely. Common to much ethics discourse is the concept of an ethical principle. An ethical principle is, most simply, a general prescriptive or normative claim. As a claim, it makes an assertion, the truth of which can be examined. For example, in biomedical ethics, the principle that patients' autonomous requests ought to be respected can be understood as true, false, or (most likely) generally or circumstantially true. One would investigate the truth of this claim by exploring more general underlying principles, the logical and practical implications of the claim, and the broader theoretical context. As prescriptive or normative, an ethical principle does not assert a factual claim but a claim that expresses values or identifies that which one *ought* to do, as opposed to what one in fact does. The description of an ethical principle as general implies two things. First, it is applicable in a broad array of situations. It does not apply merely to some specific set of circumstances but to a general variety of situations. For example, regarding the principle stated previously, it would be relevant in any case in which a patient makes a request or is given an option. To say it is applicable or relevant does not however imply that it is determinative, but rather is a factor in need of consideration—but possibly along with other relevant factors. Second, "general," in reference to the truth of a claim, is often philosophically distinguished from "universal." To assert a truth as universal would indicate that there can be no exceptions, that it is always true everywhere regardless of circumstances. To assert a truth as "general" indicates that, though in the broad array of experience it may turn out to hold as true, it may not (or cannot be demonstrated) to be true always and everywhere. That is, there may be reasonable exceptions to the principle as a guiding rule. Schwartz (1992) provides the sensational example of a patient requesting that a surgeon amputate his healthy arm. Strict adherence to the principle would demand that the surgeon comply. However, other factors and values involved in such a situation would more than likely lead to a different judgment. Further, Schwartz and we are assuming that the patient is "autonomous." If the patient is making this request as the result of a condition such as body integrity identity disorder, that would add a further layer of complication to the ethical consideration of the request (Müller, 2008).

At times in moral discourse moral rules may be referred to as well. Use of this term is not typically distinct from moral or ethical principle. And hence in much (especially nonacademic) moral discourse, "moral rule" and "moral principle" can be used fairly interchangeably. There is at least one academic use of the term "moral rule," however, that is conceptually distinct from "moral principle." In the construction of what has come to be called "principlism," Beauchamp and Childress (2013) employ a distinct use of the terms "moral principle" and "moral rule." A "moral principle," in their use, follows closely the definition given previously. A moral rule functions much the same. However, a moral rule, within principlism, is distinct from a principle in being, first, more specific or narrower in concept and application and, second, logically derived from and morally justified by the broader, more fundamental principles.

A basic concept that is fundamentally different in nature from principle or rule but is still very common in moral discourse is that of a "virtue." Whereas a principle or rule is a directive to follow (with cognitive consciousness), a virtue is a character trait or disposition to act in a moral manner, and thus is not a directive in the same way as a principle or rule. Virtues may be attended by conscious cognition or deliberation or may not, thereby merely referring to a learned behavior or reflexive act based in one's character. Virtues are also contrasted with vices, which are character traits or dispositions that tend to lead one away from moral action or toward immoral acts. When one conceives ethics in terms of virtues and vices instead of rule or principles, the focus is no longer on discrete acts, but rather on the type and quality of the person who is acting. Thus a morally good (or virtuous) person will (typically) perform morally right acts, and a morally bad (or vicious) person will (typically) perform morally wrong acts.

Discourse on ethics in the modern West is often highly analytical: Discrete acts can be broken down to essential features (consequences, inconsistencies, relationship to principle or virtues). However, there is a more holistic, less analytical approach to understanding ethics that is still part of moral discourse today but was far more prevalent in the past, particularly the classical Roman era.

Instead of focusing on discrete acts, one can view ethics in terms of the construction of an overall good life. That is, the point of ethics is not to simply affix action to justified principles but to formulate and live a life that is "good." The obvious prerequisite here is to define what "good" means in the context of a "good life." Answers to this question can range from attaining material goods to producing communal goods to cultivating spiritual goods. So, how one defines a good life and what foundation and support can be brought to any definition of the "good life" will fundamentally inform one's judgment of a good or bad person or right or wrong act.

ETHICAL THEORY

Philosophers have attempted to provide coherent understandings of ethics and the proper means of determining right and wrong through the construction of ethical theories. "Theory" can be a confusingly equivocal term. Colloquially, people often think of a "theory" as a mere guess or pure supposition with no specific support or foundation, or perhaps a little more substantially, as an educated guess. And it may make sense in lay or informal conversations to use the term in this manner. However, confusion ensues when this understanding is applied to the use of the term "theory" in academic contexts. Even in academic contexts the term can still be highly equivocal and differ based upon the specific discipline and areas of study. In the sciences, a "theory" is not simply a guess or supposition, not even simply an educated guess but an explanation for a phenomenon, typically with predictive power, for which reasonable justification exists and which has been repeatedly tested and has not yet been proven false. In science, then, theories perform an important function and are valued for their explanatory and predictive powers. In this way they are more valuable than mere facts, which many nonscientists assume are superior to theories (Dahnke & Dreher, 2016).

In philosophy, "theory" is used in a manner not exactly the same as in the sciences but closer to that conceptualization than the colloquial use. Even within the broad discipline of philosophy, "theory" can be used in various ways. In the study of ethics, an ethical theory is not merely a guess about ethics or merely an opinion from a particular person. Typically, ethical theories are given support through rational argumentation and sometimes empirical evidence as well. That is, there must be a reason that others can assess and evaluate why, according to a theorist, an ethical theory correctly describes the essence of ethics and why it provides a process for determining moral right and wrong that is the correct, most justified, or best process. An ethical theory may not be the last word about ethics (despite what many theorists may have initially believed about their theories), but neither is it merely a guess or supposition.

Another common misconception regarding ethical theories is that they are merely abstract, sterile, even alien, ways of thinking divorced from reality. This conception follows from an often overly emphasized schism between theory and practice (Dahnke & Dreher, 2016). The common thinking is that what occurs in the real world, in everyday life, is detached from the abstract theories formulated by academics in their proverbial ivory towers. Then, the less intellectualized "real world" and those who engage with it are elevated above the sterile, presumably divorced from reality, thinking of the academic. It is true that often theoretical views not only do but must rely upon a nonrealistic, sterile view of the world, or some aspect of the world. But even when this is true, that does not preclude or possibly even lessen the applicability and utility of a theory. Theories in the physical sciences, possibly the *sine qua non* of scientific theories, often presume an idealized world absent countless variables existent in the real world. Yet it is accepted that these theories present a coherent and comprehensive understanding of the world surrounding us. So, though there may be a schism between theory and reality, the distance between the two may not be as much as is sometimes assumed. And theories of physics can provide potentially accurate and useful models of reality.

Much of this analysis can be helpful when considering ethical theories in general and specifically. Rather than sterile, alien ways of thinking, ethical theories in fact draw from and build upon intuitions and ways of thinking found in how people actually think. Theorists then take these basic insights and develop them into formal and systematic models. But do these models provide us with a completely accurate picture or model of what morality is? That is a question we can probably never answer. We would need privileged, independent access to whatever the metaphysical reality of morality is in order to compare theories to them. We do not have that privileged access, which is why we theorize in the first place. But we need some standard against which to measure and evaluate our theories. Typically, this metric is some combination of intuition, experience, and reasoning. There usually is not the type of empirical evidence one finds in support of a scientific theory, but at times there are some (controversial due to the naturalistic fallacy) references to forms of empirical evidence in support of ethical theories. And often philosophers will appeal to common experience among people and presumed intuitions that most people share. So, we can have some ongoing, discursive evaluation of the accuracy and applicability of ethical theories, which can lead to deeper understanding of ethics itself and possibly an effective means of making ethical choices.

COMMON THEORIES IN APPLIED ETHICS

Over the centuries philosophers have constructed many theories to attempt to understand ethics and formulate a sound system for making ethical judgments. Some of these theories remain with us, while others have been largely shed from the philosophical canon through discursive critique. Those that remain, while each imperfect, may both reflect our thinking and intuitions about morality and aid us in deeper analysis and evaluation of the moral aspect of life. Most theories can be categorized into one of three distinct classes: consequentialism, deontology, and character theories. Consequentialist theories, as the name suggests, judge actions based upon the consequences that result from the action in question. What makes an action morally correct is that it results in a good consequence. And what makes an action morally wrong is that it results in a bad or undesirable consequence. Deontological theories eschew the moral relevance of the consequences of actions. As one theorist (Kant, 2012) argues, the consequences of our actions are not fully in our control and thus not something for which we should be praised or blamed. Also, the consequences of our actions are separate and distinct from the actions themselves, and so in order to evaluate the morality of an action, it is necessary, according to the deontologist, to investigate the action itself and not the distinct consequences that follow. Thus, in terms of moral judgment, deontological theories focus on the reality and essence of an action itself rather than the consequences that result from the action. Lastly, character theories differ from the previous categories in focusing not on the evaluation of discrete acts or general issues but on types of persons, on qualities of character. The assumption then is that a good person will perform moral actions.

Consequentialism

Consequentialist theories judge acts based upon the consequences of said acts. There can be much variation among different consequentialist theories. A particular consequentialist theory must answer an important question: What constitutes a good consequence? This question itself depends upon answers to more fundamental questions that all ethical theories must address, such as what intrinsic value or values is the theory based on and what types of beings matter morally or have moral status. Most theories identify a single (or sometimes multiple) good that is intrinsically valuable (i.e., valuable in itself) to provide a foundation for the theory.

Utilitarianism is the most lasting and influential consequentialist theory, although, arguably it is not a single theory as it has developed and fragmented into a number of variations, not all of which will be examined here but only the most general form. The theory was first formulated by British philosophers Jeremy Bentham (1748–1832) and James Mill (1773–1836) and then developed further by Mill's son John Stuart Mill (1806–1873). Bentham and the Mills identify happiness as the basic intrinsic value of ethics, which means that normatively speaking, what ultimately justifies any action is the production of happiness and the avoidance or minimization of unhappiness. In other words, all our actions should increase happiness and decrease unhappiness as much as possible. On the surface this sounds very attractive. However, the first obvious question to pose in response to this general principle is what "happiness" means. "Happiness" is a term that is open to much subjective interpretation and on that account would then seem an unlikely standard for a presumably objective approach to ethics. If our standard is fundamentally subjective, our results will similarly be subjective and thus *any* judgment would seemingly be justifiable. This would defeat the purpose of designing a uniform system of ethics. So, the architects of the theory developed a presumably objective conceptualization of happiness. Bentham (1988) first suggests this in the opening of his book *The Principles of Morals and Legislation*: "Nature has placed mankind under the governance of two sovereign masters, *pain* and *pleasure*" (p. 1). What he means here is that as a matter of human nature people seek pleasure and attempt to avoid pain. This, he argues, provides a basis for identifying the intrinsic value of pleasure. Happiness can then be defined as the net amount of pleasure over pain. That is, when one has more pleasure in one's life than pain, then one is happy. When one has more pain than pleasure, then one is unhappy. The goal of ethics then becomes to increase pleasure and to decrease pain or suffering. One can also argue for the intrinsic value of happiness by noting that people desire happiness not in order to gain anything else but only for itself. Things which people desire merely to obtain something else (such as money to obtain food, clothing, shelter, luxuries, etc.) have merely instrumental value, that is, value as instruments toward a further goal. Things which have intrinsic value are things which people value for the things themselves. The question "why do you want to be happy?" seems impossible to answer non-circularly. People want to be happy merely to be happy. Happiness is not valued for some further goal but only for happiness itself. Happiness is the intrinsic value that provides a normative base for the theory of utilitarianism and then also defines what a good or desirable consequence is. Thus, actions which result in increasing happiness will be judged as morally good actions. Actions which decrease net happiness or increase net unhappiness will be judged immoral.

This answer to the intrinsic value question then also implies an answer to the question about moral status. Any being that can experience pain and pleasure has moral status and thus is due moral consideration in decisions that affect them. This certainly includes all humans in one way or another. There are some borderline cases such as persons in vegetative states who may no longer be capable of perceiving physical pain. However, one might argue that such a state is a form of suffering (or at least inability to experience pleasure) in itself. More interestingly and controversially, moral status might also be extended to nonhuman animals—or at least many nonhuman animals. Acknowledging this implication, Bentham (1988) became one of the first philosophers to seriously consider the ethical interests of animals, noting their lack of reasoning powers as irrelevant but merely their ability to suffer as sufficient for moral status. Today, these questions are still highly controversial but not easily dismissed.

Bringing together the answers to these questions, a larger picture of the theory in general emerges. The fundamental intrinsic value of the theory is happiness. A good consequence is defined as one that increases happiness and decreases unhappiness. Moral status requires the ability to experience pleasure and pain. Bringing these together, one can more specifically answer what moral and immoral acts are. The utilitarian avers that the moral goal is to increase happiness. However, even that simple directive can be interpreted in multiple ways. The requirement for moral status is the ability to experience pleasure and pain. One can only assume that all humans are equal in this capacity. This may not be true, but there is no way to determine it is not, since one cannot directly access another's experiences. So, assuming that all humans have an equal capacity to experience pain and pleasure is true is the fairest position to take.[1] As everyone has equal capacity to suffer and the goal of ethics is to increase pleasure and decrease suffering, when making an ethical decision one must take into account, equally, the happiness of everyone who might be affected by the decision being made. This idea is then succinctly stated in the central principle of classic utilitarianism known as the principle of utility or the greatest happiness principle: Do that which will create the greatest amount of happiness for the greatest amount of people (Bentham, 1988; Mill, 2017). Unfortunately, this principle is sometimes erroneously simplified as attempting to benefit the greatest number of people, the majority. That misinterpretation neglects one of the two central aspects of the principle. One aspect is the amount of people affected. One should make as many people happy as possible. However, one must also create "the greatest amount of happiness," which many not always translate to making the most people happy. One must count not only the number of people affected by a decision but the quality of that effect. Therefore, if one option increases the happiness of a smaller population of people more

---

[1] Here, however, is where the question of nonhuman animals' moral status becomes especially complicated when we consider sophisticated forms of human suffering that nonhuman animals may not be capable of. That raises questions that while intensely interesting are outside the scope of our studies here.

than the alternative increases the happiness of a larger population, then the right choice might be the option that makes fewer people happier. For example, one context in which a utilitarian approach is commonly referred to is triage in an emergency room. If 10 patients arrive with a minor problem such as a rash or superficial lacerations, followed by a single patient with chest pain, the 10 will not supersede the single patient. Yes, with the 10 patients the happiness (as in well-being) of more persons is at stake. However, the happiness (well-being) of the single patient is at greater risk than even all the 10 put together. Thus, the 10 patients will be seen and treated, but not at the expense of the one much sicker patient.

This theory is often intuitively attractive to many who hear it for the first time. There are several reasons for that. It seems very straightforward and direct. Thus, it appeals even to those who are suspect of intellectualized theory. It appeals to a formal value most can relate to. Most learn from childhood that everyone must take responsibility for the consequences of their actions. And thus, as noted previously, rather than a completely abstract way of thinking, the theory draws upon the intuitively attractive notion that people are accountable for the consequences of their actions. However, as intuitively attractive as it may be, critics have identified shortcomings of the theory. One problem that affects all consequentialist theories is that the consequences of our actions are not certain. If one is to make decisions based upon the consequences of one's action, this speculative uncertainty can be a problem. One decides upon an action based upon a prediction of consequences, but if a harmful consequence occurs instead, that would seem to change the moral quality of the act.

Some critics point to what is sometimes called the no-rest problem or the demandingness problem. If one takes the commands of utilitarianism strictly, it seems that one would be required constantly to help others and use all one's resources for the good of others (Smart & Williams, 1973). According to the critics, this is no way to live, an unreasonable demand on our lives. A related criticism is that utilitarianism annuls the concept of supererogation (Smart & Williams, 1973). Supererogation refers to an act that is judged morally good but is not morally required. In common parlance one might say, "acting above and beyond the call of duty." If, following the utilitarian principle, one is obligated as much as one possibly can to help others, it seems there can be no action that is beyond our duties (Smart & Williams, 1973). Critics consider this a problem because supererogation is often valued itself, because it sets apart the merely good from the heroic, saintly, or morally excellent. Without this sense of supererogation, the merely good person is not completely good because that person does not do all the good that the saintly or heroic person does, and the heroic person is no longer heroic but merely meeting basic obligations.

Another criticism is represented by a popular thought experiment known as the trolley problem (Thomson, 1985). Imagine you are at the controls of a trolley with no brakes. You see five people on the tracks ahead of you, but with no brakes there is no way to stop before hitting and killing them. However, there are controls that will allow you to change tracks before reaching the five people. The problem is that there is one person on the other track. So, you can do nothing and let five people die or act and kill one person who otherwise would have been unharmed. Following a utilitarian approach, the answer appears simple: It is better for one person to die than five; therefore, divert the trolley and kill the one person. But that decision is not as simple as the utilitarian makes it out to be. The fundamental criticism is that utilitarianism creates an ethical decision-making system that while seeming to take the interests, pleasures, and suffering of all involved into account, when the decision is made, the decision-making itself is very cold and lacking in emotion and humanity. In the trolley problem, for one to be in the driver's seat of a trolley and run down and kill five people would be horrible. However, lacking brakes, the deaths are not due to your actions. If you were to take action and divert the trolley, the one person killed would seem to be the result of your own actions. If it were not for your actions, that one person would have been left unharmed. Utilitarianism seems to provide a simple, straightforward solution to difficult moral problems. However, in some cases, as illustrated in the trolley problem, the simplicity is deceptive. Other issues outside the analysis of utility arise, such as the difficulty of the agent being the cause of something bad occurring, even though something better from a utilitarian perspective also occurs.

Because of that type of neglect, some critics point out that happiness may not be the only intrinsic good relevant in moral consideration, and utilitarianism leaves no room to consider such important, possibly intrinsic, values such as justice. In the trolley problem, for example, a utilitarian analysis would lead to changing tracks to cause the death of one person rather than five. However, such an act is unfair to that one person who is not deserving of the fate that you have consigned that person to. Thus, the act appears unjust. This problem can be taken even further. Consider that there is a horrible crime rampant in your community, such as child molestation. The town leaders propose a plan to reduce the occurrence of this crime. A person will be arrested, regardless of their guilt or innocence, and be publicly punished in a torturous manner. If this plan does indeed reduce the future occurrence of child molestation, that is, if the prevented suffering of future children outweighs the suffering of the one possibly innocent person, then the punishment may be justified from a utilitarian perspective. However, this act of scapegoating is patently unfair and unjust to the person punished.

Deontological Theories

Deontological theories, like consequentialist theories, build upon a common intuition of moral thought. Most people believe on some level that despite the consequences, some actions are simply wrong in themselves, that there is something about the nature or essence of that act itself that makes it wrong. This is when we say things like, "That is simply unfair" or "The ends don't justify the means." Two deontological theories worth examining here are Kantianism and natural law theory, with a brief discussion of moral rights as well. These theories focus on the nature of actions to identify their moral value and also on the intrinsic value of human beings as opposed to the consequences of one's actions.

Kantianism or Kantian ethics is a theory developed by the 18th-century Prussian philosopher Immanuel Kant (1724–1804). Kant eschewed consequentialist approaches to ethics for a number of reasons. First, as the consequence of an action is separate and distinct from an action, to judge an action based upon its consequences is to miss the mark. Your intent is to judge one thing but then you look elsewhere. In order to judge an action, Kant argued, you must analyze and evaluate the action itself. Second, the consequences of our actions are outside of our complete control. One may perform an act in order to achieve a particular result and, due to no fault of our own, an entirely different and undesirable result may occur. It seems intuitively obvious that a person should only be judged on that which is within that person's control. Ethically speaking, according to Kant, the only element of an action that is completely within our control is what he called the Good Will. By this term Kant meant the will or motivation to do what is morally right or obligatory merely for the sake of it being right. In order to explain what is meant by this, Kant provides the example of a shopkeeper who is honest with customers (Kant, 2012). The shopkeeper may be honest with customers because the shopkeeper determines that having a good and honest reputation will be good for business. People will want to do business with someone they believe is honest, and so the shopkeeper will make more money. If the shopkeeper earns a reputation as a dishonest cheat, people will not want to patronize his shop, and the shopkeeper will not make as much money. Kant would say that though this shopkeeper is acting in accordance with morality (being honest), the shopkeeper is not acting because of morality and thus there is no true moral worth to his actions. The shopkeeper is conforming his actions to consequences rather than to the moral value of the actions themselves. So, if the shopkeeper were able to cheat customers without their knowledge (and thus make even more money), under the principle of his actions, the shopkeeper would do this. Since under his principle the shopkeeper could be honest or dishonest depending on the circumstances, he is not truly acting morally. Alternatively, the shopkeeper might be honest with customers because he cares for them or because doing so makes the shopkeeper feel good; whereas cheating them would leave the shopkeeper feeling guilty. Again, Kant would say this person is acting in accordance with morality but not truly acting morally. The shopkeeper is conforming his actions merely to his own feelings. But if the shopkeeper had different feelings, he would be seemingly justified in acting dishonestly. If the shopkeeper received a thrill from surreptitiously cheating people, the principle he is employing would seem to justify those deceptive acts. According to Kant, the only truly moral reason to act is because the action is, in itself, moral. The only truly moral reason for the shopkeeper to be honest with customers is because being honest is the right thing to do.

This leads then to the question of how to determine which acts are in themselves moral. The first thing to note on the way to answering this question is that Kant views humans as essentially rational creatures but with animal inclinations as well. As humans, we have an inherent capacity for reasoning and can conform our actions to reasoning, and it is through reasoning that we can determine what our moral duties are. We do not typically hold nonhuman animals morally responsible because they lack reasoning, which seems to support the Kantian contention that ethics is an essentially rational pursuit.[2] As rational beings we are also autonomous, which means that we have the capacity to understand the grounding of our own actions and conform those actions to reasoning. This also makes us responsible and accountable for our actions. But it also forms, according to Kant, the ground of our value as persons. Because we are rational and autonomous, we are the "valuers," the ones who determine what is morally valuable and what is not. Those beings and things without such a capacity are merely the "valued." The car I drive, the computer I work on have no capacity for reason or autonomy and thus no ability to assign value. This separates us from all other things, and establishes our intrinsic value. Whereas the "valued" only have instrumental value (value as instruments, tools, things to be used), those with rationality and autonomy have intrinsic value or dignity: "everything has either a **price** or a **dignity**. What has a price can be replaced with something else, as its *equivalent*; whereas what is elevated above any price, and hence allows of no equivalent, has a dignity" (Kant, 2012, p. 46). Our intrinsic value or dignity, then, elevates us above mere tools or instruments, making us unique and irreplaceable.

Based on this analysis, Kant develops the central principle of his ethical theory, a principle called the categorical imperative. Although Kant maintains that there is and can be only one categorical imperative, he confusingly presents several different versions of it that do not seem like the same principle. The first version is "act only according to that maxim through which you can at the same time, will that it become a universal law" (Kant, 2012, p. 34). What this means is that the underlying principles (or maxims) of our actions should be consistent in the sense that we would, as a matter of reason, agree that anyone else in a relevantly similar situation should act upon the same principle. This version of the imperative acknowledges the level playing field of all persons based upon an abstract understanding of them simply as rational, autonomous beings. Therefore, what is morally correct or obligatory for me should (in a relevantly similar situation) be morally correct for you. One cannot morally make an arbitrary exception regarding a moral principle. No one is morally privileged or has greater rights than anyone else. There should be a logical consistency in the application of the moral law. For example, if you were to shoplift a candy bar from a convenience store, application of this principle would mean that all people should shoplift when they need something or simply have desire for a chocolaty treat. But if that were a rule the world followed universally, several industries would likely collapse. We could not sustain such a rule being held universally. And if it cannot be a rule for everyone, then it cannot be a rule for just one person.

The second version of the categorical imperative is more straightforward and probably more often referred to in applied ethics: "*So act that you use humanity, in your own person as well as in the person of any other, always at the same time as an end, never merely as a means*" (Kant, 2012, p. 41). To treat someone "merely as a means" is to treat that person as a tool, an instrument, a thing; to neglect the underlying humanity, personhood, and autonomy of someone. Instead, we should treat others as ends, that is, with recognition of their dignity or intrinsic value. An "end" in this context refers to something with intrinsic value. What makes an end an end is that it is something we seek, and we seek it because it has value. It is the "end" or goal of our actions. Therefore, to say persons are ends is to say that they have intrinsic value or dignity. To treat someone as a mere tool neglects this intrinsic value, this dignity. You fail to respect a person as a person. For example, in stealing that candy bar you are neglecting the needs and interests of all who depend on such commerce. Those who work in the convenience store or work for the candy company invest their time and energy toward the sale of such products and depend on the sale of such products for their livelihood. In stealing the candy bar, you are ignoring all this and thus disrespecting the needs and interests of all involved. But note that stealing one candy bar is unlikely to have a discernible effect on any of these people. Returning us to the first version of the categorical imperative, we can see that lack of substantive consequence does not matter. If everyone did it, that would have an effect; that is, we could not sustain the principle

---

[2] This claim is certainly more controversial now than it was in Kant's time as we learn more about the intelligence of nonhuman animals, but it may still hold generally true until we learn more.

universally. And if it is wrong for people universally, it is wrong for you specifically. Regardless of the lack of discernible effect of your singular action, it is still an act of disrespect. Here we see the two versions of the principle working together, reaching the same conclusion. However, the two versions do sound quite different, and some critics have pointed out that you do not always get the same answer regarding any particular act judged from both versions of the imperative (Korsgaard, 1996). Yet the categorical imperative is still acknowledged as an important insight into morality and a contribution to our understanding of the importance of dignity and consistency in moral action.

In addition to the criticism regarding the different versions of the categorical imperative not always reaching the same judgment, critics have also pointed out the absolutism of the theory as a problem. In consequentialist theories almost any act can be morally justified, as long as the consequences merit the act. However, in Kantian ethics since consequences are irrelevant to moral evaluation and acts are either right or wrong based upon their nature, that which is immoral is immoral absolutely. For example, Kant judges that lying is wrong. Applying the first version of the categorical imperative to make it a universal rule that anyone should lie whenever it suits them would mean a breakdown in communication and a loss of the assumption that people are being honest. Thus, if it is wrong for all, it is wrong for one. And applying the second version of the categorical imperative, lying would disrespect the one being lied to. When we lie, we are attempting to control consequences and manipulate another. That act of manipulation treats the other as a mere means to our own ends, and thus denies the other's personhood. This is true, according to Kant, even of a benevolent white lie or any other well-intentioned lie. If you lie to someone to protect their feelings, you are treating them as less than a fully rational person. You are implying that the person is unable or undeserving of hearing the truth. To demonstrate the extent of rule absolutism, Kant presents a scenario in which a friend comes to you and asks you to hide him because a killer is pursuing him (Kant, 2012). You agree, but then shortly afterward the killer comes to your door and asks if your friend is there. The question then is whether you lie to the killer or tell the truth. Most people would (reasonably) say that this is a rare exception in which lying is justified. Kant, however, disagrees. Lying is wrong in itself, and it is even wrong to lie to the killer at the door. Suppose you decide to lie and send the killer elsewhere to find your friend, but unbeknownst to you your friend has snuck out and is heading directly where you sent the killer. Now you have lied and contributed to getting your friend killed. Whereas, if you had told the truth, perhaps your friend would have been killed, but that act would be on the killer, not on you. You are blameless, for you told the truth and killed no one. Many Kantian critics find this absolutism inconsistent with the complex moral life we find ourselves faced with (Varden, 2010).

One last criticism concerns the concept of moral status in relation to Kantian ethics. As ethics is a fundamentally rational pursuit according to Kant, and a person (a being with moral status) is largely understood as a rational being, this places the status of those humans with compromised, uncertain, or undeveloped cognitive states into question. What are we to say of persons in comas or vegetative states, or persons with intellectual disabilities, or even infants and children? Some of these classes of humans may have some degree of rationality or none. Some may have been rational at one point but no longer are. Are they deserving of moral treatment or not? Kant's theory seems to leave these questions at best uncertain.

Another common deontological theory, and one often appealed to in the context of bioethics and medical ethics, is natural law theory. It is difficult to attribute this theory to any single thinker. It has theoretical strands that stretch back to ancient Greek philosophy. However, the theorist most often associated with it, who perhaps developed and publicized it more than any other, is the 13th-century philosopher and Christian monk St. Thomas Aquinas (1225–1274). As a deontological theory, natural law theory identifies the moral essence of actions in terms of nature. Most simply put, that which is natural is morally right; that which is unnatural is immoral. There are various strands of this thought and also a version of legal theory with the same name and many same presumptions. However, I will stick to the most commonly referred to religious interpretation, particularly as developed by Aquinas.

According to Aquinas, there is an order in the universe instilled by God. That is, there are laws and structures that make the universe function the way that it does. Aquinas calls these laws eternal law. As mere human beings we can discern some of these laws and structures, but not all. We discern these laws through our rational faculty, but as limited beings, there is much that we do not know.

That part of the eternal law that we can discern is known as the natural law. We can look to nature and have some understanding of how it works, how things are, and, presumably, how things *should be*. Since God imbued this order in the universe, it is accepted that there is a moral correctness to it. Therefore, when we act in accordance with this natural order, we act morally; when we act contrary to this order, we act immorally. Finally, human laws are moral rules that we derive from the natural laws through rational discernment that order our behavior. Human laws, therefore, should conform to the natural law (Aquinas, 2012).

The most basic natural law, according to Aquinas, is the apparently vacuous imperative to do good and avoid evil (Aquinas, 2012). Though seemingly formal and empty, this principle expresses an important notion of human nature and morality. We, according to Aquinas, have a natural inclination to do what is good. This inclination is broken down into four more specific natural inclinations or laws: preservation of life, procreation, knowledge acquisition, and social order. That is, we naturally wish to continue living, to produce offspring, to learn, and to get along in a civil society. From these natural laws can be derived more specific human laws that help us achieve these natural goods. For example, in order to follow our inclination to preserve life, there should be rules against suicide and homicide. In order to pursue the good of procreation, we should prohibit actions contrary to or not consistent with procreation such as abortion, contraception, and homosexuality. As humans and rational beings, we naturally wish to learn, so we should establish systems that encourage education and further pursuits of knowledge. And as naturally social beings, we should have rules that help us get along together, such as rules prohibiting assault, theft, and other forms of social disorder (Aquinas, 2012).

Natural law theory is still highly influential among Catholic scholars but not common among secular ethicists. This schism points to a fundamental criticism of the theory as fundamentally religious. Although there are secular versions of natural law theory, the Christian, specifically Catholic, approach is most well known and developed. And if the theory is fundamentally Christian and even Catholic, can natural law theorists engage in discourse with nonreligious interlocutors or those of a different faith? Can it be meaningful and relevant to a nonbeliever? Another classic criticism of the theory is that it commits what is known as the naturalistic fallacy or the is–ought fallacy. According to this fallacy, originally identified by 18th-century Scottish philosopher David Hume (1711–1776), it is a logical error to infer from natural facts to a normative claim. In other words, the way things **are** does not logically imply the way things **ought to be**. Or, as Hume pithily stated, one cannot derive an ought from an is (Hume, 1974). Because natural law theory claims to locate normative truth in natural facts, it appears to commit this fallacy. And lastly, there is the problem of the "rational discernment" of natural law. Natural law theory assumes we can all look at nature and either perceive or infer the same general truths and directives from it. However, there actually appear to be a multiplicity of perceptions of nature, and even the word "natural" itself leaves itself open to a variety of interpretations. Thus, the moral objectivity that is assumed to be found in claims of nature break down into subjectivity when we acknowledge multiple reasonable perceptions and interpretations of "natural."

Before leaving the deontological theories, I want to make a few points about moral rights, since rights are an integral part of the ethics discourse in contemporary society. First, although rights are a common element of ethics discourse, the basic meaning of the concept is not always understood. Most simply, a right is a claim one has on another to be treated in a particular way. This means that with each right comes a reciprocal duty. If I have a right, this means that someone else (or multiple persons) has a duty correlative to that right. Thus, if one has a right to life, one has a claim on another such that he should not kill her. Second, one has moral rights based upon a preexisting notion of moral status, which may be based upon cognitive qualities like in Kantianism, on the reciprocal ability to respect others' rights, or another standard such as the ability to suffer or to have interests. Moral status in moral rights is still a matter of contention and debate. Third, rights exist or are assumed to exist along several different dimensions. That is, rights are recognized within the realm of ethics but also in terms of the law and civic and political life. It is important not to confuse rights along these different dimensions.

Fourth, rights can be conceived as negative or positive and as natural or social. A negative right, also known as a right of noninterference, is a right to be left alone. A negative right imposes a negative duty upon another. If we understand the right to life as a negative right, then the only duty it implies is that no one try to kill us. Positive rights, however, imply positive or affirmative duties for others. If the right to life is a positive right, then the correlative duty is not simply not to kill but to provide what is needed (food, shelter, etc.) in order to live. One common dispute regarding rights is whether rights (in general or particular rights) ought to be conceived as positive or negative. For example, the long-standing dispute about access to healthcare in the United States is often framed as whether there is a right to healthcare. More accurately, it should be framed as a debate between healthcare as a negative right or a positive right. If healthcare is a negative right, then all that one is owed is to be allowed to seek healthcare on one's own without interference. But if healthcare is understood as a positive right, then one is owed the means to access some basic level of necessary healthcare. A similar distinction exists between natural rights and social rights. Some rights theorists conceive at least some rights as natural, meaning they are universal and inalienable, based in our nature as humans and rights-bearers. Other rights, however, are considered as social rights, meaning that they apply to particular people due to particular circumstances. If Bob borrows $20 from Syadia and promises to pay her back within a week, then once the week is up, Syadia has a right to receive $20 from Bob, and Bob has a duty to pay Syadia $20. This is a right based upon a particular social agreement entered into by Bob and Syadia. This is not a right determined by human nature or one's status simply as a rights-bearer. Not all humans have a right to demand money from Bob, only Syadia. And fifth, rights can sometimes be treated as a distinct theory on its own (rights theory) or as an element of other deontological theories like Kantianism. Either way, it is important to understand the typically deontological nature of rights. Rights are held by persons as recognized rights-bearers. A violation of a right is a violation of the person himself or herself. Thus, violating a right is immoral in itself. Even absent substantive negative effects of violating a right, the wrong is still committed.

Character Theories

There is one further category of theories that focuses less on discrete actions and more on character. Instead of developing and defending principles according to which actions are to be judged as moral or immoral, these theories explore what a good person is and what it means to have good character: what type of person you should be rather than what you should do. And from a person with good character will typically come good, moral actions. Character theories present a greater challenge than principle-based theories in being adapted for applied ethics. With principle-based theories, the application seems rather straightforward. You take the principle and apply it to a case or issue and get an answer.[3] Absent applicable principles, there is not such a straightforward process for applying character theories. This points to both a problem and a possible advantage of character theories. The problem is that it is not so simple to apply the theories, but it is not impossible to do so. Philosopher Rosalind Hursthouse argues for the applicability of virtue theory with her application of it to issues such as abortion and animal rights (Hursthouse, 1991, 2006). But at the same time, character theories have the potential to provide a broader, more holistic view of ethical problems and the ethical life. Rather than breaking down issues and cases to their constituent parts in order to analytically apply a general principle, character theories force one to look at the issue or case as a whole.

The first of the two character theories I will survey is commonly referred to as virtue ethics or virtue theory. Virtue theory is arguably the oldest of the theories in Western philosophy. The moral thinking of Plato and Socrates manifests aspects of virtue, and Aristotle (1941) was the first in the West to formalize the theory in his *Nicomachean Ethics*. A virtue is a character trait or disposition that typically leads one toward morally good action. In contrast, a vice is a character trait which gives one the tendency to act immorally. A person who has the virtue of honesty, for example, will typically act honestly in situations in which one is faced with the decision to respond honestly or dishonestly. But note that virtues are not about discrete acts. A virtue is judged over the lifetime of an individual. One dishonest act does not necessarily make one a dishonest person. Further, because we are talking about dispositions, a person with the virtue of honesty will *want* to be honest. Even in cases where it

---

[3] Of course, it is never truly that simple, but that is the process in a nutshell.

is challenging to tell the truth, the honest person will be drawn to truth-telling. This is not to say that an honest person will never lie, but it is unlikely the honest person will.

Where do these virtues come from? Aristotle held that neither virtues nor vices exist in us naturally, but the potential for both does. It is through moral education that we develop either virtues or vices. A virtue in this way is similar to a skill. Just as one develops a skill such as playing a musical instrument or playing a sport through practice, one develops a virtue also through practice. One becomes honest by performing honest acts. The child learning to play baseball is directed by the coach to hold the bat in a certain way, to put the feet in a particular way, to look toward the pitcher, to point the hips in a specific direction, and so on. The child remembers maybe one of these directives the first time at bat. However, with practice and more times at bat, more of these instructions are remembered and eventually ingrained until they no longer need to be thought about. The child merely walks to the batter's box and follows the instructions as a matter of course. A child learning to play piano is instructed by the teacher to use particular fingers when playing a C scale. The child starts with the thumb on the C, then the forefinger on the D, the middle finger on the E, then cross the thumb under for the F, and so on. Again, this goes very slowly at first, with intense concentration on each finger, until ultimately after weeks of practice, the C scale is played with little conscious thought at all. Becoming an honest person works much the same way. After much time consciously choosing to be honest, one eventually responds honestly with no conscious effort.

One of the difficult theoretical and practical questions that virtue ethics has to answer is which character traits are virtues and which are vices. Aristotle answered this question by investigating the ultimate goal or good of human life. He referred to this goal as *eudaimonia*, which is often translated as happiness. However, many scholars interpret the concept more as "flourishing." This is because we moderns tend to think of happiness as a mere state, but Aristotle did not develop the concept of *eudaimonia* as a simple state but more as an activity. The idea is that the goal of life is to achieve our potential, to flourish as perhaps a garden in full bloom flourishes. Thus, virtues are those character traits that help us to flourish and pursue our potential as human beings. There are still many questions left open regarding this understanding of virtue, so this is an issue that virtue theorists have continued to explore. One of the more interesting attempts comes from 20th-century virtue theorist Alasdair MacIntyre (1985) who delineates virtues in relation to the concept he calls "practice." By practice, MacIntyre (1985) means a "coherent and complex form of socially established cooperative human activity" (p. 187). In other words, it is an activity that many people engage in cooperatively and is endorsed by society. Further, practices produce what MacIntyre calls "internal goods." These internal goods are goods that provide value to society and that can be achieved only through the practice itself. Practices also have their own standards of excellence to evaluate and police their practitioners. Examples of practices that MacIntyre provides include architecture, the game of football, farming, physics, the study of history, being a musician, and being a painter (MacIntyre, 1985). The internal goods of architecture, for example, would be the design and ultimate construction of sound (and possibly visually attractive) buildings that allow for a multitude of other useful and necessary activities. Professions such as medicine, nursing, and education would likely also qualify as practices, and the internal goods, coherence, and standards of excellence of each can easily be identified. In contrast, examples of non-practices include bricklaying and throwing a football. Notice that architecture is a practice, whereas bricklaying is not. The game of football is a practice, whereas throwing a football is not. According to MacIntyre (1985), the difference lies in the coherence of the activity and the internal goods achieved through the practice. Presumably then, merely throwing a football or laying bricks does not have such social coherence or internal goods. These discriminatory claims may be somewhat controversial and may reveal a sense of elitism in the thought of MacIntyre; however, the concept still makes for an intriguing means of objectively delineating virtues. With the concept of practice then, a virtue becomes a character trait that aids one (or a group of practitioners) in achieving the internal goods of the practice. Instead of one set of virtues applying abstractly to all humans as humans, MacIntyre fragments virtues according to socially valuable practices. But at the same time, through the connection to various goods these various virtues are also connected to the broader sense of flourishing from Aristotle. Thus, the virtues of nursing, for example, will be based upon the goods that nursing provides and will be those character traits that aid nurses in achieving these goods. The virtues of educators will be based upon the goods that education provides and will be those character traits that aid educators in achieving these goods. This approach provides an apparently concrete and objective justification for the identification of virtues, as opposed to an abstract and highly contentious list of virtues based on presumptions of human nature, yet it does not lose that grounding in flourishing.

In terms of criticism, as noted previously, some claim that without explicit principles virtue theory is difficult and even ill-suited to practical or applied ethics (Louden, 1984). But also as noted, some virtue theorists have pushed back on this criticism (Hursthouse, 1991, 2006). As just discussed, there is also the question of defining and defending which traits are virtues. That is as yet an ongoing discussion with some interesting answers to consider.

Lastly, some critics, such as philosopher Martha Nussbaum (1999), have argued that virtue ethics does not qualify as a distinct theory. Rather, virtue is better understood as an element of ethics that is integrated into other deontological and consequentialist theories, making a theory of virtue unnecessary and superfluous. Despite this criticism, virtue theory is still a vibrant part of ethical discourse. It may or may not qualify as its own distinct theory, but it is still a part of the conversation and may be helpful in future attempts to understand right and wrong.

The second character theory I wish to survey fits only controversially in this category. But it is clearly neither a deontological nor a consequentialist theory, and it does focus on particular personal traits as opposed to principles and rules. This is the theory known as ethics of care. Ethics of care has its origins in the study of descriptive ethics, particularly moral psychology. The noted moral psychologist Lawrence Kohlberg (1927–1987), after studying the manner in which people think about moral questions, hypothesized different stages people go through in the development of their moral thinking (Kohlberg, 1982). There are six stages, according to Kohlberg, beginning with the obedience/punishment stage which represents the young child's perception of moral wrong as related to punishment from authorities like parents. And the sixth ("highest") stage is the universal ethical stage in which ethical decisions are made based upon abstract, universal, rational principles. One controversial result of Kohlberg's studies on how people think about morality is that it seemed that men typically reach higher stages of moral thinking than women. There is a problem here already that the assumed hierarchy of the stages conflates descriptive and normative ethics, but I will focus on the more pertinent problem: the apparent sexism. One of his students, Carol Gilligan, was suspect of this conclusion and in her own work theorized that the problem is not with women but with the gendered presumptions of Kohlberg's model. Gilligan (1993) argued that by making the highest stage characterized by abstract, universal principles (echoing a Kantian view of ethics), Kohlberg privileged a stereotypically male way of thinking about ethics. The reason women appeared to do less well in Kohlberg's studies is because his standard reflects the presumptions of traditional, male-centered ethical theories like utilitarianism and Kantianism. By comparison, Gilligan argued, women tend to think about ethics less in terms of abstract principles but more in terms of intimate relationships, emotions, and community. That is, in women's way of moral thinking, moral obligations do not spring from abstract reasoning but develop organically from concrete relationships that form one's life. Because of historical bias against women, this way of thinking about ethics has been largely discounted and suppressed. It is not Gilligan's contention, though, that all men share one narrow form of ethical thinking and all women another, but that instead there are general tendencies that can be historically associated with gender. Neither is she asserting the claim that there is something essential (biological, genetic) about men that direct them to think about ethics in one way and women in another. The difference could be explained by socialization or any other number of factors. These are mere general tendencies, but historically identifiable and influential tendencies nonetheless.

A number of feminist philosophers, including Baier (1987), Noddings (2013), and Held (2006), picked up on Gilligan's insights to construct a new ethical theory known as ethics of care. Just as Gilligan did not claim that all men think one way about ethics and all women think a different way, the philosophers developing ethics of care were not developing an ethical theory exclusively for women. They did not assume that there should be one theory for men and one for women. Rather, the contention was that ethical theory, historically directed largely by male thinkers, overemphasized an abstract, hyperrational, supposedly "male" way of thinking and depressed, even derogated, alternative "female" ways of thinking that focus on relationships and emotions. The central ethical concept for most of these thinkers of course was care. The thinking here is that care is a fundamental human relation and an appropriate base for ethical thought to be built upon. A child is born and immediately there is a caring relationship between the child and its mother (and/or father), comprising a basic caregiver–care recipient dyad. There is no rationality to this relationship, no contractual reciprocity. There is merely natural trust and care. Despite the lack of rational foundation, these caring relationships comprise the foundation of our lives. At the very least, traditional male ethics has been negligent in failing to adequately address this fundamental aspect of life.

According to the ethics of care, ethical obligations are based not on abstract reasoning and formal principles, but based in the particular reality and relationships of our actual lives. We understand obligations as emanating from the intimate relationships that define who we are. In practical ethics the focus turns away from the general application of principle and toward analysis of specific relationships and their meaning. Although ethics of care contends to highlight a neglected aspect of the ethical life and to develop a suppressed "feminine" way of thinking, it is not without its critics, including women and feminists. Some feminist critics fear the theory perpetuates certain stereotypes about women, including that women are less rational and more emotional than men and that women are naturally subservient caregivers (Card, 1990; Puka, 1990). Traditional gendered thought in the West has often assumed a greater influence of emotion and less capacity for reasoned thought regarding women in comparison to men. This assumption has been used to disempower women, assuming insufficient intellect in women to participate in many important social roles and functions, including socially important professions, political service, and even mere voting. This type of disempowerment has also been linked to women's traditional roles of wives, mothers, nurses, secretaries, and so on (roles that are traditionally subservient, caring for a usually male authority) and have helped constrain their power and influence in society (Tronto, 1993). So according to some feminist critics of ethics of care, to emphasize and develop an understanding of women from this point of view will only strengthen this position and perception of disempowerment. In order to address this issue, some reconciliation between the apparent subjugation that aspects of care theory may manifest and the continued empowerment of women needs to be made. A further related concern is that absent a focus on rational thought, one will be less suited to engage in moral discourse and defend one's moral positions (Kuhse, 1995).

Another criticism is that the focus on intimate relationships neglects ethical concerns outside one's immediate circle of family and friends (Tronto, 1993). That is, there may be those at a distance whose ethical interests are relevant to us, as well as those proximate to us. Do we owe nothing to children starving around the world? Or is their suffering irrelevant to us merely because we lack an intimate relationship with them? And, as with virtue ethics, some theorists have argued that ethics of care does not qualify as a distinct theory itself but instead focuses on one aspect of ethics that can be developed as an element of other, broader theories (Nagl-Docekal, 1997). Have this sentence begin with Some virtue theorists have even argued that ethics of care is really a part of virtue theory (Halwani, 2003; Rachels, 1999; Slote, 1998). Whether ethics of care risks a perpetuation of stereotypes and whether it comprises a distinct theory all its own, it undoubtedly has broadened the moral discourse of the last few decades.

CODES OF ETHICS

Professional codes of ethics are utilized by discrete professions to encourage ethical action among its practitioners. Codes of ethics consolidate and coalesce the complex values, reasoning, and judgments of the broad study of a profession's ethics into a coherent, guiding statement. In addition to guiding and encouraging ethical action, codes of ethics perform several other functions. But at the same time, some ethicists and professionals have theoretical and practical criticisms of codes of ethics. In order to understand the application of codes of ethics to real-world problems, we must first understand the essence and authoritative foundation of these codes, their various possible functions and purposes, and the possible weakness and limitations identified by critics.

Essence and Authority

At its simplest, a professional code of ethics is a list of ethical principles or values that individual practitioners are expected to conform their actions to. But both theoretically and practically, codes of ethics are far more complex than that. Codes of ethics do not spring Athena-like from a high authority of professional ethics but develop as professions themselves evolve. The professions we know today were not always professions as we understand the term. They typically began as more loosely associated crafts, trades, or vocations. As practitioners organize more coherently with uniform standards and goals, professions emerge. Baker (2005) identifies three stages of professional development that lead to the introduction of a code of ethics. In the first stage, traditionalism, there are no formal and uniform standards. Instead, practitioners guide their actions according to tradition and perhaps informal rules. The second state, formalization, sees the amalgamation of these earlier traditions and rules by some organization, person, or persons into a more coherent and uniform order while attempting to provide a rational justification for these rules. And in the third stage, professionalization, an organization of allied professionals "adopts a formal code of ethics and invests its authority in its promulgation, interpretation, adjudication, revision, and in some measure of direct or indirect enforcement" (Baker, 2005, p. 33).

Once a code has developed, its nature is more complex than just a list of rules. Benjamin and Curtis (2010) identify a dual nature of professional codes of ethics. On the one hand, codes of ethics operate as a creed, a statement of regard for high ideals and commitment of professionals toward them, "a sort of oath of professional office" (Benjamin & Curtis, 2010, p. 6). On the other hand, codes of ethics operate as a set of commandments providing enforceable standards of conduct and indicating "in general terms some of the ethical considerations professionals must take into account in deciding on conduct" (Benjamin & Curtis, 2010, p. 7). As a creed, a code of ethics is a public expression of the profession's values and dedication to ethical performance within the practice, "the profession's public expression of those values, duties, and commitments," as Fowler (2008) similarly expresses (p. xiii). As a commandment, a code of ethics informs practitioners of ethical issues and concerns to be aware of and be ready to respond to according to the values and principles affirmed within. The commandment aspect of codes of ethics presents a particular challenge to their construction. In developing the principles, a middle path between two extremes must be charted (Benjamin & Curtis, 2010). If the principles are overly broad, they risk being too vague to provide any clear guidance to practitioners. But if the principles are too specific, it is likely that these principles end up being controversial, not acceptable to many within the profession. Further, a code of such specificity would be impractically lengthy, and it is likely not even possible to foresee all potential ethical problems on that level of detail.

What is the foundation or justification for a code of ethics as a ruling document? Why should a professional care about the code and comply with it? According to Fry, Veatch, and Taylor (2011), codes of ethics are binding on members "only to the text that the association can censure the member for violations" (p. 39). Having enforcement mechanisms makes a code "real" in the sense of consequences and having a reason to follow the rules that is effective on all, regardless of underlying moral commitment. In some cases legal fines could even be imposed. These types of penalties should be outlined by the professional organization beforehand in order to place practitioners on notice. To some extent, the ability to discipline members regarding the code of ethics is important. However, this is a very superficial and legalistic reason to follow a code of ethics. Such prudence does not reflect a true ethical commitment. And professions that lack licensure do not have the same ability to enforce. In some instances, suspension or expulsion from the professional organization might be a consequence of immoral action in nonlicensed professions, but that would not prevent a professional from practicing (American College of Healthcare Executives, 2019). Thus, for substantive ethical reasons among licensed professionals and for any ethical commitment at all in the case of nonlicensed professionals, a more meaningful reason to adhere to the professional code of ethics is needed.

An assumption of moral authority, that is, a legitimate right and standing to assert moral duties for others, suggests a more meaningful and substantial reason for following a code of ethics. But what is the source of this moral authority in the case of professional codes of ethics? Some might have the conception of the principles and values of a code of ethics as purely invented whole cloth by the professional organization. Under this conception, the authority of the code is based upon the authority of the architects of the code as (typically) elevated members of the profession. However, there are a number of problems with conceiving the moral authority of the code in this way.

Being an experienced physician, nurse, lawyer, or educator who has achieved some level of respect and regard within the profession does not establish one as a moral authority. That may establish one as an expert in medicine, nursing, law, or education, but not in ethics. This conception of moral authority establishes unearned privilege of moral expertise in some person or body. Further, assuming privileged moral expertise in any person or body of persons can be dangerous. The fact that the American Nurses Association (ANA) or the American Association of University Professors asserts a moral directive or principle does not in itself establish such a claim as inviolable moral truth. And lastly, assuming privileged moral expertise in some person or body of persons is intellectually lazy and an abdication of one's professional and human responsibilities to be accountable for one's own actions. So, in contrast to this, some conceive the values and principles of a code of ethics as discovered and aggregated (Baker, 2005; Dahnke, 2009) and thus "grounded in some source beyond mere convention—in reason or universal moral law or divine authority" (Fry et al., 2011, p. 39). Instead of assuming a professional organization is itself an infallible moral authority proclaiming unassailable moral truths from on high, professionals need to both recognize the moral fallibility of the code's architects and the fundamental conceptual and normative sources of the code (Dahnke, 2009).

Appealing to fallibility here might seem counterintuitive to some. One might typically assume that a normative system, in order to have force, would have to be perceived as correct, even absolutely correct. However, when it comes to moral authority, establishing absolute truth and authority is no easy task. While it is true that for some people religious authority functions as an absolute moral authority, this confidence is based upon personal faith and cannot speak for anyone outside that faith tradition. Acknowledging the fallibility of the code's architects expresses a necessary humility in ethical discourse. If we cannot assume moral perfection in any person or group of persons, we must assume and accept fallibility. However, this does not mean we surrender all confidence in the moral judgment of ourselves or others. We can have provisional confidence in the judgment of others based upon past experience and certain reasonable assumptions about those making judgments. Thus, we do not accept the moral authority of a code of ethics based upon an assumption of a privileged insight into morality by the architects of the code. We may, however, assume that such architects are experienced, well educated, and well meaning. From such reasonable assumptions we can infer a particular degree of confidence in the moral claims and directives of the code (Dahnke, 2009). The authority of the code then is grounded not in the personages of those who construct it, but in the assumption of their good will and in the reasoning they employ in constructing it. Along with this, we should realize that a code of ethics is not a replacement of ethical theory but adjunctive to it, since the principles, reasoning, and justification of codes of ethics are largely drawn from the long tradition of theoretical ethics. This establishes a theoretical foundation for the moral authority as well, but a foundation that is only as strong as the theories themselves and the reasoning drawn from those theories.

This leaves us with a reasonable presumption in the propriety of a professional code of ethics, which does not mean the code is infallible. Its architects are fallible, leaving the code itself fallible. Thus, a wise professional organization will, in its own humility, acknowledge the fallibility of its own code and undergo a process of revision from time to time (Dahnke, 2009). As one of the architects of the ANA Code of Ethics writes, the ANA Code "was never intended to be carved in stone for all eternity" [but] "evolved and developed in accord with the changing social context of nursing, and with the progress and aspirations of the profession" (Fowler, 2008, p. xiii). This openness to change does not translate into arbitrary change or moral relativism: "despite the changes over time in the Code's expression, interpretation, and application, the central ethical values, duties and commitments of nursing have remained stable" (Fowler, 2008, p. xiii). A profession can retain a central ethical core (though this too is theoretically open to question and critique) while adjusting the margins according to professional, environmental, and technological changes. Thus, an acknowledgment of fallibility allows a code of ethics to "reflect both constancy and change" and to retain stable norms while reinterpreting those norms "with the growth of the profession and changes in society" (Davis, Fowler, & Aroskar, 2010, p. 40).

In addition to this understanding of the moral authority of a code of ethics, some have also identified a social contract approach to justifying such authority (Dahnke, 2009; Fowler, 2008; Fry et al., 2011). Social contract theory is a moral and political theory that holds that a society's moral or political rules stem from the people's tacit acceptance and thus endorsement of those rules. No literal contract is involved, but in the very act of living and continuing to live in a society (and in particular, benefiting from the goods of that society), people affirm the rules of society. Change in those rules is possible, but that too requires the consent of society and a socially sanctioned means of enacting such change. Similarly, one might say that in going through the socially sanctioned process (education, degree conferral, licensure exam) of becoming a professional of a particular type, that in accepting the social privilege to practice with the title of professional, one accepts the authority of standards of practice like a code of ethics. At the same time, the code functions as a contract between the profession in general and society. It establishes, ethically and professionally, what the profession owes and promises to society in exchange for the right to practice and social sanctioning.

This question of authority, either based upon acknowledged fallibility or social contract, raises the question of violation of a code's authority. As already noted, some codes have mechanisms of enforcement for those who violate them. However, there is a deeper aspect to this question to explore. There are in fact three ways in which a professional can violate a code of ethics: negligence, willful disobedience, and moral resistance (Dahnke, 2009). The first two would unquestionably leave a practitioner open to punitive measures. It may be that a willfully disobedient act may invite a harsher punishment than an improper act committed out of pure negligence, but negligence itself may not be a complete defense. A professional may be expected to know standards of practice like a code of ethics and thus be accountable for violative acts toward it. However, the third type of violative act raises deeper, more interesting questions. Can a professional morally *violate* a code of ethics? Based on what has already been said about the fallible nature of codes of ethics, the answer here would have to be yes. In other words, it is at least theoretically possible that a code of ethics is morally mistaken or morally incomplete. However, assuming the good will, relevant experience, and sound reasoning of the architects of the code, one would be justified in presuming the moral propriety of the code until that presumption is overturned. This does not mean that one who disagrees with a code of ethics is necessarily right and the code necessarily wrong. However, that could be the case. Could one acting morally but *contrary* to a code of ethics be punished for that act? Definitely. Should they be is a more complex question. The ANA Code of Ethics asserts to be a nonnegotiable standard of ethical action. Despite the fact that, through several formal revisions, the architects of the code acknowledge the fallibility of it, these architects still characterize the authority of the Code as nonnegotiable. What this seems to mean is that the Code can be revised and improved. However, there is a proper process for this. A singular practitioner defying the provision in question is not the process, and such an action is technically immoral until decided otherwise through the proper, accepted process. This exposes the cold, procedural nature of professional ethics as expressed through the implementation of codes of ethics. Ideally, ethics is not about mere procedure. However, in guiding and maintaining the actions of an indefinitely large group of individuals, procedure may be unavoidable.

Just as there may be moral conflicts between practitioners and codes of ethics, there can also be moral conflicts between practitioners and other normative systems that confront professionals, like policy and law. Policy refers to the formal rules of an institution like a hospital or university. Ideally, policy should itself have some moral foundation and should aim to preserve the values and achieve the goals of the institution. However, again, as humans are morally fallible, policy may often fall short of these ideals. This means that practitioners with a conscience and moral awareness might have to face the possibility of morally resisting institutional policy, placing themselves and their careers at risk. Much the same could be said regarding conflicts between law and morality, but with possibly more severe consequences, which we will take a closer look at in Chapter 31, A Bad Action: Is It Ethical, Illegal, or Both?

This question of moral resistance, either to institutional policy or to a code of ethics, raises the important point of professional moral agency and helps further clarify the role of codes of ethics in ethical decision-making. The (theoretical) possibility that a professional code of ethics could be morally incorrect, while an individual professional is morally correct indicates that codes of ethics are not simply rule books to follow unquestioningly. When a professional makes an ethical decision, whether that decision is consistent with the professional's code of ethics or not, that decision is owned by that professional. Codes of ethics make no decisions themselves. It is the individual practitioner who makes and owns the decision. The code of ethics operates as a guide, not a rule book. Assuming otherwise would wrest professional autonomy from the practitioner, absolve all professionals of moral accountability, and, as noted earlier, would not even be possible, since we could not foresee all potential problems that could arise to provide a specific rule for.

Function and Purpose

From the analysis so far we see that guiding professionals in ethical decision-making is a primary and obvious purpose or function of codes of ethics. However, the social reality of codes of ethics is far more complex than this, and several more nuanced purposes of codes of ethics have been identified. Codes of ethics can function as an expression of professionalism (Biton & Tabak, 2003). The very development of a code of ethics, as implied in Baker's (2005) analysis, demonstrates the maturity of a profession and its acknowledgment of its place in society, its impact on society, and its responsibility regarding these. In a related manner, Peterson and Potter (2004) maintain that codes of ethics help to provide a group identity. Along with associations, conferences, and other forms of standards of practice, codes of ethics help to consolidate a professional identity through a common appeal to values and goals.

Noting the relationship between ethical theory and codes of ethics, Dean (1992) explains the purpose of codes of ethics as translating philosophical ethics into guidelines applied to "day to day decision-making" (p. 285). Ethical theory can often seem highly abstract and alienated from daily needs. Not every professional can be expected to have the level of philosophical training to translate this esoteric thought into practical application. Codes of ethics, according to Dean (1992), help fill this gap that the typical professional, even with some ethics education, may not be suited to fill.

Finally, somewhat cynically, one might say that a purpose of a code of ethics would be to express a professional image (Johnson, 2009; Morrison, 2011). In other words, a code acts as simple window dressing, as an attempt to appear committed to ethics without a truly substantive commitment. In an ideal world a code of ethics would not function like this, but we cannot completely discount this as a possibility. Knowing these various possible functions and purposes brings a deeper understanding of how codes of ethics can and do function. Primarily, they are understood to help in making ethical decisions, but socially they function in much more nuanced ways.

Criticisms and Limitations

As common and popular as codes of ethics are in contemporary professional ethics, some ethicists and professionals have concerns about them. Some criticisms or limitations have already been raised or implied herein. First, any code of ethics will be fallible, as it is created by morally fallible humans (Dahnke, 2009). But as argued here, this is not only a necessary quality of a code of ethics, but possibly a strength of codes as well by noting the need to acknowledge moral humility and the changing moral landscape that practitioners must confront. Related to this initial problem is the challenge of keeping up with technological, environmental, and organizational changes (Dahnke, 2009). Acknowledging moral humility and periodically revising the code of ethics is an effective means of responding to this issue.

In addition to these issues, critics have identified other problems or limitations. The interpretation problem (Eriksson, Höglund, & Helgesson, 2008) stems from the fact that specific rules for every potential problem cannot be devised and that we need to rely upon the individual reasoning (interpretation) and autonomy of practitioners. Because the principles and provisions of codes of ethics are necessarily general and based upon broader ethical theories, some degree of interpretation by individual practitioners is unavoidable. In response to this, the purpose of a code is not to make decisions for professionals but to support and guide decisions. So, of course, we must rely upon the reasoning and interpretation of individual professionals. Thus, effective ethics education should be part of the education of professionals to ensure interpretation of codes of ethics is informed and critical (Dahnke, 2014).

The multiplicity problem (Eriksson et al., 2008; Morrison, 2011) refers to the fact that some professionals might find themselves beholden to more than one code of ethics. One aspect of this problem is that there are multiple codes of ethics for some professions, such as for nurses, the ANA's *Code of Ethics for Nurses* and the International Council of Nurse's *Code of Ethics for Nurses*. A different aspect of this problem, the "bicodal" problem, arises due to professionals who operate across different distinct professions and thus may be subject to the code of ethics of each. For example, a physician or nurse who is also a healthcare administrator may be subject to the American Medical Association or ANA code of ethics but also the *American College of Healthcare Executives Code of Ethics*. This issue is only a practical problem in those rare instances in which conflicts might arise between the codes. In such cases, it may be a matter, once again (or as always), of professional autonomy and personal deliberation to determine what the correct choice is.

The legalization problem (Eriksson et al., 2008) refers to the type of superficial perception or attitude toward codes of ethics noted earlier. The very act of reducing ethics to a set of enumerated principles or provisions may lead some to view the code of ethics itself and ethics in general in terms of merely and minimally meeting published standards. One could also say that the enforcement mechanisms of licensed professions might amplify this perception. A professional may think, "as long as I don't break the rules of the code and avoid punishment, I am ethically good." This attitude may work fine in terms of the law (thus, "the legalization problem"), but ethics requires more than meeting the minimum, than merely not breaking a rule and avoiding punishment. Ethics requires a conscious and well-meaning intention to do what is right, not merely to avoid doing what will incur punishment. A correct understanding of ethics in general and correct use of a code of ethics would be a direct response to this problem.

Lastly, the futility problem (Morrison, 2011) involves "the double presumption that an appropriately ethical professional will not need a code of ethics, and an unethical professional will, as a matter of her/his character, ignore a code of ethics" (Dahnke, 2014, p. 617). This double presumption suggests a false dilemma fallacy. The broad range of character found among professionals cannot be reduced to these two simple types. There are not just those professionals who are so naturally moral or pre-professionally educated as moral that they do not need a code of ethics and those who are so immoral that no amount of support, encouragement, and education will make any difference in their action. Most professionals fall somewhere between these extremes and it is those in this middle area that are in most need of and can benefit from moral support, encouragement, and education. Also, many moral problems within the technical context of a profession are more complicated than even a highly virtuous person may be able to deal with on their own. Even they may need the support, encouragement, and education of a code of ethics when confronted by very hard cases.

These various criticisms of codes of ethics do not negate them or their usefulness in aiding ethical decision-making in a professional context. These criticisms can, however, highlight important limitations of these codes. Codes cannot and do not make decisions. Only moral agents, like autonomous professionals, can do that. However, they can do so with the assistance of the deliberation of a professional association reduced to a coherent statement of value and purpose. So, with these limitations in mind, codes of ethics can still be a valuable tool for professionals individually and also for professions as a whole to retain their reputation and their trust among the general public.

APPLIED ETHICS

Each one of the theories and the very concept of codes of ethics have been accompanied by a number of criticisms. This fact does not nullify the value of these tools of ethical deliberation. Despite the fallibility of a code of ethics, it may still help identify central values and coherently guide ethical decision-making. Despite none of the theories achieving universal assent, each may identify and develop important aspects of ethical thought and the ethical life. There are some ethicists today who subscribe to a particular theory, but most seem rather to practice some form of moral pluralism, meaning that no one theory has a monopoly on the truth of morality, but multiple theories can contribute to a broader, more comprehensive understanding of morality and a coherent, more comprehensive analysis and evaluation of specific issues and cases. In addressing an issue or case, we can learn from utilitarianism to ask about the consequences. Who is going to be harmed? Who is going to benefit? What is the extent and quality of these harms and benefits? From deontological theories, we learn that consequences are not everything. Are the means we choose to achieve these results problematic? Do they involve violation of the dignity or rights of anyone involved? We can also ask about the virtues involved in possible actions. What might someone we consider to be virtuous do in such a situation? What virtues should we draw upon or develop in addressing the issue in question? Are there important care relationships involved? Questions such as these, drawn from and inspired by the many theories that have attempted to understand what ethics is, can help us to come to a clearer understanding and possible answers to the problems that confront us.

Theories are often measured against our moral intuitions or considered moral judgments. That is not to assume that these intuitions are absolute and flawless, but they are an inherent part of our moral thinking. We also measure these theories against particular cases that we face. But this measuring or testing is reciprocal. We test our intuitions against our theories and concrete cases. We test theories and principles against our intuitions and cases. And we test cases we face against our intuitions and theories and principles. Formally speaking, this is a process introduced by political philosopher John Rawls (1971) and later developed by bioethicists Beauchamp and Childress (2013) known as reflective equilibrium. Through continuous testing of these three elements of moral thought against each other, we attempt to pursue, if not achieve, a state of coherent stability among these three elements. None of these elements is assumed to be absolute or primarily foundational. Each is accepted as fallible and corrigible. As we live life and encounter new situations, we may find one element or another does not fit or help in a new situation. This type of situation disrupts the equilibrium that holds between these elements. Through reflection (reasoned thought), we attempt to reestablish equilibrium by adjusting one of these elements. This process leaves ethical thought a continual dynamic function that never settles but is always in need of further justification and reflection and does not fall into dogmatism or unproven absolutist assumptions. Codes of ethics, as derived and justified through theoretical ethics, have a place in this process as well, in developing, testing, and revising the different elements of one's moral framework.

Are there final and objective answers to ethical questions regarding specific acts, cases, and issues? This itself is an ongoing question within the field of theoretical ethics. It seems that in applied ethics the ideal would be to reach an objectively justified answer that all reasonable people can agree with. Some might say that such an ideal answer is not possible. But others might more modestly say that it is not always possible. Above all, hopefully at the least a reason can be found to consider a search for objective answers. Most of the theories appealed to in applied ethics either assume or argue for some foundation for the reality of objective ethics. Utilitarians maintain that an objective evaluation of the benefits and harms to affected individuals will lead to an objective evaluation of a decision. Kant holds that an abstract, formal and rational evaluation of an act will lead to an objective moral judgment of it. Natural law theorists locate the objectivity of morality in the objectivity of the natural world and human nature. Virtue theorists similarly identify objective good in an analysis of human nature—or identified social goods in the case of MacIntyre. Even ethics of care theorists, whose moral evaluation appears more subjectivist and emotion based than in these other theories, engage in reasoned argumentation, defending objective truth about the value of the theory and the truth of the central place of caring in human life. In none of these are the claims of objective moral truth unquestioned or unquestionable. They all leave clear areas of uncertainty and room for veiled and unacknowledged subjectivity. This apparent failure does not disprove the existence of objective judgment in ethics but should instead point to avenues for further discussion of objective answers to be found in ethical discourse.

The assumption that there are no objective moral right and wrong often follows from the focus on "hard cases" that ethical study typically addresses. In contrast to this, what needs to be acknowledged is the mundanity of most ethical life. Many things we do in our everyday life have an ethical aspect to them. However, we typically do not recognize that, as there is little question about what is ethically proper in the situation. When a nurse compassionately and competently responds to a patient in need, she may not be consciously considering the ethics of her actions, but, when fulfilled compassionately and competently, those actions are ethical. When you shop at a store and pay for your items before leaving rather than attempting to leave without paying, you are acting ethically.

The point is that the ethical thing to do in most cases is not in question, is not something we need to commit time and thought to in order to come to a decision. It is when the moral quality of actions, cases, and issues is uncertain that we begin to think about ethics. In other words, we do not devote thought to the easy cases but to the hard cases. And so, we begin to think that ethics is only about hard cases. And if we cannot immediately come to a clear answer regarding these hard cases, we assume that there are no clear or objective answers for ethics in general.

The fact that hard cases are hard does not mean that there no objective answers to be had. However, there is no guarantee that we will come to a consensual answer either. Sometimes the most we can hope is that ethical analysis and evaluation will help sharpen the dispute and lead us to a clearer and deeper understanding of what is at stake (Strike & Soltis, 2009). Sometimes this will be enough to provide for us an answer we can successfully defend to others. Sometimes it will not. Sometimes when it comes to very difficult and complex problems, reasonable, informed, well-intentioned people will disagree. What do we do then? A practical answer to that question depends a lot on the specific situation. First, it may be helpful to remember Aristotle's (1941) counsel that we should not expect more precision from a discipline than it can provide: "for precision is not to be sought for alike in all discussions, any more than in all the products of the crafts" (p. 936). In mathematics we can expect a high level of precision. In ethics, we may learn to expect much less precision. But that is not to say there can be no clear answers. We simply have to manage our expectations in that regard. Second, if the situation is one in which the decision is ultimately yours alone, then you need to learn to trust your judgment. In that particular instance, your judgment may be right, or it may be wrong. However, if you have honestly and comprehensively analyzed the situation, if you have consulted others (especially those with potentially relevant and valuable experience and expertise), then the best you may be able to do is trust yourself and act upon that. If the situation is one in which the decision is not solely your own, the answer there too may vary. As noted, in some cases reasonable people can disagree. If possible, the discussion may have to continue, and perhaps an answer will yet be found. If it is not possible to continue discussion, you need to consider the stakes and explore the possibility of compromise or acknowledging uncertainty in letting another's judgment reign. If the stakes are too high, you may not want to surrender. But the consequences of surrendering may turn out to be worse than holding to your position. The point is, even in the midst of uncertainty, we can explore possibilities and find the best possible answer even if an ideal answer is not forthcoming. In other words, we live in a world of uncertainty. We have to accept that but not let that prevent us from doing the very best we can.

CRITICAL ELEMENTS TO CONSIDER

- Consider different ethical theories and the central elements of morality that they each focus on.
- Utilitarianism alerts us to the importance of the consequences of our actions.
- Deontological theories like Kantianism and natural law theory warn us against justifying any means to attain a desirable end. Sometimes a means may be wrong in itself and should be avoided.
- Virtue theory and ethics of care remind us of the importance of character, personal moral development, and personal relationships in the context of ethical decision-making.
- Professional codes of ethics draw upon and justify themselves through ethical theory and consolidate the values and standards of a profession as a guide toward moral deliberation and decision-making.
- Professional codes of ethics cannot answer all professional ethical questions that a practitioner might confront. Rather, it is the professional who must employ their own reasoning to make their own decision, possibly with the code providing guidance.

Helpful Resources

- Ethics Updates: A website from ethics educator and author Lawrence Hinman, Professor Emeritus of Philosophy at the University of San Diego, that provides educational resources on both theoretical and applied ethics: http://ethicsupdates.net/
- The Center for Study of Ethics in the Professions at the Illinois Institute of Technology: http://ethics.iit .edu/teaching/professional-ethics
- The American Nurses Association Code of Ethics: https://www.nursingworld.org/practice-policy/nursing -excellence/ethics/code-of-ethics-for-nurses/
- The American Association of University Professors Statement on Professional Ethics: https://www .aaup.org/NR/rdonlyres/DCB2B487-5ACF-400C-BCAA-118A27788B57/0/EthicsStmt.pdf

References

American College of Healthcare Executives. (2019). *ACHE ethics committee scope and function*. Retrieved from https://www.ache.org/about-ache/our-story/our-commitments/ethics/ache-code-of-ethics/ ache-ethics-committee-scope-and-function

Aquinas, T. (2012). *The summa theologica of St. Thomas Aquinas* (Fathers of the English Dominican Province, Trans.). London, UK: Veritatis Splendor Publications.

Aristotle. (1941). In R. McKeon (Ed.), *The basic works of Aristotle*. New York, NY: Random House.

Askitopoulou, H., & Vgontzas, A. N. (2018). The relevance of the Hippocratic Oath to the ethical and moral values of contemporary medicine. Part I: The Hippocratic Oath from antiquity to modern times. *European Spine Journal, 27*(7), 1481–1490. doi:10.1007/s00586-017 5348-4

Baier, A. (1987). Hume: The woman's moral theorist? In E. F. Kittay & D. Meyers (Eds.), *Women and moral theory* (pp. 37–55). Totowa, NJ: Rowman & Littlefield.

Baker, R. (2005). A draft model aggregated code of ethics for bioethicists 1. *American Journal of Bioethics, 5*(5), 33–41. doi:10.1080/15265160500245188

Beauchamp, T. L., & Childress, J. F. (2013). *Principles of biomedical ethics* (7th ed.). New York, NY: Oxford University Press.

Benjamin, M., & Curtis, J. (2010). *Ethics in nursing: Cases, principles, and reasoning* (4th ed.). New York, NY: Oxford University Press.

Bentham, J. (1988). *The principles of morals and legislation*. Amherst, NY: Prometheus Books.

Biton, V., & Tabak, N. (2003). The relationship between the application of the nursing ethical code and nurses' work satisfaction. *International Journal of Nursing Practice, 9*, 140–157. doi:10.1046/j.1440-172X.2003.00418.x

Card, C. (1990). Caring and evil. *Hypatia, 5*(1), 101–108. doi:10.1111/j.1527-2001.1990.tb00393.x

Catto, G. (2014). The Hippocratic Oath: Back to the future? *Medical Education, 48*, 4–5. doi:10.1111/ medu.12359

Dahnke, M. D. (2009). The role of the American Nurses Association Code of Ethics in ethical decision-making. *Holistic Nursing Practice, 23*(2), 112–119. doi:10.1097/HNP.0b013e3181a1114a

Dahnke, M. D. (2014). Utilizing codes of ethics in health professions education. *Advances in Health Sciences Education, 19*(4), 611–623. doi:10.1007/s10459-013-9484-2

Dahnke, M. D. (2015). Devotion, diversity, and reasoning: Religion and medical ethics. *Bioethical Inquiry, 12*, 709–722. doi:10.1007/s11673-015-9658-0

Dahnke, M. D., & Dreher, H. M. (2016). *Philosophy of science for nursing practice: Concepts and application* (2nd ed.). New York, NY: Springer Publishing Company.

Davis, A. J., Fowler, M. D., & Aroskar, M. A. (2010). *Ethical dilemmas and nursing practice* (5th ed.). Boston, MA: Pearson.

Dean, P. J. (1992). Making codes of ethics "real". *Journal of Business Ethics, 11*(4), 285–290. doi:10.1007/ BF00872170

Eriksson, S., Höglund, A. T., & Helgesson, G. (2008). Do ethical guidelines give guidance? A critical examination of eight ethics regulations. *Cambridge Quarterly of Healthcare Ethics, 17*, 15–29. doi:10.1017/ S0963180108080031

Fowler, M. D. M. (2008). Introduction. In M. D. M. Fowler (Ed.), *Guide to the Code of Ethics for Nurses: Interpretation and application* (pp. xiii–xx). Silver Spring, MD: American Nurses Association.

Fry, S. T., Veatch, R. M., & Taylor, C. (2011). *Case studies in nursing ethics* (4th ed.). Sudbury, MA: Jones & Bartlett.

Gilligan, C. (1993). *In a different voice: Psychological theory and women's development.* Boston, MA: Harvard University Press.

Halwani, R. (2003). *Virtuous liaisons: Care, love, sex, and virtue ethics.* Peru, IL: Open Court.

Held, V. (2006). *The ethics of care: Personal, political, and global.* New York, NY: Oxford University Press.

Hume, D. (1974). An enquiry concerning human understanding. In *The empiricists* (pp. 307–430). Garden City, NY: Anchor Books. (Original work published 1748).

Hursthouse, R. (1991). Virtue theory and abortion. *Philosophy & Public Affairs, 20*(3), 223–246. Retrieved from https://www-jstor-org.rdas-proxy.mercy.edu/stable/pdf/2265432.pdf

Hursthouse, R. (2006). Applying virtue ethics to our treatment of the other animals. In J. Welchman (Ed.), *The practice of virtue: Classic and contemporary readings in virtue ethics* (pp. 136–155). Indianapolis, IN: Hackett Publishing.

Johnson, C. E. (2009). *Meeting the ethical challenges of leadership: Casting light or shadow.* Thousand Oaks, CA: SAGE Publications.

Kant, I. (2012). *Groundwork of the metaphysics of morals* (M. Gregor & J. Timmerman, Trans.). Cambridge, UK: Cambridge University Press.

Kohlberg, L. (1982). Moral development. In J. M. Broughton & D. J. Freeman Moir (Eds.), *The cognitive developmental psychology of James Mark Baldwin: Current theory and research in genetic epistemology* (pp. 277–325). Norwood, NJ: Ablex.

Korsgaard, C. M. (1996). *Creating the kingdom of ends.* Cambridge, UK: Cambridge University Press.

Kuhse, H. (1995). Clinical ethics and nursing: "Yes" to caring, but "no" to a female ethics of care. *Bioethics, 9*(3/4), 207–219. doi:10.1111/j.1467-8519.1995.tb00356.x

Louden, R. B. (1984). On some vices of virtue ethics. *American Philosophical Quarterly, 21*(3), 227–236. Retrieved from https://www-jstor-org.rdas-proxy.mercy.edu/stable/pdf/20014051.pdf

MacIntyre, A. (1985). *After virtue: A study in moral theory* (2nd ed.). London, UK: Duckworth.

Mill, J. S. (2017). *Utilitarianism.* Mineola, NY: Dover Publications.

Morrison, E. E. (2011). *Ethics in health administration: A practical approach for decision-makers.* Sudbury, MA: Jones & Bartlett Publishers.

Müller, S. (2008). Bodily Integrity Identity Disorder (BIID): Is the amputation of health limbs ethically justified? *The American Journal of Bioethics, 9*(1), 36–43. doi:10.1080/15265160802588194

Nagl-Docekal, H. (1997). Feminist ethics: How it could benefit from Kant's moral philosophy. In R. M. Schott (Ed.), *Feminist interpretations of Immanuel Kant* (pp. 101–124). University Park: Pennsylvania State University Press.

Noddings, N. (2013). *Caring: A relational approach to ethics and moral education* (2nd ed.). Berkeley, CA: University of California Press.

Nussbaum, N. C. (1999). Virtue ethics: A misleading category? *The Journal of Ethics, 3*(3), 163–201. doi:10.1023/A:1009877217694

Pellegrino, E. D., & Thomasma, D. C. (1996). *The Christian virtues in medical practice.* Washington, DC: Georgetown University Press.

Pellegrino, E. D., Thomasma, D. C. (1997). *Helping and healing: Religious commitment in health care.* Washington, DC: Georgetown University Press.

Peterson, M., & Potter, R. L. (2004). A proposal for a code of ethics for nurse practitioners. *Journal of the American Academy of Nurse Practitioners, 16*(3), 116–124. doi:10.1111/j.1745-7599.2004.tb00382.x

Puka, B. (1990). The liberation of caring: A different voice for Gilligan's "different voice." *Hypatia, 55*(1), 58–82. doi:10.1111/j.1527-2001.1990.tb00390.x

Rachels, J. (1999). *The elements of moral philosophy.* San Francisco, CA: McGraw-Hill.

Rawls, J. (1971). *A theory of justice* (Rev. ed.). Cambridge, MA: Harvard University Press.

Schwartz, R. L. (1992). Autonomy, futility, and the limits of medicine. *Cambridge Quarterly of Healthcare Ethics, 1*(2), 159–164. doi:10.1017/S0963180100000268

Slote, M. (1998). The justice of caring. *Social Philosophy and Policy, 15*(1), 171–195. doi:10.1017/S0265052500003113

Smart, J. J. C., & Williams, B. (1973). *Utilitarianism: For and against.* Cambridge, UK: Cambridge University Press.

Strike, K., & Soltis, J. F. (2009). *The ethics of teaching* (5th ed.). New York, NY: Teachers College Press.

Thomson, J. J. (1985). The trolley problem. *Yale Law Journal, 94*(6), 1395–1415. doi:10.2307/796133

Tronto, J. (1993). *Moral boundaries: A political argument for an ethic of care.* New York, NY: Routledge.

Varden, H. (2010). Kant and lying to the murderer at the door…one more time: Kant's legal philosophy and lies to murderers and Nazis. *Journal of Social Philosophy, 41*(4), 403–421. doi:10.1111/j.1467-9833.2010.01507.x

6

The Ethics of Nursing Education

NURSING ETHICS? EDUCATION ETHICS?

When asking about the ethics of nursing education it seems that one is asking the more complicated question of the ethics of two distinct fields: nursing and education (in particular higher or tertiary education) On the one hand there exists a study of ethics that focuses on the duties and values of nursing On the other hand, a distinct study of ethics revolves around the practice of teaching and education at the college level. Thus, in considering the ethics of nursing education, one may have to examine ethics from the perspective of both fields. A further development of this complication is the dual role of most nursing professors leading to an instance of the bicodal problem of codes of ethics (Dahnke, 2014; Morrison, 2011). Most instructors who teach in nursing programs are academic professionals and also licensed nurses.[1] This implies that for the majority of nursing instructors, the ethics of nursing and the ethics of teaching, and more specifically, of tertiary education, intersect. That is, a nurse who is a nursing instructor must be mindful of the ethical values, virtues, and principles of nursing and of education as well. And more specifically, these professions also have their own statements or codes of ethics. Therefore, in this chapter I look in turn at the ethics of both nursing and of higher education, with an especial focus on established codes or statements of ethics to excavate a deeper understanding of both these and, hopefully, their intersection.

The relevance of nursing ethics, *qua* the ethics of *nurses*, to this broader study may be legitimately doubted. When one thinks of nursing in general and nursing ethics in particular, one typically thinks first, and perhaps only, of nurses' interactions with patients: acting with compassion, maintaining confidentiality, respecting autonomy, and so on. In addition, duties to patients may be perceived as having implied priority through placement in nursing codes of ethics. In the ANA's *Code of Ethics for Nurses With Interpretive Statements* (hereafter, the "ANA Code"), duties to patients are outlined in the first three provisions (2015). In the International Council of Nurses' (2012) *Code of Ethics for Nurses* (hereafter, the "ICN Code"), the first of the four elements focuses on duties to patients. Nurses who are educators do not, as educators, treat patients. They may treat patients as a possibly adventitious element of their teaching practice, but in contrast to most nurses, their primary practice is directed toward students, not patients. However, there are at least two ways in which nursing values and ethics are clearly and patently relevant to nursing education, and these can be seen expressed in major nursing codes of ethics like the ANA Code and the ICN Code. First, one can conceive a vicarious duty in that the nurse educator has a duty to protect and promote the health, safety, and dignity of the future patients a student may treat. Second, although the common understanding of

---

[1] By "most" I am acknowledging that there are instructors in specialized areas like pharmacology or ethics who teach in nursing programs but are not licensed nurses. Although these instructors may not be formally and professionally obligated to a nursing code of ethics like the ANA's code as licensed nurses are, they, in their educational activities within an academic nursing program, may still be informally obligated to duties discussed here in recognition of the goals of their teaching as preparing new, competent, and ethical nursing professionals.

nursing ethics and initial focus of codes of ethics is on the treatment of patients, that is not all there is to nursing ethics and those are not the only duties and values recognized by nursing codes of ethics. The ANA Code (2015) in its Introduction notes that "not all who are recipients of nursing care are either suffering or receiving medical treatment" (p. xi). Here, the ANA introduces the distinction between "patients" and "clients," noting the changing terminology in our culture and broader roles for nurses beyond bedside care. In addition, beyond the first three provisions the code outlines ethical values and goals much more directly related to the activities of nurse educators, especially Provisions 6 and 7, but also passing references in Provisions 2, 3, and 4. However, the moral duties of nursing in relation to education cannot be said to be exhausted by these brief mentions. The ICN Code arguably provides more developed commentary on the values and duties of the nurse educator. However, since the ANA Code is authoritative for nurses licensed in the United States, I focus on that code in the analysis to follow.

NURSING ETHICS

When investigating the ethics of a particular area of activity or professional practice, I find an Aristotelian-based approach provides a good start. In ethics, and most other areas of study, Aristotle held that understanding could be gleaned through a study of purposes. So, in attempting to understand the ethics of nursing, we need first to ask what the purposes, functions, or goals of nursing are.[2] There may be no uniform list to refer to. And if we were to ask various qualified sources (experts in nursing from various backgrounds and experiences), we would likely receive a variety of answers—though likely with some general similarities. So any answer I produce here cannot be assumed to be absolutely authoritative and final. But we are engaged in an exploration, so we can begin somewhere with at least provisional confidence. The clearest statement of nursing purpose found in the ANA Code (2015) enjoins nurses to protect, promote and restore health and well-being; prevent illness and injury; and alleviate suffering. The ICN Code (2012) identifies four similar fundamental responsibilities of nurses: "to promote health, to prevent illness, to restore health and to alleviate suffering" (p. 1). As expected, while not exactly the same, there are broad similarities among these. We could continue to investigate more sources, but these are sufficiently authoritative and clear enough to give us a place to begin.

Both of these statements of purpose include the promotion and restoration of health, the prevention of illness, and the alleviation of suffering. The ANA statement additionally conjoins well-being with health and includes injury (the prevention of) along with illness. The ANA Code also includes the restoration of health as part of nursing's purpose. In addition, the ANA Code identifies the targets of these activities. At this point we could engage in a detailed and exhaustive exegesis of the differences between these two statements and perhaps judging whether there is virtue in the relative brevity of the ICN statement or the greater overall development in the ANA statement. However, that type of textual analysis is not focus here. These statements give us a clear enough initial understanding of the purpose of nursing.

An understanding of purpose allows us to begin to explore the ethics of nursing more substantively. The ethics will consist of those values, duties, and virtues that help nurses individually and as a whole fulfill those identified purposes or can be logically derived from these purposes. In both these statements there is an implication, widely if not universally accepted around the world, that health (and well-being) is to be valued and illness is not. That is, there is a well-established assumption that health and well-being are to be sought and illness avoided. While health as a value and illness (and injury) as a detriment may seem so obvious as to be not worth mentioning, that is not entirely true. There are contexts and cultural situations in which illness and injury have been valued. In a study of medical sociology and anthropology that may be an intriguing path to follow. For us, however, we can accept, at least as a general truth, the value of health and well-being and the disvalue of illness and injury. Those rather narrow contexts in which the opposite might hold could become relevant within the context of nursing and of nursing ethics; however, their uniqueness only makes them

---

[2] Philosophically speaking, these three concepts can be importantly distinguished. However, for our purposes here those distinctions are not particularly significant. So I will elide those for now.

a hindrance to our pursuit of a general understanding of nursing ethics and they represent cases which would have to be dealt with as exceptional. Considering the question more deeply, we might realize the relativity of our judgments of good and bad (valued and disvalued) conditions. For example, many illnesses are caused by bacteria. Because we value health and well-being, we judge the conditions (illnesses) that result from these bacteria as bad and thus the bacteria themselves as bad. However, many bacteria, such as gut flora, are also necessary for our well-being, for our digestive health in the case of gut flora. What is central then is the value we place on our lives and continued existence that places a focus on our well-being. But it is not as simple as that either. Well-being itself can be an open term. It may not simply mean that one continues to exist or continues to live but also the quality of that continued existence. As persons, not merely human beings, we value particular aspects of our being: rational thought, deliberation, autonomous choice, freedom, social interaction, and so on. Thus, health and well-being, as values, come to mean something more than continued biological life but continued life of a particular kind, which leads to the need to foster and support not simply the continued metabolic functions of respiration and circulation but the ability to think for one's self, make one's own decisions, and congregate with others.

The ANA Code of Ethics

Going further, I think it will be helpful to survey statements of ethics as they apply to nurses. These statements may be morally correct or not. It is always intellectually healthy to approach any ethical claims presented to us with skepticism. And my use of these statements of ethics is primarily to examine what the commonly accepted and possibly even professionally compelled standards are and to have a rough guide rather than to presume to reinvent the wheel. I do not assume that any professional statement of ethics is a faultless moral authority. The fact that most professional codes of ethics have a formal process for revision from time to time reinforces this. However, I do approach professional codes of ethics with the assumption that they were produced by recognized experts in their field, with ethics training and study as well, who are well intentioned and have committed sincerely and assiduously to this project. Thereby, I come to a professional code of ethics with an assumption of its moral authority and rectitude but not with any assumptions of perfection or permanence. In this way, these codes can function for us as guides and learning tools.

The ANA Code (ANA, 2015) declares itself quite patently in the second line of its Preface to be nonnegotiable. It then immediately qualifies in the next sentence that it can only be revised or amended through the formal processes established by the ANA. I do not interpret this "nonnegotiable" assertion as one of moral infallibility or an assumption of *absolute* moral authority. Rather, this claim establishes a needed sense of professional and moral stability and authority (Dahnke, 2009). An absence of such stability will result in constant professional uncertainty and chaos. However, at the same time, an acknowledged process for revision communicates the recognition of fallibility and the need to adjust to a dynamic environment. This leaves open the possibility for true moral resistance in regard to the ANA Code. What I mean by this is that it is at least theoretically possible that a nurse may be morally justified in an act that contravenes the ANA Code. As stated, I begin with the assumption of moral rectitude and authority, so such an instance would be unlikely but not impossible. And because of the ANA Code's "nonnegotiable" assertion, from the perspective of accepted professional nursing ethics, such a nurse would be *de jure* morally wrong, while possibly being *de facto* morally correct. This would leave the "offending" nurse susceptible to professional censure or sanction. Stability then is purchased at the (unlikely) cost of unjust treatment of a nurse such as this. However, given the values, such as justice, affirmed in the document, such censure may be recognized as unjust and then vetoed in this particular case.[3] That would demonstrate that the ANA Code was not simply a roster of fetishized rules but a statement of sincere moral commitment. Indeed, such a reading of the ANA Code (2015) is implied further in its Preface which asserts that nurses and professional nursing organizations need to not merely adhere to the expressed values and norms but to embrace them as part of the essence of nursing. In other words, nurses must do more

---

[3] This would depend on the offending nurse being able to establish, beyond the nurse's own conscience, that the nurse's acts, not the ANA Code, were morally correct.

than simply follow rules when engaging with the ANA Code. This statement is a call for nurses to do more than simply follow rules when engaging with the ANA Code. A truly moral nurse will not just follow the rules but follow the rules because they identify with and affirm themselves the same values and ideals as are expressed in the ANA Code. These values and ideals comprise in part who they are as professionals (if not as persons) and are not just decrees obediently adopted toward the narrow end of having a means of livelihood.

In taking a look at the ANA Code, we can divide the nine provisions into three thematic sets of three provisions. The first set of three focuses on the nurse's relationship with patients:

- Provision 1: To respect the inherent dignity and worth of each person through practicing with respect and compassion.
- Provision 2: To practice with one's primary commitment to the patient.
- Provision 3: To protect, promote, and advocate for the patient's safety, rights and health.

The interpretive statements of the first provision draw largely upon deontological views of ethics as they emphasize and develop the duties of respect and justice, including respect for inherent dignity and worth of individuals regardless of individual differences (ANA, 2015). The underlying deontological basis for this is recognition of the inherent and equal value of persons as irreplaceable individuals with rationality and autonomy. Bias or prejudice based upon one's religion, culture, gender expression, primary language, and health status is to be avoided. Thus, patients are to be treated equally as persons, regardless of individual difference. Regarding prejudice in relation to health status, certain illnesses carry social stigma that can lead to different and lesser treatment by healthcare professionals. Some may attribute blame to those who suffer from so-called lifestyle diseases like obesity, heart disease, or diabetes. And the emergence of the HIV/AIDS pandemic in the 1980s presented an especially powerful challenge to this duty. Due to its infectious nature, many misconceptions of the disease in the early days of the pandemic, the lack of a cure (or even effective treatment early on), and near total fatal prognosis early on, along with association with already marginalized groups (homosexual men, IV drug abusers), the disease left many suffering from it open to discrimination—even, unfortunately by healthcare professionals (Avert, 2018). Regardless of disease, etiology, or preexisting stigma, a person suffering is simply a person suffering and in need.

Respect for patients also encompasses respect for patient self-determination. Whether or not a nurse agrees with a patient's decision about a particular issue or treatment, that decision, assuming autonomous capacity on the patient's part, should be respected. Medical decisions are comprised not just of medical facts but are a combination of medical facts and values. No one knows an individual's values better than that individual. Thus, respecting a medical decision (even or especially one that the nurse does not agree with) is a form of respecting the person. However, the provision also acknowledges a nursing duty not to deny all critical assessment of patient decisions. Choices that are "risky or self-destructive" (ANA, 2015, p. 1) should be addressed, and patients should be provided resources to change their behavior. Finally, the interpretive statements of the first provision also note the obligation to treat not just patients but colleagues and all others with whom a nurse would interact professionally in a respectful and caring manner and to cultivate kindness and civility through promotion of an ethical environment (ANA, 2015).

The second provision also draws upon deontological ethics with a focus on the principle of fidelity. This provision in part reinforces provision one but focuses especially on conflicts of interests. Of the many interests and obligations, both personal and professional, that may weigh upon a nurse, the interests and good of the patient should be primary. Thus, conflicts of interest should be avoided to ensure those interests are not put at risk due to dual loyalties. In order to ensure the primacy of patients' interests, effective collaboration with other health professionals needs to be cultivated (ANA, 2016). And finally, ensuring the primacy of patient interests requires also the maintenance of professional boundaries. There is acknowledgment of the difficulty and possible paradox of this duty, given the sometimes emotion-based description of the nurse–client relationship based upon compassion. Despite the often personal quality of the nurse–client relationship, professional boundaries are necessary to ensure the goals of health promotion, protection, and restoration. Specifically, Interpretive Statement 2.4 notes the general prohibition of gifts from patients (though it seems to leave open the possibility of the appropriate acceptance of gifts given the circumstances) and the absolute prohibition of sexual relationships with patients.

The third provision continues the focus on duties to patients and continues with a deontological basis but includes also consequentialist justifications. In outlining duties to protect the rights, health, and safety of patients, the provision addresses specifically the rights of privacy and confidentiality. According to the provision, nurses have the duty to safeguard privacy in many forms of that term. Similarly, nurses have a duty to maintain confidentiality of patients' personal information. These duties can both be seen as extensions of the duty of respect for persons and autonomy. The protection here is for information and other intimate aspects of oneself that a right to control can be interpreted as a right to one's self. And thus, a violation of these would be a violation of personhood. The provision also includes that a violation of confidentiality would risk adverse consequences to patient well-being and nurse–client trust. The provision includes as well the rights of research subjects in terms of autonomy and maintenance of health and safety.

Largely in terms of consequentialism, the interpretive statements of Provision 3 also address policing of professional standards by nurses individually and collectively, fostering a culture of safety, and responding to questionable practice and impaired practice. These all address behavior and actions that risk the health and safety of patients. To ensure health and safety, nurses must adhere to accepted professional standards and maintain competence. Clearly questionable practice which may result in patient harm needs to be addressed. And the interpretive statements identify a process for addressing impaired practice.

Provisions 4 through 6 shift the focus from the needs, rights, and interests of patients (and colleagues) to those of nurses themselves:

- Provision 4: To acknowledge and put into practice their authority, accountability, and responsibility.
- Provision 5: To recognize that the nurse is similarly an inherently valuable individual and thus is owed the same respect and care, including the maintenance of one's own moral integrity and wholeness of character.
- Provision 6: To improve the ethical environment of the workplace.

Up until the 1960s, the ethics of nursing in general, and the ANA Code in particular, emphasized a duty to obey physicians (Butts, 2020). Provision 4 acknowledges the professional development of the nursing role by explicating the authority, accountability, and responsibility of the nurse (ANA, 2015). With greater moral and professional authority and self-determination comes of course greater responsibility and accountability. This includes not just the responsibility of nurses individually but collectively as well in defining and implementing standards of practice, which defines not just nurse individuals as autonomous professionals but nursing itself as an autonomous and independent profession.

The fifth provision is unique among codes of professional ethics. The practitioners of occupations, vocations, and professions that have care as their main focus risk exploitation and self-negation and are traditionally devalued and underpaid (Tronto, 2009). These potential harms exist both due to social factors in which caregivers are often not respected on par with other professions and to personal factors like the compassion trap. It may be due to this vulnerable nature of the caring professions that the ANA in Provision 5 acknowledges the value of and need for care of nurses themselves. Just as nurses must respect their patients and colleagues, they should also respect themselves by maintaining and protecting their own health, moral integrity, and competence (ANA, 2012, p. 19). As a nurse is a person the same as any patient or colleague, the nurse's own health and safety is equally important. Thus, self-negation and effacement should be avoided in recognition of one's own value and one's own needs as a human being. This acknowledgment can be employed in consideration of the necessarily controversial issue of nursing strikes. A nursing strike may place patient welfare at risk, but if the lack of consideration and working conditions are sufficiently problematic, the needs of nurses could possibly outweigh the potential harm a strike could precipitate. A comparison with Provision 2, primary commitment to the patient, is worth a look here. Clearly, "primary commitment" does not imply "sole commitment." Nurses, as professionals, as employees, and even simply as persons will have lives defined by many commitments, even to their own selves and well-being. Thus, commitment to the patient does not include neglect of one's self or interests. Indeed, one also has a duty to ensure one's own well-being, integrity, and professional fulfillment.

As with any sufficiently complex, human-centered activity, nurses will doubtless face situations that challenge their own values. A nurse with a pro-life view on abortion may be requested to participate in an abortion. A nurse with a vitalist point of view may be involved in a case of withdrawal of life-sustaining treatment. A nurse who is a Jehovah's Witness may become involved in a case that includes a blood transfusion. While all these actions and the nursing activities that accompany them are legal and at least generally endorsed by the ANA Code, the nurses involved may find engaging in such clinical activities would compromise or violate their own personal moral values. When this happens, a nurse's wholeness of character and moral integrity are put at risk. In cases such as these, the interpretive statements of Provision 5 offer the employment of conscientious objection as a means of preserving integrity. Not all cases in which nurses finds their personal morality at odds with professional duties (and ethics) may justify claims of conscientious objection. However, in those that do, conscientious objection can help nurses retain who they are as a person in terms of character. We also see here the acknowledgment that a nurse, as a person and not just a nurse, is to be recognized and respected as such. Nurses are something more than their profession and their essence as a person matters just as much as it does for their patients.

Provision 6 addresses nursing responsibilities toward the environment in which nurses work. As with the previous two provisions, there is an appeal to virtue ethics that becomes more explicit in the interpretive statements of this provision. Virtues, following an Aristotelian model, do not exist naturally or necessarily in any particular human being. Rather, each human has the potential to develop virtues or vices. This means that the existence and maintenance of virtues, individually and collectively, depends in part on the environment in which one finds oneself. A morally good environment will help foster virtues. This implies a duty, individually and collectively, for nurses to contribute to a morally good environment, for the moral health of themselves, of others in the unit, and of those who depend upon the competent and compassionate care provided. The recognition of this duty, following a virtue ethics conceptualization is described as creating a "culture of excellence" (ANA, 2012, p. 24). Sometimes consequentialist and deontological theories are criticized for focusing largely on negative duties, meaning obligations on what not to do more than obligations outlining what one should do: affirmative or positive duties. Virtue approaches more commonly focus on affirmative duties in the pursuit of not simply avoiding immorality and the violation of moral principles but in pursuing moral excellence, building a positive vision of good (or excellent) action and practice. This is what we see most explicitly in this provision: the duty not simply to avoid moral error but to contribute to a moral environment, to build a localized moral organization, rather than the simple negative duty of not harming the working environment. Specifically, the interpretive statements include as part of this duty to develop and support policies and procedures indicating ethical expectations and consistent understand of the ANA Code and other nursing ethics positions (ANA, 2015).

The final three provisions extend the circle of influence and obligation beyond the patient and the nurse and even the workplace to the profession of nursing itself and society in general. In addition, while the first six provisions can be interpreted as defining largely perfect duties (duties which one is always obligated to conform to), the last three may generally be interpreted as imperfect duties (duties which one is not constantly expected to fulfill but still has some duty to perform them):

- Provision 7: To engage in research, scholarly inquiry, the development of professional standards, or health policy as a means to advance the profession of nursing.
- Provision 8: To work toward the goals of protecting human rights, promoting health diplomacy, and reducing health disparities through collaboration with other health professionals.
- Provision 9: To promote social justice through the work of its professional organizations. he profession of nursing, collectively through its professional organizations, must articulate nursing values, maintain the integrity of the profession, and integrate principles of social justice into nursing and health policy.

Rather than focusing on the patient or the nurse, Provision 7 addresses obligations the nurse has toward nursing itself as a practice and as a profession. These obligations can be seen both deontologically and consequentially. Deontologically, one can recognize the value the profession of nursing has brought to any individual nurse. The existence of a collective of nursing professionals that defines standards of practice and regulates education, training, and licensure, and enforces standards of excellence provides the individual nurse with the professional structure that defines their role and legitimizes their work. An obligation to advance the profession may be seen as a form of reciprocity. The profession of nursing provides the individual nurse with multiple goods through which the nurse builds a life and career. Thus, one could say the individual nurse owes the profession of nursing and can repay through actions that advance nursing itself. Further, the existence of nursing as a cohesive profession is supported by a society that provides licensing and educational opportunities, a structure in which nursing can occur. This suggests a type of social contract. In this way, a duty to improve nursing is also a duty to society and the pact that exists between nursing and society. Consequentially, the duty to advance nursing can be seen as a means of improving the state of nursing itself and the outcomes for the clients that nurses care for.

Specifically, the interpretive statements of Provision 7 identify three areas in which nurses can advance the nursing profession. The first is through research and scholarly inquiry. The typical clinical nurse may not have extensive opportunities (or indeed the time) to advance nursing in this manner. Nurse educators and nurses in other roles, especially of course education, are more likely to focus in this area. However, there may be opportunities for clinical nurses to contribute in this manner as well. Second, the nurse can contribute through the development, maintenance, and implementation of professional practice standards. These standards ensure safe, effective, and ethical treatment, and "reflect nursing's responsibility to society" (ANA, 2012, p. 28). In particular, nurse educators have a responsibility to ensure that those entering the nursing profession possess these professional practice standards. And third, nurses can contribute through the development of health policy. Nurses, along with other healthcare professionals, can help ensure health policy at all levels is ethical and aimed toward improving the health and access to health for all.

Provision 8 extends the moral circle further, beyond one's patients, oneself, or even one's profession and toward humanity itself. Acknowledging that health is a human right implies that the need for nursing is universal. Thus, nurses must advance health, welfare, and safety and more generally fight for social justice through transformation of social structures and processes that ae either unjust in themselves or breed injustice (ANA, 2015). This provision recognizes that these goals are beyond any single nurse or even nursing as a profession collectively. The only way to effectively pursue these goals is collaboratively with other healthcare professionals as well as others who work toward the goals of social justice and human rights.

Just as these last three provisions expand the scope of obligation in nursing, the last of these final three provisions expands the assumption of agency. Provision 9 addresses the obligations of the profession of nursing rather than the individual nurse. These obligations stem from the sense of social contract referred to earlier. The rights, privileges, and prestige granted to the profession of nursing is to be returned with actions that ensure nursing fulfills its obligations and retains its dignity as a profession and its "covenant between the profession and society" (ANA, 2015, p. 36). These actions include asserting and strengthening the values of nursing, maintaining the integrity of the nursing profession through adherence to ethical standards, and addressing issues of social justice.

In summary, we see the ethical values and obligations of nursing operating at three general levels: the interactions between nurses and clients (and also colleagues), the duties to oneself, and duties beyond the clinic and classroom to society. Duties to patients include largely deontological duties of respecting the personhood and dignity of patients and all others encountered in the practice of healthcare. This includes respecting patients' self-determination, rights to confidentiality and privacy, setting aside bias and prejudice, and fostering "professional, respectful, and caring relationships with colleagues" (ANA, 2015, p. 4). In addition, nurses must place patients' interests first, avoid conflicts of interest, and maintain professional boundaries. And on the more consequentialist side, nurses must protect the health and safety of patients as well as subjects of research by responding to questionable and impaired practice. Duties to self include claiming one's own moral and professional authority, accepting accountability, maintaining moral integrity, caring for one's own health and well-being, and continuing personal and professional growth. Duties beyond the clinic include the mostly imperfect duties to advance the profession of nursing through research and scholarly inquiry, collaboration with others to address issues of human rights, social justice, and health disparities, and duties of the profession of nursing collectively to seek social justice and improvements in health policy.

ACADEMIC ETHICS

As with nursing ethics, in examining the ethics of the academic world, it may also be helpful to begin with an exploration of meaning, goals, and purposes. One of the founding documents of the American Association of University Professors (AAUP), the *1915 AAUP General Declaration of Principles*, identifies three functions through which universities serve the public interest:

A. To promote inquiry and advance the sum of human knowledge.
B. To provide general instruction to the students.
C. To develop experts for various branches of the public service. (AAUP, 2002, p. 182)

Similar to nursing ethics, we see the obligations of academics falling into three general categories. Tertiary educational institutions, and their officers (faculty, etc.), have a function and responsibility to extend, produce, and advance knowledge. Universities, colleges, and other similar educational institutions have a function and responsibility to provide an education for the public in order to prepare students for future professions or simply to impart and extend knowledge within the community. And universities have duties to society to provide experts. More simply put, these are duties related to (a) advancing knowledge, (b) instructing students, and (c) benefiting society. Pursuing these goals gives value to educational institutions and helps identify the values and duties of the academic world. These three functions can provide a structure through which to explore academic ethics more closely.

Unlike nursing and most other major healthcare professions, the academic world does not have a clear and comprehensive code of ethics. The closest cognate to a fully developed code of ethics like the ANA Code would be the AAUP's *1966 Statement on Professional Ethics* (AAUP, 2009). This statement, as a code of ethics, is not comprehensive and "covers only partially the relevant topics" (Hamilton, 2002, p. 4). Also, this statement focuses largely on protecting academic freedom and does not develop much in the way of ethical duties of universities and their faculty. It would be good, as Hamilton (2002) argues, for the academic profession to develop a more comprehensive code of ethics, with each discipline providing supplementary codes specific to their own issues. However, lacking that, in attempting to develop a coherent and comprehensive understanding of academic ethics, we can appeal to the 1966 statement plus a number of other ethics-oriented statements published by the AAUP as well as the general history and culture of academia.

The Advancement of Knowledge

The notion that a key function of universities and other institutions of higher education is to advance human knowledge can be found in the earliest universities. This function also defines in part the social contract between the university and society. Society provides the systems within to work, the prestige, and so forth, and the university system improves society through the extension and production of knowledge. And key to the ability of the university to advance knowledge is the principle of academic freedom. As a normative principle regulating the relationship between society and the higher education system, academic freedom has a long history. The first university in Europe, the University of Bologna, founded in 1088 (Grendler, 2002),[4] included the importance of academic freedom in its original charter, the *Constitutio Habita* (Jarvis, 2014).

The most commonly cited defense of academic freedom is based on concepts of "freedom of opinion" and "the marketplace of ideas" from John Stuart Mill's *On Liberty* (1910). Mill argues that the only way to ensure that we, as a society, have the best and truest ideas is to encourage open discussion of *all* ideas. Mill enumerates four general and elliptical arguments for the value of open discussion and public debate of ideas for society:

---

[4] There were, however, universities in Asia and Africa predating the University of Bologna, with the University of Al Quaraouiyine, founded in Morocco in 859, possibly being the oldest (Verger, 1992).

1. We cannot know whether a silenced opinion is in fact true or false.
2. That silenced opinion may not be completely true but could still contain some measure of truth.
3. If an opinion is accepted as true, unless we leave it open to further critique, it will only be held dogmatically not with true understanding.
4. Even a true opinion, without openness to critique, will lose its value and effect if held dogmatically and will become "a mere formal profession, inefficacious for good ... preventing the growth of any real and heartfelt conviction, from reason or personal experience." (Mill, 1910, p. 112)

Mill (1910) also finds free and open critique and debate valuable personally. Lacking personal engagement with this type of thought leaves oneself open to having others make decisions for them—thereby degrading one's own humanity. In addition, the qualities fostered through decision-making—observation, reasoning, judgment, activity, firmness, and self-control—are virtues central to humanity and personal growth. Thus, freedom of opinion, including free expression, critique, and critical examination of ideas, is beneficial both for society and for individuals.

One must keep in mind Mill's utilitarian and consequentialist ideology in regard to these arguments. The overall presumption is that acknowledgment of academic freedom will lead to a better, more beneficial society and the individual. So one possible rebuke may be that some ideas are dangerous and could cause harm to society and thus their proliferation should not be encouraged, contrary to the ideal of academic freedom. Mill, however, was confident that in weighing the possible harm of these hypothetical harmful ideas against the benefits of free and open inquiry, the latter would exceed the former. However, if this is not enough we could bolster these utilitarian arguments with the deontological claims regarding freedom as central to human nature, and thus denial of freedom as a denial of personhood, humanity, and moral agency. That is, to deny free inquiry in all forms, including academic freedom, would be to demean critical thinkers (academic scholars) and deny their personhood (Strike & Soltis, 2009).

The founding of the AAUP was inspired largely by threats to academic freedom. When social scientists began to critically analyze the economic order at the turn of the 20th century, they faced attempts to quell that speech by industrialists (Hamilton, 2002). So it is not surprising that the concept of academic freedom holds a central place in one of the AAUP's founding documents: The *1915 AAUP General Declaration of Principles* (AAUP, 2002). Reflecting the three means of universities through which they serve the public interest, the statement further identifies three functions of university faculty which require the protection of academic freedom: (a) reflecting on knowledge and its sources toward achieving some result, (b) providing those results to students, and (c) providing those results to the public. And the statement then identifies three elements of academic freedom which help faculty to fulfill these functions: (a) freedom of inquiry and research, (b) freedom of teaching within the university, and (c) freedom of extramural utterance.

Corresponding to these various features and liberties of academic freedom, the 1915 statement also acknowledges correlative duties of faculty and universities. In accepting the liberties of academic freedom, faculty, individually, have a duty to meet the constraints of ethics and competency in scholarly inquiry and discourse. This implies that, yes, a faculty member is free to investigate what and as they wish and publish the results of that investigation but must do so in a professional and scholarly manner. The claim to academic freedom is held only by "those who carry on their work in the temper of the scientific inquirer" (AAUP, 2002, p. 187). The faculty collectively also have the duty to enforce the constraints of ethics and competency among its constituents. This, too, is framed as the moral price of claiming academic freedom.

In 1940, the AAUP (1940) developed these ideas further in its *Statement of Principles on Academic Freedom and Tenure*. The 1940 statement reasserts and further develops many of the same claims regarding the specific liberties of academic freedom and adds a description of the process and value of tenure and its relationship to academic freedom. The 1940 statement also identifies a number of more specific faculty obligations beyond the two general obligations from the 1915 statement, including obligations to be accurate, avoid controversial matter not relevant to course material in the classroom, respect others' opinions, alert the institution of financially compensated research, and always indicate when speaking or not speaking for the institution.

Developing a response on a more specific moral issue, in 1965, the AAUP and the American Council on Education released the statement, "On Preventing Conflicts of Interest in Government-Sponsored Research at Universities" (Hamilton, 2002). This statement expresses the importance of avoiding both actual and apparent conflicts of interest. Possible conflicts would include research that benefits a private entity without disclosure of this benefit to the institution, using institution funds to purchase from a private entity that a staff member has an interest in, and providing government-sponsored work to a private entity that are not made public (Hamilton, 2002). Conflicts of interest place one's moral integrity at risk by drawing one's goals and motivations away from the morally required direction. Even *apparent* conflicts of interest can be problematic. Although the conflict may not be actual, the appearance can result in the loss of trust and confidence.

The *1966 AAUP Statement on Professional Ethics* (revised in 1987 and 2009; AAUP, 2009) is very brief and general. It largely refers to previous published statements in expressing the proper values and duties of academics. It specifically, though briefly, identifies freedoms and responsibilities related to scholarly inquiry, students, colleagues, one's institution, and the community. These are largely ideas found in other published AAUP statements.

Students

Given that providing instruction for students is one of the primary functions of the university, the ethics of universities and their faculty will be largely informed by achieving this goal and the overall treatment of students. First, academic freedom serves not only the goal of inquiry and research but of student instruction as well. This is noted in the *1915 AAUP General Declaration of Principles*. Research will be transferred to the classroom, thus without freedom of inquiry, classroom goals of student instruction will be limited. Similarly, direct limitations on what is permitted to be presented in the classroom would limit the quality of education of students. But academic freedom also is relevant for students themselves. The AAUP addressed the need for *student* academic freedom in 1967 in a joint statement with the National Student Association (now the United States Student Association): *Joint Statement on Rights and Freedoms of Students* (see Hamilton, 2002, Appendix G). The statement acknowledges a lesser degree of academic freedom for students due to their not yet being prepared to engage in scholarly discourse. However, faculty have a duty to help prepare them in this direction. As part of this preparation, instructors should encourage free inquiry and expression of opinion in class, including the freedom to disagree with the instructor without grading retribution.

Both deontological and consequentialist defenses can be given for this acknowledgment of student academic freedom—reflecting the general moral arguments for academic freedom (Strike & Soltis, 2009). Respecting people (including students) as persons includes respecting their choices: "We cannot compel them to adopt our religion or our view of a good life, or our view of a worthy culture, even if we think we are right and they are wrong" (Strike & Soltis, 2009, p. 93). Thus, faculty should respect and encourage student expression without fear of losing points for disagreeing. However, such respect does not preclude attempts at rational persuasion toward a different view. In fact, respect may in certain contexts (like a classroom) demand such persuasion. To leave someone to languish in what you believe to be an erroneous or ignorant position is in fact more patronizing than respectful. To challenge someone's perspectives and beliefs demonstrates an acknowledgment of that person's ability to maintain and defend a reasoned position. Thus, we do not have to accept and even respect all positions *uncritically*—particularly those positions disrespectful of others. Insisting on general moral standards like a sense of justice does not violate respect for others but rather demands that respect for all. Nor does it lead us to regulating others' views of the good life, thereby leaving that respected, even if not agreed with. Consequentially, we can appeal to John Stuart Mill's defense of diversity as experiments in living to understanding the value of diversity of opinion. Diversity makes life more varied and interesting. Also, different people find happiness in different ways. Openness to different ways better ensures happiness to be found for all: "significant diversity allows people to find a way of living that fits their own concepts of happiness" (Strike & Soltis, 2009, p. 94).

The Joint Statement also outlines freedoms in relation to student affairs, including forming or joining associations that promote common interests, freedom of expression on campus but outside of class, freedom to support causes without disrupting institutional operations, the freedom to invite speakers to campus, and the freedom to participate in institutional governance. In addition to ethical freedoms and duties related to academic freedom, the AAUP 1966 professional ethics statement also identifies duties of faculty to respect students as individuals and maintain professional role boundaries, to foster honesty, to evaluate students honestly and without bias, and to avoid discriminatory treatment of students, including exploitation and harassment (2009). One issue implied here that arises commonly in the university, and is discussed elsewhere in this text, is the need for equal access to education.

It is largely acknowledged now that students should be offered equal opportunity to access the education offered to students. This can become a concern in relation to students with disabilities. The case of Elizabeth Bouvia may be instructive (Pence, 2004). In September 1983, Bouvia, a 25-year-old woman with cerebral palsy and degenerative arthritis, was driven to Riverside General Hospital in California by her father. She admitted herself voluntarily to the psychiatric unit as suicidal, stating that she just wanted to be left alone to starve to death. The hospital refused this request and sought legal orders to implement force feeding. This set off a series of legal and public battles. Study of this case often focuses on questions of quality of life, self-determination, and the right to die. Many in the disability rights community, however, saw it as a matter of discrimination and inequality. Bouvia had recently dropped out of a graduate social work program at San Diego State University (SDSU) due to resisting the school's insistence that her internship be at a site where she would work with people with disabilities. She had even been told, according to disability advocate Paul Longmore, that she would not have been admitted to the program had the school been aware of the extent of her disability (Pence, 2004). Her experience at SDSU is actually symbolic of a larger problem noted by disability rights advocates. It was argued by some that her very desire to end her life was due less to her disability itself and more to the constant obstacles encountered living in a world designed for those without a disability. The social work graduate program at SDSU, according to Longmore, thought it appropriate to professionally ghettoize Bouvia according to her difference and even admitted a willingness to exclude her and those like her from the program due to that difference. In a more just world, a woman like Elizabeth Bouvia would not feel that death was preferable to the constant obstacles she faced as a person with a disability.

Strike and Soltis (2009) present two intriguing ethical arguments in favor of equal opportunity, particularly as it relates to accommodations for students with disabilities. Before presenting these arguments, a couple points of clarification should be made. Pursuing the ideal of equality does not mean that we treat everyone exactly the same. Rather, we need to treat each individual appropriate to their situation. If a student with a disability requires more resources to benefit from instruction than most other students, that student is entitled to more resources. Equal opportunity is about achieving fairness of competition, not of results. However, the appropriate limits to the "more resources" to which a student may be entitled is not clear. In other words, how do we define and limit "reasonable accommodations"? Generally speaking, we need to balance the benefit to this student against the potential costs to other students. "We should not be willing," write Strike and Soltis (2009), "to secure marginal achievement gains … at the expense of significant losses for other students" (p. 66). This standard, which may be the best we can hope for, provides us with a general criterion in principle but will not preclude all disagreement and conflicts in practice.

The first argument for equal opportunity and reasonable accommodations begins with the assumption that we as a society would prefer a meritocratic system in which success depends on personal industry and the development of skills and talent rather than physical appearance, class or economic status. In order to achieve, or at least pursue, such a meritocratic system, equal opportunity would be necessary. And ensuring equal opportunity to succeed in society would necessitate equal opportunity to gain and develop valued skills—that is, education. The second argument begins with the reasonable assumption that most people in this society would value the creation of a democratic community: "a community in which everyone is equally valued and is treated with equal respect and dignity" (Strike & Soltis, 2009, p. 63). Providing equal opportunity to education, regardless of disability, is one strategy for achieving such a goal. To respond as the SDSU social work program is reported as responding, to a student or potential student with a disability that the student is not wanted (due to a disability) and not worth the trouble to accommodate does not contribute to a democratic community as described previously.

Society

Universities are established in the interest of the common good. Thus, universities and faculty have some responsibilities to the community, society, or possibly the government. One responsibility is stated explicitly in the AAUP's *1915 General Declaration of Principles* (2002): providing experts to advise the government and community. Related to this responsibility is the function of universities also noted in the 1915 Declaration to provide the results of research and inquiry to the public. Implicit in all this is the assumption that the production and accretion of knowledge performed at institutions of higher education is beneficial for society at large. The kinds of contributions intended can be any research or study that is disseminated to the public and may, in various ways, contribute to the public good. This covers a lot of material and most of these contributions occur without full exposure to the general public. However, sometimes these contributions break through the walls of academia in more dramatic fashion.

The most exceptional and public example of these contributions is the informal role of the public intellectual: a scholar (often though perhaps not necessarily) attached to a university whose work has especial cultural and social influence and who is recognized not just within the narrow confines of the academia or a particular field but among the general public. The phenomenon of the public intellectual is arguably more common in Europe where names like Jacques Derrida and Michel Foucault are commonly known. However, in the United States, some scholars have achieved this level of recognition and influence. One interesting recent example is Yale University history professor Timothy Snyder. In February 2017, Snyder published on Facebook what he described as "twenty lessons from the 20th century." These were brief but insightful statements, from the perspective of a historian, on the danger of democracy falling to tyranny and how to respond and resist. These lessons were later published as the book, *On Tyranny: Twenty Lessons from the Twentieth Century* (Snyder, 2017). Originally published in a nonacademic context, these lessons were highly influential beyond the academic walls. And when published as a book the text became a best seller. It is worth noting that, although the text did not explicitly target a particular political party or administration, the timing and general message of the lessons imply certain political criticism and in that way can be highly controversial. Thus, we see a university scholar, through extramural utterance, exercise as a public intellectual disseminating ideas to further his view of the public good. Certainly, this extreme example of an academic fulfilling his duties to the community is not the kind that every academic could similarly achieve. But the example may provide a type of moral exemplar of excellence achieved.

Correlative to these responsibilities is an aspect of academic freedom that the 1915 Declaration refers to as "extramural utterance." This term refers to speech and speech acts by academic professionals outside the classroom and campus, in the general public. It may be clear that in the classroom and in other on-campus contexts, professors should have academic freedom to investigate what they find interesting and important and to express their opinions and their findings related to research and scholarly inquiry. However, to what extent do such rights extend beyond the walls of the campus? The 1915 Declaration acknowledges largely the same sense and degree of academic freedom for faculty within and outside campus:

> In their extramural utterances, it is obvious that academic teachers are under a peculiar obligation to avoid hasty or unverified or exaggerated statements, and to refrain from intemperate or sensational modes of expression. But subject to these restraints, it is not … desirable that scholars should be debarred from giving expression to their judgments upon controversial questions, or that their freedom of speech, outside the university, should be limited to questions falling within their own specialties. (AAUP, 2002, p. 189)

In other words, subject to basic constraints of civility and scholarly inquiry, faculty have as much academic freedom in the general public square as within the university context. The *1940 AAUP Statement of Principles on Academic Freedom and Tenure* (AAUP, 1940) explicitly affirms the freedom from censorship that university scholars have, "[w]hen they speak or write as citizens" (p. 196). Yet at the same time, their position in the community places special obligations on them to be accurate, exercise restraint, respect others' opinions, and make transparent that they are not speaking for their institution. Without acknowledgment of extramural academic freedom, the potentially controversial (and potentially beneficial) message of a scholar like Timothy Snyder may be lost.

ETHICS OF NURSING AND ETHICS OF EDUCATION: ETHICS OF NURSING EDUCATION

In attempting to understand the ethics of nursing education, if we were to focus our study merely on explicit references to nursing education in major codes of ethics like the ICN Code and the ANA Code, our understanding would likely be severely limited. Of those two codes, the ICN Code has much more to say in an explicit manner on nursing education (ICN, 2012). Divided into four elements—Nurses and People, Nurses and Practice, Nurses and the Profession, and Nurses and Co-workers—the ICN Code identifies relevance to nursing educators and researchers within each of those elements. For example, in regard to Nurses and People, the code indicates the importance of providing an education in ethics as part of a nursing curriculum. The element of Nurses and Practice includes imperatives to provide opportunities for lifelong learning, conduct research linking continual learning and competence to practice, and promoting the importance of personal health in relation to other values. The ethical duties of educators within the Nurses and the Profession element involve providing learning opportunities in the practice setting, providing research that advances the profession, and promoting the importance of professional nursing associations to students. And, regarding Nurses and Co-workers, the ICN Code advises nurses to develop an understanding of other worker's roles, communicate the ethics of nursing to other professions, and to teach students to safeguard the individual, family, or community when healthcare personnel endanger care.

The ANA Code includes more specific and discrete explicit references to educators (ANA, 2015). Interpretive Statement 2.3 on collaboration includes educators as one of the nonclinical roles of nurses which can contribute to high-quality care of patients indirectly through influence on direct care providers (ANA, 2015). Provision 3 asserts the duty to ensure competence and commitment to professional standards before entering practice (ANA, 2015). The most explicitly relevant provision to nursing faculty is Provision 7. The focus of this provision is research and scholarly inquiry. While the bedside nurse may have limited opportunity regarding this type of activity,[5] it will be central to the role of nursing faculty. In addition to general prescriptions to advance the profession through knowledge development, the interpretive statements of this provision further indicate the necessity of educators to teach the moral standards of research methods, to maintain optimal educational standards, and to ensure that all nursing graduates possess the requisite nursing knowledge, skills, and moral dispositions—which includes developing students' commitment to nursing practice, professional and civic values, and understanding healthcare policy (ANA, 2015). And finally, the ninth provision indicates the responsibility of nurse educators to instruct students of the broader responsibility of the nursing profession to address issues of social justice.

This brief overview of the explicit references to educators (and researchers) in the ICN Code and the ANA Code provides some insight into the ethics of nurse educators. However, there is a potential for greater insight if we, through the foregoing analyses of nursing ethics and academic ethics, investigate the parallels, intersections, and overlaps between the ethics of the two disciplines. First worth noting is that in regard to educators in their role as educators, the values and duties of the ANA Code, beyond the specific references to educators, even if they cannot be perceived as directly relevant, might be reasonably interpreted as vicariously compelling. In other words, while not directly treating patients, faculty are preparing students who (the successful ones at least) will one day be caring for patients. Thus, there could be said to exist a vicarious duty of nurse educators to ensure that students understand what safe, competent, and moral care encompasses. The ANA Code implies such an idea in Interpretive Statement 2.3, indicating the interdependence and shared

---

[5] Although the first interpretive statement of Provision 7 indicates that there are means of advancing the profession through knowledge development outside of research and scholarly inquiry.

responsibility for the outcomes of nursing care (ANA, 2015). Or, as more explicitly expressed by Vanlaere and Gastmans (2007),

> When a nursing curriculum sufficiently addresses ethics, providing nurses with the tools to help them reflect critically on what nursing care implies, nursing education can contribute to the development of nurses as skilled companions. By stimulating critical reflection on nursing practice, nursing ethics education aims to encourage a virtuous attitude in nurses, forming the basis from which to provide good care. (p. 758)

And, as noted in the previous paragraph, the ANA Code explicitly identifies this duty in Provision 3. As educators, nursing faculty may not have direct effect on patient care, but their indirect influence on the quality (in terms of both competence and ethics) is indisputable. Thereby, there is a vicarious duty, in addition to the direct duty indicated in Provision 3, to ensure the same duties incumbent upon any bedside nurse are fulfilled.

An interesting parallel that emerges from the foregoing analyses of nursing ethics and academic ethics is the tripartite divisions of duties: nursing ethical duties to patients (and colleagues), to themselves, and beyond the clinic to the profession and society; academic ethical duties to knowledge, students, and society. Even individually, there are intriguing parallels. Nursing duties to patients seem parallel to teachers' duties to students, as both latter groups represent those to whom the duties of nurses and then of teachers are primarily directed. We have seen duties and value to patients and students in relation to respect, dignity, fairness, and commitment. Given the specific nature of the patient role, we see also a commitment to safety not as relevant as to the treatment of students. One as yet unexplored aspect of both relationships is that of care. The essence of the nurse–patient relationship is widely perceived to be one of caring. What this means in detail can vary widely. From the broad theory of nursing, perhaps the well-known expression of the care relationship is from Watson (2008, 2012, 2018). According to Watson (2008), a caring relationship between nurse and patient promotes healing and health, among other desirable goods. Caring acknowledges the whole person through presence and intentionality, as opposed to a reductivist view of healthcare in which the patient is a passive, reductive entity, one on whom procedures are to be performed or one reduced to their pathology (Watson, 2012). In the field of nursing ethics, a caring focus is perhaps best associated with the work of Tschudin (2004), who emphasizes the importance of a close and intimate nurse–patient relationship. Perhaps the best known critic of this focus on care is nursing ethicist Kuhse (1995, 1997) who, while accepting the inherent value of caring in nursing, questions the intensity given it by some authors like Watson and Tschudin. While, yes, she admits, a patient does not want to be treated like an object, the extent of intimacy of care implied in the language of many theorists may go too far and may result in neglecting other valuable aspects of ethical thought (Kuhse, 1995).

Caring in the teacher–student relationship is also seen as important. Noddings (2013), one of the architects of the ethical theory of ethics of care, has written evocatively on caring in the teacher–student relationship. Kuhse (1995) similarly finds the intensity implied by Noddings in the student–teacher relationship dubious. Comparing caring in the two relationships is difficult. One obvious point of comparison may be found in the distinction between "caring *about*" and "caring *for*." The former refers to "evincing concern, compassion, or empathy for the particular patient and his or her plans and projects in a particular health-related context" (Benjamin & Curtis, 2010, p. 42). The latter refers to "looking after or providing for the particular nursing-related needs of the patient" (Benjamin & Curtis, 2010, p. 42). Effective and ethical teachers will similarly "care about" their students. Clearly, of course, teachers do not "care for" students in relation to their "particular nursing-related needs." However, teachers can, and likely *should*, "care for" students' educational needs. As with nursing, though care seems an essential quality of the teacher–student relationship, the specific extent and intensity of this relationship is open to discussion. In both, one must balance care with fair and just treatment. In the ANA Code this concern is raised in relation to professional boundaries as indicated in Interpretive Statement 2.4. In relation to academic ethics, the 1967 Joint Statement alludes to this issue in relation to prejudiced evaluation. Also, since we are speaking specifically of teaching at the college level, it is worth noting that care is more often perceived as less a part of the teacher–student relationship than at the primary or secondary level of education (Barrow, 2015; Meyers, 2009). However, some studies, as indicated by Meyers (2009), appear to demonstrate the equal value of caring in teaching at the postsecondary level as at the primary or secondary level (De-Guzman et al., 2008; Foster, 2008; Straits, 2007).

Nursing ethics and academic ethics both also acknowledge an ethical duty related to knowledge production. The ethics of both nursing and academia can be interpreted as based on a contract between the profession and society. Society provides the social structures for practice and the prestige, and the professions in return provide specific goods in terms of knowledge development and problem-solving. As we have seen, knowledge production is emphasized in the ethics of both nursing and education. Thus, for nursing academics research and scholarly inquiry is doubly affirmed. We see also then the duties of both nursing and academics to society. Nursing faculty have a duty to society to prepare ethical and competent new nurses but also a duty to advance knowledge for the good of society.

The ethics of nursing education includes, then, duties and values related to both fields of nursing and academics. Some of these duties and values overlap; some are specific to each field. Nursing professors, especially the majority who are licensed RNs, may reasonably be beholden to the ANA Code (or a similarly local relevant code) in their own actions and vicariously in terms of the future (or even current in terms of clinical education) patients and others affected by their students' actions. These duties include ensuring the competency of their students but also ensuring an education in ethics as well. The healthcare field is replete with difficulties and dilemmas involving risks to the safety and dignity of patients, the rationing of healthcare resources, even ensuring the needs and interests of nurses themselves. Even instructors in nursing programs who are not licensed RNs can be said to be informally obligated to these values and goals. And both groups, as academics, need to consider the ethics related to one's role as an instructor in the higher education system. These rules, values, and goals may be less clearly defined and less authoritatively enforced, but from the perspective of a morally concerned individual, in a specialized role, they are no less important.

CRITICAL ELEMENTS TO CONSIDER

- Nursing educators may hold dual roles as nurses and college-level educators, implying moral duties following from each role.
- Even instructors who are not licensed RNs may be seen as informally obligated to the ANA Code of Ethics.
- Nurse educators can have moral duties related to nursing directly and vicariously in terms of the care of future patients that their students may treat.
- Academic freedom is central to discussions of academic ethics, but this freedom comes with correlative duties implied by these liberties.
- Overlap exists between nursing ethics and academic ethics in areas like knowledge production and duties to society.

Helpful Resources

- ANA Code of Ethics: https://www.nursingworld.org/practice-policy/nursing-excellence/ethics/code-of-ethics-for-nurses/
- ICN Code of Ethics: https://www.icn.ch/sites/default/files/inline-files/2012_ICN_Codeofethicsfornurses_%20eng.pdf
- AAUP Statement on Professional Ethics: https://www.aaup.org/report/statement-professional-ethics
- AAUP 1940 Statement of Principles on Academic Freedom and Tenure: www.aaup.org/report/1940-statement-principles-academic-freedom-and-tenure

References

American Association of University Professors. (1940). *1940 Statement of principles on academic freedom and tenure*. Retrieved from https://www.aaup.org/report/1940-statement-principles-academic-freedom-and-tenure

American Association of University Professors. (2002). *1915 AAUP general declaration of principles*. Appendix B in N. W. Hamilton, *Academic ethics: Problems and materials on professional conduct and shared governance*. Westport, CT: Praeger Publishers.

American Association of University Professors. (2009). *Statement on professional ethics*. Retrieved from https://www.aaup.org/report/statement-professional-ethics

American Nurses Association. (2015). *Code of ethics for nurses with interpretive statements*. Silver Spring, MD: Author.

Avert. (2018). *HIV stigma and discrimination*. Retrieved from https://www.avert.org/professionals/hiv-social-issues/stigma-discrimination

Barrow, M. (2015). Caring in teaching: A complicated relationship. *The Journal of Effective Teaching*, *15*(2), 45–49. Retrieved from http://web.a.ebscohost.com.proxy.library.csi.cuny.edu/ehost/pdfviewer/pdfviewer?vid=2&sid=ce6da73b-ae0e-4f85-8d86-b0e140b8fd25%40sdc-v-sessmgr03

Benjamin, M., & Curtis, J. (2010). *Ethics in nursing: Cases, principles, and reasoning* (4th ed.). New York, NY: Oxford University Press.

Butts, J. B. (2020). *Nursing ethics: Across the curriculum and into practice* (5th ed.). Burlington, MA: Jones & Bartlett Learning.

Dahnke, M. D. (2009). The American Nurses Association code in ethical decision-making. *Holistic Nursing Practice*, *23*(2), 112–119. doi:10.1097/HNP.0b013e3181a1114a

Dahnke, M. D. (2014) Utilizing codes of ethics in health professions education. *Advances in Health Sciences Education*, *19*(4), 611–623. doi:10.1007/s10459-013-9484-2

DeGuzman, A., Uy, M., Siy, E., Torres, R., Tancioco, J., & Hernandez, J. (2008). From teaching from the heart to teaching with a heart: Segmenting Filipino college students' views of their teachers' caring behavior and their orientations as care-for-individuals. *Asia Pacific Education Review*, *9*(4), 487–502. doi:10.1007/BF03025665

Foster, K. C. (2008, November). The transformative potential of teach care as described by students in higher education access initiative. *Education and Urban Society*, *41*(1), 104–126. doi:10.1177/0013124508321591

Grendler, P. F. (2002). *The universities of the Italian Renaissance*. Baltimore, MD: Johns Hopkins University Press.

Hamilton, N. W. (2002). *Academic ethics: Problems and materials on professional conduct and shared governance*. Westport, CT: Praeger Publishers.

International Council of Nurses. (2012). *The ICN code of ethics for nurses*. Geneva, Switzerland: Author. Retrieved from https://www.icn.ch/sites/default/files/inline-files/2012_ICN_Codeofethicsfornurses_%20eng.pdf

Jarvis, D. S. L. (2014). Regulating higher education: Quality assurance and neo-liberal managerialism in higher education. *Policy and Society*, *33*(3), 155–166. doi:10.1016/j.polsoc.2014.09.005

Kuhse, H. (1995). Clinical ethics and nursing: "Yes" to caring, but "no" to a female ethics of care. *Bioethics*, *9*(3), 207–219. doi:10.1111/j.1467-8519.1995.tb00356.x

Kuhse, H. (1997). *Caring: Nurses, women, and ethics*. Oxford, UK: Blackwell Publishers.

Meyers, S. A. (2009). Do your students care whether you care about them? *College Teaching*, *57*(4), 205–210. doi:10.1080/87567550903218620

Mill, J. S. (1910). *Utilitarianism, liberty, and representative government*. New York, NY: E. P. Dutton.

Morrison, E. E. (2011). *Ethics in health administration: A practical approach for decision-makers*. Sudbury, MA: Jones & Bartlett Learning.

Noddings, N. (2013). *Caring: A relational approach to ethics and moral education* (2nd ed.). Berkeley, CA: University of California Press.

Pence, G. E. (2004). *Classic cases in medical ethics: Accounts of cases that have shaped medical ethics, with philosophical, legal, and historical backgrounds* (4th ed.). New York, NY: McGraw-Hill.

Snyder, T. (2017). *On tyranny: Twenty lessons from the twentieth century*. New York, NY: Random House.

Straits, W. (2007). "She's teaching me": Teaching with care in a large lecture course. *College Teaching*, *55*(4), 170–175. doi:10.3200/CTCH.55.4.170-175

Strike, K., & Soltis, J. (2009). *The ethics of teaching* (5th ed.). New York, NY: Teachers College Press.

Tronto, J. C. (2009). *Moral boundaries: A political argument for an ethic of care*. New York, NY: Routledge.

Tschudin, V. (2004). *Ethics in nursing: The caring relationship* (3rd ed.). Waltham, MA: Butterworth-Heinemann.

Vanlaere, L., & Gastmans, C. (2007). Ethics in nursing education: Learning to reflect on care practices. *Nursing Ethics, 14*(6), 758–766. doi:10.1177/0969733007082116

Verger, J. (1992). Patterns. In H. de Ridder-Symeons (Ed.), *A history of the university in Europe. Volume 1: Universities in the Middle Ages* (pp. 35–76). Cambridge, UK: Cambridge University Press.

Watson, J. (2008). *Nursing: The philosophy and science of caring* (Rev. ed.). Boulder: University Press of Colorado.

Watson, J. (2012). *Human caring science: A theory of nursing* (2nd ed.). Sudbury, MA: Jones & Bartlett Learning.

Watson, J. (2018). *Unitary caring science: Philosophy and praxis of nursing*. Louisville, CO: University Press of Colorado.

LEGAL AND ETHICAL CASES WITH NURSING STUDENTS, FACULTY, AND ADMINISTRATORS

Neutrality, Confidentiality, and Independence: The Role of the Ombudsman When a Student Files a Complaint

Case Study 7.1
A Student Files a Complaint With the University Ombudsman

Your role: You are Dr. Hays, the Associate Dean for Graduate Nursing Programs.

Davinia Morris, CNM, is an experienced certified nurse-midwife who first earned her certificate in nurse midwifery in 1990—years before master's preparation for nurse midwives became the standard. Ms. Morris (who has a BA degree in psychology) decided to enter an MS completion program in midwifery that would allow her to obtain the MS degree but not repeat most of her previous midwifery clinical courses. Ms. Morris looked for a program that would take the least amount of time and have the lowest cost. A fellow nurse-midwife friend told Ms. Morris that she should contact a nearby university, the University of Alcoa, which all her nurse-midwife friends had attended for their MS completion degrees, indicating she could earn it quickly there. Ms. Morris made an email inquiry to the nurse midwifery program director, Ms. Anna Strauss, who informed her by email that she would need to take only 15 credits to receive her MS degree. Ms. Morris was thrilled because, although this program was not online, it required the fewest credits of any she investigated and was within easy commuting distance. Ms. Morris subsequently proceeded to take her five courses over the next 2 years.

At this same time, the College of Nursing (where this degree program resides) migrated from a paper-and-file student record system (with centralized filing in respective departments) to an online system in which paperless/electronic files are now maintained in the registrar's office. Upon completing her five courses (15 credits), Ms. Morris applied for graduation, but to her astonishment she was informed that a minimum of 30, not 15, credits must be taken *at the University of Alcoa* for any graduate student who seeks a master's degree. Ms. Morris immediately notified the program director about this issue and referred her to the registrar since it had been so long ago. To the registrar, Ms. Strauss, declared there must be some mistake, stating that "we have always awarded the MS Completion for Nurse Midwifery after 15 credits." Informed of this, Ms. Morris vehemently thought she had been wronged, and repeatedly called the registrar to bully her into awarding her the MS degree. When the registrar still would not award the degree, the registrar decided to do some historical checking and found out that at least 12 other nurse-midwife students had been awarded the completion MS degrees in the past with only 15 credits. When the registrar notified Ms. Strauss of this violation of policy, Ms. Strauss denied knowing of the policy, but blamed the registrar for her lack of oversight stating, "Don't blame me, you yourself signed off on all these degrees!" Trying to prevent widespread exposure of this violation of policy and procedure by both the midwifery department and the registrar's office, Ms. Strauss stated it wouldn't happen again, told the registrar she would work something out with the student, and said that there was no need to do anything else.

Ms. Strauss subsequently attempted to strike a deal with the student, but Ms. Morris refused to take any additional credits. Furious, Ms. Morris (and without going through any further channels) immediately notified the university Ombudsman and copied you, the Associate Dean for Graduate Nursing Programs. She was emphatic that she had a credit agreement "in writing" (the email) from the program director, and she demanded that the university own up to its commitment to her and award her the MS degree.

Questions

- As Associate Dean, how would you first proceed?
- Who should take the lead in solving this issue: The Ombudsman or the Associate Dean who was copied on the complaint?
- Independent of the student's issue with the Ombudsman, what should your course of action as Associate Dean be toward the program director who reports to you?
- What is the role of the registrar's office in this incident?

STUDENT USE OF A UNIVERSITY OMBUDSMAN: LEGAL PRINCIPLES AND REVIEW OF THE LITERATURE

Introduction

The use of some type of Ombudsman is prevalent in academia and is one of the roles in the field of *alternative dispute resolution* (ADR; Gadlin, 2000; Tauginiené, 2016). An ADR program may also lie outside a university setting; for instance, the Equal Employment Opportunity Commission (n.d.) requires one at every federal agency. Its chief function is fairness (Equal Employment Opportunity Commission, n.d.). Merriam-Webster's Online Dictionary (2010) defines *Ombudsman* as "one that investigates, reports on, and helps settle complaints" (p. 1). The first use of the role of the Ombudsman was in the early 1800s, when Sweden used the Ombudsman post to hear grievances against the government, parliament, and administrative offices (Johnson, 2013; Levin, 2009). The first college Ombudsman was established at Eastern Montana College (now Montana State University Billings) in the 1966 to 1967 academic year and by 1971 there were some 69 Ombudsman officials in colleges and universities in the United States (Stewart, 1978). There are, however, many different models of *Ombudsmanship*.

The first type of Ombudsman is the *classical Ombudsman,* which "emphasizes statutory independence from governmental control, the power to investigate complaints, and the authority to publish findings and recommendations" (Gadlin, 2000, p. 38). The classical Ombudsman's role and function are established by statute. There are some instances in which this type of Ombudsman is prevalent in the university setting, discussed later in the chapter. Gottehrer and Hostina (1998), in *Essential Characteristics of a Classical Ombudsman,* indicate the classical Ombudsman role must have the four following characteristics: independence; impartiality and fairness; credibility of the review process; and confidentiality.

The second type of Ombudsman is the *organizational Ombudsman,* whose roles are similar to those of the classical Ombudsman. However, the position or role has not been established by statute; rather, it was established by organizational forces such as a vote of a faculty senate or student body (Gadlin, 2000). Some universities also have ombudsmen that operate more organizationally than they do classically. However, both types are represented in the International Ombudsman Association (IOA; formed in 2005 with the merger of the University and College Ombudsman Association [UCOA] and The Ombudsman Association [TOA]). According to the IOA (2019) website, "The IOA is the International Ombudsman Association, the premier global professional association for organizational ombuds and their peers. IOA's mission is to 'support and advance the global organizational ombudsman profession and ensure that practitioners work to the highest professional'" (p. 1).

The IOA publishes two documents that are critical to the implementation and function of the Ombudsman role:

1. *IOA Code of Ethics* (posted January 2007)
2. *IOA Standards of Practice* (posted October 2009)

These documents are all open source and available from the IOA's Standards of Practice website at www.ombudsassociation.org/standards-of-practice-code-of-ethics-3. The *IOA Code of Ethics* is briefly summarized here and the *Standards of Practice* and *Best Practices* documents are discussed in Chapter 8, Neutrality, Confidentiality, and Independence in the Role of the Ombudsman: When a Faculty Files a Complaint.

IOA CODE OF ETHICS

There are four ethical principles—independence, neutrality and impartiality, confidentiality, and informality. First, "The Ombudsman is *independent[1] in structure, function, and appearance to the highest degree possible within the organization*" (IOA, 2007, p. 1). According to Shelton (2000), "It is intended that this independence be protected, as much as possible within the institution, by placing the appointment at the highest level of authority" (p. 84). In other words, petitioning students cannot perceive the university Ombudsman as inherently favoring faculty or university officials but as an independent agent who will review a grievance independently of the other, often more powerful individuals in the organization (Katsara, 2015).

Second, the Ombudsman must show *neutrality* and *impartiality.* The IOA (2007) states, "The Ombudsman, as a designated neutral, remains unaligned and impartial. The Ombudsman does not engage in any situation which could create a conflict of interest" (p. 1). Neutrality is essential, particularly if the Ombudsman is going to have credibility among various different agents within the university. It is obvious to both undergraduate and graduate students that individuals in the university, especially faculty with a PhD, for instance, or a department chair or Associate Dean have both personal status and power. The ability of the Ombudsman to evaluate each side equally, irrespective of status or position, is indeed one of the particular skills of an adept Ombudsman. Cornell University calls their Office of the Ombudsman a "problem-solving" campus. For them, the office does not "… take sides in any dispute, upholding their neutrality to best solve the problem presented to them" (Stimpson, 2019, para. 10). Impartiality is a slightly different concept than neutrality. Bauer (2000) favors the term *ombudsperson* (the more gender-neutral title) used at the University of Western Ontario, in London, Ontario, Canada, and indicates that impartiality "speaks to the way I behave towards different constituents within the university" (p. 61). She further elaborates, "I like the fact that impartiality is the way I behave, rather than the way I think or feel. It is clearer than neutrality, which the dictionary associates with war and adversarial conflicts" (p. 61).

---

[1] Emphasis added.

The third principle is *confidentiality*. Again, the IOA defines it as meaning that "the Ombudsman holds all communications with those seeking assistance in strict confidence, and does not disclose confidential communications unless given permission to do so. The only exception to this privilege of confidentiality is where there appears to be imminent risk of serious harm." It should be elaborated, however, that "if the complainant wishes only to talk, that will be respected. But if action is desired for a specific problem, total confidentiality becomes impossible" (Stieber, 2000, p. 53).

A differentiation should further be made between the concept of *anonymity* and *confidentiality*. Absolute anonymity, although desired by the student complainant or any other complainant, may not be feasible or practical, especially if competing parties ultimately want some form of mediation or compromise. For example, one best practice states: "Personal details that need to be disclosed for one purpose might need protection in other situations. For example, it will often be necessary to identify a complainant [student] to the staff member [faculty] whose actions have been complained about" (Commonwealth Ombudsman, 2009, p. 10).

The last IOM principle is the concept of *informality* (2007). Here, "the Ombudsman, as an informal resource, does not participate in any formal adjudicative or administrative procedure related to concerns brought to his/her attention" (p. 1). The Ombudsman will attempt to resolve conflicts or disputes through mediation and recommendation, whereas going to human resources to file a complaint for a violation of university policy, using any available ethics hotline to report a wide range of unethical behaviors, or perhaps contacting the campus-based Equal Employment Opportunity Commission (EEOC) authority (e.g., for charges of discrimination) are all alternative but *formal* dispositional ways of resolving issues.

Some university Ombudsman positions may be structured so that they see appeals made by students only, whereas some universities may have a separate faculty Ombudsman position that is aimed at protecting faculty interests, such as is the case at Ohio State University (2018). San Diego State University (n.d.) has an excellent website for their Office of the Student Ombudsman at http://go.sdsu.edu/student_affairs/ombudsman/Default.aspx and it clearly states what the Ombudsman *can do* (e.g., can provide a "safe" place for students to discuss issues, investigate your complaint if you so desire, gather information on your behalf, etc.) and *cannot do* (e.g., change grades or other university policies, give legal advice, take action without your permission, etc.). It is important for students to ask to which Ombudsman (if there is more than one type) they should direct their complaints.

DISCUSSION OF CASE STUDY

In Case Study 7.1, the first question is, as Associate Dean, how would you first proceed? Dr. Hays was flabbergasted by this incident and wondered what was really going on. The midwifery program had been independently placed in the organizational structure for a long time and had only recently been moved to Dr. Hays's portfolio of departments and programs for which she had administrative responsibility. She really was unaware that there was a post-master's option in midwifery because no one ever talked about it. Therefore, she was a little more suspicious than usual about what was going on.

The second question is, who should take the lead in solving this issue: the Ombudsman or the Associate Dean who was copied on the complaint? In Case Study 7.1, Dr. Hays communicated with the Ombudsman that he should first rule on the case of the student complaint before any further discussion took place about how to evaluate the actions of the program director.

The third question is, independent of the student's issue with the Ombudsman, what should your course of action as the Associate Dean be toward the program director who reports to you? Once she had initiated communication with the Ombudsman, Dr. Hays immediately notified Ms. Strauss that all communication between the student and herself (Ms. Strauss) must cease until the issue is resolved. Further, although not discussed with the Ombudsman, Dr. Hays also wondered to what degree the Office of the Registrar had been either complicit or negligent with the awarding of previous master's degrees in this program in violation of the university policy. Dr. Hays did notify the Dean of the college about the pending case and brought her up to date with the facts.

FINDINGS AND DISPOSITION

The university Ombudsman concluded that indeed there was evidence that the student was informed by the program director that she would receive her completion master's degree after accruing 15 semester credits or five courses. The Ombudsman ruled that this type of communication was incorrect and was not in line with standard university policy at the time of the student's matriculation. Further, although the Ombudsman was sympathetic with the student's complaint and her request to be awarded the degree because she had completed her requirements in good faith, the Ombudsman did not agree that the email communication should be upheld. Instead a compromise was made and the student was allowed to apply for graduation when she completed 30 credits, but that she would not be charged for them. In other words, a compromise was offered because of the miscommunication on the part of the program director. Although sympathetic to the student complaint, the Ombudsman ruled that it would be improper and a violation of higher education standards, including those of Alcoa University, that anyone would be awarded a master's degree after taking only 15 credit hours. The Ombudsman did not rule on any actions toward the program director, Ms. Strauss. However, upon disposition of the student complaint, the Associate Dean subsequently wrote up Ms. Strauss for her violation of the university policy and indicated that any further deviation from university policy, with regard to graduation requirements or *any other standard university policy,* would result in Ms. Strauss being terminated.

The last question is, what was the role of the Registrar's Office in this incident? Dr. Hays, in consultation with the Dean, opted not to pursue any action against the registrar mainly because in this case the registrar did rebel and refuse to award the degree. Although the Associate Dean and Dean agreed, there was obviously some sloppiness in the registrar's office; they opted to give the registrar the benefit of the doubt. They considered that only with the introduction of electronic files was it possible to ensure that all credits toward individual degrees could be absolutely accounted for. Ms. Morris accepted the Ombudsman ruling as she thought it fruitless to appeal to the president of the university. Ms. Strauss accepted her punishment, although she was angry that it would likely appear in her annual evaluation and affect her annual merit raise. The registrar contacted the Dean and assured her that their electronic systems would certainly prevent this from ever happening again.

RELEVANT LEGAL CASES

Student Files Personal Injury Lawsuit in Federal Court Over Final Grade of "C" After Negative Ruling by University Ombudsperson

---

Brian C. Marquis v. University of Massachusetts at Amherst, No. 07-30015 (D. Mass. Jan. 31, 2007).

In the fall of 2006, the plaintiff, Brian Marquis, enrolled in an undergraduate course in philosophy, Philosophy 161: Problems in Social Thought, at the University of Massachusetts–Amherst. Mr. Marquis was a 51-year-old paralegal seeking a double major in legal studies and sociology. The course was taught by a teaching assistant, Jeremy Cushing. On the first day of class, Mr. Cushing passed out a syllabus in which he indicated there would be three examinations each worth 25% of the final grade (75%); four response papers each worth 5% each (20%); and the remaining 5% for class participation. According to the lawsuit filed in the district court of Massachusetts, the syllabus read as follows: "Each paper will receive a number grade (from 0–5) in 5-point increments" (Marquis v. University of Massachusetts at Amherst, 2007, p. 4). When the semester concluded, the plaintiff had the following grades: 23%, 22.5%, and 19.5% (out of a possible 25%); response paper grades of 5, 4, 4, 4.5 (out of 5); and a 5% class participation grade that appears to be unknown, but the plaintiff calculated in the full 5%. The plaintiff therefore calculated his grade to be 92.5% and thus an A–. Upon receiving his grade report, however, he was given a final grade of 84 and thus awarded a C. After the plaintiff first appealed to the teaching assistant, Mr. Cushing claimed that "to make the grades more representative of student performances, I set a curve (or, more accurately, I drew up a new grade scale)" (Marquis v. University of Massachusetts at Amherst, 2007, p. 5). It should be noted that a curve grading scale was not mentioned in the syllabus (Elder, 2010). As written about in the *Boston Globe*: "Cushing wrote back that he graded the students more stringently on the third exam because they had a full semester to learn how to write for a philosophy class…. But the students' scores struck Cushing as too high, so he graded everyone on a curve before assigning letter grades" (Saltzman, 2007, p. 2).

Subsequently, Mr. Marquis appealed to the department chair, Phillip Bricker, who denied the appeal and who later stated, "I think suing over a grade is somewhat absurd…. It ended up just wasting a lot of people's time and money" (Saltzman, 2007, p. 2). An appeal was then made to the Ombudsperson, Catherine Porter, who also denied the appeal, writing, "I would urge you to accept this grade and continue with your course work as these are no grounds for an academic grievance" (Marquis v. University of Massachusetts at Amherst, 2007, p. 5). Porter also stated that in 30 years at the university she had never heard of a grade appeal like this one. With all appeals denied, the student's attorney filed a 15-count lawsuit in federal court claiming violation of the First, Fifth, and Fourteenth Amendments; six violations of the U.S.C. (U.S. Code); violation of Massachusetts General Law; Promissory Estoppel[2]; Breach of the Special Relationship; Breach of Contract; Intentional Infliction of Emotional Distress; and Tortuous Interference with Economic Advantage. The attorney emphasized that Marquis had suffered personal injury, because a grade of C on his transcript would hurt his chances of being admitted to law school (Marquis v. University of Massachusetts at Amherst, 2007).

After a brief hearing with the plaintiff and an attorney for the university, who asked, "Does the court really want to put itself in the business of reviewing, under some constitutional or federal statutory doctrine, the propriety of the grades which a student has received?" (Elder, 2010, p. 2). District Court Judge Michael A. Posnor dismissed the lawsuit against the university.[3]

What do you think? Do you think the judge ruled properly in this case? At some college and universities, there is no official university grading scale; however, individual colleges or departments may adopt a respective grading scale. Moreover, grading scales for nursing divisions are often higher than the ones other departments or schools use. The authors of this book worked at a university where there was a published grading scale for undergraduate or graduate grades—with a grading scale very similar to the undergraduate scale at the university in this case, whereas A– equals 3.700 points, B equals 3.00 points, and so on. Therefore, unless the individual professor prints a corresponding grading scale on the course syllabus (e.g., A– = 90–92, B = 84–87), the student may actually may not know exactly what a final grade will be if all assignments are graded with a letter grade, or in this case on a 0 to 5 scale. Indeed, as the Ombudsman in this case indicated, "faculty have their own grading scales and … one professor might view an 84 as an A minus, while another might view it as a C" (Saltzman, 2007, p. 2). Our point is that where there is no corresponding grading scale to an assigned letter grade, there is lot of room for very divergent grade calculations and in this case even the teaching assistant appeared to have instituted a grading curve (based on a review of final grades) that was not disclosed on the syllabus. What do you think about the comments of the department chair? Might you inquire as to what kind of teaching pedagogy skills the graduate teaching assistant has been given?

Although there is no indication this was the first time Mr. Cushing had taught, the decision to institute a grading scale at the end of the course without due process explanation to the students, at least in our view, seems awfully arbitrary. And most important, how do you view the decision and comments of the Ombudsperson, Ms. Porter? Did you get the sense that she was ruling with the IOA's *Code of Ethics* in mind with due attention to independence, neutrality and impartiality, confidentiality, and informality? Our concluding viewpoint is that in a country where litigation is common, in higher education an individual faculty member is perhaps more protected from charges of bias in grading if the syllabus is more precise in both grading criteria and grading scales for respective grades awarded.

---

[2] *Promissory Estoppel* —"when a person makes a false statement to another and the listener relies on what was told to him/her in good faith and to his/her disadvantage. To see that justice is done a court will treat the statement as a promise, and in a trial the judge will preclude the maker of the statement from denying it" (Wikipedia.com, 2019).

[3] Two other complementary cases include: *Stewart v. Washington State University*, Case No. C18-557-RSM (W. D. Wash. 2019). In this case, the University disciplinary actions, even if inadequate or not ideal, would be upheld as long as there was some appropriate response and due process for the victim. Following two racist attacks on the Plaintiff, the University promptly responded by mandating sensitivity training for the known parties involved, offered counseling services to the Plaintiff, and fully heard the Plaintiff's complaints. The Plaintiff contended the University did not do enough but the Court found the University's response somewhat lacking but not unreasonable. In a second case, *SS v. Alexander, No. 58335-2-I* (Wash. Ct. App. 2008), the court permitted the lawsuit, even after Ombudsmen mediation and due process, because the due process was so poor. The Plaintiff was raped by Football Player. University's response was to hold a mediation session with the Plaintiff, Football Player, Title IX Coordinator, Athletic Director, and Ombudsman. The Athletic Director and Football Player refused to accept any punishment and the University acquiesced, no punishment given. Court found this inherently unreasonable because the University was treating the rape victim and rapist the same.

SUMMARY

Although in the preceding case, the student did not have a positive outcome from use of the university Ombudsperson, at least it is notable that the student did pursue his appeal with the university Ombudsperson once there was a denial by the department chair. And although litigation in state and federal courts is almost always a legitimate possibility for most claims, courts are often wary of interfering in university activities that are in the domain of the faculty, particularly with regard to grading (Roth, McEllistrem, D'Agostino, & Brown, 2009). Nevertheless, the role of the Ombudsman or Ombudsperson is an important addition to higher education, and any student who has a legitimate claim must consider whether to consider a formal complaint to the official offices listed earlier in this chapter, or more informally to the office of an Ombudsman, where mediation, recommendation, and hopefully equitable resolutions can be sought and delivered. Remember, legal principles are still good law. Defer to the university if any reasonable process is given.

ETHICAL CONSIDERATIONS

At its best, the role of the Ombudsperson preserves and supports the ethical character of the institution by promoting a sense of justice and fairness through a mechanism and process internal to the institution but at the same time not in defense of the institution. The four ethical principles invoked by the IOA Code of Ethics—independence, neutrality and impartiality, confidentiality, and informality—help to ensure fairness toward those who depend upon the university for an education or a living and career. Independence and impartiality help to ensure that students or any complainants are respected and heard in a fair and unbiased setting. This is particularly important in a situation of power discrepancy, which typically exists between an institution and its students and employees. To dismiss the concerns (especially patently legitimate concerns) of complainants, as occurred in the *Marquis v. University of Massachusetts at Amherst* case, is to deny basic respect toward such persons. Mr. Marquis complained to the instructor, and the instructor explained his actions. However, his explanation left open further legitimate questions of fairness and propriety. The department chair did not appear to even give Mr. Marquis and his complaint as much respect and consideration as the instructor, dismissing such complaints in general as absurd. And even the ombudsperson in this case did not seem to respect Mr. Marquis or his concerns. In dismissing complaints of students or employees out of hand, the institution denies their personhood and treats them as mere means to the institution's ends. Confidentiality provides further respect to complainants and makes it more likely that those with sincere complaints will come forward. And informality removes the process from more official channels, allowing for the possibility of open mediation and resolution of conflicts, rather than authoritative, juridical decisions.

An Ombudsperson may not be an absolute necessity for all institutions, but they can help form and sustain the moral character of an institution by demonstrating and preserving respect for those subject to the power and authority of the institution. There are other means of accomplishing these goals, but the Ombudsperson role is especially suited to segregate the interests of the institution from the process of mediation. But this all assumes the Ombudsperson role is being fulfilled in the manner expected, according to values like those of the IOA Code of Ethics. Thus, faculty and administration, in supporting ethical treatment of students and employees as well as supporting the ethical character of the institution, should, in all interactions with the office of the Ombudsperson, act so as to further those particular values—to support and preserve the independence, impartiality, confidentiality, and informality of the office.

CRITICAL ELEMENTS TO CONSIDER

As was shown in the legal case but not in the nursing case presented in this chapter, students are almost always advised to follow the chain of command in an organization to pursue a complaint. If the complaint occurs within a course, then normally the student should first appeal to the course professor, then perhaps the department chair, and there may be additional levels to whom to appeal, including Associate/Assistant Dean and even Dean.

If you are a student and you believe you have a legitimate claim, you must decide to pursue either a formal complaint to the appropriate university official (e.g., human resources, confidential ethics line, office of equality officer) or an *informal* complaint if at all possible.

If there is no satisfactory resolution within the respective college or school, then identifying the Office of the Ombudsman is a proper next step. Again, because some Ombudspersons represent faculty only, make sure you have an Ombudsmperson who hears student complaints.

Put your complaint in writing and be very specific.

Try to refrain from using any derogatory terms or inflammatory language, and present your case in a precise but professional way.

Try to avoid gossip or indiscreet discussion of your issue to wide numbers of parties.

Speak confidentially only to individuals you trust whom you also believe will be discreet and offer professional, unbiased advice.

If you are called to the Ombudsperson's office to evaluate your complaint, dress professionally, present yourself in the most professional way, and communicate whether you are seeking to be completely anonymous or merely confidential. You should understand that in some cases, for an Ombudsperson to rule specifically on your case, you may have to reveal your identity. In these cases, you should seek reassurance that the defendant whom you are bringing a complaint against cannot harass you or seek reprisal. Inquire if there are any specific university policies that might protect you in these cases.

Document all conversations you have with university officials at all levels. Include dates, times, and exactly what each party said.

Go to your university or college Ombudsperson website for more information, but do not be surprised if it is not highly visible. Our review indicates many Ombudsperson websites are not as visible as we would like, and others are excellent and provide lots of details about the role of the Ombudsperson.

If you have any questions that you may want answered prior to contacting any department in an official capacity, you may be able to contact your undergraduate or graduate student government association for peer advice.

Helpful Resources

- Department of Education Student Loan Ombudsman: https://studentaid.ed.gov/sa/redirects/ombudsman-ed-gov
- Indiana University Code of Student Rights, Responsibilities, & Conduct: http://www.indiana.edu/~code/
- San Diego State University: Office of the Student Ombudsman at http://go.sdsu.edu/student_affairs/ombudsman/role.aspx
- Insidehighered.com Who will listen?: https://www.insidehighered.com/news/2015/05/21/what-kind-resources-do-colleges-provide-students-complaints
- Commonwealth Ombudsman: Ombudsman.gov.au
- How can we help? (focused on international students): https://www.ombudsman.gov.au/How-we-can-help

References

Bauer, F. (2000). The practice of one ombudsman. *Negotiation Journal, 16*(1), 59–79. doi:10.1111/j.1571-9979.2000.tb00203.x

Commonwealth Ombudsman. (2009). *Best practice guide to complaint handling.* Canberra, Australia: Author. Retrieved from https://www.ombudsman.gov.au/__data/assets/pdf_file/0020/35615/Better-practice-guide-to-complaint-handling.pdf

Elder, G. (2010). *Final grade of a "C" prompts personal injury lawsuit*. DiggFacebookRedditDel.icio
.usStumbleUponNewsvine. Retrieved from www.cc.ysu.edu/~ramcewin/LegalExamples.pdf

Gadlin, H. (2000). The ombudsman: What's in a name? *Negotiation Journal, 16*(1), 37–48.
doi:10.1111/j.1571-9979.2000.tb00201.x

Gottehrer, D. M., & Hostina, M. (1998). *Essential characteristics of a classical ombudsman*. Retrieved from
https://www.usombudsman.org/essential-characteristics-of-a-classical-ombudsman/

International Ombudsman Association. (2007). *IOA code of ethics*. Retrieved from https://www
.ombudsassociation.org/assets/IOA%20Code%20of%20Ethics.pdf

International Ombudsman Association. (2009). *IOA standards of practice*. Retrieved from https://www
.ombudsassociation.org/assets/docs/IOA_Standards_of_Practice_Oct09.pdf

International Ombudsman Association. (2020). *IOA frequently asked questions*. Retrieved from https://www
.ombudsassociation.org/ioa-faq

Johnson, A. (2013). *The role of the Ombudsman: The Swedish experience*. Retrieved from https://www
.thedailystar.net/news/the-role-of-the-ombudsman-the-swedish-experience

Katsara, O. (2015). The use of the ombudsman's services for alleviating international students' difficulties.
Journal of International Students, 5(3), 260–270. Retrieved from http://jistudents.org/

Law.com. (2020). *Estoppel*. Retrieved June, 6, 2020

Levin, P. T. (2009). The Swedish model of public administration: Separation of powers—The Swedish style.
Journal of Administration and Governance, 4(1), 1–46. Retrieved from http://www.joaag.com/

Marquis v. University of Massachusetts at Amherst, No. 07-30015 (D. Mass. Jan. 31, 2007). Retrieved from
https://loweringthebar.net/wp-content/uploads/2007/10/Marquis_v_UMass.pdf

Merriam-Webster. (2010). *Definition of Ombudsman*. Retrieved from http://www.merriam-webster.com/
dictionary/Ombudsman?show=0&t=1284575547

Ohio State University. (2018). *Faculty Ombudsman* Retrieved from http.//Ombudsman.osu.edu/

Roth, J. A., McEllistrem, S., D'Agostino, T., & Brown, C. J. (2009). *Higher education law in America* (10th ed.).
Malvern, PA: Center for Education & Employment Law.

Saltzman, J. (2007, October 4). Student takes his C to federal court. *The Boston Globe*. Retrieved from http://
www.boston.com/news/local/articles/2007/10/04/student_takes_his_c_to_federal_court/

San Diego State University. (n.d.). *Office of the Student Ombudsman*. Retrieved from http://go.sdsu.edu/
student_affairs/ombudsman/role.aspx

Shelton, R. L. (2000). The institutional Ombudsman: A university case study. *Negotiation Journal, 16*(1),
81–98. doi:10.1111/j.1571-9979.2000.tb00204.x

Stewart, K. (1978). What a university ombudsman does: A sociological study of everyday conduct. *Journal of
Higher Education, 49*(1), 1–22. doi:10.1080/00221546.1978.11776595

Stewart v. Washington State University, Case No. C18-557-RSM (2019).

Stieber, C. (2000). 57 varieties: Has the Ombudsman concept become diluted? *Negotiation Journal, 16*(1),
49–57. doi:10.1111/j.1571-9979.2000.tb00202.x

Stimpson, J. (2019, February 22). Office of university ombudsman focuses on "problem solving" campus
issues. *Cornell Daily Sun*. Retrieved from https://cornellsun.com/2019/02/22/office-of-university
-ombudsman-focuses-on-problem-solving-campus-issues/

Tauginiené, L. (2016). Embedding academic integrity in public universities. *Journal of Academic Ethics, 14*(4),
327–344. doi:10.1007/s10805-016-9268-4

U.S. Equal Employment Opportunity Commission. (n.d.). *Alternative dispute resolution (ADR)*. Retrieved
from https://www.eeoc.gov/federal/fed_employees/adr.cfm

8

Neutrality, Confidentiality, and Independence: The Role of the Ombudsman When a Faculty Files a Complaint

Case Study 8.1
A Faculty Member Files a Complaint With the University Ombudsman[1]

Your role: You are the Department Chair.

Dr. David Riles makes an appointment to see you. Although he does not report directly to you, he does teach 50% of his load (pediatrics) in the BSN programs that you oversee. You've heard that the pediatric nursing faculty members are concerned about a suddenly announced resignation of one of their own members. You have also heard rumors about their fury that they were not involved in choosing her replacement. As the department chair, you are in a serious predicament; the faculty member who resigned was the senior coordinator of the pediatric clinical nursing course, and she had a course reduction for these administrative responsibilities. She unfortunately resigned just 2 weeks before the fall term was to begin. Given that time span and with large sections of pediatric courses about to commence, there was no time for a search committee to be appointed. You knew you needed to find a replacement quickly, and in fact you already have. Before doing so, you consulted with the Associate Dean for your division and shared your judgment that none of the undergraduate faculty in this specialty really has the leadership skills (and perhaps the work ethic, as this is a very time-consuming endeavor) to undertake such a large responsibility. You considered appointing a highly qualified graduate nursing faculty member (a proven and experienced leader), but she is nearing retirement and likely does not want this huge responsibility (although you did not ask her). The Associate Dean informed you she has a resume from a brand-new DNP

---

[1] Note: In Chapter 7, Neutrality, Confidentiality, and Independence: The Role of the Ombudsman When a Student Files a Complaint, which deals with a student's use of the Ombudsman, there is a note about dissatisfaction with the term Ombudsman. It is used here for the reasons indicated there.

graduate who is very experienced, has undergraduate teaching experience, and has exhibited strong leadership qualities in her previous position—something the pediatric core lacks depth in from your observations and evaluation of them. You agree with the Associate Dean, that due to the urgent time constraints, you personally inquire if she would be interested in this position. Learning that she was, you quickly interviewed her, was very impressed, offered her the position, and she accepted. She is currently in the process of becoming a new employee. Somehow, word got out before you were able to manage the announcement and spread like wildfire, and not just among the pediatric core faculty. You believe you have made the right decision, but now know you are going to likely be met with resistance.

When Dr. Riles meets you, and he expresses his personal offence, and that of his other colleagues, that there was no search committee and no search at all. You had already heard he was upset that one of his best friends on the pediatric core team was not offered the position. In your meeting, you indicate that the resignation was sudden and close to the beginning of the term and that a formal search was not possible. You inform him that you are well aware of all the pediatric faculty's credentials and that the new hire was best positioned to undertake this new role. You further tell Dr. Riles that the hire was known to be a "workhorse" and at the top of her graduating class. Dr. Riles was not interested in your rational for the decision; instead he begins to advocate vigorously for his friend, but you interject noting that his friend had never expressed any interest in the position, nor had he stepped up to inquire about the position as soon as he knew the position was vacant. You civilly inform Dr. Riles that his advocacy, although perhaps well meaning, was nonetheless inappropriate (advocating for someone who could not speak for herself); you reinforce that the position has been filled. The meeting ends, but not well. The next day you receive notification from the university Ombudsman that Dr. Riles filed a complaint against you for not following due process in hiring a new faculty member.

Questions

- How would you first proceed?
- Have you followed the university policy on hiring or violated a required faculty hiring protocol? You wonder why Dr. Riles skipped the chain of command and gone directly to the Ombudsman?
- When you either meet with the Ombudsman or provide your side of the case in writing, what will you say or write?

FACULTY USE OF A UNIVERSITY OMBUDSMAN: LEGAL PRINCIPLES AND REVIEW OF THE LITERATURE

Introduction

Chapter 7, Neutrality, Confidentiality, and Independence: The Role of the Ombudsman When a Student Files a Complaint, presented a common definition of an Ombudsman and identified two primary types: classical and organizational, with the former instituted by statute and the latter instituted by other agents or bodies. The International Ombudsman Association (IOA) is the leading international organization for establishing common global standards and best practices, and these are discussed in this chapter, as they emanated from the IOA's first developed Code of Ethics (2007). According to Alcover (2009), "University and academia are, due to its nature, its structure and its inside relationships, a perfect breeding ground for the conflicts, disputes, problems, and grievances. In these settings, mediation is one of the dispute resolution mechanisms most used by University" (p. 275).

Whereas Chapter 7 discussed the Ombudsman or the Ombudsperson who works with university students, staff, and faculty (in other words, the full university community), this chapter will focus on the role of the Ombudsman who is specifically assigned to work with faculty. Clivikly Powell, a

Professor Emerita from the University of New Mexico and now Ombudsman, has stated, ""I'm kind of blatantly subversive in that what I'm trying to do is move the campus to a culture of resolving difficulties at the least adversarial level in a constructive way," and "I've been a faculty member, so I have strong credibility" (June, 2019, p. 1).[2]

IOA STANDARDS PRACTICE AND CODE OF ETHICS

The IOA's Standards of Practice (2009) were developed from the aforementioned Code of Ethics. According to the Standards of Practice preamble, "Each Ombudsman office should have an organizational Charter or Terms of Reference, approved by senior management, articulating the principles of the Ombudsman function in that organization and their consistency with the IOA Standards of Practice" (p. 1). In many ways, the Standards of Practice are extensions of the Code of Ethics and provide more direction to each of its four principles: independence, neutrality and impartiality, confidentiality, and informality. Table 8.1 describes the principles of the Code of Ethics as represented by the Standards of Practice. The Code of Ethics is intended to provide guidance to Organizational Ombudsmen in practicing according to IOA Standards of Practice to the highest ethical and professionalism levels possible.

The second primary document of the IOA is the Standards of Practice guide which is "… based from the ethical principles stated in the IOA Code of Ethics" and is intended to provide guidance to Organizational Ombudsmen in practicing according to IOA Standards of Practice to the highest level of professionalism possible. As the *Standards of Practice* are broad explanations of the *Code of Ethics,* similarly the *Best Practices* document provides more detail to the *Standards of Practice,* but *only* to the organizational Ombudsman.

Recall from Chapter 7, Neutrality, Confidentiality, and Independence: The Role of the Ombudsman When a Student Files a Complaint, that the classical Ombudsman is organized by statute and operates by the direct language of that statute. The organizational Ombudsman's role is probably therefore more loosely structured. According to Howard (2013):

> An Organizational Ombuds provides confidential, informal, independent and neutral assistance to individuals through dispute resolution and problem-solving methods such as conflict coaching, informal mediation, facilitation, and shuttle diplomacy. An Organizational Ombuds can also serve as a resource to help you identify ways in which you surface any concerns about possible misconduct. The Organizational Ombuds responds to concerns and disputes brought forward by visitors to the office and may report trends, systemic problems, and organizational issues to high-level leaders and executives in a confidential manner. He or she does not advocate for individuals, groups or entities, but rather for the principles of fairness and equity. (p. 3)

Who is qualified to be an Ombudsman? Gadlin (2000) indicates that the first university ombudsmen were "truly amateurs" (p. 40). However, there is general consensus that anyone who is serving as an Ombudsman should possess "integrity, ability to be fair and sympathetic, willingness to be critical of the powers that be, etc., along with knowledge of the rules, procedures, and culture of the institution within which they were assuming the Ombudsman role" (p. 40). These individuals also need to be skilled at neutrality, confidentiality, independence, dispute resolution, and mediation (Exhibit 8.1). One question often asked is whether an individual serving as an Ombudsman should be an attorney. The usual answer is no, unless there are specific guidelines that require someone with a law degree, usually a state statute. For example, in Indiana the new Ombudsman for the Department of Child Services was required to have either a law degree or a master's degree in social work (Evans, 2009). This Ombudsman position, because it is created by state statute, is therefore an example of a classical Ombudsman. Similarly, Fallberg, Mackenney, and Övretreit (2004) indicate having legal

---

[2] In fact, most ombudsmen are simply faculty members who are generally well respected and therefore trusted to "have the right instincts" and "do the right thing." Few ombudsmen are first trained experts, but often grow into the role.

[3] Some university Ombudsman see faculty, staff, and students. There have been discussions in one Faculty Senate whether an Ombudsman can fairly represent equally when either a faculty and student or faculty and staff (and other dyads), if each has contacted the Ombudsman regarding the same issue. In our case, very often a university or college Ombudsman is also a faculty member and there at least seems to be an altered balance of power certainly from the student/staff perspective. Other universities have agreed that a specific Ombudsman may better serve the faculty, and for example, at Duke University, the Faculty Ombudsman is a 2-year appointment and is elected by the faculty (Duke Today, 2010).

Exhibit 8.1 General Job Description Requirements for Position of Ombudsman

CRITICAL SKILLS AND CHARACTERISTICS

1. Communication and problem-solving skills
2. Decision-making/strategic-thinking skills
3. Conflict resolution skills
4. Organizational knowledge and networking skills
5. Sensitivity to diversity issues
6. Composure and presentation skills
7. Integrity

ACCOUNTABILITIES

1. Dispute resolution/consultation and referral
2. Policy analysis and feedback
3. Community outreach and education
4. Establish/maintain office of the Ombudsperson

EDUCATION AND WORK EXPERIENCE

1. Varies, usually mostly a bachelor's degree, but an advanced degree is often desired and based on the setting of the Ombudsperson
2. A work history that indicates the above characteristics and function of this job have been previously demonstrated

training is very important because it is necessary to arrive at settlements between parties. Stanford University (2019) also employs a lawyer as the Ombudsman, but this person does not provide legal services, Nevertheless, understanding the concept of due process and having some alacrity and familiarity with the law are likely very valuable and helpful. Above all else, an irreproachable reputation and the highest ethical standards are two character traits that are essential in individuals serving in these roles (Harrison, 2004). Finally, it should be mentioned that the American Association of University Professors (AAUP), founded in 1915, remains the leading organization dedicated to the promotion and protection of the academic freedom and rights of university faculty (AAUP, n.d.). Most colleges and universities follow general AAUP guidelines found in the 11th edition of its Redbook –AAUP's Policy Documents and Reports (AAUP, 2015), especially its procedures for hiring, promotion, and tenure; other institutions use the Redbook as a resource even if they do not follow it.

America society is fluid, and able arbiters are necessary to address organizational disputes that need skilled mediation, not just policies that aim first to reprimand and then punish. Adjudication need not predominate in higher education in this text, but of course there are academic rules, and regulations that must be in in compliance with various stakeholders and particularly, accreditors, and often many of them both local, state and federal.

Finally, it should be mentioned that the American Association of University Professors (AAUP), founded in 1915, remains the leading organization dedicated to the promotion and protection of the academic freedom and rights of university faculty (AAUP, n.d.). Most colleges and universities follow general AAUP guidelines found in the 11th edition of its *Redbook—AAUP's Policy Documents and Reports* (AAUP, 2015), especially its procedures for hiring, promotion, and tenure; other institutions use the *Redbook* as a resource even if they do not follow it.

DISCUSSION OF CASE STUDY

Case Study 8.1, although quite complex, in reality is an example of the layers of detail that ordinary academic nursing administrators encounter every day. Indeed, this author was once queried by a new interim academic department chair who was requesting a very straightforward answer to a question, and my response began with "rarely ever is the decision-making process of a department chair very black and white." In this case study, the levels of complexity are not surprising, especially in a very

Table 8.1 Principles of the IOA Code of Ethics			
Independence	**Neutrality/Impartiality**	**Confidentiality**	**Informality**
The Ombudsman Office and the Ombudsman are independent from other organizational entities.	The Ombudsman is neutral, impartial, and unaligned.	Communications between the Ombudsman and others (made while the Ombudsman is serving in that capacity) are considered privileged. The privilege belongs to the Ombudsman and the Ombudsman Office, rather than to any party to an issue. Others cannot waive this privilege.	The Ombudsman functions on an informal basis by such means as: listening, providing and receiving information, identifying and reframing issues, developing a range of responsible options, and—with permission and at the Ombudsman's discretion—engaging in informal third-party intervention. When possible, the Ombudsman helps people develop new ways to solve problems themselves.
The Ombudsman holds no other position within the organization that might compromise independence.	The Ombudsman strives for impartiality, fairness and objectivity in the treatment of people and the consideration of issues. The Ombudsman advocates for fair and equitably administered processes and does not advocate on behalf of any individual within the organization.	The Ombudsman does not testify in any formal process inside the organization and resists testifying in any formal process outside of the organization regarding a visitor's contact with the Ombudsman or confidential information communicated to the Ombudsman, even if given permission or requested to do so. The Ombudsman may, however, provide general, nonconfidential information about the Ombudsman Office or the Ombudsman profession.	The Ombudsman, as an informal and off-the-record resource, pursues resolution of concerns and looks into procedural irregularities and/or broader systemic problems when appropriate.

Source: Adapted from International Ombudsman Association. (2009). *Standards of practice.* Retrieved from https://www.ombudsassociation .org/assets/docs/IOA_Standards_of_Practice_Oct09.pdf

large nursing organization. The first question asked was, how would you first proceed? Certainly, administrators knew the department chair must adhere to a few key leadership/managerial tenets if they were to be both ethical and responsible in the conduct of their administrative duties: (a) there are always two sides to any story—wait until you hear both before you jump to conclusions; (b) faculty members may disclose what they want you to know, and not disclose what they want to hide or not reveal or keep private (not public); (c) your job is to serve the good of the organization, treat everyone fairly, and ensure they obtain whatever process if "due"; and finally, (d) you are being paid to exercise your best judgment, otherwise there would be someone else in your position, or it would not exist.

Here, all pediatric faculty (both undergraduate and graduate) knew of this resignation, and yet no one formally expressed a personal interest in the position to the Department Chair or even Associate Dean. Instead, a senior faculty member went to advocate for another, a process often observed in academia, with faculty members not asking *directly* for what they want and instead expressing their desires or wishes *indirectly* and even through others. In the absence of anyone stepping forward to volunteer for this position (and the work involved), the administrators were challenged to fill the position quickly and ensure a smooth transition to a new academic term. Expressing these facts to Dr. Riles demonstrated honesty and a certain transparency, and Dr. Riles possibly may have agreed with them, if not with the way the emergency was resolved.

The second question was, have you followed the university policy on hiring or violated a required faculty hiring protocol? What do you think?

In this case, the university human resource policy does not direct that Senior Nursing Coordinator positions be posted, as these are not line administrative positions, such as Department Chair or Associate Dean. Further, even with a faculty resignation there is no assumption that there is a budget allocation for a new hire. That would need to be determined by the Dean. That there was a formal announcement of the resignation (although not required in this case) was at least arguably sufficient notice for any interested candidates to express their interest in the position to the respective academic nursing administrator.

Although Dr. Riles had the right to file a complaint with the university Ombudsman, the question remains whether he was exercising good judgment in doing so. Academia is no different from the corporate world when it comes to give-and-take in the workplace. There are often consequences of being or not being a team player or in being an agent who helps maintain or improve organizational morale or one who tends to contribute to negative organizational morale. The indirect, but underbelly reality of this situation is that Dr. Riles is going to need the support of the Department Chair and the Associate Dean for promotion, and he is not using good emotional intelligence if he thinks he can act without consequence. This is not to insinuate that he should not report violations of due process[4] if they are indeed founded, but he should evaluate very seriously if the charges have real merit and how the issue is best addressed without damaging his own institutional reputation. More important, there is a strong case that Dr. Riles was acting very independently and even interfering.

By the same token, there is reason for the faculty to protect its interests in shared governance and its place at the hiring and appointments tables per the bylaws of the University. Going to an Ombudsman does not require the process to be nasty or adversarial; it can create a better process for *the next time* an emergency like this occurs. If that had been the way that Riles presented the issue, it would have demonstrated maturity and commitment to the organization. If this had been his objective, however, the better option would have been to have reflected on whether he should have raised that point with the Department Chair directly—and only petitioned the Ombudsman if the Chair declined to consider the issue, period.

WHEN TO CONSULT THE UNIVERSITY COUNSEL

University counsel is available to answer questions about the law, to provide guidance and interpretations about dispute resolution processes, and to help university clients resolve problems. But university counsel is counsel for the university, not for any particular member of the faculty, and not "for" one member "against" another. Typically, requests for legal assistance are best made by a Department Chair or Associate Dean, so faculty members should think about going to their supervisors first. If you view your issue as serious and rising above

---

[4] As noted in several other chapters, the words "due process" mean different things and can vary greatly in meaning between private and public institutions. The implications are more formal in public institutions because of constitutional prohibitions on "the state" depriving people of "property or liberty" interests "without due process of law. Private institutions can also commit themselves to fair procedures, and those procedures are what is "due," but they are not protected by the constitution.

the specific jurisdiction or powers of the Ombudsman (remember, this is not a legal course of action), you will need to consider where your complaint is best heard by going through the chain of command or even using an ethics hotline most universities maintain. With most confidential or anonymous ethics hotlines, your claim can be reviewed by someone with independent authority to decide whether it ought to be reviewed by university counsel.

FINDINGS AND DISPOSITION

In this case, it was unfortunate that Dr. Riles did not choose instead to report his complaint to the school's or department's faculty affairs committee—first, because a complaint to the university Ombudsman can take the issue away from those who should "own" it, involve an outsider unnecessary to resolution, and complicate the process by injecting different processes and even participants. Perhaps he should have also consulted with some of his other senior colleagues to determine what the proper action should be. Perhaps he could have asked the dean (or another senior confidant) if he or she felt this was a due process violation or if the appointment followed accepted university procedures for "emergency" hiring. It is unknown whether this was done, but it might have allowed him more time to reflect on a course of action and to more carefully weigh the impact of a variety of strategies to communicate displeasure.

The third question posed in the case study was, when you either meet with the Ombudsman or provide your side of the case in writing, what will you say or write? What do you think you should say about how you handled this complaint?

In this case, there was no formal meeting between the Ombudsman and the Department Chair. Instead the Ombudsman called the Department Chair and agreed the human resource policy on faculty hiring was definitive; this was not an administrative level appointment that required a formal posting procedure. The Department Chair informed the Ombudsman that they did disclose that an email had gone out to all faculty about the individual's resignation but due to the emergent nature of a replacement with just weeks before the beginning of the term, an administrative decision was made by the Dean and the Chair to not convene a formal search committee. However, if anyone had expressed formal interest in the position, the Chair would have evaluated that candidate. With that, the Ombudsman thanked the Department Chair and made a note to personally check with Human Resources and the Associate Dean to verify if there really were specific policies on emergent faculty hiring.

As for the disposition of this case, the DNP graduate was hired and was ultimately very successful in the role, but was not welcomed warmly. It took longer than it should have to become integrated, and they experienced ongoing resentment from the other pediatric faculty. Although the new hire's competency allowed some breathing room, residual individual issues remained to some extent with the other pediatric faculty. The Ombudsman later asked Human Resources and the Associate Dean whether there was any internal policy regarding the appointment of senior course coordinators. Upon the Associate Dean's reply (and Human Resource's confirmation that no procedural hiring policies were violated) that these appointments were always made internally and that formal search committees are rare and not the ordinary process by which these positions are filled, the Ombudsman concluded that the appointment had not violated any rule or procedure, and in a meeting with Dr. Riles explained all of this. The Ombudsman did indicate he was not "the decider" in this issue and that if a formal Ombudsman hearing was requested, he would facilitate that using the processes of the Office of the Ombudsman. Dr. Riles declined, and the Ombudsman called the Department Chair and Associate Dean, advising them he was closing his file. He cautioned them that they must guard against taking any action that could be interpreted as retaliation against Dr. Riles, especially as he would soon be considered for promotion. Last, a senior colleague of Dr. Riles (after the fact) did mention to him in a conversation that he really must be more careful about "stirring up trouble," and although Dr. Riles was defensive, he realized that perhaps he was the only one damaged in this altercation. He subsequently decided to request a delay in his application for full professorship by a year to help heal his relationships with the administrators who would evaluate him.

The way this case ended serves to remind those who utilize the Ombudsman must be assured that there will not be any adverse consequences (retaliation) toward those who choose it. The fact that Dr. Riles was not comfortable with proceeding with his application for promotion was his decision; but if he had decided to proceed with his candidacy for promotion, the Associate Dean and Department Head would have had to be scrupulously fair. Any "no" vote by them could well have been alleged to be retaliation for having filed the charge.

RELEVANT LEGAL CASES

DePree v. Saunders, 80, No. 08-60978 (5th Cir. 2009).

Dr. DePree, a tenured professor at the University of Southern Mississippi, sued the university's president and various administrators and faculty members after he was removed from teaching duties in August 2007 and evicted from his office in the College of Business. The Interim Dean of the College of Business had written to the president and stated Dr. DePree had contributed, according to court records, to "an environment in which faculty members and students do not feel safe to go about their usual business." He was accused of engaging in negative and disruptive behaviors and criticized as the only accounting professor who had failed to "engage in the scholarly or professional activities necessary to be labeled 'academically-qualified' or 'professionally-qualified' by the University's accrediting agency, AACSB [Association to Advance Collegiate Schools of Business]." Eight letters from other faculty in the department confirming these allegations accompanied the interim dean's letter. Upon receipt of the letter, the president notified Dr. DePree that he was relieved of all his teaching duties and service requirements to the university, not permitted to enter the College of Business except to retrieve personal items, and to continue his scholarship with continued access to the university computer system and library. The president then instructed the provost to investigate the charges and requested the university Ombudsman investigate the charges and submit a report.

DePree filed a lawsuit with the district court within 3 weeks of the letter and complained these actions were in retaliation for maintaining a website critical of the university and some of its administrators and faculty and because he complained to the College of Business' accrediting agency (AACSB) about the school. In his suit, DePree claimed First Amendment retaliation, due process violations, and various state law claims. The Ombudsman delivered a report to the president in December 2007 and recommended that DePree have a mental health examination to assess his fitness to teach, that he had to produce sufficient scholarly work to the satisfaction of independent evaluators, and that the restrictions by the president remain in place.

The district course granted summary judgment in favor of the defendants and denied DePree's motion for temporary and permanent injunctive relief. Further, the district court denied a temporary restraining order against the defendants in suit. On appeal to the Fifth Circuit Court, the issues of First Amendment retaliation, due process violations, and various state law claims were again evaluated.

On the First Amendment retaliation, the appeals court indeed remanded DePree's injunctive claim based on First Amendment retaliation for further development chiefly because the appeals court could not determine whether the president could impose discipline on the plaintiff if indeed the discipline was retaliatory and the website comments and letter to the AACSB were protected speech. Second, the actions by the president preceded the late report by the Ombudsman. However, the First Amendment charges against all parties aside from the president were dismissed because recommendations for a course of action against DePree were not described and the president alone enforced the penalties on the plaintiff. In discussion, the court admitted that these issues of protected speech were complex. Is website material or a letter to an accrediting body written by a tenured professor "protected speech," and did the university indeed retaliate because of these behaviors? There is no access to the eight written letters, but there is a statement of the court that this issue was difficult to ascertain.

On the due process claim, DePree claimed a violation of the due process clause because the university prohibited him from teaching and denied him further access to the College of Business. As stated in this ruling, "The threshold requirement of any due process claim is the government's deprivation of a plaintiff's liberty or property interest" (*DePree v. Saunders 80*, 2009, p. 1). This claim was rejected because the plaintiff's salary and title continued and there was nothing contractual that indicated every professor had to teach as part of his or her professorial role, and therefore the court ruled he had no constitutional property right to teach. Although it is unclear whether the plaintiff had a right to enter the building, the court did affirm the university had a right to reassign or transfer an employee. It is this temporary and permanent restriction to the building that may have been evaluated as potentially retaliatory as part cause for the remand on the First Amendment retaliation claim, but there is no certainty. There is no indication that the plaintiff was provided office space (normally accorded to a tenured professor) somewhere else to conduct the scholarly work he was required to produce.

On the alleged state violations, all were dismissed for various reasons. Because his salary continued, he could not claim breach of contract, and because this claim appeared in a later legal response, not the original brief, it was dismissed. Further, state charges of tortuous interference with business relations, intentional infliction of emotional distress, breach of contractual duty of good faith and fair dealing, defamation, and assault were all dismissed against all defendants mostly from lack of genuine material fact to support the allegations. The assault charge was interesting. From the court record, according to the plaintiff, the associate dean "aggressively walk[ed] toward [DePree], yelling at [him], repeatedly referring to [him] as a 'son-of-a-bitch,' and shaking papers in his face creat[ing] an apprehension in [DePree] of an imminent harmful or offensive contact." The court did not find evidence of any imminent or harmful contact, and there was no claim of personal injury. Indeed, the court indicated there was evidence these two individuals had squared off like this before, and there was no indication that DePree was harmed merely because someone was cursing at him and waving papers in his face. Other cases found, like *Cutcliffe v. Wright State University* (2019) and *Blessing v. Ohio University* (2011), came out similarly.

SUMMARY

In *DePree v. Saunders 80* (2009), we do not know the ultimate outcome of this case. It appears, however, the plaintiff maintained his salary and title, but there was acknowledgment by the court that at this appeal there was some concern that there *may* have been retaliation against the tenured professor for activities that were protected speech. We are likewise concerned that severe penalties were enacted *before the Ombudsman's report,* and barring the faculty from entering the College of Business building permanently without any indication of alternate office space seemed extreme.

Overall, as this chapter is focused on the role of the Ombudsman for faculty, we are faced with a few questions. Could the Ombudsman have been better utilized? Why did it take 4 months for the Ombudsman to conduct an investigation and prepare a final report? Could the President have taken some intermediary disciplinary measures while the investigation was ongoing? Could the plaintiff have gone to the Ombudsman himself? How would that have operated? Could the Ombudsman have fairly done both tasks (serve the faculty member by hearing his complaint and conduct the investigation as requested by the President)? We do worry about this when we see models in which one Ombudsman sees faculty, students, *and* staff. Is it possible there was someone else better prepared to conduct this investigation, perhaps one of the university's staff attorneys? The better strategy might have been to have used the Ombudsman to prepare a report *before* the severe penalties were first enacted.

If you are a faculty member or seeking to become a faculty member, it is wise to find out if your respective university or college has an Ombudsman and what type—one who serves faculty only or one who serves the full university community. It may also be important to consult your university website or faculty handbook and determine the functions of the Ombudsman. If you are a faculty member and you have an issue that you believe needs to be resolved, you will need to decide what is the best avenue for your claim—human resources, office of equality, the next person on your administrative chain of command, the university attorney, or the Ombudsman. Determining who is best to handle your issue is critical. Each has its own timetable, process, and consequences. It is worth taking the time to consider all your options and consult individuals who will give you confidential, wise counsel and consider your best course of action.

ETHICAL CONSIDERATIONS

The cases from this chapter show that appealing to an Ombudsman may not always be the best way to resolve a conflict, but they do provide important service maintaining the ethical character of the institution for many difficult to resolve cases. The IOA Code of Ethics evokes the ethical principles of independence, neutrality and impartiality, confidentiality, and informality in order to best ensure fair resolutions and fair treatment of all parties that come before the ombudsman (IOA, 2007). In addressing conflicts among faculty or between faculty and administration in a fair and substantive manner, the institution demonstrates respect for the faculty as persons. Failing to respond in such a manner would reduce the faculty to cogs for the institution's ends. In addition, respecting the concerns and complaints of faculty and having a reputation for doing so will create a more pleasant and attractive working environment, which will help the institution achieve its overall goals.

CRITICAL ELEMENTS TO CONSIDER

- Do you have a university Ombudsman? What kind? Whose claims do they hear?
- What is the best office to hear your claim—office of the Ombudsman, equality, another person in your administrative chain of command (Dean or Provost perhaps), or Human Resources? Or does your issue require hiring your own attorney?

Helpful Resources

- International Ombudsman Association: http://www.ombudsassociation.org/
- The National Long-Term Care Ombudsman Resource Center Ombudsman Training: https://ltcombudsman.org/omb_support/training
- International Ombudsman Association About the CO-OP Credential and Other Levels of Designation: https://www.ombudsassociation.org/about-the-co-op-credential
- Consumer Financial Protection Bureau Ombudsman resources: https://www.consumerfinance.gov/cfpb-ombudsman/ombudsman-resources/
- CMS.gov (Centers for Medicare and Medicaid Services) Ombudsman Center: https://www.cms.gov/Center/Special-Topic/Ombudsman-Center

References

Alcover, C.-M. (2009). Ombudsing in higher education: A contingent model for mediation in university dispute resolution processes. *Spanish Journal of Psychology*, *12*(1), 275–287. doi:10.1017/S1138741600001682

American Association of University Professors. (2015). *AAUP's policy documents and reports* (11th ed.). Washington, DC: Author.

American Association of University Professors. (n.d.). *History of the AAUP*. Retrieved from http://www.aaup.org/AAUP/about/history/

Blessing v. Ohio University, Case No. 2:09-CV-0762 (S.D. Ohio 2011).

Cutcliffe v. Wright State University, Case No. 3:17-cv-222 (S.D. Ohio 2019).

Duke Today. (2010). *Dawson elected faculty Ombudsman. Professor to serve two-year term*. Retrieved from https://today.duke.edu/2010/05/ombudsman.html

DePree v. Saunders 80, No. 08-60978 (5th Cir. 2009).

Dunn, A. (2010). Officials consider creating Ombudsman office: Proposed ethical concerns department to take legal requests from faculty. Seattle, WA: Seattle University.

Evans, T. (2009). DCS Ombudsman codified, but that's just the beginning. Indianapolis, IN: Indy.com.

Fallberg, L., Mackenney, S., & Øvretreit, J. (2004). Protecting patients' rights? In S. Mackenney & L. Fallberg (Eds.), *A comparative study of the Ombudsman in healthcare*. Cambridge, MA: Radcliffe.

Gadlin, H. (2000). The Ombudsman: What's in a name? *Negotiation Journal*, *16*(1), 37–48. doi:10.1111/j.1571-9979.2000.tb00201.x

Harrison, T. (2004). What is success in ombuds processes? Evaluation of a university Ombudsman. *Conflict Resolution Quarterly, 21*(3), 331–335. doi:10.1002/crq.65

Howard, C. (2013). *The organizational ombudsman*. Chicago, IL: The American Bar Association.

International Ombudsman Association. (2007). *Code of ethics*. Retrieved from https://www
.ombudsassociation.org/assets/IOA%20Code%20of%20Ethics.pdfl

International Ombudsman Association. (2009). *Standards of practice*. Seattle, WA: Author.

June, A. W. (2019, July 20). Meet your campus troubleshooter, *chronicle.com*. Retrieved from https://www
.chronicle.com/article/Meet-Your-Campus/246797

The Ombuds Blog. (2014). *Texas Tech University to appoint first faculty Ombuds*. Irving, TX: Author.

Stanford News. (2019). *New university ombudsperson talks about her role in resolving conflicts*. Palo Alto,
CA: Author.

9

Due Process Issues
for the Student

Case Study 9.1
Due Process for Students

Your role: You are Dr. Jill Mahoney, Course Coordinator for Fundamentals of Nursing course. You are responsible for the oversight of two theory/didactic sections of 40 students each as well as the oversight of 10 clinical rotations with eight students in each clinical group.

You receive an email from a BSN-accelerated nursing student, Eric Johnson, who is in his first semester of study (out of three semesters), contesting his clinical failure. He states he is being held to a higher standard because he is a male student and Professor Connelly does not like him. The clinical faculty member, Jennifer Connelly, told you that Mr. Johnson was unprepared for medication administration, does not engage in a therapeutic manner with patients, has anger management issues, and is defensive with constructive feedback. Professor Connelly reports that Mr. Johnson has not met the clinical objectives and she has awarded Mr. Johnson a clinical grade of Unsatisfactory for unprofessional behavior. She also states that he had an anger management issue in the post-clinical conference and during a medication calculation exam where he failed to follow the proctoring policy. He responded in an uncivil manner when Professor Mahoney held him accountable.

Questions
- What questions do you need to ask Professor Connelly?
- What documentation do you need to review?
- What is your best course of action?

DUE PROCESS: LEGAL PRINCIPLES AND REVIEW OF THE LITERATURE

Given a proper understanding of due process, nursing faculty can appropriately address student clinical performance or behavior that is not meeting expectations. Therefore, it is crucial that clinical faculty understand the student's right to due process (Walker, 2016; Whitney, 2009). *Due process* is one of the most complicated subjects in American law: It fills casebooks and is the subject of semesters of study in law schools. The two simple words *due process* express the notion that whenever a state agency does something that results in harm to an individual, it must first follow a process that is fairly designed to produce a fair result to that person. Exactly what process is due to the individual varies from case to case and depends on many different factors. But in very general terms, the right of due process equates to fairness (Johnson, 2009; Kaplin & Lee, 2013).

The Fifth and Fourteenth Amendments of the United States Constitution guarantee citizens "due process of law" and seek to ensure fairness in the application of governmental authority to citizens. *Substantive due process* is fairness on the merits of the subject, and *procedural due process* is fairness in the way that the merits are addressed. The Constitution does not protect every interest that citizens may have. For example, we have no right to a job, nor do we have a right to be protected from people who are mean or who upset us. In fact, just the opposite is true: The right of free speech means that other people have the right to say things that make us unhappy, and most of us (e.g., those without collective bargaining agreements or tenure) can be fired for no reason at all. What the Constitution protects are *property and liberty interests,* and in actual *cases and controversies*—and as you might expect, lawyers have been fighting about the meaning of those words for centuries.

The Constitution has another limitation in that it only protects citizens from government action. This means it applies to public universities, but whether it applies to private universities "depends" (as lawyers say)—for example, on whether the conduct involved government funding or a specific federal right (e.g., the right to be free of racial discrimination). In the private university context, however, there is a complex matrix of state laws—codified in constitutions, statutes, and administrative codes, or expressed in judicial decisions—that in general terms result in the same bottom line. One of the principles judges use to examine corporate behavior is called the Business Judgment Rule. It is a principle of deference. It recognizes that judges do not know as much about a business as the person doing that job, and means that a judge will not substitute their judgment for that of the businessperson as long as the businessperson reached the decision through a reasonable process. In the context of a university, the test is frequently whether the faculty's decisions have been careful and deliberate (Smith, McKoy, & Richardson, 2001; Walker, 2016).

What a due or "reasonable" process is often depends on the outcome: The greater the impact on a third person, the better the process should be. Grading performance in a single class can be more subjective and involve fewer protections (perhaps no process is due for that) than deciding to expel a student from the program. The process does not have to be perfect and the decisions do not have to be right, but the process must be fair. The two concepts that are fundamental and always looked to are *notice* and *opportunity to be heard:* Did the student know it was happening, and did they get the chance to tell their side of the story to someone who was independent and had no stake in the outcome?

In education, the nursing program or college satisfies these essential requirements by stipulating in writing—in the form of policies and procedures—what performance is expected, what constitutes misconduct, and the process that will be followed in imposing a punishment—a deprivation of liberty or property. Students have these interests. They have paid money and given up their time for an education, and they have the expectation (based on written and oral promises from the university) that they will receive a degree as long as they perform satisfactorily. Applied to students, *due process* means that before their interest in earning a degree is injured, they will know why. In particular, the procedural guidelines should ensure that students are given the opportunity to be heard, the opportunity to review the charges and evidence against them, the opportunity to appear before an impartial decision-maker, and the opportunity to appeal the decision (Lindsay, 2012; Roth, 2007).

Applied to a university's clinical settings, *due process* has been interpreted to mean that a student has ample opportunity of notice of misconduct, is given suggestions for improvement, and is advised of the consequences for failure to improve (Gaberson & Oermann, 2010; Gallant, McDonald, & Higuchi, 2006; Johnson, 2009). It is to be predicted that there will be disagreement about whether this process was followed, and that is why documentation is essential. Lawyers like to say, "If it's not in the record, it didn't happen." They do so because writing something down at the time it happens is considered by everyone to be proof (a) that it was important and (b) that it happened. It is far easier to conclude that a punishment was properly imposed (and due process accorded) when there is ample documentation by the faculty and notice to the student with recommendations for improvement and information regarding the student's right to appeal (Gardner & Suplee, 2010; Suplee, Lachman, Siebert, & Anselmi, 2008). Recording students' activities on each clinical day by keeping meticulous anecdotal notes concerning accomplishments, performance issues, and discipline conferences clearly satisfies the obligation (Gardner & Suplee, 2010; Smith, McKoy, & Richardson, 2001).

The considerations for *substantive* due process are the same: They specify what is expected and the rules by which performance will be judged. Standards for theory, clinical objectives, and performance must be provided to students at the start of each semester. Students must be informed that their student status is analogous to all nurses in maintaining a professional standard of care as delineated in the American Nurses Association's Code of Ethics (Chunta, 2016; Johnson, 2009). Students' practice expectations should be addressed in the course syllabus to include respectful behavior, communication, and clinical preparation, as well as professional responsibility to faculty, professional nursing staff, ancillary clinical employees, patients, and families (Anselmi, Glasgow, & Gambescia, 2014; Whitney, 2009). Conduct that is not within acceptable limits should also be addressed in the nursing student handbook, course syllabi, and clinical evaluation tools. Students and faculty reflect the image of the educational institution. A breach of expected conduct, whether covert or overt, reflects poorly on the nursing program and can place the institution in a precarious predicament (Johnson, 2009).

Universities are free to define what constitutes misconduct—that's the so-called business of education in which courts do not want to get involved. Misconduct can range from emotional outbursts, incivility, and lack of integrity to acts of poor judgment. In the clinical setting, students may demonstrate misconduct by being unprepared for clinical assignments, disrespecting staff and patients, and displaying an inability to manage the stressors related to clinical performance (Ahn & Choi, 2018; Smith et al., 2001). Misconduct by student nurses may jeopardize the health and welfare of patients. To ensure that the college or university pass students who provide safe nursing care, faculty have a legal responsibility to convey unsatisfactory grades to students who are not capable of meeting standards of nursing practice; in doing so, faculty must also remember to provide due process to students at the same time (Smith et al., 2001; Walker, 2016).

Students must know the expected behaviors as well as the consequences if they fail to meet them in the very beginning of their clinical rotation (Ahn & Choi, 2018; Kolanko et al., 2006). Faculty versed in the concept of fairness and just decisions regarding clinical evaluations are responsibly acting for the public they serve (Smith-Glasgow & Dreher, 2007). When misconduct failures or dismissals are enacted, several steps must be taken by the clinical faculty to ensure the student's right to due process is maintained (Johnson, 2009). The steps are as follows:

1. The college or university must have clear policies regarding the student conduct and appeals processes.
2. The student is entitled to written notice of any charges against them.
3. The student is provided sufficient opportunity to rebut the charges.
4. The student has a right to select an adviser (if stipulated in the program or college policy).
5. The student has a right to confront their accusers.
6. The student has a right to present evidence to an impartial body.
7. The student has a right to have an adequate and accurate record of the proceedings.

This is the full panoply of procedures that *could* apply to a deprivation. Whether all of the procedures *should* apply is a matter of discretion for each university to decide on its own. The key point is that there should be something in writing to describe the fair process that a student can follow when they contest the fairness of a decision and that the process is fair given the importance of the decision to that student.

DISCUSSION OF CASE STUDY

In Case Study 9.1, the consequences to the student are severe, a clinical failure, and the process of reviewing the imposition of the penalty needs to be scrupulously fair. This requires a thorough investigation of the facts. In this situation, Dr. Mahoney, the Course Coordinator, would need to meet with Professor Connelly, the clinical faculty member, to get the full story. The key facts are what actually happened during clinical, post-conference, and the medication calculation exam, what parts of it Professor Connelly personally observed, and who were independent witnesses to it. Dr. Mahoney would also need to review the clinical evaluation form and related clinical documentation to see if it was both accurate and adequate. If Professor Connelly was present for the incidents in question, then Dr. Mahoney would ask her to explain the behaviors that she witnessed in detail and to summarize all of her verbal and written communications with the student since that time. Dr. Mahoney would also note if Mr. Johnson had any other incidents of clinical or academic misconduct. She would carefully review the nursing program student handbook, clinical course failure policy, syllabus, and clinical evaluation form for clarity and the student appeal policy. Dr. Mahoney would also meet with Mr. Johnson again to ask follow-up questions and remind him of his ability to consult the office of equality if he felt that he was the victim of improper discrimination because of his gender, as well as the appeal process if warranted.

WHEN TO CONSULT THE UNIVERSITY COUNSEL

Consult the university attorney when you are confronted with a new and difficult situation, or if you want to review high-stakes policies such as clinical misconduct, clinical failure, or clinical dismissal policies.

FINDINGS AND DISPOSITION

After conducting an investigation, it was found that Professor Connelly was present when Mr. Johnson had his alleged "anger management incidents" and was ill-prepared for medication administration. Professor Connelly wrote a detailed account of her observations on the Professional Violation Form and shared it with Mr. Johnson after each incident. Mr. Johnson responded to Professor Connelly's written feedback with a long narrative response disputing her findings essentially taking no accountability for his actions. Professor Connelly had documented what she observed on the clinical evaluation form and clinical warning form. Furthermore, Professor Connelly met with Mr. Johnson to hear his account of the incidents.

There were anecdotal records delineating acts of clinical unpreparedness and misconduct. Furthermore, Dr. Mahoney reviewed the nursing program student handbook, syllabus, and clinical evaluation tool in reference to the incident. Dr. Mahoney inquired if Mr. Johnson had any other conduct issues from his other faculty and learned that Mr. Johnson refused to follow the Testing Protocol during another exam and was uncivil to the faculty member.

After considering the facts and consulting with the department chair, Dr. Mahoney affirmed Professor Connelly's decision to fail Mr. Johnson and deny his appeal on the basis that he had been afforded due process. She determined that Mr. Johnson's behavior did warrant a clinical warning and failure, as well as a counseling session related to professional conduct. Dr. Mahoney met with Professor Connelly and explained how her actions were reasonable and the student's due process rights were afforded. Although Dr. Mahoney was aware of some aspects of Mr. Johnson's clinical performance and conduct issues, she fully investigated the situation. Dr. Mahoney acknowledged that Professor Connelly was a seasoned clinical faculty member but nevertheless she was counseled to consult the course coordinator before issuing a clinical failure to any student on clinical performance or conduct grounds in the future. Dr. Mahoney also agreed that Mr. Johnson should be permitted to retake the course rather than be dismissed from the program because the infractions occurred in the introductory clinical course but that the student receive counseling with respect to professional behavior expectations in a clinical program. Mr. Johnson will also receive a formal letter that will refer him to the professional behavioral expectations in the student handbook and the consequences should he fail to adhere to them.

Prevention Tips

- *Offer faculty development sessions on clinical evaluation and due process.*
- *Remember the importance of first finding out all the facts.*
- *Follow written policies and guidelines outlined in the student handbook.*
- *Have evidence that students have read clinical expectations—such as a signed statement indicating that they have read the handbook.*
- *When an incident occurs, document deviations from policy and have faculty and students develop a plan with specific follow-up date and consequences of failure to satisfactorily complete the plan.*
- *Have students read the documentation, have a chance to put their version in writing, and sign the form indicating they are aware of the documentation—they do not have to agree with the documentation; however, there does need to be evidence that they have read it.*

RELEVANT LEGAL CASES

Board of Curators of the University of Missouri v. Horowitz, 435 U.S. 78 (1978).

Regents of the University of Michigan v. Ewing, 474 U.S. 214 (1985).

Landmark cases have set precedents for misconduct dismissals and adherence to due process. In 1978, the U.S. Supreme Court found for the University of Missouri, sustaining dismissal of a medical student for clinical deficiencies (*Board of Curators of the University of Missouri v. Horowitz*, 1978). In this particular precedent case, a medical student was dismissed for deficiencies in clinical performance. The Court determined that clinical evaluation of inadequacies was sound because the university adhered to standards of due process. The Court applied the principle of judicial deference in this case, respecting the authority of the university's decision regarding the deficiency misconduct. This landmark case situated universities in authoritative posture, imposing that no court should intrude into academic decisions regarding student performance (Parrot, 1993). The Court did not overturn the clinical evaluation, given that the university granted the student cumulative information of academic deficiencies and consequences of same (*Missouri v. Horowitz*, 1978).

> In cases of academic dismissal from a state educational institution, when the student has been fully informed of the faculty's dissatisfaction with the student's academic progress and when the decision to dismiss was careful and deliberate, the Fourteenth Amendment's procedural due process requirement has been met. (*Missouri v. Horowitz*, 1978)

Substantive due process was supported in Ewing's case, when the evaluation process of the student to meet clinical performance was upheld and deferred to the faculty member's judgment (*Regents of the University of Michigan v. Ewing*, 1985). In this case, the student filed suit to stay a dismissal on the grounds that the university did not grant him due process privileges. The Court found that the university did not depart from accepted academic norms (Smith et al., 2001). The above two cases were decisive contributors to the *Morin v. Cleveland Metro General Hospital*, 516 N.E.2d 257 (Ohio, 1986). Morin's case challenged dismissal of the nursing student for misconduct and unsafe clinical practices. The student's case was filed complaining the dismissal was arbitrary and capricious; however, the court of appeals upheld the student's dismissal, citing precedence of case law set by *Missouri v. Horowitz*, 1978 and *Michigan v. Ewing*, 1985. In *Rogers v. Tennessee Board of Regents, 273 F. App'x 458* (6th Cir. 2008), a nursing student dismissed from the program alleged both substantive and due process violations. The court determined that the plaintiff's interest in nursing education was not protected by substantive due process—that is nursing education is not a fundamental right.

SUMMARY

When a student receives feedback and evaluation of clinical misconduct, clinical faculty members will be held to a standard of fairness when investigations are made concerning whether a fair process was followed. In Case Study 9.1, the clinical faculty member was reasonable and did not rush to quick and unfair judgment of clinical misconduct. The faculty member actually provided the student with an opportunity to be heard and improve his clinical performance. In the appeals process, the course coordinator followed a thoughtful process that resulted in evidence that supported the clinical failure. The extensive documentation in the student's record provided evidence to impose remedial action fairly, and confirmed that there was evidence that formative evaluations had taken place. As a result, the record demonstrated that due process had been provided to the student. Dr. Mahoney did decide to require the student to undergo additional training in appropriate behavior. You may have noticed that the record did include another incident of "improper anger management" in another course during an exam. Dr. Mahoney's decision was reasonable, and the decision to affirm the clinical failure was appropriate. For that reason, it is extremely unlikely that any judge or jury would interfere—rather, the law would support the business judgment that Dr. Mahoney had made, because she followed a process that was due. Courts do not typically intervene if the program and faculty have not acted in an arbitrary and capricious manner—faculty have followed all published policies and procedures and all students are held accountable to the same academic standards (Smith, 2012).

Imagine what would have happened in this case if Professor Mahoney had not afforded the student due process. The student failed the course, was dismissed, and filed a lawsuit. A judge or jury would viewed Professor Connelly's actions as careless and the university actions as arbitrary if the university had allowed Mr. Johnson to fail without appropriate due process. It is not difficult to predict the outrage that the court would have expressed—and that means the verdict and award of money damages against Professor Connelly and the university, compensating the student for the university's defective and unfair conduct, could well have been high.

Due process, in short, protects not just the student. It protects the faculty member and the university as well.

ETHICAL CONSIDERATIONS

Poor academic and clinical performance should and must be addressed by academic nursing programs. Nursing faculty have an ethical obligation to ensure safe patient care and have the right to set and maintain academic standards. Nursing faculty are integral to educating nurses who are deemed safe to enter practice (Walker, 2016). As "gatekeepers" to the profession, clinical faculty have a duty to ensure that only students with the appropriate knowledge, skills, and ethics care for patients and be allowed to graduate from a nursing program, and be admitted to the profession, thereby protecting society from unsafe clinicians (Hunt, McGee, Gutteridge, & Hughes, 2012). Regardless of the setting, the nurse's primary commitment is to the patient (American Nurses Association, 2015).

CRITICAL ELEMENTS TO CONSIDER

- As a faculty member, you must provide the student with an opportunity to be heard before rushing to summary judgment.
- Consult academic policies related to clinical failure prior to informing the student verbally or in writing.
- If you are a novice faculty member, consult an experienced faculty member to review your documentation.

- If you are an experienced faculty member or academic administrator, educate new faculty about students' due process rights.
- Provide the student advance notice of a clinical failure.
- Maintain daily evidence-based anecdotal documentation.
- Document student behavior in an objective manner including date, time, location, witnesses, and action taken.
- Remember: Most cases related to clinical misconduct or performance issues have been upheld by the courts as long as due process has been afforded to the student and the nursing program followed its own policies.

Helpful Resource

- The American Nurses Association's Code of Ethics can be found at www.nursingworld.org. Click on the **Nursing Ethics** header, and then **Code of Ethics for Nurses**.

References

Ahn, Y. H., & Choi, J. (2018). Incivility experiences in clinical practicum education among nursing students. *Nurse Education Today, 73*, 48–53. doi:10.1016/j.nedt.2018.11.015

American Nurses Association. (2015). *Code of ethics for nurses with interpretive statements.* Silver Spring, MD: Author.

Anselmi, K. K., Glasgow, M. E. S., & Gambescia, S. F. (2014). Using a nursing student conduct committee to foster professionalism among nursing students. *Journal of Professional Nursing, 30*(6), 481–485. doi:10.1016/j.profnurs.2014.04.002

Board of Curators of the University of Missouri v. Horowitz, 435 U. S. 78 (1978).

Chunta, K. (2016). Ensuring safety in clinical: Faculty role for managing students with unsafe behaviors. *Teaching and Learning, 11*, 86–91. doi:10.1016/j.teln.2016.03.001

Gaberson, K., & Oermann, M. (2010). *Clinical teaching strategies in nursing* (3rd ed.). New York, NY: Springer Publishing Company.

Gallant, M., McDonald, J., & Higuchi, K. S. (2006). A remediation process for nursing students at risk. *Nurse Educator, 31*(5), 223–227. doi:10.1097/00006223-200609000-00010

Gardner, M., & Suplee, P. (2010). *Handbook of clinical teaching in nursing and health sciences.* Sudbury, MA: Jones and Bartlett Learning.

Hunt, L. A., McGee, P., Gutteridge, R., & Hughes, M. (2012). Assessment of student nurses in practice: A comparison of theoretical and practical assessment results in England. *Nurse Education Today, 32*(4), 351–355. doi:10.1016/j.nedt.2011.05.010

Johnson, E. G. (2009). The academic performance of students: Legal and ethical issues. In D. M. Billings & J. A. Halstead (Eds.), *Teaching in nursing. A guide for faculty* (pp. 33–52). St. Louis, MO: Saunders.

Kaplin, W. A., & Lee, B. A. (2013). *The law of higher education* (5th ed.). San Francisco, CA: Jossey-Bass.

Kolanko, K., Clark, C., Heinrich, K., Olive, D., Serembus, J. F., & Sifford, K. S. (2006). Academic dishonesty, bullying, incivility, and violence: Difficult challenges facing nurse educators. *Nursing Education Perspectives, 27*(1), 34–43. Retrieved from https://pubmed.ncbi.nlm.nih.gov/16613130/

Lindsay, C. L., III. (2012). *The college student's guide to the law.* Dallas, TX: Taylor Trade Publishing.

Morin v. Cleveland Metro General Hospital, 516 N.E.2d 257

Parrott, T. E. (1993). Dismissal for clinical deficiencies. *Nurse Educator, 26*(1), 33–38. doi:10.1097/00006223-199311000-00013

Regents of the University of Michigan v. Ewing, 474 U. S. 214 (1985).

Rogers v. Tennessee Board of Regents, 273 F. App'x 458 (6th Cir. 2008).

Roth, J. (Ed.). (2007). *Higher education law in America* (8th ed.). Malvern, PA: Center for Education and Employment Law.

Smith, M. (2012). *The legal, professional, and ethical dimensions of higher education in nursing* (2nd ed.). New York, NY: Springer Publishing Company.

Smith, M. H., McKoy, E., & Richardson, J. (2001). Legal issues related to dismissing students for clinical deficiencies. *Nurse Educator, 26*(1), 33–38. doi:10.1097/00006223-200101000-00015

Smith-Glasgow, M. E., & Dreher, H. M. (2007). Legal issues in student supervision. *Advance for Nursing, 9*(18), 37–41. Retrieved from https://www.researchgate.net/publication/256843327_Student_supervision_Legal _issues_can_include_discrimination_and_grade_appeals

Suplee, P., Lachman, V., Seibert, B., & Anselmi, K. K. (2008). Managing nursing incivility in the classroom, clinical setting, and on-line. *Journal of Nursing Law, 12*(2), 68–77. doi:10.1891/1073-7472.12.2.68

Walker, S. Y. (2016). Due process in nursing education. *Teaching and Learning, 11*, 126–127. doi:10.1016/j. teln.2016.03.005

Whitney, K. M. (2009). Managing the learning environment: Proactively responding to student misconduct. In D. M. Billings & J. A. Halstead (Eds.), *Teaching in nursing. A guide for faculty* (pp. 227–237). St. Louis, MO: Saunders.

10

A Critical Explanation of What "Academic Freedom" Really *Is* and What It *Is Not!*

Case Study 10.1

An Undergraduate Nursing Faculty Member Claims It Is a Violation of Her Academic Freedom to Be Forced to Use a Certain Textbook for Class

Your role: You are Dr. Onish and you are the course chair for NURS 101: Holistic Care of Self and Others, taught during the sophomore year in a BSN program at State University.

As the fall semester is about to begin, you are informed that that there will be four sections of NURS 101 taught with 25 students in each section. A new faculty member has been hired, Dr. Roy, and so as course chair you send an email in early July informing the four faculty teaching this course (including Dr. Roy) that you have gone ahead and ordered the textbook for the course. You also tell them that in the next few weeks you will be scheduling a course meeting so the group can plan for the logistics of the course in the fall. You subsequently receive an email from Dr. Roy informing you that she has selected an alternative text for her section. You politely email her that the standard policy of the undergraduate nursing program is that all nursing sections have the same textbook and that more than one text confuses students and has implications for testing. Dr. Roy replies that it is her academic freedom to choose her own text and that as long as she meets the objectives of the course, there really should not be a problem with her using a separate text.

Questions
- How would you first proceed?
- Is Dr. Roy correct that a faculty member's right to an individual course textbook selection falls within the domain of academic freedom?
- What do you think is the rationale for the policy of using the same text for all sections of one course?
- Can this issue be resolved to avoid discord among the teaching faculty for this course?
- If this were a collective bargaining environment, would academic freedom have any different guidelines?

UNIVERSITY FACULTY AND THEIR ACADEMIC FREEDOM: LEGAL PRINCIPLES AND REVIEW OF THE LITERATURE

As Kaplan and Lee (2013) write in *The Law of Higher Education* (perhaps the leading text on the law in higher education):

> Academic freedom traditionally has been considered to be an essential aspect of American higher education. It has been a major determinant of the missions of higher educational institutions, both public and private, and a major factor in shaping the roles of faculty members as well as students. (pp. 247–248)

However, they also further elaborate: "Yet the concept of academic freedom eludes precise definition…. It draws meaning from both the world of education and the world of law" (p. 248). Questions of academic freedom, often interpreted as issues of free speech, are therefore common in academia. Typically, the most public issues surround an individual faculty member's right to free speech,[1] but there are still occasions when student free speech or academic freedom is debated. For example, whom does the First Amendment (free speech amendment) protect? Does it protect those in both public and private institutions equally? Remember what Kaplan and Lee write: "It has been a major determinant of the missions of higher educational institutions, both public and private…" (pp. 247–248). Under a strict interpretation of the First Amendment:

> The freedom of expression and speech guaranteed by the First Amendment **does not fully protect academic freedom**. Under the state action doctrine, the First Amendment applies only to government actors. Therefore, while the First Amendment applies to all public universities, it does not apply to private or religious institutions. (Vile & Hudson, 2017)

Sometimes religious institutions avoid these issues surrounding academic freedom by having faculty/staff adhere and sometimes sign a Testament/Statement of Faith in order to be employed. Two examples of institutions that use this procedure are Wheaton College in Wheaton, Illinois[2] and Eastern University, an evangelical Christian university in St. Davids, Pennsylvania.[3]

The issue of Academic Freedom constitutionally falls under the First Amendment and is aimed at protecting verbal, written, and symbolic communication. In the U.S. Constitution, the First Amendment reads:

> Congress shall make no law respecting an establishment of religion, or prohibiting the free exercise thereof; or abridging the freedom of speech, or of the press; or the right of the people to peaceably assemble, and to petition the Government for a redress of grievances.

Regarding whom the First Amendment protects, it is important to note that the legal system treats high school students under age 18 and college students age 18 and over very differently, with high schools having greater authority to regulate the speech of their students than universities.

The tenets of academic freedom have been mostly associated with university faculty, but we must acknowledge these issues are pertinent for college-age students as well. However, this chapter examines the often confusing issues surrounding what actually constitutes faculty "academic freedom."

The American Association of University Professors' (AAUP) classic "1940 (Revised in 1970 & 1990)[4] Statement of Principles on Academic Freedom and Tenure with 1970 Interpretive Comments" states the following:

1. Teachers are entitled to full freedom in research and in the publication of the results, subject to the adequate performance of their other academic duties; but research for pecuniary[5] return should be based upon an understanding with the authorities of the institution.

---

[1] In a technical sense, universities have a right to determine who may teach, what may be taught, and who may be admitted to study, and so it is the university that has academic freedom more than an individual professor, and this was affirmed in 2008 in *Stronach v. Virginia State University* (Roth, McEllistrem, D'Ogostino, & Brown, 2009).

[2] "At Wheaton, our first and foremost priority is to ensure our faculty and staff are strongly grounded in their faith. All employees of Wheaton College are expected to affirm our Community Covenant and Statement of Faith" (2019, p. 1). Retrieved from https://www.wheaton.edu/about-wheaton/offices-and-services/human-resources/for-job-seekers/

[3] "Faculty must be willing to endorse by signing the Eastern University's doctrinal statement." Retrieved from https://www.eastern.edu/about/offices-centers/human-resources/employment-opportunities

[4] The 2007 and 2009 revision, published in 2010, does not supercede the 1940 version but does offer new cases that were thoroughly investigated by AAUP and has new published findings.

2. Teachers are entitled to freedom in the classroom in discussing their subject, but they should be careful not to introduce into their teaching controversial matter which has no relation to their subject. Limitations of academic freedom because of religious or other aims of the institution should be clearly stated in writing at the time of the appointment.

3. College and university teachers are citizens, members of a learned profession, and officers of an educational institution. When they speak or write as citizens, they should be free from institutional censorship or discipline, but their special position in the community imposes special obligations. As scholars and educational officers, they should remember that the public may judge their profession and their institution by their utterances. Hence, they should at all times be accurate, should exercise appropriate restraint, should show respect for the opinions of others, and should make every effort to indicate that they are not speaking for the institution. (AAUP, 2006, pp. 3–4)

Underlying these three principles is the central thesis that teachers (in this case they are speaking about university or college professors, regardless of their rank) are entitled to freedom in the classroom in discussing their subject. This principle does not indicate that controversial statements cannot be made in the classroom, but that they should have some direct context to the course and the relevant course readings.

As the First Amendment is interpreted, *speech* is not just the spoken word (including the right *not* to speak), but the written word and symbolic acts (Lindsay, 2005). Although subject to interpretation through numerous legal decisions and commentary, the actual text of the First Amendment is quite short:

> Congress shall make no law respecting an establishment of religion, or prohibiting the free exercise thereof; or abridging the freedom of speech, or of the press; or the right of the people peaceably to assemble, and to petition the Government for a redress of grievances.

The First Amendment was one of 10 amendments adopted in 1791 that make up what is commonly referred to as the "Bill of Rights." These were not included in the original Constitution proposed for ratification. Rather, the Bill of Rights originated from the debates that occurred in individual states over whether to adopt the proposed Constitution. Opponents argued the new Constitution gave the federal government too much power at the expense of the states and did not adequately protect people's individual rights. The debate over whether to ratify the Constitution in several states hinged on the adoption of a Bill of Rights (History, 2009) that would safeguard basic civil rights under the law. Advocates for adoption of the new Constitution promised the Bill of Rights in order to secure votes in favor of passage.

What you will need to determine in Case Study 10.1 is whether freedom of speech can somehow be determined to also extend to an individual faculty member's right to select a respective textbook for their course.

As made clear elsewhere in this book, even the First Amendment is not absolute. There are kinds of speech that are not protected, and reasonable regulations can be imposed in certain circumstances. Speech that can be "banned" includes that which is intended to incite lawless actions or panic or threat of public safety—for example, one cannot stand in an auditorium and jokingly yell "Fire!" (*Gitlow v. People*, 1925),[6] obscenity (*Roth v. United States*, 1957),[7] or speech that is judged to be defamatory or libelous (*New York Times v. Sullivan*, 1964).[8] Finally, the term *commercial speech*, which first entered the judicial vernacular in 1971, is different from *public speech* and can be regulated to ensure it is not false (Cásarez, 1998).

---

[5] Pertaining to money.

[6] In *Gitlow v. People* (1925), it was determined one could not falsely yell "Fire!" if there was no fire and if such speech would cause panic and potential injury to others.

[7] In *Roth v. U.S.* (1957), the first real legal standard for judging obscenity, it was determined whether, to the average person, applying contemporary community standards, the dominant theme of the material, taken as a whole, appeals to prurient interest. However, as seen in the courts since this ruling, communities are not monolithic and what perhaps is obscene in one community may not be in another.

[8] In *New York Times v. Sullivan* (1964), a constitutional prohibition was announced in which for the first time it was codified that a public official could not recover damages for a defamatory falsehood relating to their official conduct unless the public official could prove that the statement was made with "actual malice"—that is, with knowledge that it was false or with reckless disregard of whether it was false or not. Defamation or libel, although both serious, remain difficult ultimately to prove.

One case that received both national and international attention concerned the University of Colorado Department Chair and Ethnic Studies Professor Ward Churchill. Mr. Churchill was a tenured professor but without a doctorate—facts that would become important in his later dismissal case. He wrote an essay on September 12, 2001, very critical of the United States in light of the attacks on New York City on September 11, 2001. Although the essay at the time did not draw much attention, his expanded comments were included in his 2003 book, *On the Justice of Roosting Chickens: Reflections on the Consequences of U.S. Imperial Arrogance and Criminality.* In 2004, Churchill was supposed to give a speech at Hamilton College in upstate New York, but after a political science professor saw his name on a roster of future speakers, a maelstrom arose, particularly after the student newspaper reprinted Churchill's 2001 essay (Schreker, 2010). His speech was eventually canceled by university officials, and thereafter the controversy surrounding Churchill's printed comments led to the cancellation of most of his other university speaking tour events, often for expressed reasons of "safety and security of our students, faculty, staff, and the community in which we live" and for "credible threats of violence" (Schreker, 2010, p. 3). Lost in the debate was Churchill's overriding thesis that the promise of equality as prescribed in the Declaration of Independence had largely gone unfilled (Briley, 2005).

A great debate took place in the United States and abroad about whether Mr. Churchill had a right to free speech (academic freedom) or not. Ultimately, the University of Colorado (a state-funded institution) came under enormous pressure from politicians and constituents in that state, and a committee was empaneled to investigate the quality of his scholarship and research, arguably in response to the allegations of a few about plagiarism and research misconduct. In May 2007, the President of his university set in motion the procedures to dismiss or fire Mr. Churchill, on the grounds of plagiarism and research misconduct; but Mr. Churchill claimed that was subterfuge for the attack on his right to free speech and institutional guarantee of academic freedom (Jaschik, 2007). After reviews by two separate committees—a Committee on Scientific Misconduct and a second committee required to address his tenure—the University's Board of Trustees voted 8-1 to terminate his employment. Mr. Churchill immediately filed suit in state court, and after almost 2 years, a jury rendered a verdict in his favor of $1 (yes, $1) on April 2009 for violation of his First Amendment right to free speech. This verdict was set aside a year later by the Court of Appeals on the grounds of immunity. Later, on November 29, 2010, the Colorado Appeals Court ruled that the University of Colorado Board of Regents was largely immune from being sued by Mr. Churchill either for (a) its handling of his case, and (b) for any First Amendment violations; and the court specifically stated that it did not see its ruling limiting the rights of other faculty members.

On September 12, 2012, the Colorado Supreme Court upheld the Court of Appeals' decision in this case. It upheld the decisions of the appeals and trial court which both held that Professor Churchill was not entitled to any of the remedies that he sought. Churchill brought a claim under 42 U.S.C. § 1983 claiming that the University of Colorado at Boulder opened an investigation into his academic integrity in retaliation for the publication of a controversial essay, and that both the investigation and resulting termination of his employment violated his free speech rights. The proceedings against Churchill took more than 2 years and included five separate opportunities for Churchill to present witnesses, cross-examine adverse witnesses, and argue his positions. The Colorado Supreme Court found that it possessed the characteristics of an adversary proceeding and was functionally comparable to a judicial proceeding. The Court held that the Regents' termination proceeding was a quasi-judicial proceeding, and the Regents were entitled to absolute immunity. The Court also affirmed the trial court's ruling denying Churchill request to be reinstated and to receive front pay. The trial court accepted as fact that the two University's investigation found that Churchill had plagiarized his academic writings, fabricated evidence, and violated the University's academic standards. The trial court ruled that reinstating Churchill would not be appropriate because the relationship between Churchill and the University has been irreparably damaged. Reinstating Churchill, the trial court ruled, would harm the University's ability to enforce its standards of academic integrity and could impair the University's ability to attract good students and faculty. The Colorado Supreme Court affirmed the trial court's rulings and findings holding that they did not constitute an abuse of discretion by the trial court.

More than 5 years after the University of Colorado Board of Regents fired him, the U.S. Supreme Court declined to hear his appeal in 2013 (Jaschik, 2013, p. 111).

What is often lost in the discussion surrounding academic freedom is that the courts almost always rule that "the right to academic freedom belongs to universities and not to individual professors." It is this principle that is most likely to affect the discussion between Dr. Drayton and Dr. Joy. A few recent cases illustrate the point.

In *Stronach v. Virginia State University Dist. Court*, ED Virginia, 2008, mentioned briefly in Chapter 9, Due Process Issues for the Student, a physics professor's grade of D assigned to a student was overturned by the Department Chair when the Chair sided with the student, who claimed the professor had in error given him higher grades on two quizzes (the student sent in faxed copies of his quizzes). The professor claimed the student had doctored the grades on the quizzes. He sued in federal district court, claiming violation of his academic freedom because administrators had retaliated against him for testifying for another professor who had sued the university. Virginia State University officials asserted that they had a right to change the grade without the professor's input or consent and the court agreed, dismissing this claim. It did so, saying "Significantly, the Court has never recognized that professors possess a First Amendment right of academic freedom to determine for themselves the content of their courses and scholarship, despite opportunities to do so." An *untenured* professor's right to assign grades was rejected in *Lovelace v. Southeastern Massachusetts University* (1986) and similarly, the claim of a *public* university professor that the First Amendment right to expression gave him personally the right to assign grades was rejected in *Brown v. Amenti* (2001). While not precisely on point, the courts' logic in these cases is almost certainly fatal to a professor's claim to have the "First Amendment Right" to select the textbooks for their class or section thereof.

Discussion of Case Study

Let's consider our first question: How would you first proceed? Remember, your new faculty member is resisting using the same textbook as the rest of the team. Dr. Onish was very displeased that this issue had surfaced. Many years ago, faculty were individually choosing their own texts, pledging that they would all adhere to covering the same course objectives. However, Dr. Onish recalled there was dissension among students who on course evaluations panned one text and praised another. Dr. Onish also recalled those course team meetings were always disjointed because different texts presented information in different ways, so that developing a coherent outline of content was always a cumbersome process. Aside from the different textbooks (and complaints about their variable cost), Dr. Onish also had to deal with complaints about how *Professor X* gave three tests whereas *Professor Z* gave only two.

Despite the practical difficulties, Dr. Onish and other faculty members had always subscribed to the belief that these faculty choices and decisions about teaching and conducting their respective courses were all sound issues of pedagogy, important for the faculty members individually to decide, and therefore a matter of academic freedom. In short, Dr. Onish was sympathetic with Dr. Roy on a personal level, if not an administrative one.

Is Dr. Roy correct that a faculty member's right to an individual course textbook selection falls within the domain of academic freedom? Arising out of this long-standing discord, a faculty decision had been made years ago that to increase the quality of the nursing program and increase NCLEX scores, the faculty must work more closely together and move toward consensus on the standardization of the curriculum.

Actually, discussions concerning the standardization of nursing curriculum have been ongoing for years. In 1981, Nichols called for more standardization but it was in the context of requiring a baccalaureate degree for entry level into professional nursing. Koithan (1994) later documented nursing's obsession with standardizing both baccalaureate and associate degree education that resulted in an overemphasis on training rather than educating nurses. More recently, Clavreul (2008) has written: "A nationwide, standardized nursing curriculum at both the associate and bachelor levels would allow nursing students to move effortlessly between schools, and in turn, allow nursing schools to fill vacant seats where appropriate. Far too often, a student drops out and that seat remains vacant" (para. 12).

Clavreul's (2008) concerns are geared toward better upward mobilization of nurses from lower educational ranks to higher ones, particularly when Aiken, Cheung, and Olds (2009) have documented that only 6% of nurses having an associate degree go on to achieve a master's or doctoral degree, whereas 20% of nurses prepared at the BSN level do. Further, more upward mobility of nurses (which would likely be enhanced by more national standardization of curricula) is necessary to realize the goal for nursing recently announced by the Institute of Medicine (2010) in *The Future of Nursing: Leading Change, Advancing Health*. The report calls for an increase in the number of nurses prepared at the baccalaureate level from 50% to 80% by 2020 and for doubling the number of nurses having a doctorate by 2020. Much of the necessary standardization of nursing that will be needed to achieve these goals can be still be done in the context of innovation and by close alliance to the strategies also recently outlined in *Educating Nurses: A Call for Radical Transformation* (Benner, Sutphen, Leonard, & Day, 2010). In 2013, the Robert Wood Johnson Foundation and American Association for Retired Persons (AARP) partnered to establish The Future of Nursing: Campaign for Action, and published some of the actions taken since the publication of the report. A few of these indicated that there has already been progress toward 80% of RNs achieving the BSN by 2020 and several colleges and universities have recently announced new programs to facilitate academic progression (Robert Wood Johnson Foundation & AARP, 2013).

Dr. Onish was fortunate that, years before Dr. Roy joined the faculty, a policy was developed and approved by full nursing faculty vote. The policy called for individual course chairs to oversee the text selection for each respective required baccalaureate nursing course in consultation with the other faculty team members who were teaching the course. In other words, this policy did not give the course chair unilateral power, but enabled the course chair to lead the textbook review process, moving the group faculty team to consensus, and end by taking a vote on which text or texts to select. It was also determined that for required courses in which there was more than one faculty member teaching the course, each semester one syllabus template would be agreed upon.

The third question in Case Study 10.1 is: What do you think is the rationale for the policy of using the same text for all sections of one course? Subsequent implementation of this policy immediately changed the dynamics of the students in various course sections, and having one group of students prefer one professor's syllabus requirements (or different text) over another ceased almost immediately. A common syllabus and common text also gave faculty more flexibility and allowed for seamless opportunities for faculty to take over a class when one faculty member was traveling to a conference to present a paper or was to be absent for a short period.

Last, although previous NCLEX scores had traditionally been excellent, the baccalaureate nursing program administrators worried that the faculty would become complacent and "sit on their laurels" and that this might result in a decline in the scores. This policy was therefore created to ensure more standardization and stability in the program, necessary components if there was to be more psychometric microanalyses of individual course outcomes rather than just on exit HESI scores or NCLEX performance.

Findings and Disposition

Dr. Onish, being an experienced course chair and longtime nursing faculty member, wanted to solve the problem expeditiously while maintaining the cohesiveness of her course team. This leads to the fourth question: Can this issue be resolved to avoid creating discord among team teaching faculty in this course? Instead of choosing to email Dr. Roy again and inform her of the standing policy on textbook selection, Dr. Onish thought a more personal approach would be best. Lots of literature (Cheese, 2015; Martin, 2007) discusses how even in a climate in which email is predominant, often face-to-face communication is essential and may be more effective. And while certainly not appropriate in this case, there are even times in today's modern society where social media may be more appropriate than face-to-face communication (Kokemuller, 2019).

Dr. Onish therefore called Dr. Roy and left a message on her voicemail that that they should instead meet so she could go over some of the background of the reason that textbook selection is handled as a group faculty decision and not an individual one. Dr. Roy agreed to a meeting. After an explanation by Dr. Onish and a review of the policy, Dr. Roy stated that she honestly did not agree with the policy. And while in her previous position this was certainly not the practice, she would willingly comply. She was also glad to hear that the policy did not apply to elective nursing courses. She did ask whether the policy applied to master's and doctoral courses, and Dr. Onish informed her that although there was no set policy for graduate courses, most of the faculty did work together to use common texts, especially for core cognate courses and for specialty courses in which one textbook might be used for a series of courses. But she could not assure Dr. Roy that if by some chance she was to teach one of two sections of an advanced practice course, a standard text, used over several semesters, would be selected. Dr. Onish was glad she handled this issue with a personal touch, and she was proud of her own leadership abilities in handling the matter without involving the department chair. Moreover, Dr. Roy seemed amenable to the new institutional policies she would now be expected to follow.

But would these academic freedom issues be different in a collective bargaining faculty environment, where academic freedom policies may be contractual in a union environment? This author has worked in both environments and the first comment is that every contract is different in some way so there are no template faculty-collective bargaining templated contracts. To further examine this issue, two contemporary Collective Bargaining Agreements were reviewed and the search word used was "text(s)." In the first case reviewed,[9] in the document the word was only used twice and it was in reference to the teaching course defined as "Laboratory Courses" and the agreement did include the following: "The laboratory course requires the instructor to see that it is related to and correlated with lectures on professional/technical skills, and supplemented with [appropriate assigned texts][10] (such as textbooks and program manuals)" (p. 59). In the second Collective Bargaining Agreement reviewed,[11] there is actually an entire section devoted to Textbook Selection (Article 20). Three sentences stand out: (a) "The selection of textbooks and supplementary materials to be used are the prerogative and responsibility of the full-time faculty member and shall be determined according to departmental guidelines" (p. 33); (b) "Textbooks to be used for a non-sequential, college credit course shall be selected by each faculty member from a list of textbooks agreed upon by the faculty"; and (c)

> A committee, with equal representation from the Union and the Administration, shall be jointly established to annually develop non-binding recommendations addressing textbook affordability. The initial meeting of this committee shall be no later than September 30, 2016 with initial recommendations delivered to the Provost and the President of the Faculty Senate by the end of each academic year. (p. 33)

The entire policy is quite interesting and can be reviewed on p. 33 of Article 20.[11]

WHEN TO CONSULT THE UNIVERSITY COUNSEL

If you believe your academic freedom has been or is being violated, document thoroughly first, and then go through all the appropriate channels, especially the chain of command. Again, many faculty members are very confused about what academic freedom actually entails. It should be possible to contact the university attorney for a simple query, but even university attorneys are likely going to operate from a context of what is in the best interest of the university, since that is their first client, not the individual member.

---

[9] Collective Bargaining Agreement Between the Board of Trustees of the Miracosta Community College District and the Miracosta College Academic Associate Faculty CCA/CTA/NEA for the period July 1, 2015 to June 30, 2017. Retrieved from http://www.miracosta.edu/hr/downloads/2014-17contractFINAL_002.pdf

[10] My emphasis.

[11] Collective Bargaining Agreement between District Board of Trustees of Florida State College at Jacksonville and United Faculty—Florida State College at Jacksonville, Effective August 16, 2016. Retrieved from https://www.fscj.edu/docs/default-source/hr/faculty-instructor-resources/collective-bargaining-agreement.pdf?sfvrsn=be37b5d5_0

RELEVANT LEGAL CASE

Sheldon v. Dhillon, No. C-08-03438 RMW (N.D. Cal. 2009)

June Sheldon was a master's-prepared biology and microbiology instructor at San Jose/Evergreen Community College. Having taught at San Jose/Evergreen Community College since 2004, Sheldon received a student complaint in August 2007 about a class discussion 2 months earlier regarding the Mendelian basis of homosexuality. After an internal investigation in December 2007, the vice chancellor notified Sheldon in December 2007 that her contract for the spring term 2008 was rescinded, she was to be removed from the senior adjunct faculty roster, her employment terminated, and that this was being done with the approval of the District Board of Trustees.

Sheldon contested much of the findings of the internal investigation committee. According to Sheldon, after taking a quiz, the student questioned the theory of the heredity of homosexual behavior. Sheldon answered the student, using the assigned textbook as a guide for her discussion, and indicated there was a stronger biological basis for homosexual behavior in men than in women. She also indicated in class that there was substantial debate over the question of nature versus nurture and did not believe she had engaged in any kind of polemic at all. According to the student, however, she had made "offensive and unscientific" (p. 3) statements including saying that "there aren't any real lesbians" (p. 3) and that "there are hardly any gay men in the Middle East because the women are treated very nicely" (p. 3). Having been made aware of the student's complaint in September 2007, Sheldon agreed to meet with the biology faculty to discuss mainstream scientific thought on the issue and was subsequently offered a spring teaching contract without mention of the incident. With a teaching contract renewed, Sheldon declined teaching opportunities at other institutions.

On December 6, 2007, Sheldon received a letter from the Dean of the math and science division accusing her of teaching misinformation in science and stating that the seriousness of the complaint warranted her dismissal. This was followed by a letter from Human Resources on December 18, 2007. On July 16, 2008, Sheldon filed suit in federal court for retaliation in violation of her First Amendment rights (stating her answer to a student question was protected), for violation of her First Amendment rights of her protected content and viewpoint of her speech, and for Fourteenth Amendment guarantees of equal protection and due process.

In its ruling the court held that free speech as a private citizen is protected but not necessarily the speech of public employees in their work capacity, citing the case of *Ceballos v. Garcett* (2004). "There is some argument that expression related to academic scholarship or classroom instruction implicates additional constitutional interests that are not fully accounted for by this Court's customary employee-speech jurisprudence" (*Ceballos v. Garcett*, 2004, p. 425). The court allowed the professor to pursue her First Amendment claims, and in July 2010 the case was settled, with the community college district agreeing to pay her $100,000 and to remove from her file any reference of her dismissal (AAUP, 2010).

SUMMARY

This chapter has demonstrated that the domain of faculty academic freedom is not nearly as expansive as is sometimes presumed. It is actually *private citizen speech* that is protected by the First Amendment and not necessarily speech conducted by employees, even when the employer is a university or college. Furthermore, it is likely the university, not the faculty member, that is entitled to the freedom from constraints. The courts give great deference to educational institutions to conduct their educational enterprise without great interference from the courts, and that includes deciding what is taught in the classroom.

The AAUP historically has been a great advocate for the rights of academic freedom for faculty, but even that organization did not intervene formally in the Ward Churchill case because in the end he was not dismissed (technically) for his September 11 essay, but instead for faulty scholarship. However, it is not implausible that he was indirectly fired for his speech, and the actions that took place (analogous to a witch hunt, perhaps) occurred in a highly politicized environment. However, several faculty bodies did meet, investigated charges extensively, and all produced lengthy summaries and findings, all of which indicate some degree of due process did take place (Fourteenth Amendment protection).

Finally, in the case of Sheldon, it is perhaps comforting to know that there is some legal precedence by which the content of scholarship of an individual faculty member is protected (even to a nontenured faculty member), particularly if the classroom speech directly pertains to the content of the course directed. Although the court could not determine (indicated this in the ruling) whether the student claim in this case was truthful or the faculty claim was truthful, nonetheless, it seems logical to us that if the community college could have provided confirmation of the professor's classroom speech by other students in the classroom at the time, then the defendant's case would have been much stronger.

If you are taking courses in a history or political science department, it is not uncommon to see political flyers on faculty office doors and bulletin boards. Rarely has an individual faculty member been required to remove the flyers. However, political flyers on nursing faculty offices are likely less common, and there have been directives seen by this author in which nursing faculty have been particularly discouraged to do this. Is this right or wrong? Do you think a nursing faculty member has a right to put something that is not obscene, defamatory, or libelous but that is political on an office door? Having an expert or a lawyer with higher education or particular First Amendment expertise come to a faculty meeting and discuss exactly what faculty and student freedom is might be a very valuable faculty development topic, especially in our high litigation country (U. S. Chamber Institute for Legal Reform, 2013).

ETHICAL CONSIDERATIONS

The *1915 AAUP General Declaration of Principles* identifies three functions through which universities serve the public interest:

A. To promote inquiry and advance the sum of human knowledge.
B. To provide general instruction to the students.
C. To develop experts for various branches of the public service. (AAUP, 2002, p. 182)

Conceiving these functions as ethical imperatives, we can see that academic freedom is a necessary prerequisite for fulfilling these. Mill (1910) argued for the open discussion and inquiry of all ideas to ensure that society has the best and truest ideas. Without open discussion and critique of all ideas, we cannot know which are true or false. Even a false idea may have some degree of truth which could not be known absent open critique. Further, we cannot as autonomous, intelligent, self-aware beings sincerely affirm an idea without exploring it fully. To do so absent such critique would be mere dogmatism. And without continuous critique of even a true idea, the idea will lose its value and efficacy without sustained examination. Open critique and debate is also valuable personally, for lack of freedom to explore and examine ideas degrades one's humanity by forcing one, through default, to submit to the thoughts and judgments of others. Regarding the function of providing instruction to students, academic freedom enhances this function as direct limitations on what is permitted to be presented in the classroom would limit the quality of education of students. Finally, universities are established in the interest of the common good, implying fundamental responsibilities to the community, society, or possibly the government: to increase the body of knowledge in order to improve society and provide experts for dealing with social problems. The assumption is that the production and accretion of knowledge performed at universities is beneficial for society. Academic freedom better guarantees the achievement of this fundamental ethical function.

Yet academic freedom is not completely free. The 1915 statement also acknowledges correlative duties of faculty and universities. Each faculty member is duty bound to restrain their expression and examination of ideas within the bounds of ethics and the standards of competent scholarly inquiry. Collectively, faculty body is also obliged to enforce those standards among members of the faculty. Both these obligations are framed as reciprocal to the assumption of academic freedom. The acceptance and employment of the liberties of academic freedom morally oblige one to engage in research and expression of ideas according to the standards of scholarly research. The rights one has according to academic freedom and the status and the recognition of expertise afforded to academics create expectations that may not hold to those outside the profession.

CRITICAL ELEMENTS TO CONSIDER

■ First, remember at its most rudimentary interpretation, the First Amendment right to free speech mostly pertains to the speech of private citizens speaking on public issues, not employees talking about work issues.

■ Second, the courts have mostly ruled that freedom of speech rests more in the hands of the institution, not of the individual faculty. Your classroom response to questions and classroom commentary is likely protected as long as it is relevant to the course content.

■ Departmental policies almost always need to be followed unless there are extenuating circumstances or if you can prove the policy is improper for some reason.

■ Collegial faculty relationships are important, and it takes good leadership skills to problem-solve effectively. Email has become our default form of efficient communication, but often problem-solving will require personal interaction.

■ Faculty handbooks can become very important legal contracts. Read yours. Know what is in it. Individual or groups of faculty can request that certain procedures become codified as policy. Informing a new faculty member that some practice is policy rather than a generally accepted practice is more organizationally sound.

Helpful Resources

● American Association of University Professors (AAUP): http://www.aaup.org/aaup
● American Association of University Women: http://www.aauw.org/about/
● American Civil Liberties Union (ACLU): http://www.aclu.org/
● First Amendment Law Prof Blog: http://blogs.law.unc.edu/falr/
● *Journal of Academic Freedom* [online]: http://www.academicfreedomjournal.org/

References

Aiken, L., Cheung, R. B., & Olds, D. M. (2009). Education policy initiatives to address the nurse shortage in the United States. *Health Affairs, 28*(4), w646–w656. doi:10.1377/hlthaff.28.4.w646

American Association of University Professors. (1915). *APPENDIX I 1915 Declaration of Principles on Academic Freedom and Academic Tenure.* Retrieved from https://www.aaup.org/NR/rdonlyres/A6520A9D-0A9A-47B3-B550-C006B5B224E7/0/1915Declaration.pdf

American Association of University Professors. (1940). *Statement of Principles on Academic Freedom and Tenure with 1970 Interpretive Comments.* Retrieved from https://www.aaup.org/file/1940%20Statement.pdf

American Association of University Professors. (1970). *1940 Statement of Principles on Academic Freedom and Tenure with 1970 Interpretive Comments.* Retrieved from https://www.aaup.org/file/1940%20Statement.pdf

American Association of University Professors. (2006). 1940 statement of principles on academic freedom and tenure. In *AAUP's policy documents and reports* (10th ed.). Washington, DC: Author.

American Association of University Professors. (2010). *Legal cases affecting academic speech: Sheldon v. Dhillon.* Retrieved from https://www.aaup.org/get-involved/issue-campaigns/speak-speak-out-protect-faculty-voice/legal-cases-affecting-academic

Benner, P., Sutphen, M., Leonard, V., & Day, L. (2010). *Educating nurses: A call for radical transformation.* Stanford, CA: Carnegie Foundation for the Advancement of Teaching.

Briley, R. (2005, February 10). Ward Churchill's comments—and the general's. *HHN: History News Network.* Retrieved from http://hnn.us/articles/10146.html

Brown v. Amenti, 247 F.3d 69 (3d Cir. 2001).

Cásarez, N. B. (1998). Don't tell me what to say: Compelled commercial speech and the First Amendment. *Missouri Law Review, 63,* 929. Retrieved from https://papers.ssrn.com/sol3/papers.cfm?abstract_id=2436731

Ceballos v. Garcetti, 361 F.3d 1168, 1180 (9th Cir. 2004).

Cheese, A. (2015). Email vs. phone vs. in-person: What's best for workplace communication? *Strategic America.* Retrieved from https://www.strategicamerica.com/blog/2015/05/email-vs-phone-vs-person-whats-best-workplace-communication/

Churchill, W. (2003). *On the justice of roosting chickens: Reflections on the consequences of U.S. imperial arrogance and criminality.* Edinburgh, UK: AK Press.

Clavreul, G. M. (2008). Should nursing school curriculum be standardized? *Workingnurse.com.* Retrieved from https://www.workingnurse.com/articles/Should-Nursing-School-Curriculum-Be-Standardized

Eastern University. (2019). *Employment opportunities.* Retrieved from https://www.eastern.edu/about/offices-centers/human-resources/employment-opportunities

Gitlow v. People, 268 U.S. 652 (1925).

History. (2009). *Bill of rights.* Retrieved from https://www.history.com/topics/united-states-constitution/bill-of-rights

Institute of Medicine & Committee on the Robert Wood Johnson Initiative on the Future of Nursing, at the Institute of Medicine. (2010). *The future of nursing: Leading change, advancing health.* Washington, DC: National Academies Press.

Jaschik, S. (2007). Colorado moves to fire Churchill. *Inside Higher Ed.* Retrieved from https://www.insidehighered.com/news/2006/06/27/colorado-moves-fire-churchill

Jaschik, S. (2013, April 2). Final loss for Ward Churchill. *Inside Higher Ed.* Retrieved from https://www.insidehighered.com/news/2013/04/02/supreme-court-rejects-appeal-ward-churchill

Kaplan, W. A., & Lee, B. A. (2013). *The law of higher education* (5th ed.). San Francisco, CA: Jossey-Bass Publishers.

Koithan, M. (1994). Incorporating multiple modes of awareness in nursing curriculum. In P. L. Chinn & J. Watson (Eds.), *Art and aesthetics in nursing* (pp. 145–162). New York, NY: National League for Nursing.

Kokemuller, K. (2019). What are the benefits of social media vs. face to face? *Small Business—Chron.* Retrieved from https://smallbusiness.chron.com/benefits-social-media-vs-face-face-80091.html

Lindsay, C. L., III. (2005). *The college student's guide to the law.* Lanham, MD: Taylor Trade Publishing.

Lovelace v. S.E. Mass. Univ., 793 F.2d 419, 425 (1st Cir. 1986).

Martin, C. (2007). The importance of face-to-face communication at work. *CIO.* Retrieved from https://www.cio.com/article/2441851/the-importance-of-face-to-face-communication-at-work.html

Mill, J. S. (1910). *Utilitarianism, liberty, and representative government.* New York, NY: E. P. Dutton.

National Academies of Medicine. (2019). *The future of nursing 2020-2030.* Retrieved from https://campaignforaction.org/

New York Times v. Sullivan, 376 U.S. 254 (1964).

Nichols, B. (1981). Standardized education for nursing. *American Journal of Hospital Pharmacy, 38*(10), 1455–1458. doi:10.1093/ajhp/38.10.1455

Robert Wood Johnson Foundation & AARP. (2013-2019). *Future of Nursing: Campaign For Action.* Retrieved from https://www.rwjf.org/en/how-we-work/grants-explorer/featured-programs/future-of-nursing–campaign-for-action.html

Roth, J. A., McEllistrem, S., D'Ogostino, T., Brown, C. J. (2009). *Higher education law in America* (10th ed.). Malvern, PA: Center for Education & Employment Law.

Roth v. United States, 354 U.S. 476 (1957). Retrieved from https://supreme.justia.com/cases/federal/us/354/476/

Schreker, E. (2010). Ward Churchill at the Dalton Trumbo Fountain: Academic freedom in the aftermath of 9/11. *AAUP Journal of Academic Freedom (Vol. 1).* Retrieved from https://www.aaup.org/JAF1/ward-churchill-dalton-trumbo-fountain-academic-freedom-aftermath-911

Sheldon v. Dhillon, No. C-08-03438 RMW (N.D. Cal. 2009).

Stronach v. Virginia State University, No. 3:07CV646-HEH, 2008 WL 161304 (E.D. Va. Jan. 15, 2008).

U.S. Chamber Institute for Legal Reform. (n.d.). *About ILR: Restoring balance. Ensuring justice.* Retrieved from https://www.instituteforlegalreform.com/about-ilr

U.S. Institute for Legal Reform. (2013). *International comparisons of litigation costs Canada, Europe, Japan, and the United States.* Retrieved from https://www.instituteforlegalreform.com/uploads/sites/1/ILR_NERA_Study_International_Liability_Costs-update.pdf

Vile, J. R., & Hudson, D. L., Jr. (2017). Academic freedom. *The First Amendment Encyclopedia.* Retrieved from https://mtsu.edu/first-amendment/article/17/academic-freedom

Wheaton College. (2019). *Job seekers.* Retrieved from https://www.wheaton.edu/about-wheaton/offices-and-services/human-resources/for-job-seekers/

11

Intellectual Property: When Faculty Members Misrepresent a Work Product as Their Own

Case Study 11.1
An Undergraduate Faculty Member Discovers a Graduate Faculty Member Has Used Her Intellectual Property Without Her Permission

Your role: You are Professor Bose, an undergraduate faculty member teaching a junior-level medical–surgical nursing course, and you share an office with Professor Davis, a graduate faculty member teaching in the nurse practitioner program.

As a new faculty member, you are interested in increasing your scholarly productivity. You agree to write a pharmacology chapter for a new medical–surgical text. You are excited because you are working on your PhD and this will be your first publication. You have to research all the latest drug therapies; in addition to writing a narrative, you must also compile very intricate tables that list the drug, its indications, special nursing considerations, and prominent side effects. Professor Davis, who shares an office with you, is teaching in the graduate nurse practitioner program and has an upcoming lecture to give on oncology-focused primary care.

Professor Davis one day notices the impressive, detailed tables on oncology/cancer drugs that you have compiled for your chapter, and she asks you if she may borrow your tables and take a look at them. As it was a simple request and you wanted to be collegial, you agreed to let Professor Davis review your pre-publication materials. Two months later, you are in your joint office and need a paper clip. You wander over to Professor Davis's desk to look for one and see something that looks very familiar. You reach down to more carefully examine the item on Professor Davis's desk, and you are stunned to discover that it is a graduate nursing handout on oncology drugs that is almost an exact copy of your own detailed tables. Further, it has Professor Davis's name on it but no attribution that the tables are your original work. Astonished, you are certain that you had not given Professor Davis permission to use the tables in her graduate course (although you almost certainly would have, had Professor Davis asked). And as you previously taught in an Associate Degree program, you are certain that

Professor Davis could not make a case that this was "fair use" of your intellectual property by any stretch of the imagination.

Questions

■ How would you first proceed?

■ Do you believe that you have been the victim of theft of intellectual property, or was it "fair use" by Professor Davis?

■ If indeed intellectual theft has occurred, what should be the action against Professor Davis?

UNIVERSITY FACULTY INTELLECTUAL PROPERTY: LEGAL PRINCIPLES AND REVIEW OF THE LITERATURE

This chapter focuses on three issues: (a) chiefly grievances between faculty when accusations of intellectual property theft of original work are made by one faculty against another; (b) work-for-hire issues, in which the university that pays the salary of individual faculty may claim or have ownership of intellectual property that is authored or invented while the faculty is employed by the university; and (c) how co-authorship between student and faculty may be challenged.

LEGAL PRINCIPLES AND REVIEW OF THE LITERATURE

What exactly is meant by the term *intellectual property*? According to the World Intellectual Property Organization (WIPO, n.d.), "Intellectual property (IP) refers to creations of the mind: inventions, literary and artistic works, and symbols, names, images, and designs used in commerce" (para. 1). It can be divided into two categories:

> Industrial property, which includes inventions (patents), trademarks, industrial designs, and geographic indications of source; and Copyright, which includes literary and artistic works such as novels, poems and plays, films, musical works, artistic works such as drawings, paintings, photographs and sculptures, and architectural designs. (para. 2)

In most universities, particularly research universities, issues surrounding intellectual property rights, especially patent rights, are highly regulated activities because new patentable inventions by work for hire[1] faculty have the possibility to result in enormous royalties for not only the inventor personally but also for the university itself. The specifics surrounding university faculty intellectual property rights are discussed in the beginning of this chapter, but the issues surrounding a student's right to their own creative ideas, inventions, and even prose while enrolled at a university are also discussed.

Faculty or Colleague Theft of Original Work

Intellectual property disputes in academia often surround legal challenges to copyright, patents, trademarks, and original work that may not yet have reached the copyright, patent, or trademark application stage. In the case of original work, one of the hallmarks of being a faculty scholar employed by a university is that the faculty member engages in the production of creative, original endeavors—whether the faculty member is a fine arts instructor, a chemist, an English professor, or a nursing professor. The 2018 update of the 2006 Carnegie University and College Classifications adds more institutional information (including for the first time "professional doctorates" which includes the DNP or PharmD and others) but still considers the respective mission of the university and rank them as (a) a university with very high research activity, (b) a university with high research activity,

---

[1] The concept of *work for hire* is an important legal term. It is a concept in intellectual property law in which the work of an employee is considered to be owned by the employer. Operationally, work for hire is an exception to **the copyright concept that the creator of a work is its owner.**

or (c) a doctoral/research university, all depending on the amount of aggregate scholarship expected of the individual faculty and number of PhDs awarded (p. 120).[2] At research universities, the number of publications is associated with an increased likelihood of securing federal research grants, and therefore the institutional pressure on faculty to produce creative endeavors (publications, books, grants, other sources of funding, etc.) is substantial (Ali, Bhattacharyya, & Olejniczak, 2010). It is this kind of institutional pressure on the production of scholarship that can lead to aggressive, unethical, and even nefarious conduct and intellectual dishonesty up to and including theft.

One of the most public cases of charges of intellectual property theft occurred in 1996 in the Department of African American Studies (the first PhD program in the then-new discipline founded in 1988) at Temple University. In that case, the founding Department Chair, Dr. Molefi Kete Asante, who first articulated the concept of Afrocentric Theory, was accused of misappropriating the intellectual work product of Assistant Professor Ella Forbes, a junior untenured faculty member in his department. According to Boynton (2002), "During his 12 years as chairman, Dr. Asante built the department into a nationally recognized center that promoted his popular ideology, and he enjoyed unchallenged autonomy" (p. 1). Boynton further writes, "He stepped down in 1996 amid charges that he misappropriated a professor's work for a textbook and then denied her tenure when she complained. The conflict was deemed a book contract dispute, not misconduct, and the junior professor was granted a new tenure review, minus Dr. Asante" (p. 1).

The case received international attention because Dr. Asante was regarded as a prodigious scholar and chief architect of this new discipline. The notoriety of the case was inflamed by Dr. Asante, who was reported in the press as having given a speech at a meeting of the United Africa Movement in which he characterized the controversy as a "racist plot" by "White people" and "their agents within our department" for an authorship dispute that was threatening his scholarly reputation (Goodman, 1996).

Although it was not disputed that Asante first recruited Forbes to help him cowrite a high school textbook, Asante and his publisher claimed Forbes had agreed her name would not appear as a coauthor of the textbook unless more than 30% of text was her own work product and that this benchmark was not met (Goodman, 1996). For its part, Temple University concluded that this was a contractual dispute and not a claim of intellectual property theft (although it did grant Forbes a second full-tenure review).

Work for Hire

More typically, intellectual property or work product disputes by faculty are with their employer—the university. In this case, the concept of *work for hire* is usually central to the dispute. As defined in the 1976 Copyright Act (U.S. Copyright Office, 1976) as amended,[3] "work for hire" in the copyright context is:

> (1) a work prepared by an employee within the scope of his or her employment; or (2) a work specially ordered or commissioned for use as a contribution to a collective work:
> - as a part of a motion picture,
> - as a part of other audiovisual work,
> - as a translation,
> - as a supplementary work,
> - as a compilation,
> - as an instructional text,
> - as a test,
> - as answer material for a test, or
> - as an atlas. (Title 17, Section 101 of the United States Code)

---

[2] The criteria and formula used to categorize a university in one of three categories include the following: research and development spending (in science, engineering, and other areas); the number of postdoctoral and nonfaculty research staff members with doctorates, doctoral degrees conferred, number of disciplines in which the doctorate is conferred; and a per capita calculation to judge the relative importance of research within institutions.

[3] All the amendments to the Copyright Act of 1976 made since 1976 through June 30, 2009, can be found at www.copyright.gov/title17/92preface .pdf.

The most important point is to determine whether a given work product fits with this definition, and a key factor in making that determination is the relationship between the parties. However, the statutory definition is complex, and circumstances under which the principle can be applied vary, which is where university counsel can be very helpful. Certain work for hire principles may also apply to patentable subject matter. For instance, what if a professor claims his work on a patent took place in his off-hours and not while he was at work (Jassin, 2010)? The current definition of *work for hire* in a copyright context was established by the United States Supreme Court in *Community for Creative Non-Violence v. Reid* (1989). In this landmark case, the Court held that to determine whether a work is made for hire, one must first ascertain whether the work was prepared by (a) an employee or by (b) an independent contractor.

As it would be somewhat unusual for a full-time faculty member to be employed as an independent contractor (there are cases in which adjunct faculty may be technically hired as independent contractors), overwhelmingly the work product of a faculty member derived as part of their employment or role likely falls into the work for hire category (Borstoff & Newton, 2006). To resolve some of the complexity surrounding work for hire principles for employees (in this case, faculty), particularly for a group of individuals who are encouraged to create, design, invent, and publish all types of works that would fall under copyright, patent, or trademark law, royalty policies are usually established under which the individual faculty directly benefits from the creative work product. In the case of revenue-producing inventions or products, the university may also benefit. At Drexel University, the following formula currently applies[4] to most revenue-generating intellectual property that falls within certain work for hire boundaries which can be found at https://drexel.edu/provost/policies/intellectual_property.

It is best to be proactive when there are potential revenue sources for an individual faculty member's intellectual property. Faculty members are encouraged to be very familiar with their university's policies on intellectual property. In particular, research universities are certain to have one (and, e.g., a technology transfer office or division of technology licensing), as university faculty-generated ideas and inventions can become enormous lifelong revenue sources for colleges and universities (Johnson, 2010). If there is ambiguity and/or reason to create a relationship more appropriate to a particular project, we encourage faculty to reach (negotiate) an understanding with the university as early in the process as possible.

Copyright and "Fair Use" Guidelines for Faculty

University and college faculty are often faced with confusion over what is proper "fair" and free use of copyrighted works. For instance, if an individual faculty member wants to assign a chapter in a book for students to read but does not want students to have to buy the book for a single chapter, can the professor simply make copies of the chapter and distribute them in class? Educators and others can make "fair use" of copyrighted materials under certain guidelines established in Title 17 of the United States Code.

In *Stewart v. Abend* (1990), the Supreme Court ruled that the principle of fair use relies on the potential for that use to negatively affect the work's potential market or value. In this case, a story, written in 1948, became a famed Alfred Hitchcock movie, *Rear Window* (1954). The author of the original story, Cornell Woolrich, had first sold the short story rights and then the movie rights to that short story. He died in 1968 before the copyright renewal of the book reverted back to the original author, which, according to the first copyright law of 1909 (Sixtieth Congress, 2d Session, 1909) would have done so after a period of 28 years. When the movie was subsequently shown on television, the new copyright holder of the movie rights (which had passed on and were sold after Woolrich's death) sued the production company of *Rear Window*. Mr. Abend, the new owner of the movie rights, sued because the movie was a derivative work of Woolrich. In other words, although the first production of *Rear Window* in 1954 was legal, the subsequent television broadcast in 1971

---

[4] As the law evolves and as new fact patterns and discoveries arise, so university policies have to change. Intellectual property policies are likely to become the subject of significant interest (and perhaps contest) on campuses as universities look to increase "alternative revenue sources" (nontuition revenues), including commercialization of intellectual property.

was not deemed "fair use" of the derivative work even though the author had died and there was a new owner of the original literary rights. In principle, what this 1990 Supreme Court ruling established was that the control of an original piece of work reverts back to the author—or the author's designee or successors[5]—when renewal comes up. This, therefore, protects the author (and the heirs) from being deprived of any future value of the work.

As for faculty, fair use can be evaluated, or tested, based on the following four factors:

1. *The purpose and character of the use, including whether such use is of a commercial nature or is for nonprofit educational purposes* (Roth, 2009, p. 350). In this example, the proposed use is for a nonprofit, educational purpose, which weighs in favor of this being a fair use.
2. *The nature of the copyrighted work* (Roth, 2009, p. 350). Works that are primarily collections of facts are typically afforded greater fair use protection than creative works. The type of book that the faculty member proposes copying would need to be looked at in more detail from this perspective to determine if the use weighs in favor of, or against, fair use.
3. *The amount and substantiality of the portion used in relation to the copyrighted work as a whole* (Roth, 2009, p. 350). This directive can be somewhat vague. Can one-third of the book be copied legally and distributed to the class? Possibly. Can over one-half of the book be copied— likely not. But a case can also perhaps be made that several chapters would be considered "substantial" and thus be disallowed. It may also depend on how many total chapters there are in the book and whether the faculty member copies the same chapters of the book year after year for each section of the class, likely arguing against fair use. Reasonable and prudent judgment must be carefully exercised.
4. *The effect of the use upon the potential market for or value of the copyrighted work* (Roth, 2009, p. 350). Is the photocopying by the faculty member depriving the copyright owner of royalty income, for example? This is often an issue that will prompt a lawsuit from a publisher and should be considered very carefully.

These four factors must be considered as a whole in determining whether a particular use is fair use. Applying rules based purely on the percentage of a work being copied, for instance, without due consideration of all four factors is a dangerous proposition. Overall, faculty members are encouraged to be very cognizant of fair use legal principles and to be wary of violating them, as such conduct can be reported by anyone, including a student. The very public prosecution of students who illegally downloaded music from the Internet is clear proof that the force of law in the area of copyright infringement can be perilous (Morley & Parker, 2009).

DISCUSSION OF CASE

Consider the first question in Case. How would you first proceed? Recall that you are Professor Bose and you have just discovered your original work was reproduced under the name of your office colleague, Professor Davis. Bose was shocked by the disregard for her hard work that was apparently being passed off as the work of Davis, and Bose immediately thought she had been the victim of intellectual property theft again so early in her academic career. Having moved to Buffalo from Alabama only months earlier, a colleague at Bose's previous employer (a large community college nursing program) had notified her that a poster of a human caring program that she had conceived and developed had just been presented by the current community college nursing dean as the dean's own work product. When she heard this, she was shocked and could not understand how anyone could simply take the work product of another and pass it off as their own, without any attribution at all. This practice is not so uncommon, and a quick visit to the "Harvard Plagiarism Archive," which has tracked allegations of Harvard faculty accused of plagiarism since 2002, highlights this pervasive issue, even at a leading university such as Harvard (*Harvard Plagiarism Archive*, 2010).

Nonetheless, it seemed only months earlier Bose had sworn to herself that she would never again be the victim of intellectual property theft, but here she was confronting almost the very same situation. However, Bose was also very confused about what her best course of action should be. Consider

---

[5] That is, if the original author has died and willed all intellectual property rights to their heirs.

the second question: Do you believe Dr. Bose has been the victim of intellectual property theft? Or do you think that this was instead a case of unethical misrepresentation (but not illegal taking) of another author's work because the work was unpublished?

WHEN TO CONSULT THE UNIVERSITY COUNSEL

When it comes to faculty disputes between or among faculty about authorship or percentage of effort on grants or other similar types of concerns, it is best to try to resolve the issue with the individual in question. If one-on-one discussion cannot resolve the issue, then we suggest using the usual department procedures (Chair and then Dean) and then seeking assistance from the university Ombudsman. It is unlikely that the university attorney would be an agent who would be consulted for interfaculty disputes. If using the Ombudsman is not an appropriate or effective strategy, then going through normal university departmental strategies is suggested. If that fails, try securing your own personal attorney for legal advice. Some inventions or patents (and sometimes creative authorship) can generate huge revenues; therefore, making sure one's own intellectual property interests are protected is essential.

FINDINGS AND DISPOSITION

This chapter's Case Study 11.1, like most accusations of intellectual property theft that go unreported, was not resolved in a public way (Siegel, 2008). Professor Bose, as a newly hired untenured assistant professor without a doctorate, was very afraid of what might be the result of such a public accusation of intellectual property theft and was not at all certain that she would receive the administration's support. After all, her previous dean had just committed intellectual property theft as soon as she left the community college, and she wondered if perhaps the stakes were higher for her now in this new position. She further suspected there was some favoritism by the current dean toward Professor Davis, and Bose was further cautious about taking a very public course of action. Still, she also wondered if she should confront Davis about the work product and see what she had to say. As Bose was still new to academia, she chose perhaps a more painful path, to keep the incident to herself, but she did acknowledge personally that she would never again trust Professor Davis. However, by sharing an office with Davis, it was quite challenging for Bose to keep her feelings hidden, but she did.

Years later, circumstances took a circuitous turn, and despite both professors leaving the small college where the intellectual property theft had occurred, Bose and Davis (now both holding doctorates) wound up being employed in the same college in New York City. Dr. Bose had never forgotten what had happened to her years earlier, and she thought her best course of action was simply to maintain some professional distance from her previous colleague, who she still thought had engaged in intellectual dishonesty. As you read the ending to this case, do you think Dr. Bose (then Professor Bose) could have handled her situation differently?

RELEVANT LEGAL CASE

Board of Trustees of Leland Stanford Junior University v. Roche Molecular Systems, Inc., Nos. 08-1509, -1510 (Fed. Cir. Sept. 30, 2009)

In this case, Stanford University undertook a lawsuit against the pharmaceutical giant Roche, claiming that a laboratory method to detect HIV antibodies was discovered by one of its faculty members on their campus and was owned by Stanford. However, Roche claimed that researcher Mark Holodniy signed a contract with Roche giving the company the rights to the intellectual property. Again, this is another complicated legal case, and what is important here is who owns the rights to the patent. Is it the inventor in this case, Mark Holodniy? Is it his employer, Stanford University (under original work for hire principles and intellectual property policy principles as the primary employer), where he was employed as a research fellow? Or was it Centus (later bought out by Roche), the company with which Mr. Holodniy signed certain contracts that may relate to the work? As an indication of the importance and complexities associated with *Stanford v. Roche* and related cases, the matter made its way to the U.S. Supreme Court. In November 2010 the Supreme Court agreed to hear the case. The decision was "largely moot" as the majority, led by Chief Justice Roberts, held that U.S. patent rights have always (since 1790) initially vested in "the inventor" and that the nonspecific language of the Bayh–Dole Act does nothing to change that arrangement. As a result, the Supreme Court's decision certainly reassured inventors, as well as all those involved in the practice of law involving inventions, that their established belief that the ownership rights in inventions belong first and foremost to inventors is correct.

From a different prospective, we have a case of a professor who claimed her contributions to a student's work was misrepresented by the undergraduate nursing student as solely her own. In that case, the student claimed it was her academic freedom to determine whether her instructor deserved co-authorship on the student's paper, and clearly, she did not think so. Although this case could be discussed as a form of an individual student's academic freedom, this case is similar but will be approached from the perspective of intellectual property rights. As mentioned previously, cases of faculty accused of misappropriating the intellectual property of their students (especially graduate students) are unfortunately not uncommon.

SUMMARY OF CASE

Intellectual property theft is not necessarily common or uncommon. It does happen (as evidenced by the Harvard Plagiarism Archive), and most of the cases never reach the level of publicity, much less a lawsuit, but are settled quietly. Any accusation of intellectual property theft, be it a copyright, trademark, or patent dispute, is inherently damaging not just to the individual involved but also to the reputation of the institution. Any faculty member who engages in any creative endeavor that might generate revenue (*any revenue*) is encouraged to read, understand, and be very clear about the institution's intellectual property policy. Further, collaborations with other faculty on projects (written or otherwise) need to be clearly negotiated, written, and signed. If significant revenues are possible, consider having a witness and the signatures notarized.

It is easy to be sympathetic with Bose's actions in Case Study 11.1, but it was perhaps the path of least resistance, and therefore the real ethical issues surrounding the actions of Davis went unchallenged. Who gains here? Does society gain when ethical lapses, even potential ethical lapses, are overlooked and individual rights are blurred? Was Bose at fault for not trying, even politely, to address the issue with her officemate? If, upon confrontation, Davis had become defensive and denied using the tables without proper authorization, should Boise have pursued relief within her department or college? What if Davis had profusely apologized and their relationship possibly healed, leading Bose to never to have to distance herself and act as though nothing had happened between them? Would either of these actions have been preferable to what Bose ultimately decided to do? Or did she have too much to risk by employing one of these alternative actions? Some nursing programs have been particularly vigorous about sensitizing nursing students and faculty to ethical issues and encouraging that they be addressed as early as possible. The question has always been, will a cheating or dishonest student (or faculty member, in this case) always act ethically (and differently) with their patients?" It is actually a very disturbing question to pose, as it is thought that all nurses (including nursing faculty) should act with the highest ethical standards, and faculty are bound to model this behavior if they are going to be authentic in their own professional and academic roles.

CRITICAL ELEMENTS TO CONSIDER

- Before entering into a joint authorship or creative project, negotiate the percentage of effort by all parties and determine what authorship order is agreed on.
- Review any college or university intellectual property policy and determine whether you agree with the said stipulations.

■ Determine whether all classroom materials are being used according to proper fair use policies.

■ Our recommendation is that if you have ever had an unsatisfactory collaboration with another colleague (a dispute over authorship order or perhaps a colleague not participating equally in a collaborative effort), you should resolve never to collaborate with them again.

■ Before working with a colleague on a large project, first strategize to work together on a smaller project to see if the work chemistry is satisfactory and if the colleague's work ethic is agreeable to you.

Helpful Resources

● Copyright Act of 1976: http://www.copyright.gov/title17/
● "Harvard Plagiarism Archive": http://authorskeptics.blogspot.com/
● Fisher, W. (n.d.). *Theories of intellectual property*. Cambridge, MA: Harvard Law School. Retrieved from http://www.law.harvard.edu/faculty/tfisher/iptheory.html
● Washington University Law School. (n.d.). *Faculty plagiarism guidelines*. Retrieved from http://law.wustl.edu/students/pages.aspx?id=1000

Case Study 11.2
A Master's Nursing Student Discovers Her Faculty Mentor Has Presented Their Joint Work at a Conference Without Giving the Student Authorship

Your role: You are Dr. Goings, the Assistant Dean and supervisor of the accused faculty mentor, Dr. Perpetua.

As Assistant Dean for Graduate Nursing Programs, you get an email one day from Ms. Ray, a student in the MSN in Community Health track. According to the student, she was assigned to Dr. Perpetua for her master's practicum. The student had conceived the idea to open up a nonprofit women's advocacy center in economically deprived neighborhoods to inform women of their rights and services, particularly surrounding healthcare and personal safety. As her faculty mentor, Dr. Perpetua had assisted Ms. Ray with the development of the project and the supporting business proposal. Unknown to the student, Dr. Perpetua had submitted an abstract to a national conference outlining the proposal, but without giving acknowledgment to Ms. Ray as the primary creator of the idea. Ms. Ray would have possibly never known about this had she not heard about the conference and discovered Dr. Perpetua was actually listed as a conference presenter of her project. In this email, the student indicates that she is shocked and upset and is afraid to confront Dr. Perpetua, but she is asking you to do something about the situation.

Questions
■ How would you first proceed?
■ How will you investigate this case?
■ Do you believe the student has been the victim of theft of intellectual property?
■ If indeed theft of intellectual property has occurred, what should be the action against Dr. Perpetua?

At first glance, it might appear that this is a very simple issue: "If the student invents or authors it, it belongs to the student!" However, what if the invention took place in a laboratory, very likely the laboratory of a faculty mentor or often a dissertation adviser? What if there were collaborators on the creative project, extremely likely especially in a laboratory setting? Science is no longer a solitary enterprise and therefore it is very unlikely that most graduate student work can be labeled as completely independent, thus resulting in the complexities of authorship and invention.

This is what happened to Eugene Aserinsky, who was a graduate student in 1952 at the University of Chicago. Now he is officially recognized as the individual who discovered rapid eye movement (REM) sleep when he noted and documented the cyclic occurrence of eye movements during sleep every 90 to 100 minutes in adults (Brown, 2003). However, at the time of the discovery it was co-attributed to his PhD adviser (and department chair of physiology) Nathaniel Kleitman, and that incorrect attribution remained common understanding until recently. According to the corrected obituary for Dr. Aserinsky that the *Los Angeles Times* published on August 14, 1998—20 days after it had incorrectly identified him as the co-discoverer of REM sleep—he alone discovered REM. Kleitman was listed as the second author because he was the professor who supervised Aserinsky's doctoral thesis.

The fascinating story of Aserinsky and Kleitman is told by Lamberg (2004) in her short article, "The Student, the Professor, and the Birth of Modern Sleep Research." This story did not include litigation (as many others have), chiefly because the discovery of REM did not result in the invention of a commercial product or a literary work. The discovery resulted in publication in the prestigious peer-reviewed journal *Science* (Aserinsky & Kleitman, 1953), where Kleitman was erroneously given credit for the discovery as second author. As mentioned, current intellectual property is divided into industrial property which includes, but is broader than inventions and copyrighted artistic expressions. Another case of an alleged intellectual property theft by a professor of a student's creative capital[6] took place in 2010 when Seung Won Lee, a graduate student at Parsons, the New School for Design in New York City, claimed he spent 3 years working on a social networking gaming application called Jump-Cell for his graduate thesis (Markos, 2010). His professor, Jinsook "Erin" Cho, had encouraged him to develop a marketing plan for his idea, and he traveled to his home in Korea to do so. Shortly thereafter, he read a newspaper account of a new application very similar to his, called Rat Busters, which had been developed by his thesis adviser, Professor Cho, with an $80,000 institutional grant from Parsons. After reading that the invention was attributed to Professor Cho and one of his friends, Lee returned to the United States and filed his lawsuit in the New York Supreme Court in Manhattan. Subsequently, Professor Cho filed countercharges, admitting that Mr. Lee had come up with the idea, but arguing that he and his colleague had indeed done all the development work at great expense to put the invention to market (Markos, 2010).

At the time this book was published, the case of *Lee v. Cho* had not been litigated, but the questions for academic faculty are clear: (a) Is it legal to appropriate another's idea (even if it is not yet fully developed) and refine it (as Professor Cho has admitted) for a patent; (b) is it ethical that, although the professor admits he borrowed the idea, there was absolutely no acknowledgment of the student's contribution; (c) did the university have a policy on intellectual property that applied to this dispute; and (d) what could university counsel advise regarding the applicability of U.S. patent law to an inventorship dispute such as this? These questions are considered in the following.

Copyright is a particular form of intellectual property that is a core concept in academia because it applies to writing (scholarship) and other forms of expression (e.g., software, courseware), and it is the most likely source of misappropriation by students, who claim authorship in prior manuscripts (e.g., course papers). According to the Berne Convention for the Protection of Literary and Artistic Works[7] most of whose signatory countries belong to the World Trade Organization, copyright extends to the following:

- Books, pamphlets, and other writings;
- Lectures, addresses, sermons;
- Dramatic or dramatico-musical works;

---

[6] Students can also be accused of stealing each other's creative concepts, as the movie *The Social Network* vividly demonstrates.

[7] The Berne Convention principles were actually instigated by Victor Hugo, author of *Les Misérables* among other works, who was concerned about the *droit d'auteur* ("right of the author"), which at the time of his writings meant authorship rights, and copyright did not extend beyond an individual country's borders. Signed in 1886, this agreement has been updated over the years and as of 2007 some 163 countries have signed this document, which is essentially an international trade agreement (Bouchoux, 2008).

- Choreographic works and entertainments in dumb show;
- Musical compositions with or without words;
- Cinematographic works to which are assimilated works expressed by a process analogous to cinematography;
- Works of drawing, painting, architecture, sculpture, engraving and lithography;
- Photographic works, to which are assimilated works expressed by a process analogous to photography;
- Works of applied art; illustrations, maps, plans, sketches and three-dimensional works relative to geography, topography, architecture or science;
- Translations, adaptations, arrangements of music and other alterations of a literary or artistic work, which are to be protected as original works without prejudice to the copyright in the original work; and
- Collections of literary or artistic works such as encyclopaedias and anthologies which, by reason of the selection and arrangement of their contents, constitute intellectual creations, are to be protected as such, without prejudice to the copyright in each of the works forming part of such collections. (WIPO, n.d.-a, Art. 2)

Although students (undergraduate and graduate) may not often be involved in issues of patent rights from inventions, Arizona State University's Master's in Healthcare Innovation (MHI) in Healthcare Innovation (a joint degree between nursing and business), Ohio State University's MHI, and Drexel University's MSN in Innovation are degree programs in which graduate nursing students may actually invent and seek patents through their respective universities. An important point about copyright is that ideas themselves cannot be copyrighted; however, the expression of ideas can be copyrighted, as was first derived in *Story's Executives v. Holcombe* (1847).

In a 2009 copyright case at San Jose State University, an undergraduate student was taking a course titled Data Structures and Algorithms. Emanating from a class assignment, the student posted his class work product, in this case computer code, on the Internet (Stripling, 2009). His professor claimed that the student had committed copyright infringement by publishing work product (code) that was connected to his class.[8] In this case the professor argued the purpose of the code was for his class, under his instruction, and therefore he had at least partial claim to it (Stripling, 2008). A commentary on this case provides a good summary of the impact of copyright laws on university or college students:

> Students own the copyrights in the works they create at our institutions. As the digital age offers new opportunities to disseminate scholarship, including student scholarship, we need to remember that students own their copyrights (just as professors own theirs) and formulate appropriate policy to respect those rights. (Smith, 2009, para. 3)

Whether in fact the student had any claim to ownership, as university counsel would tell you, depends on the facts; for example, whether the invention or creative work was made possible by substantial use of the university's resources, what the university's IT policies state, and whether there was a contractual agreement with a funder/sponsor of research.

DISCUSSION OF CASE STUDY 11.2

Recall the first question: How would you first proceed? Remember, you are Dr. Goings, and you are confronted by an accusation from a student against Dr. Perpetua. One of the more central tenets of management and leadership, especially when dealing with conflict resolution, is that there are always two sides to a story. It is easy to be seduced by a salacious story or to come to quick judgments about a claim when you are first presented information or evidence, which at first glance appears convincing and true. However, in any given individual case in academia, what first seems obvious is untrue or far different from the actual reality. Therefore, fact finding directed at both sides (or in some cases there may be additional sides) is essential. This leads to the second question: How will you investigate this case?

---

[8] There were other issues as well, including whether the student had breached the honor code by posting answers (code) to an examination that was already due.

The next step Dr. Goings will take is fact finding. She or an appropriate university designee will need to investigate this claim thoroughly before she can best establish to her satisfaction the actual details and facts of the case, which would then lead her to a conclusion and a course of action. Although she already has the initial student claim, Dr. Goings asks the student to provide greater detail and any supporting documents or other evidence that relates to her claim. Once she receives this further explanatory documentation from the student, Dr. Goings knows she will have to do the same with Dr. Perpetua, including having a private meeting with Dr. Perpetua to present her with the accusation, hear her side of the story, and obtain her documentation.

In the meantime, Dr. Goings sends a confidential email to her Associate Dean, outlining the situation. She opts, however, not to copy or blind-copy any email correspondence (an often-overused practice in academia) between the student or Dr. Perpetua and herself. It is important for Dr. Goings to be confident that she can handle this situation properly. Moreover, this Associate Dean has confidence in Dr. Goings, and knows that Dr. Goings will seek her counsel at any point that she decides she needs further administrative assistance. But there is a very important legal reason not to send email at all, or at least to use it carefully and judiciously. This is because claims often lead to litigation, and litigation *always* leads to extensive "discovery," meaning that copies of relevant documents and other evidence must be turned over as part of the litigation.

 WHEN TO CONSULT THE UNIVERSITY COUNSEL

If a student believes that he has been a victim of intellectual property theft, the best course of action is to follow the chain of command: approach the professor first, make the case, then go to the department chair and dean if there is no resolution. Sometimes, obtaining advice from the ombudsman can be helpful. If there are real disagreements about "rights," then university counsel can be consulted. Note, however, that the university counsel's client is *the university*, and counsel will say so at the start of the meeting, as giving legal advice to both sides of a dispute could result in later disqualification if the case goes to court. In that case, however, the student will need to retain personal counsel, and if the professor claims a personal interest in the proceeds (separate from the institution), the professor might have to do so as well.

FINDINGS AND DISPOSITION

After Dr. Goings received the more formal student complaint, she discerned it was a serious charge. Recall the third question: Do you believe the student has been the victim of intellectual property theft? Dr. Goings brought Dr. Perpetua in for a meeting, and Dr. Perpetua did confess that she had sent the abstract in without the student's permission and without properly acknowledging her efforts on it. Incredulous, Dr. Goings asked why she had done this. Dr. Perpetua indicated that she exercised poor judgment, but that the student's work was similar to her own and that the student had developed her work in great part from her direction and supervision. Dr. Goings dismissed these rationalizations and handed Dr. Perpetua a copy of the authorship guidelines of the college which Dr. Perpetua's conduct clearly violated.

Recall the fourth question: If intellectual property theft has occurred, what should be the action against Dr. Perpetua? With the admission of misconduct, Dr. Goings informed Dr. Perpetua that she would consult with the Associate Dean and Dean to formulate a penalty for this violation. In the meantime, she requested that Dr. Perpetua write the student a letter of apology (with a copy to Dr. Goings) and offer to meet with the student to discuss the issue. After consultation with both the Associate Dean and Dean, it was decided that Dr. Perpetua would receive a written letter of reprimand that would be placed in her permanent file and would be noted on her annual evaluation. She was further warned that any additional violation of this nature could result in further action against her, up to and including termination.

RELEVANT LEGAL CASE

S. R. Seshadri v. Masoud Kasraian, No. 97-1610 (7th Cir. 1997)

In this case, Mr. Kasraian was a PhD electrical engineering student at the University of Wisconsin. Professor Seshadri was an electrical engineering professor and Kasraian's dissertation supervisor. From court records it is documented that the two individuals had previously published four joint articles, with Kasraian as first author and Seshadri as second author. Subsequently, Seshadri had requested that Kasraian sign up for a course he was teaching, but the student refused. Whether Seshadri considered the course essential to the program of study for Kasraian or whether the course was to be canceled without adequate enrollment (thus causing anger at the student for refusing to take the class) is unknown. However, shortly thereafter, the two individuals submitted a paper to the *Journal of Applied Physics,* with Kasraian again as first author and the professor as second author, and they both signed a copyright form to the journal in the event the article was accepted and published. A dispute ensued, and the professor wrote the journal editor and requested his name be removed from the article and that the article be rescinded. The professor claimed the submission "was based on certain erroneous information given by" Kasraian ("Student Is Joint Author," 1997, para. 1), and the article was returned to the student.

The student proceeded to revise the article and resubmitted it to the journal, with the professor given an acknowledgment but not second authorship, and the article was accepted for publication. The professor filed academic conduct charges against the student, claiming he (the professor) was the sole author of the manuscript, but the charges were dismissed when the student showed evidence that he (the student) was actually the sole author, not just on the manuscript in question but on the four previous articles as well. For his part, the student alleged the professor committed academic misconduct, and the professor was suspended from the university for a year without pay and not allowed to supervise graduate students for a year.

The professor then filed suit against the student in federal court in Wisconsin, alleging copyright infringement and theft of intellectual capital.[9] Ruling in favor of the student, the court dismissed the case on summary judgment, holding that there was probably joint authorship, but the professor had declined authorship on the paper in question and thus there was no copyright infringement. Further, there was no finding that there was a basis for the charge that the manuscript contained erroneous information. The plaintiff appealed to the federal appeals court, which affirmed the dismissal despite the professor's argument that his copyright claim was still valid with respect to future publications.

SUMMARY

Disputes over intellectual property between students and faculty can be anticipated to involve graduate students and their faculty supervisors, often thesis or dissertation chairs. Conflicts can easily arise when university policies are nonexistent or ambiguous, and when clear directions about authorship are not fully addressed (the more proper term is "negotiated") at the beginning of any joint scholarship enterprise. Students are understandably not well versed in the protocols and procedures, common courtesies and laws that govern the generation of knowledge or intellectual property, but faculty members—even research faculty—are often surprisingly uninformed. A more serious problem is presented by faculty, who may take unethical advantage of their position of power and authority over the student.

Clear college or university policies and guidelines are the first line of defense that protects faculty and students as well as the institution. A best practice is to include a link to the institution's policy on intellectual property on a course syllabus, in order to set a standard for academic integrity, and how joint authorship relationships should proceed and under what criteria. It is

---

[9] The professor also sued the university, claiming that his suspension violated Title VII of the Civil Rights Act of 1964, which prohibits employment discrimination based on race, color, religion, sex, or national origin. He claimed the adverse action was taken against him because of his "creed [which] requires scrupulous honesty in the scholarly pursuit of scientific knowledge." The claim was dismissed because this "creed" did not constitute a "religion." This footnote is provided to show that, when litigation occurs, you can expect the claims to be many and varied and that lawyers are willing to make all kinds of arguments.

often the professor who says, "This is good work. I think it could get published. Would you like me to help you?" It is at that point that a whole host of questions arise and should be addressed: (a) Will the professor suggest he or she be second author? (b) Will the professor procure the college's authorship policy and discuss it with the student? (c) Will the professor decline second authorship even if in the end the professor's contribution is significant? Unfortunately, it often happens that faculty members are discouraged into minimizing their own contributions to student work. If an instructor is giving substantive feedback, and if that instructor's guidance on revisions is shaping the structure of the manuscript, and if in the end the instructor's contribution to the work product is significant, then the student should understand that it would be unethical to submit the work as solely their own. That is what academic integrity is all about. Of course, some faculty may simply decline authorship because they do not need the publication or have particular reasons for removing themselves from co-authorship. However, a faculty member should not decline co-authorship simply because they do not think it is the right thing to do. Good science and well-articulated ideas (and manuscripts) are often best produced by having multiple sources of input. Finally, lacking the gravitas of a faculty member (particularly one with a doctorate) to help them, students will often find editors very uninterested in publishing their work, especially if they sense it is simply a classroom work product. In the end, student scholarship is copyrighted at its creation and inception, but the tangled web of who owns what then evolves as other individuals add their input to the ideas and words written for possible publication.

CRITICAL ELEMENTS TO CONSIDER

- Student work (intellectual property) is copyrighted at its creative inception. Unlike patents, there are no specific forms to complete, unless copyright registration, which is optional and affords certain additional rights to the copyright holder, is desired.
- If a student is seeking publication of his work or joint work, usually copyright is relinquished to the publisher unless negotiated otherwise.
- Students should procure the authorship policy in their college or university if seeking co-publishing with a faculty member.
- Remember, co-publishing with a faculty member is a good thing, and if the professor/faculty member is particularly reputable or has a national or international reputation, these kinds of joint scholarly ventures can enhance a student's career immensely.
- If an author's name is to be included on an abstract or manuscript or any document submitted for peer review, it is that person's ethical responsibility to review the materials with all parties (coauthors) before it is submitted for review and to attest that the authorship (and authorship order) attributed to the respective author(s) is valid.
- Publishing is the best way nursing science can be transmitted in a permanent way. It is the most influential form of showcasing one's ideas and possibly making an impact on the discipline. Nursing students (both undergraduate and graduate) are encouraged to seek out publishing opportunities as they arise.

Helpful Resources

- American Bar Association Section. *Intellectual Property Law—Law Student and Outreach Programs.* Retrieved from http://www.abanet.org/intelprop/law_student.html
- Harrington, T. (2010). Intellectual property on campus: Students' rights and responsibilities. Carbondale: Southern Illinois University Press.
- Whittaker, Z. (2010). Students: All your intellectual property belongs to us. *ZD Net.* Retrieved from http://www.zdnet.com/blog/igeneration/students-all-your-intellectual-property-belong-to-us/4648
- World Intellectual Property Organization. (2019). *Intellectual Property Basics: A Q&A for Students*, Retrieved June 8, 2020 from https://www.wipo.int/publications/en/details.jsp?id=4410&plang=EN

References

Ali, M. M., Bhattacharyya, P., & Olejniczak, A. J. (2010). The effects of scholarly productivity and institutional characteristics on the distribution of federal research grants. *Journal of Higher Education, 81*(2), 164–178. doi:10.1080/00221546.2010.11779047

Aserinsky, E., & Kleitman, N. (1953). Regular occurring periods of eye motility, and concomitant phenomena, during sleep. *Science, 118,* 273–274. doi:10.1126/science.118.3062.273

Board of Trustees of the Leland Stanford Junior University v. Roche Molecular Systems, Inc., Nos. 2008-1509, 2008-1510 (Fed. Cir. Sept. 30, 2009).

Borstorff, P., & Newton, S. (2006, April). Independent contractor classification: The challenge of doing it right. *Entrepreneurial Executive*. Retrieved from https://www.questia.com/library/journal/1G1-166778406/independent-contractor-classification-the-challenge

Bouchoux, D. (2008). *Intellectual property for paralegals: The law of trademarks, copyrights, patents, and trade secrets* (3rd ed.). Florence, KY: Cengage Learning.

Boynton, R. (2002, April 14). Black studies today; Out of Africa, and back. *The New York Times, Education Life*. Retrieved from https://www.nytimes.com/2002/04/14/education/black-studies-today-out-of-africa-and-back.html

Brown, C. (2003, October). The stubborn scientist who unraveled a mystery of the night. *Smithsonian*. Retrieved from https://www.smithsonianmag.com/science-nature/the-stubborn-scientist-who-unraveled-a-mystery-of-the-night-91514538/

Carnegie Classification of Institutions of Higher Education. (2018). *2018 update: Facts and figures*. Retrieved from https://carnegieclassifications.iu.edu/downloads/CCIHE2018-FactsFigures.pdf

Community for Creative Non-Violence v. Reid, 490 U.S. 730 (1989).

Copyright Act of 1909, Pub. L. 60-349, 35 Stat. 1075, H.R. 28192 (1909). Retrieved from http://www.copyright.gov/history/1909act.pdf

Copyright Act of 1976, Pub. L. No. 94-553, 90 Stat. 2541 (1976). Retrieved from http://www.copyright.gov/title17/92appa.pdf

Goodman, H. (1996, July 21). Professor depicts dispute as a racist plot. *The Philadelphia Inquirer*, p. Bl.

Harvard Plagiarism Archive. (2010). *Authorskeptics* (blog). Retrieved from http://authorskeptics.blogspot.com/

Jassin, L. J. (2010). Working with freelancers: What every publisher should know about the "work for hire" doctrine. *Copylaw.com*. Retrieved from http://www.copylaw.com/new_articles/wfh.html

Johnson, J. (2010, November 1). Stanford patent suit heads to U.S. Supreme Court. *Newsfix: KQED's Bay Area News Blog*. Retrieved from https://www.kqed.org/news/3644/stanford-patent-lawsuit-heads-to-u-s-supreme-court

Lamberg, L. (2004, Spring). The student, the professor, and the birth of modern sleep research. *Medicine on the Midway*, pp. 17–25.

Markos, K. (2010, July 28). Fort Lee man says professor, former friends stole his game design. *NorthJersey.com*. Retrieved from https://nl.newsbank.com/nl-search/we/Archives?p_widesearch=yes&p_multi=BE|NWNW|&p_product=NJMNP&p_theme=njmnp&p_action=search&p_maxdocs=200&s_dispstring=Fort%20Lee%20man%20says%20professor,%20former%20friends%20stole%20his%20game%20design&p_field_advanced-0=&p_text_advanced-0=(Fort%20Lee%20man%20says%20professor,%20former%20friends%20stole%20his%20game%20design)&xcal_numdocs=20&p_perpage=10&p_sort=YMD_date:D&xcal_useweights=no

Morley, D., & Parker, C. S. (2009). *Understanding computers: Today and tomorrow* (12th ed.). Boston, MA: Course Technology.

Roth, J. (2009). *Higher education in America* (10th ed.). Malvern, PA: Center for Education and Employment Law.

Seshadri v. Kasraian, No. 97-1610 (7th Cir. 1997).

Siegel, L. J. (2008). *Criminology* (10th ed.). Belmont, CA: Thomson Higher Education.

Smith, K. (2009, June 26). Openness and academic values. *Scholarly Communications @ Duke*. Retrieved from https://blogs.library.duke.edu/scholcomm/2009/06/26/openness-and-academic-values/

Stewart v. Abend, 495 U.S. 207 (1990) (Supreme Ct, No. 88-2102)

Story's Executives v. Holcombe, 23 F. Cas. 171, 175 (C.C. Ohio 1847).

Stripling, J. (2009, June 16). Code warrior. *Inside Higher Ed*. Retrieved from https://www.insidehighered.com/news/2009/06/16/code-warrior

Student is joint author, not liable for infringement in suit by professor. (1997). *Mealey's Litigation Reports: Intellectual Property*. Retrieved from http://cyber.law.harvard.edu/metaschool/fisher/joint/links/articles/mealey.html

Sullivan, K. J. (2011, February 23). *U.S. Supreme Court to hear arguments Feb. 28 in Stanford v. Roche*, Retrieved from https://news.stanford.edu/news/2011/february/supreme-court -lawsuit-022311.html

World Intellectual Property Organization. (n.d.). *What is intellectual property?* Retrieved from https://www .wipo.int/about-ip/en/

(top right chapter marker)

12

The Tenure Process

Case Study 12.1
The Tenure Process

Your role: You are Dr. O'Hara, the new dean in the college of nursing.

You have three faculty candidates applying for tenure and promotion this academic year. One of the candidates, Dr. Dorothy Sullivan, is wife of the Provost and Vice President for Academic Affairs. You report directly to the Provost, Dr. Hines. Due to the spousal relationship, you review Dr. Sullivan's personnel file to determine what arrangements were made for the evaluation of Dr. Sullivan's candidacy. No letter related to this matter exists in her file. You address the matter with Provost Hines and he informs you that Dr. Mason, the Vice Provost for Academic Affairs will review and serve as chair in Dr. Sullivan's case in lieu of the Provost. Dr. Mason also reports directly to Dr. Hines. The members of the College Tenure Committee request how Dr. Sullivan's case will be evaluated at the Provost's level. In scanning Dr. Sullivan's third review at the college level, you note that the former dean, department chair, and third year committee all focused on Dr. Sullivan's lack of scholarly and service productivity and poor collegiality. They found her quality of teaching record to be adequate. You are concerned because you have another faculty candidate who is borderline with respect to tenure and promotion. You worry Dr. Sullivan is more likely to receive tenure and promotion because of her spousal relationship.

Questions
- What are the potential conflicts in this case?
- Are the other nursing faculty receiving a fair review?
- What is best practice with respect to this case?

TENURE PROCESS: LEGAL PRINCIPLES AND REVIEW OF THE LITERATURE

The notion of tenure has been in place since the 12th century. Tenure protects faculty members by safeguarding academic freedom, ensuring a fair process prior to dismissal, and providing job security (Adams, 2006). The process of awarding academic tenure typically requires review of three key areas of participation within the academy: publishing, research, and program funding; service to the institution and community; and teaching. The emphasis and relative weight placed on each of these categories vary by academic institution.

The decision to award or deny tenure is perhaps the single most important decision in the career of a member of the faculty. Negative tenure decisions can cause extreme stress for tenure candidates, ill will in departments, and costly lawsuits for universities. Because careers can be broken by denials, challenges to denials are to be anticipated; and because fairness is both promised and demanded, all involved in the process (including judges who are often called in to review it at the end) are very sensitive to how fairly the candidate was treated. The tension arises when everyone agrees that on the merits the candidate does not deserve tenure, but also agrees that the college did not do what it should to hold up its end of the bargain. In a field such as nursing in which the faculty have spent their careers rendering aid and assistance to people, there may perhaps be even greater empathy and emphasis on protecting the candidate.

Most colleges and universities have well-articulated tenure policies. Tenured faculty and administrators have collaborated on developing standards and procedures that match their unique institutional circumstances. However, some aspects of a tenure policy may be unclear or incomplete, creating the potential for ambiguity or conflict. If a step is missed in the process, or if the tenure denial is based on a criterion that does not specifically appear in the written policy, or if the criteria changed after the candidate was initially hired on the tenure track, then the unsuccessful candidate may argue that the decision was unfair or improper.

Some courts are sympathetic to these claims. Other courts give universities latitude in interpreting, for example, research as including the ability to attract external funding, or teaching as including social skills in relating to students. The safest course for colleges and universities is to articulate written standards that reflect the major criteria that are actually used. The evaluators at all stages in the tenure process should know—and apply—the criteria (American Association of University Professors, American Council of Education, & United Educators Insurance Risk Retention Group [AAUP, ACE, & United Educators], 2000).

The AAUP, ACE, and United Educators (2000) issued a report that provides guidance on conducting tenure evaluations. The report, *Good Practice in Tenure Evaluation: Advice for Tenured Faculty, Department Chairs, and Academic Administrators,* recommends that tenure decisions be guided by four principles:

- *Clarity in standards and procedures.* Institutions should ensure that both the criteria and the process for tenure decisions are clearly delineated in writing, that they are communicated to candidates, and that they are followed in practice.
- *Consistency in decisions.* Tenure criteria should be applied consistently to all candidates regardless of personal characteristics—such as race, gender, disability, or national origin—that are protected by law or by university policy. It is also important that individual candidates be given consistent information and feedback during the probationary period.
- *Candor in evaluations.* Senior faculty should not back away from offering constructive criticism and a realistic assessment of how well a tenure candidate is meeting tenure requirements.
- *Caring for unsuccessful candidates.* Faculty and academic administrators should treat unsuccessful tenure candidates in a respectful and professional manner, making sure that they do not become isolated during the terminal year and providing whatever assistance possible to assist them in finding a new position.

The report stresses that faculty and administrators must collaborate to clarify tenure guidelines and adhere to tenure processes. In addition to following these principles, faculty and academic administrators should review their past tenure evaluations and ask the following questions: Have candidates who have been denied tenure been surprised by the decisions? Have lawsuits or disputes over tenure arisen? If so, what was learned as a result, and how can the policy or procedures be changed to reduce those risks in the future? It should also be made clear to candidates at the beginning of their appointment that annual evaluations may not be the same as tenure evaluations: The criteria for receiving a lifetime appointment are not the same as for receiving an annual pay increase. Negative tenure decisions that are preceded by positive evaluations and optimistic departmental promises are particularly problematic.

Faculty committees that hold tenure-granting rank are also considering collegiality when they make their tenure decisions. *Collegiality*—the spirit of collaboration and cooperation—recognizes important aspects of a faculty member's overall performance (AAUP, 1999, 2006). According to the AAUP (2006), collegiality does not have a distinct capacity to be assessed independently of the established three-part tenure test but is a quality whose worth is expressed in the successful implementation of three criteria—teaching, scholarship, and service. The AAUP (1999) also reminds members that collegiality is not simply enthusiasm, dedication, or a display of deference for the sake of harmony; rather, "such expectations are flatly contrary to elementary principles of academic freedom, which protect a faculty member's right to dissent from the judgments of colleagues and administrators" (p. 2). In essence, the AAUP has recommended against including collegial behaviors in faculty evaluations stating that the inclusion could hinder academic freedom by not allowing for dissent and that the construct of collegiality is vague and thus an effective tool to evaluate collegial behavior is not pragmatic (Johnston, Schimmel, & O'Hara, 2012).

That said, faculty members do have a duty of collegiality in the fulfillment of their job responsibilities and in satisfying their dual role as employees and managers in self-governance (Adams, 2006). As noted by Pertnoy (2004), "Each of us decides, depending on our individual interpretive mechanisms, whether being collegial means having a personality trait that suits ours, being able to disagree without being disagreeable, or having to forfeit one's contrary opinion to another's for the sake of keeping peace" (p. 202). With that said, universities are not insisting on congeniality but rather collegiality, which is generally viewed as promoting and participating in supportive interactions among colleagues. Despite concerns that collegiality is counter to a culture of thoughtful debate and a lively exchange of ideas and opinions in the academy, faculty exchanges should be conducted in a culture of mutual respect (Tacha, 1995). Collegiality plays an essential role in maintaining a respectful, supportive climate that supports the teaching, research, and service mission of the university.

The point is that if universities do want to use collegiality as a criterion in the consideration of a tenure candidate, it is only fair (and smart) to include it in the list of essential factors, so that candidates have notice in advance of what will be on the test, so to say. When it is included as a factor, the decisions that are made will be left alone. Courts recognize that the tenure decision is among the most personal decisions that a university can make, and therefore give significant deference to universities' tenure decisions, recognizing the subjective and evaluative nature of the decision. This applies to interpreting what is meant by the word *collegiality*. In fact, Connell and Savage (2001) state that "there is no case in which a court rejected consideration of collegiality unless there was evidence of discrimination or a violation of free speech or academic freedom" (p. 833).

DISCUSSION OF CASE STUDY

The avoidance of conflict of interest in a Tenure and Promotion review committee is an important consideration in the tenure review process, and the failure to adhere to policy is a violation of tenure process. This is more than just a checklist item. Although it could be argued that some tenure candidates have strong professional and social relationships with colleagues, a spousal or familial reporting relationship is prohibited in most settings, a spouse or family member cannot have direct supervision or evaluative authority over one's spouse or family member in most university settings. The university would not have followed its own personnel policies should they have allowed a spouse to evaluate one of their employees as in the case of a faculty member.

Conversely, tenure policies are not designed to be tests that the administration must pass at the end of the tenure review process or a game by which candidates can avoid harsh decisions by finding missteps. The tenure track is intended to be a pathway to learning as well as evaluation, and tenure candidates have duties as well as rights. If a step is missed or a conflict exists, the tenure candidate or other faculty should be expected to point it out and correct the issue. In Case Study 12.1, Dean O'Hara rightly contacted Legal Counsel to discuss her concerns and the concerns of her faculty. She would be under immense pressure to provide a favorable review to Dr. Sullivan or compromise her own relationship with the Provost and possibly her career in this situation. The nursing faculty had already recognized the serious conflict of interest.

As per AAUP, ACE, and United Educators (2000) in *Good Practice in Tenure Evaluation: Advice for Tenured Faculty, Department Chairs, and Academic Administrators,* tenure criteria should be applied consistently to all candidates regardless of personal characteristics—and certainly without regard to such factors as race, gender, disability, sexual preference, national origin, or other factors that the law defines as illegal. It is also important that individual candidates be given consistent information, feedback, and treatment during the probationary period. In Case Study 12.1, the university's tenure criteria could have been compromised because Dr. Sullivan had a distinct political advantage because of her relationship with the Provost, as his spouse. Other faculty could have filed grievances or lawsuit if they did not obtain tenure because of this conflict of interest and perceived advantage. Even the substitution of the Associate Provost for Academic Affairs, Dr. Mason, for the Provost's role in the discussions of Dr. Sullivan's case, is questionable as the Associate Provost for Academic Affairs reports directly to the Provost. Dr. Mason could feel immense pressure to sway the University Tenure and Promotion Committee and/or recommend the granting of tenure to the President.

WHEN TO CONSULT THE UNIVERSITY COUNSEL

- Consult counsel with tenure policy changes and implementation.
- Consult counsel if violations in the tenure policy occur.

FINDINGS AND DISPOSITION

In Case Study 12.1, a conflict of interest exists if the Provost weighs in on his wife's candidacy for tenure and promotion. The involvement of the Provost in a ruling on his wife's case would have deleterious effects on the integrity of the tenure process at the university. To avoid the appearance of a conflict of interest, the Associate Provost for Academic Affairs, Dr. Mason was originally asked to "step in" for the Provost at the University Committee level. Dean O'Hara consulted Legal Counsel to discuss her and her faculty's concerns about the situation. In the current organizational structure, the Dean and Associate Provost were in precarious political positions, responsible for writing evaluative letters for the Provost's wife and possibly damaging their future employment relationship with their supervisor if the letters are not favorable in nature or conversely potentially losing the trust of the faculty if they support the candidate. Legal Counsel consulted with the President in this matter and developed an alternative process whereby the case would be reviewed by an external dean at a comparable university. The President would meet with the University Tenure Committee with respect to this case in an effort to maintain the integrity of the tenure process and protect the dean of the college. The Associate Provost for Academic Affairs was removed from the process since he reports directly to the Provost. At its end, the College Tenure and Promotion Committee did not recommend Dr. Sullivan for tenure and promotion by a unanimous vote. She received poor evaluations by her department, by the external dean, and University Committee, and was denied tenure. One can only imagine the outrage if Dr. Sullivan had obtained tenure despite the college faculty's objections because of a spousal relationship. Faculty who denied tenure could file lawsuits because of these perceived injustices.

RELEVANT LEGAL CASE

University of Baltimore v. Iz, 716 A.2d 1107 (Md. Ct. Spec. App. 1998)

University of Baltimore v. Iz (1998) was a lawsuit against the University of Baltimore for sex and national origin discrimination under Title VII, violation of equal protection and breach of contract, which Dr. Iz filed following the denial of her tenure candidacy. The steps in the tenure review process were as follows:

- In 1989, the University of Baltimore hired Dr. Iz as a visiting assistant professor under a 1-year contract. Her appointment was in the Department of Information and Qualitative Sciences in the Merrick School of Business.

- In 1990, Dr. Iz accepted the university's offer of a tenure-track position. Based on credit for a prior faculty appointment at Miami University, her initial tenure review date was the 1994 to 1995 academic year, but the applicable policy permitted early tenure review. Against the advice of senior departmental colleagues, Dr. Iz decided to undergo tenure review 1 year early, in 1993 to 1994. Although the policy on early review does not require a vote, the tenured members of her department voted (5 to 1, with one abstention) to recommend against early tenure review. Dr. Iz appealed to the university's central administration, and the president informed her that she could seek early review but, if she were denied tenure, then she would not receive another review. She decided to proceed with the early review, and the provost instructed the Merrick faculty to consider her for tenure with promotion to the rank of associate professor.
- At the first stage of review, Dr. Iz's tenured colleagues in the department voted 3 to 2 against tenure, with one abstention. Relying on a recent review of her teaching, research, and service, which had been required at the end of her third year, her colleagues noted in a written report that Dr. Iz "has been showing progress and would have a stronger case next year." In addition, the former department chair, who had held the position for 17 years and had hired Dr. Iz, emailed his vote while he was away on sabbatical; providing one of the three recommendations against tenure, he stated that she was a good teacher, had publications, and was involved in professional service activities, but he expressed concern about "her attitude and collegiality."
- The current department chair, however, recommended in favor of tenure and promotion, judging her as meeting or exceeding the necessary qualifications for teaching, research, and service.
- Next, the school's Tenure and Promotion Committee voted 6 to 4 in favor of awarding tenure to Dr. Iz.
- After receiving these three recommendations, the dean voted against tenure and promotion. In his opinion, Dr. Iz met or exceeded the qualifications for research and service but not for teaching. He also observed that she was reluctant to accept "peer evaluation" and that her colleagues had "strongly recommended that she not apply early for tenure and promotion."
- Before making his final determination, the provost met separately with Dr. Iz and the department chair to give them an opportunity to be heard on the points where Dr. Iz's performance had been found inadequate in the process. In a follow-up letter, the department chair confirmed that Dr. Iz was inflexible, defensive, and unwilling to take constructive advice, including peer evaluation. Further, he explained that he had not included this information in his recommendation because he had not regarded it as a pertinent criterion in the tenure and promotion process.
- Subsequently, the provost recommended against tenure and promotion. Although acknowledging Dr. Iz's strengths in research and service, he found significance in her difficulties with her departmental colleagues.
- Dr. Iz filed an internal appeal. The Tenure Appeals Committee was split and could not reach an agreement on whether or not to uphold the provost's tenure denial.
- The president accepted the provost's recommendation against tenure.
- Dr. Iz sued the university on the basis of sex and national origin discrimination under Title VII, violation of equal protection and breach of contract. The breach of contract claim was based on Dr. Iz's assertion that the university could only use criteria that were specifically listed in the university tenure policy, and that collegiality was not one of those factors.
- The jury determined that the university had breached Dr. Iz's contract and awarded $425,000 in compensatory damages.
- The university filed an appeal.

The only issue before the appellate court was whether the university had the right to use collegiality as a criterion for tenure, even though it was not specifically referenced. "We are persuaded that collegiality plays an essential role in both teaching and service" (716 A.2d at 1122). The court held that the trial court should have ruled, as a matter of law, that the university could use collegiality as a tenure criterion.

Among other things, it is worth noting that the appellate court's decision was rendered 4 years after the tenure process had occurred. The amount of time, expense, and disruption this process caused cannot be underestimated. Simply including collegiality among the factors that would be considered for tenure would have prevented it all. In fact, several courts have ruled that the lack of civility or collegiality can be used as a legitimate basis to terminate a full-time faculty member (*Bresnick v. Manhattanville College, Stein v. Kent State University*).

SUMMARY

Consideration for tenure is a fundamental moment in an academic's career. Therefore, it is imperative that tenured faculty and administrators use best practices discussed in this chapter as well as the advice outlined in *Good Practice in Tenure Evaluation: Advice for Tenured Faculty, Department Chairs, and Academic Administrators* (AAUP, ACE, & United Educators, 2000). A consistent, fair, and transparent process is in the best interest of the tenure candidate, faculty, administrators, and the university. Knowledge of the promotion and tenure process is essential to success for nursing faculty. The majority of nursing faculty come to the academic setting from the clinical environment. Consequently, the tenure and promotion process may not be familiar to junior nursing faculty prior to their entry into the academy, so it is important for faculty to familiarize themselves with the tenure requirements and institutional culture (O'Connor & Yanni, 2013).

For the nursing professor entering the academic arena, knowledge of promotion and tenure is essential. O'Connor and Yanni (2013) address eight important lessons for nurse academics pursuing tenure and promotion:

1. Know the institutional requirements.
2. Know the department's available resources (human and material).
3. Find a mentor or mentors.
4. Systematically collect cumulative evidence to support your case with knowledge of institutional perspectives and priorities.
5. Establish the importance of teaching and how it is measured.
6. Establish the importance of service and how it is measure.
7. Identify and develop a research/scholarly agenda.
8. State your case convincingly and present your evidence persuasively. (pp. 84–86)

Prevention Tips

- *Institutions should ensure that both the criteria and the process for tenure decisions are clearly delineated in writing, that they are communicated to candidates, and that they are followed in practice (AAUP, ACE, & United Educators, 2000).*
- *Offer development sessions to department chairs and academic administrators on offering constructive feedback during the annual faculty review process.*
- *If universities wish to use collegiality as a criterion in the consideration of tenure candidates, it is only fair (and smart) to include it in the list of essential factors, so that candidates have notice in advance concerning what will be used as a criterion for tenure.*

CRITICAL ELEMENTS TO CONSIDER

- The tenure policy should comprehensively list all the major criteria used for evaluation.
- The policy and procedures should be reviewed by the university attorney to determine areas in which they are unclear or might not fully express the university's expectations for tenured faculty.
- The evaluators at all stages in the tenure process should know—and apply—the criteria.

- The tenure policy should address whether tenure evaluators will consider positive events occurring after the tenure application has been submitted.

- The tenure policy should indicate what steps the institution will take if a faculty member under consideration for tenure is charged with misconduct or if other negative events emerge.

- The tenure policy should indicate times when the "clock" will stop, slow, or otherwise be adjusted (e.g., leave for disability or pregnancy, maternity, military service).

- The tenure policy should address the voting protocol when an evaluator serves at more than one level of review (e.g., department chair in the same discipline).

- Individual faculty members may wish to express their own opinions about a tenure candidate to members of the campus-wide promotion and tenure committee or to the administration. The tenure policy should address how the recipients should treat these individual opinions.

- All reviewers should meticulously follow tenure procedures. The probationary faculty members should also be instructed as to their obligation to be a full participant in the process, and their duty to call errors to the attention of the dean (or other appropriate official).

  - Take conflicts of interest in promotion seriously—any conflict of interest needs to be brought to the attention of the University Legal Counsel and Provost for review and consideration. The Provost will then render a decision and inform all parties in writing about changes in the tenure and promotion process. If the Provost has a conflict of interest, the President will stipulate in writing any changes in the Tenure and Promotion process.

  - Recognize the power tenured faculty have over junior faculty and monitor for abuses.

- Conduct workshops for department chairs on the appointment and evaluation of tenure-track faculty.

- Conduct workshops on tenure procedures for faculty serving on the tenure and promotions committee (AAUP, ACE, & United Educators, 2000).

ETHICAL CONSIDERATIONS

The job protection afforded with tenure is unique—termination only for "good cause" is not the norm in America, where at-will employment contracts are the standard (meaning workers can be fired for any reasons, except those specifically prohibited by antidiscrimination laws). The termination for cause has ethical implications as do the ethical issues that arise in tenure decisions. Let's be candid, tenure in the United States has not been helped by the fact that universities regularly fail to undertake proceedings for termination when good cause actually does exist (sexual harassment, incivility, low productivity; Leiter, 2017), due to political cowardice, legal exposure, or negative press. Tenure does play a distinct role in academia because of the unique function of universities in the discovery of truth and knowledge development and therefore should be safeguarded. Faculty should be protected from political interest groups and corporate entities to pursue knowledge free of political interference (Leiter, 2017). However, when the protection (tenure) intended to promote the specific social good (discovery of truth and knowledge development) of academic professions is corrupted in order to protect misbehaving individuals whose actions do not clearly further the profession's goals, not only are the profession's goals at risk but so is the integrity of the tenure system and even the profession itself.

The integrity of the tenure system is critical to the protection of tenure, which is critical to the furtherance of the professional goals of academics. Nursing faculty need to be cognizant of potential ethical violations, which include discrimination—age, gender, race/ethnicity, religion, or sexuality, in addition to equity in workload and expectations. Fewer nursing academics successfully achieve tenure than other disciplines outside of allied health. There is speculation that these low numbers have been attributed to underperformance in the area of scholarship by nursing faculty, who are predominantly female and socialized to be service oriented (O'Connor & Yanni, 2013). However, issues of gender equity and gender bias are ethical concerns that warrant consideration, close observation, and action. Is the nursing faculty workload higher than male-dominated disciplines? Do nursing faculty receive the same benefits as other faculty disciplines (start-up packages, mentoring, conference support, grant peer review, editorial support, compensation levels, restricted service obligations, etc.)? As a predominantly female profession, academic nursing needs to pay close attention to the rates of promotion of nursing faculty.

References

Adams, M. L. (2006). The quest for tenure: Job security and academic freedom. *The Catholic University Law Review, 56*(67), 189–190. Retrieved from https://papers.ssrn.com/sol3/papers.cfm?abstract_id=1133641

American Association of University Professors. (1999). *On collegiality as a criterion for faculty evaluation.* Retrieved from http://www.aaup.org/AAUP/pubsres/policydocs/contents/collegiality.htm

American Association of University Professors. (2006). On collegiality as a criterion for faculty evaluation. In *Policy Documents and Reports* (10th ed.). Washington, DC: Author.

American Association of University Professors, American Council of Education, & United Educators Insurance Risk Retention Group. (2000). *Good practice in tenure evaluation: Advice for tenured faculty, department chairs, and academic administrators.* Retrieved from https://www.aaup.org/sites/default/files/files/Good%20Practice%20in%20Tenure%20Evaluation.pdf

Bresnick v. Manhattanville College, (SDNY, 1994) 864 F. Supp. 327, 95 Ed. Law Rep 121.

Connell, M. A., & Savage, F. G. (2001). The role of collegiality in higher education tenure, promotion, and termination decisions. *Journal of College and University Law, 27*(2), 833–843.

Johnston, P.C, Schimmel, T., & O'Hara, H. (2012). Revisiting the AAUP recommendation: The viability of collegiality as a fourth criterion for university faculty evaluation. *College Quarterly.* Retrieved from https://files.eric.ed.gov/fulltext/EJ976454.pdf

Leiter, B. (2017). Academic ethics: Rethinking the justification of tenure. *The Chronicle of Higher Education.* Retrieved from https://www.chronicle.com/article/Academic-Ethics-Rethinking/238888

Pertnoy, L. (2004). The "C" word: Collegiality real or imaginary, and should it matter in a tenure process. *St. Thomas Law Review, 17,* 201–224.

O'Connor, L. G., & Yanni, C. K. (2013). Promotion and tenure in nursing education: Lessons learned. *Journal of Nursing Education and Practice, 3*(5), 78–88. doi:10.5430/jnep.v3n5p78

Stein v. Kent State University Board of Trustees, 994 F. Supp. 898 (N.D. Ohio 1998) aff'd181 F.3d 103 (6th Cir. 1999).

Tacha, D. R. (1995). The "C" word: On collegiality. *Ohio State Law Journal, 56,* 585–587.

University of Baltimore v. Iz, 716 A.2d 1107 (Md. Ct. Spec. App. 1998).

13

Harassment

Case Study 13.1
Harassment

Your role: You are the Chair of the Undergraduate Nursing Program, Dr. Ashley Miller.

You assumed the Chair position when the NCLEX-RN® scores were in the low 80s with respect to first-time NCLEX-RN pass rate. The State Board of Nursing (in your state) requires an 80% first-time pass rate or the nursing program is placed on probationary status. Dr. Miller developed a comprehensive curricular approach with the faculty, which included the integration of standardized exams and a comprehensive standardized exam at the end of the program. NCLEX-RN pass rates have increased in an incremental fashion to most recently, 92%. This year, 21 students out of 200 students (11%) did not pass the comprehensive exam after two attempts. Dr. Miller arranged for the students to get free remediation in the summer and free campus housing until they were successful. She also arranged for remedial tutoring, both individual and group sessions by the BSN Success Coach, Mr. Hunt. Dr. Miller is concerned that an 11% failure rate for the end of the program is higher than other years. She also notes that this class has a higher percentage of borderline students with grades of C in clinical courses. Once the grades are officially released, Dr. Miller is bombarded with phone calls from angry parents—demanding that Dr. Miller pass their children. Some express an interest to meet with Dr. Miller in person; others call the Dean, Provost, and President. Dr. Miller meets with the course faculty again to examine the issue—the students are clearly weaker than other students with respect to nursing content. The affected students missed classes in some cases, and did not complete remediation and other assignments. Dr. Miller continues to receive threatening phone calls from parents, one of which is a university administrator, Dr. Johnson, who appears to be the leader of the parents. Dr. Miller consults the Dean for advice and assistance as she is feeling harassed. During this time, it is discovered that the parents (many of whom are wealthy) have hired a public relations firm to embarrass Dr. Miller and pressure the school to forego the course requirement and pass their student in various ways. Dr. Miller is barraged with emails, appeal letters, and phone calls. A group of parents develops a social media page stating they are going to get Dr. Miller fired. Dr. Johnson, the University Administrator, has posted on the social media page, making derogatory and racist remarks about Dr. Miller and the nursing program. He has also posted derogatory remarks on other nursing websites.

Questions

- How would you proceed?
- What are the implications for the university administrator, Dr. Johnson?
- What actions should you take in your role as the Chair? Does the school have any jurisdiction over the social media page?

DEALING WITH WORKPLACE HARASSMENT: LEGAL PRINCIPLES AND REVIEW OF THE LITERATURE

Dr. Miller is in a difficult position—balancing the health and welfare of the public and maintaining the reputation of the program by graduating knowledgeable nurses with unreasonable parental demands to forego graduation requirements, one of which is a university administrator. Nursing faculty and administrators can receive intense pressure from nursing students and parents in these instances. In some cases, the incivility escalates creating faculty and administrator distress.

Foremost, administrators are responsible for maintaining the quality of the workplace environment, as well as the performance quality of employees. Those who are responsible for the educational mission must also protect and enhance the quality of the academic and research missions, for both students and faculty. However, administrators may also be members of the faculty themselves, and entitled to enjoy the benefits and protections that are awarded to faculty. When one member of the faculty attacks others (including an administrator), the situation can become very complex.

Broadly speaking, *harassment* occurs whenever offensive or unwelcome conduct affects the performance of a person or persons. If it is expressed against a person in a protected class, harassment can also constitute discrimination that violates local, state, and/or federal laws. The prohibitions are meant to combat decision-making based on stereotypes, and typically include race, sex, age, national origin, religious belief, and sexual orientation. The harasser can be in the same protected class as the victim and can be the victim's supervisor, coworker, or even a nonemployee (e.g., a student or a student's parent). Federal law is often very specific in prohibiting discrimination, as with this statement from the U.S. Department of Education Office for Civil Rights (OCR), which is charged with enforcing Title IX:

> No person in the United States shall, on the basis of sex, be excluded from participation in, be denied the benefits of, or be subjected to discrimination under any education program or activity receiving Federal financial assistance.

The OCR (2019) recognizes two types of gender-based sexual harassment in academic institutions: quid pro quo harassment and hostile environment harassment.

> Under the law, there are two kinds of discriminatory harassment—quid pro quo harassment of a sexual nature where someone is threatened with a negative consequence unless certain favors are granted or where someone is seduced by the promise of a positive consequence. The second kind of discriminatory harassment is called hostile environment. Hostile environment harassment, may occur whenever someone's offensive conduct has the effect of interfering with another's performance. For example, words or behaviors that put down an individual by insulting an aspect of the person's identity (race, sexual orientation, gender, national origin, etc.) can create a hostile work or study environment for that individual. It is easy to recognize quid pro quo harassment, but hostile environment harassment frequently goes unrecognized or is not acknowledged either by the victim or by the one who is causing the problem.

Words or behaviors that are considered severe enough to create a hostile environment may be determined by such factors as the nature of the conduct (physical or verbal); the frequency of the conduct; and the degree of offensiveness (U.S. Equal Employment Opportunity Commission [EEOC], 2018).

Federal and state laws exist to make sure that employees do not have to endure prejudice at the workplace that is based on age, sex, race, national origin, pregnancy, religion, sexual preference, veteran status, and disability. These laws include Title VII of the Civil Rights Act of 1964, the Age Discrimination in Employment Act of 1967 (ADEA), and the American Disabilities Act of 1990 (ADA; EEOC, 2018), among others. The law protects everyone, regardless of whether the prejudice arises from the administration, from superiors, from colleagues, or from third parties. Employers have the obligation to protect their employees from such discrimination, and from any form of illegal harassment.

There is liability when the conduct is severe or pervasive enough to create a work environment that a reasonable person would consider intimidating, hostile, or abusive. Such conduct may include slurs, physical assault or threats, intimidation, insults, or interference with work performance. Isolated examples of improper comments, especially made by those who are in no position to affect someone's compensation or conditions or work, typically do not rise to the level of illegality. They can become so when the comments become frequent, managers are aware of them, and management fails to respond and stop them. At that point, the management can be deemed to have "accepted" them and allowed them to "be" the workplace environment.

The American Association of University Women (AAUW; 2005) published a report on sexual harassment at colleges and universities, which defined sexual harassment as "unwanted and unwelcome sexual behavior, which interfered with your life" (p. 8). Sexual harassment may occur throughout the campus, including in student housing and classrooms. Student-to-student harassment is the most common form of sexual harassment on campus. The #Me Too movement has increased awareness about sexual assault that dates back over 10 years ago and has garnered widespread media attention after dozens of women in the film industry alleged that Harvey Weinstein had engaged in a myriad of acts of sexual misconduct. As these accusations surfaced, conversations have shifted to the broader issue of institutional sexism and gender discrimination against women in other industries, including the academy. The #Me Too and Time's Up movements have created a platform for women to challenge inappropriate gender-related treatment in the workplace (Soklaridis et al., 2018).

Because employers bear the burden related to harassment in the workplace, it is in the employer's best interest to educate employees concerning workplace harassment. There should be unambiguous communication regarding both the types of behaviors that constitute harassment and the specific behaviors that will not be tolerated in the work environment. In the event that workplace harassment is suspected, harassment-reporting mechanisms and harassment policies and procedures need to be clearly identified, including associated reporting documentation required by the university. The university should also conduct faculty education that teaches faculty how to identify behaviors that are consistent with harassment, and it should emphasize its zero tolerance for workplace harassment (EEOC, 2020).

Prevention Tips

Prevention is the best action to obviate workplace harassment. Preventive measures are usually in the form of "Workplace Violence Prevention Programs," new faculty orientation, and human resources policies that prohibit workplace harassment (Kelleher, 1996; Nelson, Anis-Abdellatif, Larson, Mulder, & Wolff, 2016). To help prevent harassment at your university or college, it is important to establish a code of conduct for faculty and students so that everyone is clear as to what does and does not constitute harassment. Publish the code of conduct both in print and on the website so that student and faculty can easily access the information. Hold seminars in which the harassment policy is reviewed, and provide anti-harassment training to all administrators and faculty.

Failure to address problem behaviors could give the harasser, the victim, and other in the organization the impression that the harassing behavior is tolerated. It is suggested that the faculty member speak to the harasser directly regarding the unwanted behavior and ask for the conduct to cease immediately (Kolanko et al., 2006; Mansfield, Beck, Fung, Montiel, & Goldman, 2017). However, supervisors and faculty need to be familiar with their institution's policies on sexual harassment and nondiscrimination and the reporting obligations they have under those policies. Most colleges and universities have now established written policies and procedures to govern the handling of discrimination and harassment allegations and complaints. These policies and procedures will usually assign specific offices and administrators with the responsibility for investigating and adjudicating these claims. Faculty may have a mandatory obligation under the school's policy to report the hostile work environment to a supervisor so that an investigation can take place and prevent the situation from further escalation.

The entire academic community should be educated concerning the triggers that may prompt a hostile work environment. These triggers may include feeling uncomfortable or threatened when a colleague makes a personal, racial, or ethnic slur. The development and implementation of a code of conduct for faculty and students will assist in alerting the academic community what behaviors constitute harassment and of the associated consequences for such behaviors; the code of conduct will emphasize that the university has zero tolerance for harassment by any member of its community (Kolanko et al., 2006). The code of conduct should clearly communicate to the academic community that unwelcome harassing conduct is not tolerated. Universities can achieve this objective by establishing an effective complaint or grievance process, providing anti-harassment training to all faculty and administrators, and taking immediate and appropriate action when an employee or student complains. Universities should strive to create an environment in which students, faculty, and staff feel free to raise concerns and are confident that those concerns will be addressed (Kaplin, Lee, Hutchens, & Rooksby, 2019).

It is important that all employees, especially those who are faculty and administrators, recognize their obligations to report improper conduct and take appropriate measures to stop the harassment. Failure to act in accordance with these obligations may result in disciplinary action against the employee and should also be noted in evaluating their job performance.

Social media has become the way that people communicate. Some seem to live on their Facebook pages. What they do there is not what they do in the classroom or on campus. Few universities actively monitor student speech, not just because of constitutional protections (free speech), but also because universities do not want to put themselves into the role of Internet police, searching for and responding to instances of improper conduct. However, this does not mean that universities do not have to respond when social media activities that violate the law or institutional policies are reported to them. It should be noted that employees are generally held to a higher standard if they identify oneself as a university employee.

> Employee Use – When using social media as a part of their official duties, and/or when presenting oneself in social media settings as a university representative, employees must comply with applicable University policies governing employee behavior and acceptable use of electronic and information resources. (University of Houston, 2019)

DISCUSSION OF CASE STUDY

As Department Chair, you report the incident to legal counsel, public relations, and the Dean of the School of Nursing, alerting all of them to the problem and asking them to review the situation and respond as appropriate. You provide the transcripts, a record of completed assignments in the capstone course, and attendance records for the capstone class and remediation sessions to the Dean and legal counsel. You also share the Undergraduate Student Handbook and course syllabi for the capstone course in addition to the electronic signatures of the 21 students attesting that they understood that they were responsible for understanding and abiding by the current policies in the Student Handbook for the last 4 years. As a member of the faculty, you file a formal grievance against Dr. Johnson so that there is a record on file of your dissatisfaction with his behavior. The office of legal counsel does send Dr. Johnson, the University Administrator, an email to desist all communication on social media and other websites disparaging Dr. Miller. A copy of the letter is also sent to the Provost, Dr. Johnson's direct supervisor.

WHEN TO CONSULT THE UNIVERSITY COUNSEL

Consult the university counsel if you directly observe or receive secondhand reports or information about conduct or behavior that may be illegal harassment or discrimination.

FINDINGS AND DISPOSITION

Dr. Miller is shaken from the bombardment of angry emails, calls, and meetings with parents. She is particularly concerned with the racist remarks posted on the social media site and the petition that calls for her firing. The Provost and legal counsel meet with Dr. Johnson, a University Administrator who heads the Center for History and Politics and whose daughter is in the nursing program. During the meeting, Professor Johnson is suspended pending further investigation of the situation and is informed to cease and desist all derogatory and racist remarks about Dr. Miller. He is also referred to the appropriate policies for all personnel including faculty. The resolution of the issue will be conducted in accordance with the guidelines, policies, and procedures of the university. He is also informed that Dr. Miller has filed a grievance against him. Legal counsel also sends a letter to the 21 parents to cease and desist *harassing* communication with Dr. Miller; they are permitted to engage in collegial discussions about their student's remediation. The Public Relations Department prepares a press release to the media addressing the importance of graduating safe, knowledgeable nurses who are going to care for sick patients in the community. This is especially important because graduate nurses can practice without an RN license for 1 year in the area. The press release reads:

> The University takes its responsibility to graduate knowledgeable safe nurses very seriously. Although the university regrets that 21 nursing students are inconvenienced for 6 weeks while they prepare for their comprehensive exam, patient safety is our priority. In an educational philosophy consistent with our mission, tuition and student housing is free for these students while they work diligently to complete their studies. We stand behind our curriculum and graduation requirements that all of nursing majors are required to meet.

After an investigation by the Faculty Grievance Committee, Dr. Johnson is demoted from his administrative position by the Provost (as he served at the Provost's discretion) and returns to the faculty in the history department with a strict warning that any future racist remarks or verified harassing behaviors will be considered "good cause" for the removal of tenure and termination. The 21 students successfully passed the comprehensive exam in the summer with additional remediation and study time and the NCLEX-RN on the first attempt. The university also developed communication guidelines for faculty and university employees who have children enrolled in the university, especially in light of the fact that university employees receive tuition remission for their children.

RELEVANT LEGAL CASE

Gupta v. Florida Board of Regents, 212 F.3d 571 (11th Cir. 2000), cert, denied, 121 S.Ct. 772 (2001)

Dr. Srabana Gupta joined Florida Atlantic University's faculty as an assistant professor of economics in August 1994 on the university's Davie campus. Her position was within the social sciences division of the College of Liberal Arts. During the 1994 to 1995 academic year, Dr. Rupert Rhodd was the coordinator of the social sciences division for the Davie campus, and Dr. Gupta reported to him.

In *Gupta v. Florida Board of Regents,* Dr. Gupta alleged that Dr. Rhodd sexually harassed her during a 7-month period of time following her arrival at the campus. The supervisor's behavior included twice touching the professor's leg and dress (making comments to her, such as "women are like meat" and "men need a variety of women"; and calling her at home two to three times a week).

One morning after a bad thunderstorm the night before, Dr. Rhodd called Dr. Gupta and asked if she needed a ride to a university seminar. During that conversation, he said, "Oh, you were all by yourself on a dark and stormy night? Why didn't you call me? I would have come and spent the night with you." Dr. Gupta understood Dr. Rhodd's suggestion to mean "that he wanted to [have a] sexual relationship with me." She told him, "Don't talk to me that way. You are talking nonsense." Dr. Gupta complained to several people about his inappropriate conduct, and instituted an informal dispute resolution process in January 1995 through one of the university's sexual harassment counselors; however, that process was discontinued in September 1995 as a result of Dr. Gupta's failure to participate.

Dr. Gupta filed suit in the spring of 1996 against Dr. Rhodd for sexual harassment, and against the board of regents for allowing the harassment and permitting a hostile work environment. She later amended the complaint to allege that the university had retaliated against her (made her working conditions more difficult) after she had complained to the university about Dr. Rhodd's conduct. The jury found that Dr. Rhodd had not harassed her, but found the board liable both for having permitted a hostile environment and for retaliation.

The board appealed the decision. The appellate court began by noting there are two types of sexual harassment claims: (a) quid pro quo, which are "based on threats which are carried out" or fulfilled, and (b) hostile environment, which are based on "bothersome attentions or sexual remarks that are sufficiently severe or pervasive to create a hostile work environment" (Kaplin et al., 2019). The court of appeals found no evidence at all in the record to support a claim of quid pro quo sexual harassment. It found that Dr. Rhodd had engaged in conduct that was "bothersome and uncomfortable" for Dr. Gupta, but it was not "physically threatening or intimidating," nor of the type that would "unreasonably interfere with the plaintiff's job performance"; rather, the court termed his conduct "the ordinary tribulations of the workplace." Most of the conduct that was offensive to her was not explicitly sexual in nature, though she interpreted it as such; they also found that it was not "so frequent, severe, or pervasive" that a reasonable person would have found it to constitute sexual harassment or to have felt it created a "hostile environment."

With respect to the retaliation claim, "Dr. Gupta presented testimony that she was subject to the following actions, which she contends are adverse employment actions: (1) she was not given a pay raise despite an above satisfactory evaluation by her supervisor; (2) she was denied an extension on her tenure clock; (3) she was placed on the search committee for a position at the university's Boca Raton campus, which prevented her from applying for that position; (4) she was assigned to teach more credit hours than other professors and to teach classes on three different campuses in the fall 1997 session; (5) she was not assigned to teach a desired class in the summer 1995 second session; (6) Dean White's office intentionally delayed her visa application to the Immigration and Naturalization Service; and (7) the informal resolution process involving her sexual harassment claim was terminated without notice after she missed one deadline."

The court held that charges (3) through (7) did not constitute "adverse employment actions." None of those actions were "objectively serious and tangible enough" to alter Gupta's "compensation, terms, conditions, or privileges of employment, deprive … her of employment opportunities or adversely affect … her status as an employee." In particular, the court held that a university has the right to assign its professors to teach the classes it needs them to teach and that an action cannot be termed *adverse* if it is corrected as soon as the proper official is made aware of it and before it goes into effect. The court did hold that the first two charges would, if supported, constitute "adverse employment actions" but also found that the university had demonstrated the decisions were made on the merits.

Requiring the plaintiff to prove that the harassment is severe or pervasive ensures that Title VII does not become a mere general civility code. The court had no doubt that Dr. Gupta subjectively perceived the alleged harassment to be unwelcome, inappropriate, and threatening. However, a court will consider four factors in determining whether statements and conduct are sufficiently severe and pervasive from an objective standpoint to alter an employee's terms or conditions of employment: "(1) the frequency of the conduct; (2) the severity of the conduct; (3) whether the conduct is physically threatening or humiliating, or a mere offensive utterance; and (4) whether the conduct unreasonably interferes with the employee's job performance."

The case of *Gupta v. Florida Board of Regents* illustrates that uncomfortable or bothersome remarks are not considered liable. The conduct complained of must be "sufficiently severe or pervasive to alter the conditions of employment and create an abusive work environment." It is this element that tests the spirit of most sexual harassment claims.

In the case of *Finke v. Purdue University*, Finke, the dean of the College of Health and Human Services, raised the following claims: (a) sex discrimination in violation of Title VII against all Defendants; (b) hostile work environment in violation of Title VII against all Defendants; (c) age discrimination in violation of the Age Discrimination in Employment Act against all Defendants; (d) violation of the Equal Pay Act against all Defendants; and (e) disparate treatment on the basis of sex in violation of the Fourteenth Amendment (made applicable against the state by 42 U.S.C. § 1983), after her demotion as dean. Finke agreed to dismiss all of these claims other than the Equal Pay Act claim against the Provost and Chancellor. In doing so, Finke must show that she was a member of a protected class, she was meeting her employer's legitimate expectations, she suffered an adverse employment action, and the university treated a similarly situated man more favorably. There is ample evidence that Finke was not meeting her employer's legitimate performance expectations, and thus, her claim fails there. Second, even assuming that Finke could establish a clear case, Purdue has proffered a legitimate reason for the disparity: The median salary in the marketplace, according to the CUPA, for a position like Finke's, Dean of the College of Health and Human Services, is lower than her other dean colleagues.

SUMMARY

People can say bad things—even things that are racist—without it creating a legal liability for the university or its administrators. For a liability to occur, either the actor must be in a position to influence or affect the individual's quality of employment directly (through punishing behavior such as adverse work assignments or deprivation of benefits) or the conduct must be of such significance and persistence that it adversely affects the workplace to the point at which a supervisor should have done something to stop it. However, just because the conduct does not qualify as illegal discrimination or harassment does not mean that the university is powerless to stop such behavior. Employees may still be subject to disciplinary action if the conduct is considered objectionable in not meeting performance standards, unprofessional or in violation of another university policy like a code of conduct.

Universities should note the value that the court's decisions have placed on the existence of accessible harassment policies and complaint procedures. To minimize liability for harassment, colleges and universities should make their anti-harassment policies and procedures clear, publish and disseminate them as widely as possible, and provide training to potential complaint handlers and faculty, staff, and students (Kaplin et al., 2019).

Complainants should be treated with respect and compassion, and be given anonymity when possible and protection from retaliation. Respondents should receive due process during the investigation. It should be the intent of all colleges and universities to offer a place where students and faculty can pursue knowledge independent of threats or assaults; at the same time, free speech and the ability to criticize, even unfairly, is core to the mission. Universities are not responsible for what students do off campus, but social media knows no geographic boundary. When what is being done online is adversely affecting the academic mission, a court may hold a university responsible for getting involved. What those duties and liabilities are has not yet been determined. However, it is likely that a university will not be found liable if it acts reasonably under the circumstances to address the situation as it affects the university community according to standards that are appropriate for its mission (e.g., codes of conduct that require civility among classmates). The university must fairly and impartially review all harassment charges and deal with such matters in a confidential and professional manner. The college/university should also prohibit any behavior that is in retaliation to an individual who files a harassment complaint. University administration is responsible for publicizing and implementing a stringent sexual and racial harassment policy in addition to educating all constituencies in promoting a zero tolerance for student harassment.

CRITICAL ELEMENTS TO CONSIDER

- Consult human resources.
- Establish an effective complaint or grievance process.
- Respond immediately when faculty or staff (employees) or student makes a harassment claim.
- Consult the appropriate university official (dean of students, office of equality officer, office of public safety, or legal counsel) based on your university policy.
- Educate students about the dangers of social networking sites and the requisite professional behavior that is required on such sites.
- Offer a web-based method for submitting complaints.
- Have a designated person or office to contact if someone is a victim.
- Provide information about the college's student/sexual harassment policy on the university's website.
- Educate faculty and university officials concerning sexual and other forms of harassment.
- Consult your respective State Board of Nursing with respect to any guidelines or policy advisories related to existing standardized testing.

Helpful Resource

- Consult the Equal Employment Opportunity Commission website (www.eeoc.gov) for information regarding harassment and employer liability.

ETHICAL CONSIDERATIONS

There is no doubt that Dr. Miller's university colleague and the parents of the students (who failed their comprehensive exam) treated Dr. Miller poorly. As a diverse (African American) female administrator, Dr. Miller has been subject to an increased level of harassment and threats most likely because she is a female and minority, and possibly a member of a female-dominated profession. Academic contra power harassment (ACPH) occurs when someone with seemingly less power in an educational setting (e.g., student) harasses someone more powerful (professor, administrator). In a 2017 study, women faculty reported that students were more likely to challenge their authority, argue or refuse to follow course policies, and exhibit disrespectful or disruptive behaviors (Lampman, Crew, Lowery, Tompkins, & Mulder, 2016). Lampman (2012) reported several other significant predictors of greater bullying from students, including being a racial or ethnic minority, being younger, or degree held. One can only imagine what would have happened to Dr. Miller if the university leadership had not stepped in and addressed the harassing behaviors against Dr. Miller. She was already distressed that the parents were attempting to tarnish her academic reputation. Demand and consumer-driven higher education has contributed to a rise in aggressive behavior by students and parents. Have we seen this level of parental harassment in male-dominated majors? The answer is probably no. There are studies that have looked at student harassment from a sexual harassment perspective (Lampman, 2012; Lampman et al., 2016; Lee, 2006). As nursing academics, if we do not deal with gender and ACPH, from an ethical perspective, nursing faculty will be less likely to stay in academia, thus exacerbating an already significant nursing faculty shortage (Christensen, White, Dobbs, Craft, & Palmer 2019). Role modeling gender equality to our students is an ethical obligation of universities. As a final matter, the concern for public safety in a nursing program is high and outweighs any student, parent, or faculty objections to completing program requirements and assessments. The department chair has an ethical duty to graduate knowledgeable, safe clinicians; therefore, requiring additional remediation for students in need of this continued professional support.

References

American Association of University Women. (2005). *Drawing the line: Sexual harassment on campus.* Retrieved from https://files.eric.ed.gov/fulltext/ED489850.pdf

Christensen, M., White, S., Dobbs, S., Craft, J., & Palmer, C. (2019). Contra-power harassment of nursing academics. *Nurse Education Today, 74,* 94–96. doi:10.1016/j.nedt.2018.12.002

Gupta v. Florida Board of Regents, 212 F.3d 571 (11th Cir. 2000), cert, denied, 121 S.Ct. 772 (2001).

Finke v. Purdue University, 1:12-CV-124-JD, United States District Court, N.D. Indiana, Fort Wayne Division.

Kaplin, W. A., Lee, B. A., Hutchens, N. H., & Rooksby, J. H. (2019). *The law of higher education: A comprehensive guide to legal implications of administrative decision making* (6th ed.). San Francisco, CA: John Wiley & Sons.

Kelleher, M. (1996). *New arenas for violence: Homicide in the American workplace.* Westport, CT: Praeger.

Kolanko, K. M., Clark, C., Heinrich, K. T., Olive, D., Serembus, J. F., & Sifford, K. S. (2006). Academic dishonesty, bullying, incivility, and violence: Difficult challenges facing nurse educators. *Nursing Education Perspectives, 27*(1), 34–43.

Lampman, C., Crew, E. C., Lowery, S., Tompkins, K. A., Mulder, M. (2016). Women faculty distressed: Descriptions and consequences of academic contrapower harassment. *Journal of Women in Higher Education, 9*(2), 169–189. doi:10.1080/19407882.2016.1199385

Lampman, C. (2012). Women faculty at risk: U.S. professors report on their experiences with student incivility, bullying, aggression, and sexual attention. *NAPSA Journal about Women in Higher Education, 5,* 184–208. doi:10.1515/njawhe-2012-1108

Lee, D. (2006). *University students behaving badly.* Stoke on Trent, UK: Trentham Books.

Mansfield, K. C., Beck, A. G., Fung, K., Montiel, M., & Goldman, M. (2017). What constitutes sexual harassment and how administrators should handle it? *Journal of Cases in Educational Leadership, 20*(3), 37–55. doi:10.1177/1555458917696811

Nelson, A., Anis-Abdellatif, M., Larson, J., Mulder, C., & Wolff, B. (2016). New faculty orientation: Discussion of cultural competency, sexual victimization, and student behaviors. *Journal of Continuing Education in Nursing, 47*(5), 228–233. doi:10.3928/00220124-20160419-09

The Office of Civil Rights. (2019). *Sexual harassment guidance.* Retrieved from https://www2.ed.gov/about/offices/list/ocr/docs/sexhar00.html

Soklaridis, S., Zahn, C., Kuper, A., Gills, D., Taylor, V. H., & Whitehead, C. (2018). Men's fear of mentoring in the #Me Too era—What's at stake for academic medicine. *The New England Journal of Medicine, 379*(23), 2270–2274. doi:10.1056/NEJMms1805743

University of Houston. (2019). *Social media policy.* Retrieved from http://www.uh.edu/marcom/guidelines-policies/social-media/index

U.S. Equal Employment Opportunity Commission. (2018). *Harassment.* Retrieved from https://www.eeoc.gov/laws/types/harassment.cfm

U.S. Equal Employment Opportunity Commission. (2020) Retrieved from https://www.eeoc.gov/harassment

14

Managing Issues of Student Complaints of Discrimination

Case Study 14.1
An Undergraduate Faculty Adjunct Uses a Racial Slur in a Clinical Agency

Your role: You are Dr. Roam, the department chair for the undergraduate nursing program, and Professor Wiley is an undergraduate faculty adjunct teaching her third clinical community health clinical course and this time to senior students. Although you have ultimate responsibility for the department, the adjunct faculty (because so many of them are hired each semester) are largely managed by the undergraduate clinical coordinator, Professor Vision.

Professor Vision's job each semester is to assess the adjunct clinical needs for all the undergraduate clinical sections, hire or rehire the proper number of adjuncts from the available adjunct pool, and monitor their performance in the clinical agencies in which they supervise students (including doing their annual evaluation and making decisions to rehire or simply not offer a subsequent semester contract based on poor performance). Professor Wiley's evaluations have been satisfactory, but not necessarily above average, and there are no complaints or disciplinary actions in her personnel file. Professor Vision does not necessarily make site visits to assess the adjuncts, but she is always available to handle any issues that arise, particularly when course coordinators (full-time nursing faculty who have the ultimate responsibility for each clinical course and who directly oversee clinical faculty on a day-to-day basis during the semester) email her or call her about a problem with a particular adjunct faculty member.

On this day, you have just received a text message from Professor Vision, indicating that she urgently needs to speak to you about an incident in the community health clinical course. She says there are no safety issues involved, but as the issue is confidential in nature, she did not want to discuss it via email. The next day you meet with Professor Vision, and she informs you that one of the students emailed her with a complaint against Professor Wiley. The student claims Professor Wiley used the term wetbacks in reference to Hispanics in a conversation with another staff member at the community health agency. The student further claimed that two other Hispanic students in the group feared that by reporting this incident they might face retaliation (or even clinical failure) from the clinical instructor.

Questions

- How would you first proceed?
- Do you believe Professor Wiley should be punished for this incident if indeed it is found to be true?
- Do you think this incident is essentially rare, or do you believe the adjunct faculty (or even the faculty at large) ought to undergo workplace sensitivity training?
- How will you bring this incident to a close and circumvent any rumormongering that might take place?

COMPLAINTS OF UNIVERSITY STUDENT DISCRIMINATION: LEGAL PRINCIPLES AND REVIEW OF THE LITERATURE

Any discussion of harassment is likely to include discrimination, and vice versa. According to most federal and state laws, discriminatory motives or harassing behaviors due to race, national origin, religion, age, gender, and disability (some locales include sexual orientation) are illegal. Discrimination based on race, color, or national origin is actually prohibited by Title VI of the Civil Right Act of 1964 to any institution that receives federal assistance in this case higher education (U.S. Department of Education, 2016). Colleges and universities may also have policies that prohibit discrimination or harassment in categories not currently covered by federal and state law such as gender identity or expression, or sexual orientation or socioeconomic status. This chapter addresses both discrimination and harassment complaints by students in the university setting.

Discrimination

Discrimination can take many forms. An individual can be discriminated against based on gender, race, religion, ethnicity, sexual orientation, marital status, and disability, but also on weight, height, smoking status, accent, dress, political beliefs, and an endless number of other factors that are not necessarily prohibited by law. In the university setting, the following are federal laws that prohibit a variety of forms of discrimination: Title VI of the Civil Rights Act of 1964 (discrimination based on race, color, or national origin); Title IX of the Education Amendments of 1972 (sex discrimination); Section 504 of the Rehabilitation Act of 1973, as amended and the Americans with Disabilities Act (both prohibit disability discrimination); Age Discrimination Act of 1975 (age discrimination).

In the university setting, charges of discrimination by students generally fall into the category of an individual student claiming that a university employee with power or authority over them, such as a professor, perhaps a department chair or adviser, has discriminated against them. However, discriminatory behavior by students, visitors, contractors, and other members of the university community can also be covered. The following is a discussion of various types of student discrimination based on a protected class, including examples of sexual orientation discrimination that is law in eight states and the District of Columbia.[1] Disability discrimination is discussed in Chapter 21, Individual Rights and Public Safety: Addressing Conduct and Mental Health Issues Among Students.

There are two main types of discrimination: disparate treatment and disparate impact (Lindsay, 2005). *Disparate treatment* is sometimes called *intentional discrimination,* and it occurs when a teacher treats a student differently because of their status as a member in a protected category—for example, if a faculty member gave higher grades to females than males in a college course. In this case, Dr. Kelly, a tenured Ohio University professor charged with having inappropriate relationships with staff and students for over a decade, resigned instead of facing dismissal and tenure revocation

---

[1] The states include California, Connecticut, Massachusetts, Minnesota, New Jersey, New York, Vermont, and Wisconsin.

procedures (Pyle, 2010). The final charges that led to the resignation included complaints by female Indian students (the university had an MBA program in India) that Dr. Kelly was giving higher grades to an Indian student with whom he was involved. The other type of discrimination, *disparate impact,* is more difficult to prove because it involves a seemingly neutral action or practice whose effects are discriminatory on members of a protected category even though there is no direct evidence of discriminatory motive or intent.

The Harvard case is a good example of *disparate impact* as the qualified Asian students (Harvard disputes the case, period) may suffer from career opportunities by not having access to perhaps the most prestigious university in the country (Walsh, 2019). Another very public charge of disparate impact discrimination is the long-standing argument that the SAT college entrance examination is biased against minorities, and the lower scores they receive bars them from admission to leading universities or colleges (Freedle, 2003). To mitigate this concern, the College Board recently piloted a "diversity index" score to the SAT, to place the individual applicant in the context of their socioeconomic advantages or disadvantages, and they had plans to expand it (Jaschick, 2019). However, a public outcry over the use of this additional score to admissions decisions led the College Board to drop the idea of an additional score (Hammell & Boyette, 2019). Instead, while a score will not be used, they haven't exactly abandoned the idea. Instead, they have eliminated the score and created an Environmental Context Dashboard and renamed it "Landscape," which will transparently allow students, families, and schools to view statistics on crime rates and poverty in their neighborhoods. The intent is that admission offices can discern the kinds of obstacles these students have faced "... doing well with less" (Hammell & Boyette, 2019, p. 1) according to David Coleman, the College Boards Executive Director.

Title VII of the Civil Rights Act of 1964, which covers employers, prohibits both gender and racial discrimination against employees, graduate students who are serving in any kind of student–employee classification (e.g., teaching assistant) have additional protections under the Equal Employment Opportunity Commission (EEOC) regulations, where complaints can be filed but only within 180 days of the harassment or discrimination charge. Every university or college has a designated administrator responsible for overseeing the institution's compliance with these laws and regulations. At Drexel University in Philadelphia, Pennsylvania, those duties are handled within the Office of Equality and Diversity. According to the EEOC guidelines, there are four steps in a complaint process: informal/counseling, formal complaint, appeal, and the final phase which starts the judicial process (U.S. Department of Transportation, n.d.). Today, some literature has pointed out that racism has been shifting from open violent behavior and aggressive racism to unconscious forms of racism (Lin-Sommer & Lucek, 2015). Soyer also states that "explicit racism is not common any more in modern colleges and universities. The cultures in these institutions often have certain values that reduce the ethnic inequalities, and the assimilation pressure on the students of color" (Soyer, 2008, p. 2). However, Soyer (2008) also indicates the dominant White culture still retains racial hierarchies, addresses apparently racial matters, but resists addressing genuine diversity. Whether this last assessment is centrally valid or merely the interpretation of the author is probably a good discussion point. Finally, there is also the concept of *reverse discrimination.* It is defined as "policies or habits of social discrimination against members of a historically dominant group with an implication of unfairness" (U.S. Legal, 2010, p. 1). Often these charges are brought by individuals who believe that affirmative action or quota practices are inherently unfair or illegal. The first and most notable reverse discrimination case ruling by the Supreme Court was *Regents of the University of California v. Bakke* (1978) (No. 7811) 18 Cal.3d 34, 553 P.2d 1152. In this historic case, Allan Bakke (a 35-year-old White male applicant to the University of California–Davis medical school) was denied admission although his benchmark admission score was higher than some applicants admitted through a special program that gave preference to those from economically or educationally disadvantaged backgrounds or who were members of a minority group. Writing for the majority in a 5 to 4 vote, Justice Powell wrote:

1. *Title VI proscribes only those racial classifications that would violate the Equal Protection Clause if employed by a State or its agencies.*

2. *Racial and ethnic classifications of any sort are inherently suspect and call for the most exacting judicial scrutiny. While the goal of achieving a diverse student body is sufficiently compelling to justify consideration of race in admissions decisions under some circumstances, petitioner's special admissions program, which forecloses consideration to persons like respondent, is unnecessary to the achievement of this compelling goal, and therefore invalid under the Equal Protection Clause.* (pp. 287–320)

3. *Since petitioner could not satisfy its burden of proving that respondent would not have been admitted even if there had been no special admissions program, he must be admitted.* (p. 320)

The issue was again addressed in 2003 when the degree to which race (as an affirmative action remedy) could be used in the university admissions process was again litigated. In two separate rulings, the Supreme Court ruled that race *could be used* in the admissions process, but that it could not be the overriding factor. By a 6 to 3 (*Gratz v. Bollinger*, 2003) vote, the University of Michigan undergraduate admission program was ruled unconstitutional because it used a point system for race in its admissions process. By a 5 to 4 (*Grutter v. Bollinger*, 2003) vote, the university's law school admissions process was upheld as it used a much narrower race factor in its admissions procedures. The last Supreme Court ruling on affirmative action in higher education was in 2016. In the case of *Fisher v. University of Texas*, ruled "… admissions officials may continue to consider race as one factor among many in ensuring a diverse student body" (Liptak, 2016, p. 1). Every case that makes it to the Supreme Court always has unique circumstances or differences from other cases heard by the Court. In Texas, the top ranked students from "all" high schools in the state were awarded admission to the University of Texas, replacing a system where the top ranked students, regardless of what high school they graduated from, were awarded admission. The old system was thought to depress minority (Hispanic and Black students) attendance due to one prevailing argument, the quality of high schools many minority students attended were poorer and students lacked access to any wealthier school districts and high schools. The suit was filed by a white student, who believed the new system discriminated against her because she was White and had a high ranking at her school (Wolf, 2016).

Harassment

Harassment on university campuses has been reportedly mostly based on sex or race; the case of an assistant attorney general in Michigan who very publicly cyber-harassed and bullied the University of Michigan student body president student because he was openly gay is an example that stretches the contemporary definition and scope of sexual harassment (Jones, 2010). In 2014, a lawsuit was filed against Harvard University for discriminating against Asian students in the admissions process (Anderson, 2018). Essentially the plaintiffs claimed Harvard surreptitiously tried to decrease the number of Asian students admitted because they believed that Asian students were overrepresented. It is certainly a controversial issue but Li (2018) states you can both be for affirmative action and make the case for the Asian students' legal standing. Moreover, these claims against Harvard are not singular. A lawsuit was filed in 2018 against the University of California state system, where, for instance at UCLA, 29% of students are Asian American, 27% are White, 22% are Hispanic, and 3% are Black. The allegation was that while California voters in 1996 passed Proposition 209, barring state institutions from considering race and ethnicity in admissions, the U.S. system was still "… considering race and ethnicity in admissions, in ways that favor Black and Latino students and hurt Asian Americans" (Jaschick, 2018, p. 1). While the Harvard case has now been argued before the Court, no ruling has been made.

By current definitions, the legal term *harassment* can be defined as physical or verbal hostility toward someone with legally protected status. *Nolo's Plain-English Law Dictionary* (2010, p. 340) defines protected status or class as "a group of people protected by law from discrimination or harassment based on their membership in the group. For example, under federal law, race, national origin, sex, and age are examples of protected classes" (p. 1). There are also state and local laws as well as university policies that prohibit discrimination on the basis of sexual orientation (Lassek, 2010). While a poll conducted by YouGov/Huffington Post in 2014 reported 62% of Americans believed discrimination based on sexual orientation was illegal (Moore, 2014), in reality there are 30 states where there is no full protection of discrimination based on sexual orientation or gender identity (Freedom for all Americans, 2018).

Sexual harassment is defined by the U.S. Department of Education as "unwelcome [verbal, non-verbal, or physical] conduct of a sexual nature" (U.S. Department of Education, 2001). Sexual harassment is prohibited by Title VII of the Civil Rights Act of 1964 and by Title IX of the Education Amendments of 1972. Sexual harassment is generally broken into two types: *quid pro quo* harassment and hostile environment harassment (Lindsay, 2005). Using the revised Department of Education Guidelines, the two categories are defined as follows:

> Quid pro quo harassment occurs if a teacher or other employee conditions an educational decision or benefit on the student's submission to unwelcome sexual conduct, [regardless of whether] the student resists and suffers the threatened harm or submits and avoids the threatened harm....
>
> By contrast, [hostile environment] harassment ... does not explicitly or implicitly condition a decision or benefit on submission to sexual conduct [but does nevertheless] limit a student's ability to participate or benefit from the school's program based on sex. (U.S. Department of Education, 2001)

Because students do not ordinarily have control over other students, only faculty and other university employees are charged with *quid pro quo* harassment, and fellow students are more frequently charged with hostile environment harassment. According to the American Association of University Women (AAUW, 2006), sexual harassment is pervasive on college campuses today. From the AAUW's 2006 report, *Drawing the Line: Sexual Harassment on Campus,* statistics indicate 62% of female college students and 61% of male college students report having been sexually harassed at their university, and more than 35% do not tell anyone or report these incidents. A more recent massive study of 150,000 women at 27 research universities conducted by the Association of American Universities (with a response rate just over 9%) reported 11.4% sexual assault involving penetration or oral sex due to a lack of affirmative consent. Study also included the largest sample of LGBTQ students whose assault rate was higher at 14.8%. Moreover, no university had fewer than 49% of women in the survey who had experienced sexual harassment (Cantor et al., 2015). It may also alarm some that in 2017 the current Secretary of Education, Betsy DeVos, softened the threshold reporting sexual assault (possibly in violation of Title IX guidelines instituted in 1972) by re-writing the 2011 guidance letter on sexual assault based on the Obama administration's an unjust system for handling college sexual assault (Gambee, 2017). Nevertheless, the preceding statistics are alarming, and indicate that despite the enactment of numerous laws and university polices prohibiting sexual harassment and an apparent "ethic" of equality among the most educated, it is still a significant problem and more campus-based educational programs to protect students need to be pursued.

DISCUSSION OF CASE

Recall from Case Study 14.1 that you are Dr. Roam and your undergraduate clinical coordinator, Professor Vision, has just informed you that Professor Wiley has made an ethnic slur in conversation. How would you first proceed? The first question to ask is does your university have an office where you must or should report this complaint or allegation. If so, you and your department should know that *their* first call should be made to that office and not to you. The office should be regarded as the experts and its advice sought from the start, as it is likely the office will know best how to proceed. Therefore, you would begin by asking Professor Vision if she had made that call. But assume for the moment that your university does not have that infrastructure in place.

Dr. Roam was very disturbed by the "alleged comment," and although she understood the students' fear of exposure and being potential targets of retaliation, she reminded Professor Vision the incident should be phrased as alleged until the facts of the case could be fully investigated. Dr. Roam was very adamant that this be handled in the most professional and confidential manner. As posed in the second case study question, do you believe Professor Wiley should be punished for this incident if indeed it is found to be true?

WHEN TO CONSULT THE UNIVERSITY COUNSEL

It is unlikely that a student would contact university counsel for allegations of harassment or discrimination as the EEOC office is specifically charged to hear such complaints. However, it is common for administrators and/or faculty to consult with university counsel as these types of matters arise. Even after consulting with university counsel for advice, the ultimate business decision remains the responsibility of the administrator/faculty.

FINDINGS AND DISPOSITION

Not being a trained investigator, Professor Vision was uncertain whom she should interview first, and so she recontacted Dr. Roam, who said the faculty member should certainly be contacted first and simply, calmly, and constructively questioned whether she had indeed made the comment or not. Dr. Roam told Professor Vision that any word (or hint) of an investigation being conducted without having first given the accused faculty member a chance to present her side of the case would be detrimental to faculty due process. Professor Vision subsequently asked Professor Wiley to meet so they could discuss the alleged remark she made. Almost immediately Professor Wiley acknowledged her use of the term "wetbacks" in a casual conversation, said it was not intentional and certainly not indicative of the kind of person she is. She apologized profusely for this indiscretion. She stated it was not meant to be a public but a private conversation but that she was indeed sorry any student had overheard her and had been offended. She also acknowledged that the term was racially charged and inappropriate for a nursing faculty member to use. She offered to personally apologize to the student and if requested, to the entire clinical group, assuming the comment probably had been now discussed by the entire clinical group. Professor Vision could clearly see that Professor Wiley was anguished by the incident. Nevertheless, Professor Vision informed Professor Wiley that the students involved are somewhat fearful of being harassed by her for reporting this incident. Professor Vision reminded Professor Wiley that school policy prohibits retaliation against any person who brings a complaint of discrimination or who participates in investigations of these complaints. To this, Professor Wiley strongly stated that she would never do such a thing. Professor Vision concluded the meeting and informed Professor Wiley that she would have to speak to Dr. Roam about how this incident should be handled further and that she would get back to her. She did encourage Professor Wiley to write up her side of the story for the record and to include the comments she had just shared with her. What kind of punishment should Dr. Roam enforce, or is the offer by Professor Wiley to personally apologize to the student(s) sufficient?

Upon hearing the facts of the case, Dr. Roam encouraged Professor Vision to complete her interview with the accusing students and to forward her any new information from the meeting. She would then make a decision. She contacted the university counsel and informed her that if there were no additional, extenuating circumstances presented by the student (it was unlikely based on the trajectory of the story) then she would fire Professor Wiley for her conduct. The university counsel agreed but informed her it was best to first receive the written statement from Professor Wiley admitting to the act. Within 2 days, Professor Vision forwarded the statement to Dr. Roam (there were no substantive changes from the facts first admitted to by Professor Wiley), and so Dr. Roam called Professor Wiley in and terminated her contract because the conduct violated the school's nondiscrimination policy and did not meet the professional standards expected from faculty members in the program. Dr. Roam was very professional in her delivery and informed Professor Wiley that she had done the ethical and honest thing by admitting to the incident and, although she appreciated the offer of a public apology, the incident in her view was severe. She believed Professor Wiley's credibility in the clinical agency was now significantly damaged and would interfere with the educational mission of the current student and perhaps others in the future who might hear of the incident. She wished Professor Wiley well and Professor Wiley moved on with her life and career without any further action or appeals. Do you think that termination was an appropriate disciplinary action to take under the circumstances?

Recall the third case study question, do you think this incident is essentially rare, or do you believe the adjunct faculty (or even the faculty at large) ought to undergo Workplace Sensitivity Training? Discuss this in class now.

Recall the fourth case study question, how should Dr. Roam bring this incident to a close and circumvent any rumormongering that might take place? Indeed, Dr. Roam was concerned about this, and as the department chair, she felt it important for her (not Professor Vision) to bring the incident to a close and try to prevent any further gossip or rumormongering to persist. Professor Vision was able to find a last-minute clinical replacement for Professor Wiley, and then she emailed the students in the clinical group and informed them that a new faculty member would be taking over the class without going into the reasons for the change. Dr. Roam met with the three accusing students and informed them the school's investigation found that Dr. Wiley's conduct was not acceptable under university policy. Dr. Roam said they would have a new clinical faculty the following week and that she appreciated the students coming forward. She further reiterated she was always dedicated to safe, ethical, and respectful clinical/work environments, and she hoped they would move forward with their clinical rotation with those values in mind. She told the students that they should contact her immediately if they ever felt they were being treated differently in the program because they came forward with their complaint about Dr. Wiley. She asked if the students had any questions or concerns. As the students had none, the meeting was concluded. On her way out, one student came over and said, simply and quietly, "Thank you." Dr. Roam later thanked Professor Vision for the excellent and professional manner in which she had conducted the case and its resolution.

RELEVANT LEGAL CASE

Underwood v. LaSalle University, No. 07-1441, 2007 WL 4245737 (E.D. Pa. Dec. 4, 2007)

In this case, Starling Underwood, a former undergraduate nursing student at LaSalle University, filed a lawsuit against the university alleging the nursing program had dismissed him based on race, and he claimed violations of the Title VI of the Civil Rights Act of 1964 as well as gender and disability discrimination claims under Tide IX of the Civil Rights Act, the Rehabilitation Act, and Title II of the Americans with Disabilities Act.

Mr. Underwood had initially passed nine nursing courses between 2003 and 2004; however, in the spring semester 2005, he received a grade of D in a pediatrics class and an F in a nursing research course. He had initially asked for permission to withdraw from the nursing research class, but he waited until the last day of class to do so, thereby violating the policy on withdrawals and so his request was denied, resulting in an F for the course. LaSalle had a policy to dismiss a student who received two grades lower than a C in any given semester; therefore, Mr. Underwood was dismissed and he subsequently sued the university. The university initially moved to pre-trial summary judgment, and it was only at this time that Mr. Underwood added claims of gender and disability discrimination based on his claim of poor vision that was not severe enough to qualify him for an accommodation (nor was his disability claim of discrimination from using Ebonics seen as valid).

The court ultimately granted LaSalle University summary judgment as Mr. Underwood had already denied racial discrimination at a previous deposition. His claim to gender discrimination had a 2-year statute of limitations in Pennsylvania, despite being added at the twelfth hour as a frivolous claim, according to the court, and the disability claims were likewise dismissed.

SUMMARY

Harassment and discrimination persist in society—and as is clear from the press accounts of attacks on Muslims following terrorist attacks, not far beneath the surface. It may also be inferred that the mass murder of nine African Americans in 2015 at a mostly Black church in Charleston South Carolina, the 2018 mass murder of 11 Jews in Pittsburgh, Pennsylvania, and the most recent August 3,

2019 mass murder in El Paso, Texas, of 22 persons at a Walmart, where the assailant was thought to be targeting Hispanics, were first motivated by an embedded sense of racial and religious discrimination. Because universities and colleges are microcosms of society at large, it is not surprising that these issues continue to arise in higher educational settings.

As for sexual assault, despite all the public focus on sexual assault in the military, it is still a plague, with report of assault reaching its highest level in 2016. Reports of sexual assault in Service members jumped to 6,172 cases reported in 2016 versus in 2012 when only 3,604 were reported (Applewhite, 2017; Cohen, 2018). There are widely known long-standing records that high percentages of sexual assault of both women and men in the military go unreported, and often these events coincide with high levels of alcohol consumption and because cadets (in one of major service academies, the U.S. Air Force Academy) fear reprisals for the disclosure (Associated Press, 2019). In 2017 it was even reported that 38 men are raped every day in the U.S. military (thedailybeast.com). Again, these are alarming numbers, and as the military (perhaps like most work environments) is a "top-down" organization, it is obvious that cadets are taking their cues from what is apparently being tolerated in the environment. These statistics make one wonder: What are the statistics *outside the military academies,* and is it possible they are similar or perhaps even higher?

We have administratively dealt with numerous allegations of harassment and discrimination in our tenure as nursing academic administrators. Although this chapter's Case Study 14.1 did not advance to actual charges of harassment, the students felt vulnerable as a racial minority and their fears of discrimination (or harassment) were well founded. It is prudent not to rush to judgment in any case, and make sure all sides are heard. Students who have very strong feelings that they have been harassed or discriminated against should go to the Office of Equality and Diversity. This does not mean there should be an investigation of very obvious frivolous charges, however. But even here, who should best ascertain that a student's charges are frivolous or groundless? Administrators in respective Offices of Equality and Diversity should be more familiar with the federal due process rights that students from a protected class have when claiming any form of discrimination or harassment. Often it is more efficient for these offices to handle these situations, and they should be skilled at detecting the merits of a complaint. It is also important to note that some complaints are made informally and only made formal when a student seeks to fully document an incident and follow through with all the normal investigative procedures. In the LaSalle University case, it became very obvious to the court that the plaintiff only added gender and disability claims in his lawsuit at the 12th hour as an addendum to his original claim of racial discrimination.

CRITICAL ELEMENTS TO CONSIDER

- Students do not have to be subject to harassment or discrimination. There are laws at the federal, state, and local levels and university/college policies that are designed to protect students and effectively deal with illegal conduct.
- Any faculty member should be familiar with the on-campus office that handles EEOC complaints and be ready (even as an adviser) to steer students to that office when appropriate.
- Because charges of discrimination are so antithetical to the academy, so deeply personal, and so easy to make, it is unfortunately the case that faculty members need to be prepared for having such charges made against them unfairly. It is difficult to prepare against them (and not worth the energy or effort) except by acting with respect to all at all times. However, in the event that you sense a particular "agenda" being advanced by a student, sharing your concern with your supervisor and preserving that communication in an email can later document what was really going on.

- If there is discrimination based on sexual orientation, it is important to understand that there are some state and local laws and university policies that prohibit this.
- If a student does not feel safe going through normal academic channels for whatever reason (e.g., sexual harassment), the student can contact the university's public safety office, the university's Ombudsman, or the university's counseling center.

Helpful Resources

- American Association of University Women: http://www.aauw.org/
- American Civil Rights Association: http://www.aclu.org/
- Americans with Disabilities Act: http://www.ada.gov/pubs/ada.htm
- Equal Employment Opportunity Commission (EEOC): http://www.eeoc.gov/
- Human Rights Campaign: http://www.hrc.org/
- National Association for the Advancement of Colored People (NAACP): http://www.naacp.org

References

American Association of University Women. (2006). *Drawing the line: Sexual harassment on campus.* Retrieved from http://www.aauw.org/learn/research/upload/DTLFinal.pdf

Anderson, N. (2018). Harvard admissions trial opens with university accused of bias against Asian American, *Washington Post.* Retrieved from https://www.washingtonpost.com/education/2018/10/15/harvard-admissions-goes-trial-university-faces-claim-bias-against-asian-americans/

Applewhite, S. J. (2017). Sexual assaults in U.S. military reach record high: Pentagon. *NBC News.* Retrieved from https://www.nbcnews.com/news/us-news/sexual-assault-reports-u-s-military-reach-record-high-pentagon-n753566

Associated Press. (2019, January 31). At military academies, sexual assault reports are on the rise and often go unreported. *CPR News.* Retrieved from https://www.cpr.org/2019/01/31/at-military-academies-sexual-assault-reports-are-on-the-rise-and-often-go-unreported/

Cantor, D, Fisher, B., Chibnall, S., Townsend, R., Lee, H., Bruce, C., & Thomas, G. (2015). Report on the AAU campus climate survey on sexual assault and sexual misconduct. *Washington Post.* Retrieved from http://apps.washingtonpost.com/g/documents/local/association-of-american-universities-campus-survey-on-sexual-assault-and-sexual-misconduct/1747/

Cohen, Z. (2018). From fellow soldier to "monster" in uniform: #MeToo in the military. *CNN.* Retrieved from https://www.cnn.com/2018/02/07/politics/us-military-sexual-assault-investigations/index.html

Fisher v. University of Texas, 14–981 (2016).

Freedle, R. O. (2003). Correcting the SAT's ethnic and social-class bias: A method for reestimating SAT scores. *Harvard Educational Review, 73*(1), 1–43. doi:10.17763/haer.73.1.8465k88616hn4757

Freedom for all Americans. (2018). *LGBT Americans aren't fully protected from discrimination in 30 states, today.* Retrieved from https://www.freedomforallamericans.org/states/

Gambee, R. (2017). Betsy DeVos and Title IX changes. The Dartmouth Review. Retrieved from http://dartreview.com/betsy-devos-and-title-ix-changes/

Gratz v. Bollinger, 539 U.S. 244 (2003).

Grutter v. Bollinger, 539 U.S. 306 (2003).

Hammell, K., & Boyette, C. (2019). Remember that SAT "adversity score"? That's no longer happening. *CNN.* Retrieved from https://www.cnn.com/2019/08/27/us/college-board-sat-adversity-score-trnd/index.html

Hill, C., & Silva, E. (2005). Drawing the line: Sexual harassment on campus, *American Association of University Women Educational Foundation,* Retrieve June 7, 2029 from https://files.eric.ed.gov/fulltext/ED489850.pdf

Jaschick, S. (2018). New front in fight over racial discrimination. *Inside Higher Ed.* Retrieved from https://www.insidehighered.com/admissions/article/2018/11/19/new-lawsuit-suggests-u-california-has-been-considering-race-admissions

Jaschick, S. (2019). New SAT score: Diversity. *Inside Higher Ed.* Retrieved from https://www.insidehighered.com/admissions/article/2019/05/20/college-board-will-add-adversity-score-everyone-taking-sat

Jones, M. T. (2010, November 8). Anti-gay assistant attorney general in Michigan fired for cyber-bullying. *change.org.* Retrieved from http://gayrights.change.org/bg/view/anti-gay_assistant_attorney_general_in_michigan_fired_for_cyber-bullying

Lassek, P. J. (2010). Sexual orientation added to protected-classes list. *Tulsa World.* Retrieved from https://
    www.tulsaworld.com/news/local/government-and-politics/sexual-orientation-added-to-protected
    -classes-list/article_58176268-5eb3-55a0-9293-d9f934da0d83.html

Li, M. (2018). I support affirmation action. But Harvard is really hurting Asian American.
    Vox. Retrieved from https://www.vox.com/first-person/2018/10/18/17995270/
    asian-americans-affirmative-action-harvard-admissions-lawsuit

Liptak, J. (2016, June 23). Supreme Court upholds Texas affirmative action program. *New York Times.*
    Retrieved from https://www.nytimes.com/2016/06/24/us/politics/supreme-court-affirmative
    -action-university-of-texas.html

Lindsay, C. L., III. (2005). *The college student's guide to the law.* Lanham, MD: Taylor Trade Publishing.

Lin-Summer, S., & Lucek, S. (2015). The dangerous mind: Unconscious bias in higher education.
    Brown Political Review. Retrieved from http://www.brownpoliticalreview.org/2015/04/
    the-dangerous-mind-unconscious-bias-in-higher-education/

thedailybest.com. (2017, April 14). 38 men raped in the U.S military every day. Retrieved June 7, 2020 from
    https://www.thedailybeast.com/cheats/2014/09/10/38-men-raped-in-u-s-military-each-day

Moore, P. (2014). Poll results: Discrimination. *YouGov.* Retrieved from https://today.yougov.com/topics/legal/
    articles-reports/2014/06/18/poll-results-discrimination

Nolo's Plain-English Law Dictionary. (2010). Protected class. *Nolo.* Retrieved from http://www.nolo.com/
    dictionary/protected-class-term.html

Pyle, E. (2010, April 17). OU professor retires after ultimatum. *The Columbus Dispatch.* Retrieved from https://
    www.dispatch.com/article/20100417/NEWS/304179895

Regents of the University of California v. Bakke, 438 U.S. 265 (1978).

Soyer, M. (2008, July). *Factors affecting racial discrimination among college students.* Paper presented at the
    Annual Meeting of the American Sociological Association, Boston, MA.

thedailybest.com. (2017, April 14). 38 men raped in the U.S. military every day. Retrieved from https://www
    .thedailybeast.com/cheats/2014/09/10/38-men-raped-in-u-s-military-each-day

U.S. Department of Education. (2001, January). *Revised sexual harassment guidance: Harassment of students by
    school employees, other students, or third parties, Title IX.* Retrieved from https://cdn.atixa.org/website
    -media/atixa.org/wp-content/uploads/2013/11/12194226/OCR-2001-Revised-Sexual-Harassment
    -Guidance-Title-IX.pdf

U.S. Department of Education. (2016). *Overview of Title VI of the Civil Rights Act of 1964.* Retrieved from
    https://www.justice.gov/crt/fcs/TitleVI-Overview

U.S. Department of Transportation. (n.d.). *Equal employment opportunity complaint process.*
    Retrieved from https://www.transportation.gov/civil-rights/complaint-resolution/
    equal-employment-opportunity-complaint-process

U.S. Legal. (2010). *Reverse discrimination law and legal discrimination.* Retrieved from http://definitions
    .uslegal.com/r/reverse-discrimination/

Walsh, C. (2019). Final arguments in admissions suit. *Harvard Gazette.* Retrieved from https://news.harvard
    .edu/gazette/story/2019/02/final-arguments-in-admissions-suit-against-harvard/

Wolf, R. (2016). Supreme Court upholds affirmative action in university case. *USA Today.* Retrieved from
    https://www.usatoday.com/story/news/politics/2016/06/23/supreme-court-university-texas
    -affirmative-action-race/83239790/

15

Academic Dishonesty Among Students

Case Study 15.1
Academic Dishonesty

Your role: You are Dr. Regina Morgan, a faculty member for the Role Transition Capstone course.

You teach two sections of a BSN Role Transition Capstone Course for seniors. Monica Drake, a senior student with predominantly grades of C in major clinical courses, achieves the highest score on the comprehensive standardized exam, 1226 (A), and is the first student in the class to complete the exam in 88 minutes and 51 seconds. Students have 4 hours to take the exam, most students requiring approximately 3 hours to complete the exam. You check Monica's previous score in your grade book and Monica obtained a 683 (F) on the first attempt. Given her previous score, you are concerned that there is an academic integrity issue as her grade increased by 543 points on a standardized exam. You have never seen such a large increase in 4 weeks. You consult the department chair for advice and she refers you to the Comprehensive Exam Testing Policy. As a result, you write the following letter to Monica Drake.

Dear Monica,

I am writing to inform you that your comprehensive score was flagged due to a score 1226 (an increase of 543 points since your last comprehensive exam version) in addition to a testing time of 88 minutes and 51 seconds to complete the exam on April 30, 2019. As per our policy, the comprehensive exam is a highly structured and widely adopted standardized test. As such, there are a great deal of data available on the thousands of students who have taken the exam and their performance. We expect that students' scores will improve over time, and we commit a great many resources to facilitating that kind of student success. Modest increases, appropriate to time in the program, are anticipated. Occasionally, a student may have a dramatic increase in score (300 points or greater) in a relatively short period of time, and those are considered to be statistical outliers. These large increases will be investigated by faculty and administration for both potential breaches in security and for concerns about accurate assessment of student performance (such as a "cramming" session that resulted in a huge jump, but not in learning that can be retained over time). We reserve the right to require students who have scores that increase more than 300 points since last testing to retest using another version, so they can sufficiently demonstrate content mastery (Undergraduate Student Handbook, 2019–2020, p. 13).

Based on these data and consistent with the Comprehensive Exam Testing Policy, the faculty will require you to re-take the exam with a score of 900 or greater on the exam in order for you to successfully pass the Role Transition Capstone course. If you do not achieve a score of 900 or greater, you will be required to engage in additional remediation and retest using another version, so you can demonstrate content mastery. I would like to meet with you to discuss this issue. Please contact me so we can arrange a mutually convenient time for you to re-take your exam and discuss this matter.

Dr. Morgan

Based on the policy, you inform Monica that she must re-take the exam. Monica does not arrange a time to re-take her exam. A few weeks after you notify the student, Dean Connelly contacts you and informs you that Monica has retained an attorney and filed an Equal Employment Opportunity Commission (EEOC) complaint, claiming discrimination based on race. She also requested to re-take the exam at an approved testing center.

Questions
- How would you proceed?
- Do you have sufficient evidence for an academic dishonesty violation? What other information would you need?
- What evidence would you need to testify at the student conduct committee hearing?

ACADEMIC DISHONESTY: LEGAL PRINCIPLES AND REVIEW OF THE LITERATURE

"Academic dishonesty" is a relatively simple term that covers a very wide variety of offenses against the spirit and substance of academia. It can include cheating, collusion, fabrication, false information or misrepresentation, falsification, forgery, plagiarism, and any type of fraudulent academic misconduct. It includes intellectual property theft of published or unpublished materials (Lindsay, 2005; McCabe & Trevino, 1993). Technology has provided more efficient, highly sophisticated and complex methods for cheating, thus facilitating academic misconduct (Kolanko et al., 2006). But "academic dishonesty" is not limited to intentional misconduct: it also includes less serious errors, even "innocent mistakes" such as failing to give someone credit for an idea or for assistance in writing an article; failing to note where an image, a table, or other data came from; or backdating a work that is entirely original. It's not about the actor's state of mind or intentions; it is only about the integrity of the act.

Academic dishonesty challenges faculty and institutions of higher education because it threatens the core value of the academy: the creation of knowledge. Whatever a person says or writes must be that person's own, unless it is building on or using someone else's idea as a springboard, in which case that other person's contribution must be noted. Any form of dishonesty to obtain a degree or certificate, or even to complete a homework assignment, constitutes a breach of the core value and compromises the integrity of the specific institution and the academic community at large. It is both an absolute and a "slippery slope." "No matter the prevalence of cheating, the educator's professional duty remains the same: to identify the deviant behavior, to resolve unethical issues, and develop policies and processes that prevent or correct unacceptable behaviors. Unfortunately, faculty often learns misconduct deterrent strategies by trial and error" (Stonecypher & Willson, 2014, p. 167).

There is a very important social purpose at work here. Universities certify personal achievement and ability. The public relies on those certifications. As a result, universities have a responsibility to the public to ensure that individuals who receive educational credentials from their institutions have met the established criteria and standards to deal with the complexities and challenges in the subject area for which they are credentialed. Awarding a degree to someone who has not earned it and does not deserve it will allow that person to misrepresent their abilities to an unsuspecting public, in essence allowing fraud to be perpetuated on innocent consumers. That's why the rule is so strict and the student's intention not an issue: The purpose is to protect the public (and the institution). That is all the more important in areas such as healthcare, where mistakes can cause severe, long-lasting, and often permanent harm to people.

In an effort to eliminate academic dishonesty, institutions of higher education typically have policies that explain the core values of academia, specify the forbidden deviations, and make it easy to punish students who cross the lines. However, what happens when individual teachers "take pity" on a transgressing student and do not act in accordance with the university code? Because academia is a community in which all expect to be (and should be) treated the same, the uneven or ineffective execution of honor codes may result in litigation against the university and its faculty when they are applied according to their terms. It is therefore imperative that universities pay attention to laws relevant to academic misconduct codes when designing institutional policies and executing disciplinary actions against students who violate those policies.

Nursing faculty must be diligent in holding nursing students accountable to higher standards of integrity because empiric findings suggest that nursing students who cheat are more likely to fall short in meeting professional standards or, at worst, place the health and safety of their patients at risk (Schmitz & Schaffer, 1995). Bavier (2009) underscored the need for nursing faculty to view academic dishonesty among nursing students as a matter of life and death because cheating on the part of a nurse can result in the demise of human life. The implications of cheating should prompt nursing faculty to accept their legal and ethical responsibilities as the gatekeepers of the profession very seriously. Strategies to curtail cheating include taking proactive steps to prevent academic dishonesty, teaching and applying ethical standards, acting quickly and with serious purpose to address transgressions, and imposing appropriate sanctions to hold students accountable for acts of academic misconduct.

When considering cases of academic misconduct, it is important for the nursing administrator and faculty member to recognize that courts distinguish between academic and disciplinary cases. Although the line between academic and disciplinary issues can sometimes be murky, the vast majority of courts hold that cases involving accusations of cheating, plagiarism, or other forms of academic dishonesty require the school to provide the more extensive procedural protections that are offered for disciplinary matters or misconduct (such as notice and opportunity for a hearing) rather than the less burdensome ones required for decisions based on academic performance or evaluations.

DISCUSSION OF CASE STUDY

In Case Study 15.1, the student's standardized test score was not consistent with usual increases in standardized tests or the student's academic profile according to the testing company and literature. Dr. Morgan had a duty to question the score and address the matter. Ms. Drake could have been caring for patients as a graduate nurse without the adequate knowledge to do so safely. Ms. Drake was in her fourth year of study in the undergraduate nursing program and should recognize the seriousness of the cheating if she did in fact hack or have someone hack into the testing site. Dr. Morgan and the dean called the testing company and asked if anyone had accessed the exam other than the date and time of the comprehensive exam. The testing company reported that someone accessed the exam prior to the date of the exam through Ms. Drake's account. The dean consulted with IT and Legal Counsel and determined the best course of action was to allow Ms. Drake to re-take a different version of the exam at a testing center since the school could not *absolutely* prove that Ms. Drake changed her score. The testing centers are used for the NCLEX-RN®, ensure identity verification, and secure proctoring. Dr. Morgan then requested an appointment with the student, to make her aware of the issues, allow the student an opportunity to be heard, and present the dean's decision to allow her to take a different version of the exam at a testing center. If Dr. Morgan had not reported the suspected grade, we would not have known of the issue or been able to investigate it.

WHEN TO CONSULT THE UNIVERSITY COUNSEL

Consult the university counsel in the development and management of academic honesty or academic misconduct policies, including when instances of academic honesty or misconduct may overlap with issues regarding academic performance or evaluations.

FINDINGS AND DISPOSITION

The Dean received notice that Ms. Drake achieved a 700 on the comprehensive exam (a 900 is passing) and notified Ms. Drake that she failed the course. The EEOC complaint found no evidence of discrimination especially in light of the fact that Ms. Drake obtained a 700 on the re-take exam at the testing center and a student came forward to report Monica Drake for cheating. One student, Kenya Moore, came forward and confessed that Ms. Drake had asked her if she wanted the answers to the comprehensive exam, but she had declined to participate in the cheating scandal. Ms. Moore had a copy of the texts from Ms. Drake as evidence. Based on this evidence, Ms. Drake's case was forwarded to the School of Nursing Academic Standing Committee (ASC) with a written statement from Kenya Moore and screenshots of the texts of Ms. Drake asking Ms. Moore if she wanted the answers. Based on the evidence, the ASC made a recommendation to the Dean that Ms. Drake should be dismissed for academic integrity violations as per their policies. Monica Drake was dismissed from the BSN program in her senior year for cheating on her comprehensive final exam. Kenya Moore recognized (albeit later) that she had an ethical duty to report Ms. Drake for cheating. Faculty reminded Ms. Moore what she would do as a professional nurse if she observed unethical behavior, such as diverting narcotics, wrongly noting a chart, or abusing a patient. She needs to report any transgressions in a timely manner.

Prevention Tips

To prevent cheating during a test, faculty members can do the following:

- *Offer different course examinations to different sections.*
- *Prohibit cell phones and personal items from the testing area.*
- *Require academic honesty tutorial early in the student's academic program.*
- *Require that students sign an academic honesty statement for each examination (Figure 15.1).*
- *Assign seats to students during the test.*

RELEVANT LEGAL CASES

Matthew Coster v. Cristina Duquette, AC 30601 (Conn. Super. Ct. 2008)

Nancy Jones v. The Board of Governors of the University of North Carolina, 704 F.2d 713 (W.D. N.C. 1983)

Academic honesty and fairness are core values in the university setting. Although public safety is a core public value, courts will not allow university administrators to rush to judgment in punishing students for cheating unless the record proves that there was in fact cheating. Very few cases of academic dishonesty ever get to court, and even fewer get to the point in court at which a judge issues an opinion; however, in those cases, the courts have made it clear that universities must not rush to judgment when they seek to protect the core value of academic integrity. Two reported cases show how the problem can develop.

In the case of *Nancy Jones v. The Board of Governors of the University of North Carolina* (1983), a nursing student was accused of cheating on an exam. The Dean was very upset by the charges and

---

Intellectual Honesty Certification

All nursing students, both undergraduate and graduate, are now required to attach the following signed statement to every paper they submit in every nursing course they take. Papers that do not have this signed statement attached will not be graded.

I certify that:

- *This paper is entirely my own work, without any words and/or ideas from other sources (print, Web, other media, other individuals, or groups) being properly indicated (words with quotation marks), cited in text, and referenced. I have not submitted this paper to satisfy the requirements of any other course.*

Student's Signature _____

Date _____

Figure 15.1 Sample of an intellectual honesty certification.
Source: Drexel University College of Nursing and Health Professions.

pushed hard for punishment. The student judicial court found the student guilty, largely because of the pressure they received from the Dean. The student appealed this decision by filing a Section 1983 lawsuit for the violation of her civil rights in U.S. District Court, arguing that the state of North Carolina had deprived her of property without due process of law. The judge found that there had been substantial procedural flaws in how the university had handled the charges, including the facts that the student had not been told the identity of her accusers, or what the evidence against her was, or even the specific charges against her. Holding that the "balance of hardship" favored the student and ordered her immediate reinstatement pending the final resolution of her case, the judge also held that the Chancellor denied the student due process of law by unilaterally imposing punishment without complying with any established procedures. The court's decision was affirmed by the U.S. Court of Appeals when the university took the appeal. The student was not only allowed to complete her course, but was vindicated at a fair hearing and was awarded her degree; the university was forced to pay all of the attorneys' fees and costs of the trial, as well as pay damages to the student for having mistreated her.

The case of *Matthew Coster v. Cristina Duquette* (2008) highlights the fact that university internal review boards sometimes get it wrong and underlines that fact that universities need to proceed with care, especially when imposing severe sanctions. Mr. Coster and Ms. Duquette were classmates in a course taught by Dr. Moss at Central Connecticut State University. The final exam was a paper about the Holocaust, and students were to place their completed papers in Dr. Moss's mailbox. Dr. Moss concluded that approximately 80% of the papers submitted by Mr. Coster and Ms. Duquette were similar. Professor Moss then met with both students about the similarities, and each denied plagiarizing anyone else's work. Believing Ms. Duquette to be the more able student, he then filed a charge of academic misconduct against Mr. Coster. A detailed comparison of the writing style, grammar, and references used in both papers confirmed the professor's charge of plagiarism, and the university accepted the professor's assignment of fault, charging Mr. Coster with stealing Ms. Duquette's paper from Professor Moss's mailbox, copying it, and then lying to Dr. Moss at the meeting.

A student judicial hearing was held before a three-person panel, which found Mr. Coster guilty of academic dishonesty and recommended expulsion from the university. Mr. Coster appealed the panel's decision to the director of student affairs, who denied the appeal.

Mr. Coster did not appeal the university's decision to the courts. Instead, he filed a civil lawsuit against Ms. Duquette, alleging that she in fact had copied his paper. As part of the litigation, experts were hired and used to examine the electronic evidence of when documents were created and worked on; other documents were produced that supported Mr. Coster's claim that he had in fact worked on the paper. Negative inferences were drawn against Ms. Duquette because she was not able to do the same. On the basis of the evidence submitted, the trial court decided that Ms. Duquette, not Mr. Coster, had cheated, held her liable for conversion, and awarded compensatory and punitive damages against her. Ms. Duquette appealed the decision to the court of appeals, which affirmed the trial judge's decision.

SUMMARY

Empiric findings have identified that contextual factors influence the amount of academic dishonesty that occurs in universities (McCabe & Trevino, 1993). For example, students are less likely to violate academic codes in an environment in which the institution creates a climate that is supportive of academic integrity and has requisite codes and polices in place that affirm those principles. In addition, faculty members need to implement and employ such codes and policies and hold students accountable when there is academic dishonesty. It is imperative that faculty prevent academic misconduct/dishonesty in a proactive manner rather than address academic misconduct in a reactive manner—for example, by discussing the importance of doing one's own work, by making students read and sign an integrity code at the beginning of a course, and by requiring students to sign an integrity warranty whenever they submit a paper or take a test. Detailed policies related to proctoring, academic honesty, standardized exams, and the testing environments will assist with the deterrence of academic misconduct, as will publication of what penalties the student will receive whenever an act of academic dishonesty is discovered. In the event of an academic misconduct charge, the faculty needs to follow the institution's policy while being fair to the students involved.

ETHICAL CONSIDERATIONS

To create a just culture that views cheating as unacceptable, faculty and students must work together to create a culture of academic integrity (Stonecypher & Willson, 2014). Standalone ethics courses and integration of ethics content is important in a nursing curriculum. The formation of an ethical framework for practice is an essential aspect of nursing students' development to engage in professional nursing practice. Students learn how to apply theory to specific cases and to use moral reasoning to establish justified ethical stances about what a student *should do*. The faculty's role with respect to ethical development is to serve as a role model and instill moral character in students (Koharchik, Vogelstein, Crider, Devido, & Evatt, 2017). Academic dishonesty needs to be addressed from an ethical perspective and linked to patient safety. Faculty should use real cases to demonstrate unethical behavior's negative effect on patient outcomes. The stakes are high when a nursing student cheats and cares for patients without a strong command of the content. Nursing faculty need to enforce policies related to academic honesty to ensure patient safety.

CRITICAL ELEMENTS TO CONSIDER

- Develop an academic integrity policy.
- Develop a testing/proctoring policy for faculty (with student assigned seating, escorts for breaks, student personal belongings secured or in front of room).
- Develop a testing policy for students.
- Have students complete an academic honesty online tutorial early in their academic program.
- Consider the use of a software program to detect plagiarism.
- If you are an academic administrator, hold faculty development sessions related to managing and documenting acts of academic dishonesty.
- Provide the student with due process.

- Develop a rubric on how to manage specific academic dishonesty violations so that students are dealt with consistently and fairly in terms of sanctions.
- Establish a student conduct committee to investigate cases of academic dishonesty.
- Develop a test review policy that would include the academic program's position on audiotaping test review, note-taking, test question appeal process, and the like.

References

Bavier, A. R. (2009). Holding students accountable when integrity is challenged. *Nursing Education Perspectives*, *30*(1), 5. Retrieved from https://www.ncbi.nlm.nih.gov/pubmed/19331031

Koharchik, L., Vogelstein, E., Crider, M., Devido, J., & Evatt, M. (2017). Promoting nursing student's ethical development in the clinical setting. *American Journal of Nursing*, *117*(11), 57–60. doi:10.1097/01. NAJ.0000530227.40835.24

Kolanko, K. M., Clark, C., Heinrich, K. T., Olive, D., Serembus, J. F., & Sifford, K. S. (2006). Academic dishonesty, bullying, incivility, and violence: Difficult challenges facing nurse educators. *Nursing Education Perspectives*, *27*(1), 34–43.

Lindsay, C. L., III. (2005). *The college student's guide to the law*. Dallas, TX: Taylor Trade Publishing.

Matthew Coster v. Cristina Duquette, AC 30601 (Conn. Super. Ct. 2008).

McCabe, D. L., & Trevino, L. K. (1993). Academic dishonesty: Honor codes and other contextual influences. *Journal of Higher Education*, *64*(5), 522–538. doi:10.2307/2959991

Nancy Jones v. The Board of Governors of the University of North Carolina, 704 F.2d 713 (W.D. N.C. 1983).

Schmitz, K., & Schaffer, M. (1995). Ethical problems encountered in the teaching of nursing: Student and faculty perceptions. *Journal of Nursing Education*, *34*(1), 42–44. doi:10.3928/0148-4834-19950101-10

Stonecypher, K., & Willson, P. (2014). Academic policies and practices to deter cheating in nursing education. *NLN Nursing Education Perspectives*, *35*(3), 167–179. doi:10.5480/12-1028.1

16

Academic Freedom and Speech: Examining the Student Perspective

Case Study 16.1
A Student Claims the Academic Freedom to Deny Her Professor Co-authorship on Class Paper Submitted for Publication

Your role: You are Dr. Fontana, the faculty member who is teaching this RN/BSN course.

Dr. Fontana has been teaching full time in the undergraduate nursing program for 8 years. She has mentored several undergraduate and graduate nursing students who have published their classroom papers in peer-reviewed nursing journals, the student as the first author and—on most occasions—Dr. Fontana as the second author. Dr. Fontana discloses her authorship policy to every class at the beginning of the year: If a student receives critiques, comments, and feedback on one or two drafts of any paper, and if the paper is then ready for publication, that student is free to seek publication as the sole author. However, if a student writes a paper that still needs work after two drafts, and if the student is willing to work with Dr. Fontana on the paper after the course is formally over, then Dr. Fontana requests second authorship.

At the beginning of the new semester, Dr. Fontana was assigned to an RN/BSN course and she disclosed verbally her authorship policy. One of the students decided to write a paper on female circumcision, a subject that Dr. Fontana had studied years ago. Enthusiastically, Dr. Fontana encouraged the student to seek publication of the work and by the end of the term, Dr. Fontana had provided two substantive reviews of the paper and a third review that was more modest, but that did provide additional feedback. As the semester drew to a close, Dr. Fontana was discussing the most appropriate journal to which the article might be submitted when the student announced to her that she had reconsidered and thought she should be the sole author. Dr. Fontana, startled, did reiterate her standing policy, but the student countered that she thought the feedback was minor and did not warrant second authorship. Dr. Fontana disagreed with her assessment and told the student so; the semester came to a close with no resolution of the issue.

Questions

- How would you first proceed?
- Are there any university or departmental guidelines on student/faculty collaboration and co-publication?
- Did the student have the academic freedom to seek sole authorship and publication of the article?
- Is there any possible recourse for the faculty member should the student indeed seek publication of the article as sole author?

UNIVERSITY STUDENTS AND THEIR ACADEMIC FREEDOM: LEGAL PRINCIPLES AND REVIEW OF THE LITERATURE

As Kaplin, Lee, Hutchens, and Rooksby (2019) write in *The Law of Higher Education* (perhaps the leading text on the law in higher education):

> Academic freedom traditionally has been considered to be an essential aspect of higher education in the United States. Academic freedom has been a major determinant of the missions of higher educational institutions, both public and private, and a major factor in shaping the roles of faculty members as well as students. (p. 751)

However, they also further elaborate: "Yet the concept of academic freedom eludes precise definition.... It draws meaning from both the world of education and the world of law" (p. 248). Questions of academic freedom, often interpreted as issues of free speech, are therefore common in academia. Typically, the most public issues surround an individual faculty member's right to free speech,[1] but there are still occasions when student free speech or academic freedom is debated. For example, whom does the First Amendment (free speech amendment) protect? Does it protect those in both public and private institutions? And does it protect verbal, written, and symbolic communication? Recall what the First Amendment says:

> Congress shall make no law respecting an establishment of religion, or prohibiting the free exercise thereof; or abridging the freedom of speech, or of the press; or the right of the people to peaceably assemble, and to petition the Government for a redress of grievances.

Regarding whom the First Amendment protects, it is important to note that the legal system treats high school students under age 18 and college students age 18 and over very differently, with high schools having greater authority to regulate their speech than students at universities.

As early as 1965, Schodde wrote advocating for a free student press, freedom of speech, the rights of students to hear controversial speakers on campuses from any sides of a respective issue, the right of due process *for students* when accusations of university policies' violations are alleged, and even a rebellion to the principles of in loco parentis[2]—in which the college student's right to privacy (and academic freedom) and the rights of the parents intertwine, especially when parents are providing financial support in whole or in part. To Schodde, actions supporting in loco parentis were improper for college-age adults. To this day there are still ongoing residual issues despite the erosion of in loco parentis, as the social pendulum swings toward individual college student rights and away from parental rights and parental notification.

Another critical issue when determining whether a college student's First Amendment freedom of speech is breached is to return to a founding principle that exists within the amendment itself:

---

[1] In a technical sense, universities have a right to determine who may teach, what may be taught, and who may be admitted to study, and so it is the university that has academic freedom more than an individual professor, and this was affirmed in 2008 in *Stronach v. Virginia State University* (Roth, McEllistrem, D'Ogostino, & Brown, 2009).

[2] The doctrine of in *loco parentis* is a time-honored legal opinion borrowed from English common law, which "by placing the educational institution in the parents' shoes, the doctrine permitted the institution to exert almost untrammeled authority over students' lives" (Kaplan & Lee, 2007, p. 16).

"The rules in the U.S. Constitution only apply to *government actors*. Private entities, and therefore private colleges, don't have to live by them" (Lindsay, 2005, p. 121). In other words, the constitutional protections on freedom of speech for a private college are not codified as they would be at a state-supported college (thus a government entity). Nevertheless, any university, private or not, is usually reticent to abridge constitutional rights that might lead to very negative publicity. Further, as most private colleges and universities usually are recipients of some types of federal monies or aid, they can voluntarily become subject to government regulation.

What sorts of communication does the First Amendment protect in academia? One of the most highly visible high school student free speech cases was *Tinker v. Des Moines Independent Community School District* (1969), in which students were found to have the right to wear black armbands to a public school as an expression of opposition to the Vietnam War. The Supreme Court concluded this was a form of "symbolic speech" and "closely akin to pure speech" and that this form of speech in high school students was protected unless school administrators could show that it would cause a substantial disruption of the school's educational mission. The court ruled that high school students do not "shed their constitutional rights when they enter the schoolhouse door." But the Court did note that school administrators have far greater ability to restrict free speech than governments do.

Another widely publicized case involving freedom of verbal speech of college students occurred in 1993 and received national attention. In this case, Eden Jacobowitz, a freshman at the University of Pennsylvania, was trying to write an English paper in his dorm room, but he was disturbed by noise from below his window coming from a group of female African American students celebrating their sorority's Founders Day. His first response was to yell out "Please keep quiet!" (Kors & Silvergate, 1998, p. 1). As the noise continued, 20 minutes later he yelled out, "Shut up, you water buffalo. If you want a party, there's a zoo a mile from here" (p. 1). Within weeks the university administrative judicial inquiry officer filed charges of racial harassment against Jacobowitz. He was given an option of a settlement or an academic plea bargain or of facing a judicial hearing and possible penalties up to and including expulsion. After very contentious public charges and countercharges, Penn officials later offered to dismiss the charge of racial harassment if Jacobowitz would apologize, attend a racial sensitivity seminar, agree to dormitory probation as long as he lived on campus, and accept a temporary mark on his record (until his junior year if he had no further infractions) that would brand him as guilty. Jacobowitz claimed his use of the phrase *water buffalo* was not used as a racial epithet, and for that reason he declined the settlement, and Penn went forward with the formal charges that he had violated its code of conduct.

What Penn did not expect was the intense national spotlight that would shine on the university, putting its speech code (and the conduct of all the Penn administrators) under severe scrutiny. The American Civil Liberties Union (ACLU) became involved, and a federal lawsuit was filed by Jacobowitz against certain Penn officials, including the school's president. With a highly publicized, now international case causing harm to the reputation of this Ivy League school, an offer was made to Jacobowitz that he simply apologize for the remarks. In turn, the women would drop the case. The case thus came to a close, and Penn conducted an investigation concerning why this episode escalated so. The code of conduct regulating freedom of speech was subsequently dropped and later reissued in a revised form. Penn established a Committee on Open Expression with very specific guidelines, and the current PennBook (2019–2010) states that individuals or groups violate the Guidelines on Open Expression if:

a. *They interfere unreasonably with the activities of other persons. The time of day, size, noise level, and general tenor of a meeting, event or demonstration are factors that may be considered in determining whether conduct is reasonable;*
b. *They cause injury to persons or property or threaten to cause such injury;*
c. *They hold meetings, events or demonstrations under circumstances where health or safety is endangered; or*
d. *They knowingly interfere with unimpeded movement in a University location.*

Finally, people are constantly reminded not to take academic freedom and First Amendment protections to *write freely* for granted or to minimize their importance. Remember the case of the

Jordanian university student who was jailed for writing a poem (which he denied doing) that was critical of Jordan's king (Joyce & Kevlin, 2010). In the United States, the right to criticize leaders dates to before the Constitution and the case of John Peter Zenger, the printer, who criticized the King of England. But it is routinely tested, on a variety of grounds, and always, always for "good reasons."

As evidenced by the issue of the black arm band, the shouts from a college dorm window, and an undergraduate student's writing, these are all forms of expression that warrant a discussion of whether they are protected by the First Amendment and the principles of academic freedom or not. Whether the undergraduate student in Case Study 16.1 was exercising her constitutional right to publish her paper without her professor is actually another example of both the complexity of this First Amendment case that is addressed in *DePree v. Saunders* (2009) and Kaplan and Lee's admonition that the principles of academic freedom both traverse the social system of higher education and jurisprudence (2007).

DISCUSSION OF CASE STUDY

In Case Study 16.1, Dr. Fontana learned that her student intended to publish her class paper independently. At first, Dr. Fontana was quite distressed by the student's decision, as she had given the student substantive feedback on two drafts, including a significant restructuring of the paper. Subsequently, the student had asked for a third round of assistance, which triggered the policy and her right to be identified as a coauthor. In Dr. Fontana's view, she had provided feedback on three drafts, was very pleased with the progress of the work, and was looking forward to the student publishing the work with her coauthorship. This had never happened before, and so Dr. Fontana was concerned whether she had done anything to make the student react, in her view, so unprofessionally. She asked herself whether her standing policy could in any way be perceived as improper. Dr. Fontana decided to search the Internet to see if she could find any publishing guidelines that could instruct her. She did realize, however, that communicating her policy orally to students might not have been "strong enough," even though it was announced so early in the year, before the paper-writing process started.

The second question in Case Study 16.1 is, Are there any university or departmental guidelines on student/faculty collaboration and copublication? In this case, Dr. Fontana's college did not, and this episode later compelled her to spearhead the development of such a guideline. A quick literature review search on the Internet found very little direction for nursing faculty facing copublishing issues, but an article by two biology professors, "To Co-Author or Not to Co-Author: How to Write, Publish, and Negotiate Issues of Authorship With Undergraduate Research Students" (Burks & Chumchal, 2009), did confirm that there are real negotiating strategies to take with undergraduate students and also risks to faculty who undertake this kind of scholarship. The American Mathematical Society (Karp, 2016) has advocated for copublishing in research journals with undergraduate students, but they take the issue from a different approach—the *adding* of students to a paper where the content they contributed was part of the faculty member's research. There certainly were no signs during the semester that there were any relationship issues between the student and Dr. Fontana and so, with the semester at an end and the manuscript graded and returned, Dr. Fontana contemplated what the best course of action would be.

 WHEN TO CONSULT THE UNIVERSITY COUNSEL

It would be unlikely that a student who claims their academic freedom has been violated by a professor would contact the university attorney, but there is absolutely nothing that would prevent the student from asking. University counsel is likely to get involved if the question is related to an article that is being readied for publication (when intervention and advice can solve a situation before it becomes a problem) and also when an alleged violation *has already occurred* (e.g., the student and faculty are fighting over a journal submission); even here, university counsel will perceive the adverse effects of claims and litigation and will be inclined to intervene to protect the university's interests.

In Case Study 16.1, it is recommended to negotiate with the individual professor if there are co-authorship disputes. If that does not resolve the issue, the student has the option of going through regular administrative channels (e.g., Department Chair, Associate Dean, or Dean) or going directly to the Ombudsman. Filing a lawsuit directly against the faculty is an option, but that should be a last resort, for which university counsel will provide advice.

If the case of alleged academic freedom violation has already taken place, the decision tree is more complex. If it involves ideas or a product that has led to patents or inventions (less common in nursing), then the stakes (and future possible income) are higher. If the student claims plagiarism of something in print, first contact the alleged offending faculty member, and ask them to contact the journal editor in question, and either retract the paper or acknowledge the authorship omission and request adding the student as co-author (even as first author). It is unlikely that the student will only request an addition of an acknowledgment. If the faculty member refuses, the student can contact the journal or file a complaint. Most universities have a committee on scientific misconduct, and the student can file a claim with that committee. The functions of the Committee on Scientific Conduct for the University of Maine, for example, can be found at https://umaine.edu/research-compliance/research-misconduct/committee-scientific-misconduct/. A simple Internet search will provide the procedures of similar committees at various universities. If the alleged action has already taken place (an article is under review, but it has not been published) and the student has subsequently graduated, it is unlikely that departmental channels can effectively resolve the issue or whether the Ombudsman office can technically still be used (i.e., the student is now a graduate), but those avenues could be considered. In case of loss of royalties and revenues from patents, individual legal recourse is likely an option.

FINDINGS AND DISPOSITION

If Dr. Fontana had not thought much about her efforts on this manuscript or had not believed in its potential for publication, she might have just let the issue go. However, Dr. Fontana genuinely felt her effort and direction were substantive, and in the end decided it would actually be unethical for the student to submit the work to the journal, falsely representing the work as solely her own. Dr. Fontana, therefore, emailed the student to inquire whether she was still committed to publishing the article and whether she had given her argument that indeed she (as the teaching faculty) had met her guidelines for co-authorship. After about two months with no answer from the student, Dr. Fontana emailed the student again and finally got a response.

The student informed her that she had considered what Dr. Fontana had said at the beginning of class about co-authorship, but reminded her that her guidelines were not written on the syllabus. She further declared in her email that she had given the situation much thought and determined that the amount of feedback given did not warrant co-authorship, despite Dr. Fontana's feedback on the first two drafts and the "most minor of feedback" on the third draft, as she put it. She said she had already submitted the paper for publication and had listed Dr. Fontana in the acknowledgments and stated she thought that was a better representation of Dr. Fontana's efforts. This leads to the third question: Did the student have the academic freedom to seek sole authorship and publication of the article?

Dr. Fontana was convinced that the student was unethically misrepresenting the work as her own, and she simply could not accept the student's actions. True, her policy was not contained in the syllabus, where, in retrospect, it might better have been, but the student never denied being made fully aware of the policy. After much thought and consultation with a fellow colleague (who did not necessarily agree with Dr. Fontana's proposed course of action), Dr. Fontana decided to mail a certified letter to the student declaring that if the student did not contact the editor and request that the article be pulled, she would contact the state board of nursing in which the student was licensed and file an ethics complaint against her. After that, she wrote that she would also contact the editor and declare the submission unethically submitted, an action that would certainly cause the editor to pull it. Shortly thereafter, Dr. Fontana received a curt email from the student simply stating that she had pulled the article. To confirm this, Dr. Fontana contacted the editor and indeed verified that the article had been rescinded by the student. Without disclosing any further information, Dr. Fontana thanked the editor for the information.

The fourth question is, do you agree with the actions or recourse that Dr. Fontana took? Would you have acted differently? If so, what different recourses would you have taken when the student sought sole authorship of the article?

Dr. Fontana decided that in the future she would always include her copublishing guidelines on her syllabus and thought it might be in the college's best interest to devise a publishing policy that would protect both faculty and student intellectual property interests. Several months later, Dr. Fontana did an Internet search to see if the manuscript had been published elsewhere. It had not.

It is also important to note that the actions taken by Dr. Fontana were not supported by the colleague she spoke to. It is entirely debatable whether the actions of this RN would constitute an ethical charge against her right to practice according to the respective state nurse practice act. It is entirely possible that the student could also pursue countercharges. Although the strategy taken by Dr. Fontana worked in this case, it seems a high-risk course of action. If the paper were publishable, the result of the way this misunderstanding was handled resulted in important, new knowledge that was not shared with the nursing scholarship community.

RELEVANT LEGAL CASE

Ogindo v Binghamton University et al, No. 3:2007cv01322

In this complicated legal case, the argument that a doctoral student had the academic freedom to publish his work without crediting his dissertation adviser became a point of contention and litigation. In *Ogindo v. Binghamton* (2007), a doctoral student in chemistry sued his professors over intellectual theft. In 2007, Charles Ogindo filed a suit seeking $200 million in compensatory damages and $2 million in punitive damages and attorney fees against Binghamton University; his former dissertation adviser, John J. Eisch; the former and current chemistry department chair; and the director of graduate studies.

After successfully completing his oral examinations and all coursework toward his PhD in chemistry, Ogindo never completed his dissertation. His adviser, Dr. Eisch, had disciplined him and ultimately went through the internal policies of the Graduate Progressions Committee (GPC) to have him dismissed from the program for poor performance in the laboratory and unacceptable scholarship.

Ogindo filed the lawsuit only when he later discovered that two papers on two experiments he participated in had been published without naming himself as co-author, or acknowledging his contributions (Swartz, 2007). One of the experiments was his dissertation experiment, for which Dr. Eisch had criticized his results, only to reverse himself later and admit the student was right after all.

This story is complex, but charges of academic theft or plagiarism of graduate students by professors, and specifically academic advisers (in this case, the doctoral student's dissertation chair), are not uncommon, according to the prestigious *Chronicle of Higher Education* (Bartlett & Smallwood, 2004). Generally, lawsuits or formal complaints stem from the following:

1. Questions over jurisdiction, mainly from state-funded universities
2. Questions over internal processes, especially due process
3. Fear of reprisal and professional fallout, especially when the accused is a well-known professor (Bartlett & Smallwood, 2004)

In this case, there was a very tenuous relationship between the student and his graduate adviser. Around April 2005, the student, having had completed all requirements for his doctorate except his dissertation, alleged that his adviser would not approve his proposed dissertation experiments, and instead wanted him to forge data on another experiment led by Eisch and Dutta (another doctoral student). Ogindo attempted to replicate Dutta's experiment, but was unable to do so. Ogindo alleged he was being asked to forge unreplicable results, and Eisch subsequently attempted to get Ogindo removed from the laboratory. An appeal to the director of graduate studies allowed Ogindo to return under probationary status, and eventually Eisch confirmed Dutta's data indeed could not be replicated, and Ogindo agreed to work with another former student. In January 2006, Ogindo applied for a part-time teaching position at another state university, but needed Eisch's permission to take the job because he was in dissertation advisement and was being funded under a Clark Fellowship. Eisch refused to support the job offer, indicating it would interfere with the struggling student's full-time commitment as a doctoral student. In late January, Ogindo requested his probationary status be repealed because his initial claims about the viability of Dutto's data had been confirmed. Eisch denied the appeal but affirmed that Ogindo's work product had improved but that he would have to sustain this progress.

In July 2006, Eisch sought to terminate Ogindo's participation in Eisch's research program. Ogindo again appealed to the director of graduate studies and sought possession of his laboratory notebooks, which was granted. Ogindo proceeded to submit several manuscripts to various journals based on his experiments, but without his adviser's approval. Because it is unusual for graduate student work in chemistry to be authored without the graduate adviser, the editors of these journals contacted Eisch, who confirmed he had not authorized the manuscript submissions. Eisch filed a complaint against the student with the GPC who ruled that "Mr. Ogindo on three instances submitted work for publication or presentation without Professor Eisch's knowledge or consent" (Justia US Law, 2010, p. 5). The GPC believed these acts constituted serious professional and ethical transgressions. The GPC recommended termination from the PhD program, but the chemistry department faculty tabled the recommendations and worked out a compromise whereby an outside reader would independently evaluate the student's dissertation work. If the evaluator affirmed the quality of the work, then the student would be allowed to defend the dissertation. If not, he would be offered to resubmit it as a master's thesis. The student agreed to drop his grievance against his adviser and accept these terms, but retained the right to renew his claim.

In September 2006, Ogindo requested that a new dissertation committee be reconstituted, and in November he submitted another draft of his dissertation. In December the dissertation committee rejected the dissertation and gave the student until February 22, 2007, to revise it. Ogindo submitted a new draft on February 5, 2007, but his new adviser found it unacceptable and wanted a complete rewrite rather than a corrected copy. Subsequently, the Cornell University professor (the selected outside reader) completed his evaluation of Ogindo's work but found "the dissertation in no way constituted a PhD thesis" (Justia US Law, 2010, p. 6). On May 25, 2007, Ogindo was informed his work did not constitute a PhD, and he was offered the opportunity to complete a master's thesis. Ogindo refused the offer, and requested his grievance be reinstituted and he be allowed to defend his dissertation. He was informed he could not reinstate the grievance because the terms of the grievance had been completed and his insistence that he be allowed to defend his dissertation was again denied.

In July 2007, Ogindo became aware that his adviser Dr. Eisch had co-authored a paper published in the *European Journal of Inorganic Chemistry* that mirrored his own work. As Ogindo's name was not included as a co-author or contributor, he filed a lawsuit against the defendants in New York State Supreme Court alleging breach of contract, fraud, and promissory estoppel, but his lawsuit was dismissed on October 24, 2007.

Later that fall, Ogindo requested registration for one credit of independent study to maintain the continuous registration required of doctoral candidates. Because his fellowship funding had been discontinued, the student was obligated to pay the one credit tuition himself, which he ultimately failed to do. In December, Ogindo refiled his lawsuit in the federal court, alleging federal causes of action including substantive due process, copyright infringement, and patent infringement as well as discrimination and retaliation. In March 2008, he was warned by the graduate director that he was in danger of being formally dropped from the university (remember, the offer for the master's thesis was still on the table) if he did not maintain his continuous registration with a full tuition payment. As he could not technically register for spring courses because he had not paid his fall tuition bill, he was dismissed from the university on March 26, 2008, for nonpayment and noncontinuous graduate registration. In June 2008, Ogindo amended his federal court complaint. On October 17, 2008, the court dismissed all claims of substantive due process, copyright infringement, patent infringement, breach of contract, promissory estoppel, educational malpractice, and fraud claims. The plaintiff's remaining claims alleging (a) discrimination on account of his race and/or national origin; (b) retaliation for plaintiff's assertion of a right protected by 42 U.S.C. § 1983; and (c) a violation of his right to due process of law, were reviewed and also summarily dismissed in January 2010.

SUMMARY

This chapter examines how academic freedom is much more than just a professor's right to express unpopular points of view, in public or in the classroom. The principles of academic freedom extend to students, too, and apply broadly to words, symbols, dress, lifestyle, and actions—to newspapers, the "public square," and to the Internet. But the right to speak is not without bounds.

Although the court ruled against the graduate student, it remains obvious that these issues are very difficult for students to win (although certainly not impossible) because of the power differential between student and professor or student and university. Complicating all this is the academy's need for alternative revenue sources, and the desire to control what "results from" the exercise of inquiry on campus. In the case of *Ogindo v. Binghamton* (2007), the findings of the contested experiments and the revenue from possible patents in the biotech industry might have been significant, meaning that the financial stakes for both student and university could have been high. The student made one major mistake, which turned out to be fatal: initially seeking independent publication of the experiment articles himself and without his adviser. This procedural error caused him to "lose" on the merits. Finally, as mentioned in Case Study 16.1, Dr. Fontana did not have a published standard college/department co-authorship policy at the time of this case. Other subsequent and similar cases led to the development of a co-authorship policy.

ETHICAL CONSIDERATIONS

In 1967, the American Association of University Professors (AAUP), along with the National Student Association (now USSA) and the Association of American Colleges (now Association of American Colleges and Universities), published a Joint Statement on Rights and Freedoms of Students (Hamilton, 2002). In this statement, the groups collectively acknowledge that while some measure of academic freedom ought to be afforded to students, it would not be a lesser concept of freedom. Students, it is noted, *qua* students, are not yet fully prepared to engage in scholarly discourse. However, it is the duty of the institution and faculty to encourage and prepare students to develop the relevant capacities for scholarly discourse and the pursuit of truth. The statement enumerates several specific freedoms to be afforded students in the context of the classroom, student affairs, and off-campus activities that all speak to the degree and extent of student academic freedom, sometimes with corresponding student obligations (see Hamilton, 2002, Appendix G). The three freedoms in the classroom include the freedom of expression, including the ability to disagree with presented information or views while still being responsible for learning the course content. Secondly, students should be free from biased evaluation based upon disagreeing views, while also being responsible for meeting the standards of academic performance. Thirdly, students have a right to confidentiality regarding their views, beliefs, and political associations. Regarding student affairs, students have a freedom of association, allowing students to join or to organize associations to promote or engage in common interests. But these organizations should also meet certain criteria, such as avoiding discrimination in its membership (with some exceptions for religious organizations). Secondly, as in the classroom, in other activities on campus students should enjoy freedom of inquiry and expression, including the freedom to support, in an orderly and nondisruptive manner, causes they believe in and the ability to invite speakers of their own choosing to campus. Thirdly, students are free to express views on institutional policy and participate in the governing of the institution. And fourthly, students have the freedom to produce their own publications without censorship or prior restraint and protection from institutional reprisal. Regarding off-campus activities, firstly, students have the same rights of any other citizen, including rights of speech, peaceful assembly, and the right to petition for grievances absent attempts to inhibit the exercise of these rights by institutional powers. And secondly, when students violate the law, institutional authority should only be employed when the institution's interests are clearly involved. What is within this statement may not fully define the extent and import of academic freedom for students, but the statement does present a thoughtful framework within which to consider these issues.

CRITICAL ELEMENTS TO CONSIDER

- College-age students 18 and above have a constitutional right to freedom of expression, but that freedom only limits government actors. Private institutions have greater rights to limit free speech.
- There is no "academic freedom" for students to publish work product independently of their professors who have had substantive input into that intellectual work product. If a student is going to turn a class assignment or paper into a publication, the student should first ask this question: "Is this work completely my own or have I had assistance with it in first draft or revision?"
- The next step is to consider whether there is an official co-authorship policy for student and faculty in your university, college, department, or in the course syllabus. That should be the best guide for how to next proceed.
- Our view is that co-authorship between student and faculty ought to be encouraged and welcomed, not discouraged or resisted by the student. The best science today is team science and not the product of a single individual, viewpoint, or effort.
- Further, editors, especially nursing editors, really do not want to publish student papers unless they reach a very high bar. A journal editor would not publish anything that looks as though it is a class assignment. Journals have very specific guidelines and missions, and all successful submissions ultimately published in respected journals have met the standards set by the editor and the journal's editorial board. Having faculty review and participate helps students exceed this bar. In short, two heads are typically better than one.
- Nursing students (particularly undergraduate students, but also graduate students) are often at an advantage when their submission is co-authored by a faculty member, especially one with a doctorate. It gives the manuscript gravitas that otherwise may be missing, especially when the student is technically not a licensed nurse.
- Students are encouraged to question professors, civilly and constructively, who profess the policy that anything written in their class may warrant the option that the professor be listed as second author. These policies, unless they adhere to acceptable co-authorship standards and policies, may be unethical, and for this reason knowing what co-authorship policies exist is very important. Challenges to policies should be made up the chain of command, and in a respectful way, with the argument that the university's intention should be to encourage and reward (by recognition, when deserved) innovation and creative thinking, not burden it.
- There are also guidelines for co-authorship that are found on journal websites, and when a manuscript is submitted, often each author's exact contribution must be attested to. For example, the *Journal of Clinical Nursing* has very specific guidelines that state the following:
  1. Have made substantial contributions to conception and design, or acquisition of data, or analysis and interpretation of data;
  2. Been involved in drafting the manuscript or revising it critically for important intellectual content;

3. Given final approval of the version to be published. Each author should have participated sufficiently in the work to take public responsibility for appropriate portions of the content; and

4. Agreed to be accountable for all aspects of the work in ensuring that questions related to the accuracy or integrity of any part of the work are appropriately investigated and resolved (Authorship, 1999–2019, p. 1).

- Further, the *Journal of Clinical Nursing* and many others adhere to the definition of authorship designated by the International Committee of Medical Journal Editors (ICMJE). According to the ICMJE criteria, established authorship or co-authorship must be based on substantial contributions to conception and design of, or acquisition of data or analysis and interpretation of data; drafting the article or revising it critically for important intellectual content; and final approval of the version to be published (ICMJE, 2010, p. 1).

- Our view is that co-publication between students and faculty ought to be a positive experience, but students should not be taken advantage of in the scholarship of publishing enterprise, and adherence to best practices in co-publishing will ensure this. Academic freedom of students (not just faculty) must be protected.

- Last, respective faculty guidelines (that do not, of course, violate any institutional policy) should appear in any course syllabus.

Helpful Resources

- The First Amendment in Schools. http://www.ascd.org/Publications/Books/Overview/The-First-Amendment-in-Schools.aspx
- Student Press Law Center: Test Your Knowledge of the First Amendment: http://www.splc.org/falawtest/
- Freedom With Limitations: How the Supreme Court Has Limited Students' Freedom of Speech Over the Past Five Decades. https://commons.trincoll.edu/edreform/2017/05/freedom-with-limitations-how-the-supreme-court-has-limited-students-freedom-of-speech-over-the-past-five-decades/
- Foundation for Individual Rights in Education (FIRE): http://www.thefire.org/
- American Civil Liberties Union (ACLU): http://www.aclu.org/

References

Authorship. (1999–2019). *Journal of Clinical Nursing*. Retrieved from https://onlinelibrary.wiley.com/page/journal/13652702/homepage/forauthors.html#editorial

Bartlett, T., & Smallwood, S. (2004, December 17). Four academic plagiarists you've never heard of: How many more are out there? *Chronicle of Higher Education*. Retrieved from https://www.chronicle.com/article/Four-Academic-Plagiarists/31890

Burks, R. L., & Chumchal, M. M. (2009). To co-author or not to co-author: How to write, publish, and negotiate issues of authorship with undergraduate research students. *Science Signals, 2*(94), 3. doi:10.1126/scisignal.294tr3

DePree v. Saunders 80, No. 08-60978 (5th Cir. 2009).

Hamilton, H. W. (2002). *Academic ethics: Problems and materials on professional conduct and shared governance*. Westport, CT: Praeger Publishers.

International Committee of Medical Journal Editors. (2010). *Uniform requirements for manuscripts submitted to biomedical journals: Ethical considerations in the conduct and reporting of research: Authorship and contributorship*. Retrieved from https://www.ncbi.nlm.nih.gov/pmc/articles/PMC3142758/

Joyce, R., & Kevlin, N. (2010). Jordan: Student jailed for writing poem. *University World News*. Retrieved from https://www.universityworldnews.com/post.php?story=20100911064405442

Kaplin, W. A., Lee, B. A., Hutchens, N. H., & Rooksby, J. H. (2019). *The law of higher education: A comprehensive guide to legal implications of administrative decision-making* (6th ed.). San Francisco, CA: John Wiley & Sons.

Karp, D. (2016). Publishing research with undergraduate co-authors. *American Mathematical Society*. Retrieved from https://blogs.ams.org/mathmentoringnetwork/2016/12/23/publishing-research-with-undergraduate-co-authors/

Kors, A. C. & Silvergate, H. A. (1998). The water buffalo affair. In *The Shadow University: The betrayal of liberty on America's campuses*. New York, NY: Free Press. Retrieved from http://movies2.nytimes.com/books/first/k/kors-university.html

Lindsay, C. L., III. (2005). *The college student's guide to the law*. Lanham, MD: Taylor Trade Publishing.

Ogindo v. Binghamton, No. 07-CV-1322 (N.D.N.Y 2007). Retrieved from https://law.justia.com/cases/federal/district-courts/new-york/nyndce/3:2007cv01322/70116/100/

PennBook. (2019–2020). *Guidelines on open expression*. Retrieved from https://catalog.upenn.edu/pennbook/open-expression/

Roth, J. A., McEllistrem, S., D'Ogostino, T., & Brown, C. J. (2009). *Higher education law in America* (10th ed.). Malvern, PA: Center for Education & Employment Law.

Stronach v. Virginia Stale University, No. 3:07CV646-HEH, 2008 WL 161304 (E.D. Va. Jan. 15, 2008).

Swartz, D. (2007). Binghamton University doctoral student sues professors over intellectual theft. *Africa Resource*. Retrieved from https://www.africaresource.com/essays-a-reviews/race-watch/448-binghamton-university-doctoral-student-sues-professors-over-intellectual-theft?showall=1

Tinker v. Des Moines Independent Community School District, 393 U.S. 503 (1969).

17

Incivility: Faculty on Faculty and Academic Nursing Administrator on Faculty, Their Subordinates

Case Study 17.1
When Faculty Flout Normal Procedures

Your role: You are Dr. Fowler, the Associate Dean for the division of nursing at State University.

There has been much discussion among your faculty concerning a proposal to offer more teaching credit for undergraduate courses that typically average 53.2 students; the typical graduate course averages only 18.6 students. This disparity has long existed, and faculty members who primarily teach graduate students have enjoyed teaching significantly fewer students in each annual review over the past 5 years. The undergraduate faculty members feel as if they are carrying a heavier and unfair teaching load compared with members who teach in the master's or doctoral program. The Curriculum Committee At-Large, which represents faculty members who sit on the baccalaureate, master's, and doctoral curriculum committees, has decided to use a blog for faculty members to express their viewpoints on a proposal to give more credit for classes of more than 50 students and also to reduce credit (except a doctoral seminar or doctoral advisement) for any course with fewer than 10 students. Blogs have been used for faculty voting for years, but no specific instructions for using the blog have been established.

The blog has been up now for 10 days, and although many undergraduate faculty members have posted their views, which are largely supportive of the change, very few of the graduate faculty members have posted on the blog. In a previous full nursing faculty meeting, one of the tenured faculty members, Dr. Isherwood, stood up and declared it took more preparation to teach graduate students which startled and disturbed the undergraduate faculty. One of the undergraduate faculty members, Dr. Alami, asked her to prove her statement and to back it up with data. Since this confrontation in the full nursing faculty meeting took place, the graduate nursing faculty members have been very defensive but have never put forth the data to support Dr. Isherwood's statement.

After 10 days of the open blog being posted, a full nursing faculty meeting is scheduled for final discussion and a vote taken on the new credit system. One hour before Dr. Fowler is to convene the meeting, open the discussion, and conduct a vote, he receives a letter signed (scanned and sent by email) by six of the eight tenured faculty members, stating their vehement opposition to the proposal. They also write that because they are tenured, their views should carry extra consideration. The Dean is copied on the letter to Dr. Fowler. Dr. Fowler is flabbergasted by this last-minute ploy and is furious at what is perceived to be an unprofessional and uncivil act. Dr. Fowler knows there is a faculty meeting in only an hour, and ponders what the best course of action should be.[1]

Questions

- Are the six tenured nursing faculty members being uncivil in their submission of this last-minute letter?
- How should Dr. Fowler first respond?
- What should Dr. Fowler say at the full nursing faculty meeting?
- Should graduate faculty members receive *more* credit for their courses (as some institutions practice) than for teaching undergraduate courses, or should they receive the same or less credit (as this proposal suggests) for teaching small graduate courses on average?
- Should tenured faculty members have a larger or more influential voice than the non-tenured or non-tenure-track faculty?
- How can the contribution of every faculty member, regardless of position and rank, be valued in any respective nursing division or college?

MANAGING FACULTY INCIVILITY: LEGAL PRINCIPLES AND REVIEW OF THE LITERATURE

Although the incivility of students appears to have garnered the most attention in the literature, the problem with faculty incivility cannot be ignored or minimized. The deterioration of student civility has real parallels to what is happening among faculty in general and nursing faculty in particular. Everyone has likely experienced excessive gossip; faculty members who are very egocentric and overly focused on their own careers or teaching schedules at the expense of the teaching mission of the department, college, or university; too much passive-aggressive behavior and avoidance of real conflict resolution; and disparaging comments made about administrators, even though few nursing faculty members have any desire to become a department chair or an academic nursing administrator (Glasgow, Dreher, Cornelius, & Bhattacharya, 2009). In other words, all too often, there are many critics but few faculty members who want to serve in the very demanding job of an academic nursing executive at any level.

Faculty on faculty incivility has many implications. Wright and Hill (2015) write "Faculty-to-faculty incivility is especially relevant to academic medical centers because many faculty within health professions schools have responsibilities for both student education and patient care. They educate students in classroom and clinical settings, fellow health professionals, and patients" (p. 12). Problems with incivility in this and other academic centers risk the deterioration of their academic mission, and may impact health and patient care in a negative way. Clark and Springer (2010) define "academic incivility" as "disruptive behavior that substantially or repeatedly interferes with teaching and learning. Incivility on college campuses jeopardizes the welfare of all members of the academy" (p. 319).

Clark and Springer (2010) further write that "the challenge of demanding workloads [for nursing faculty], maintaining clinical competence, advancement issues, and a perceived lack of administrative support, contribute to faculty stress" (p. 322), which is characterized by problematic students; long-standing salary inequities; and faculty-to-faculty incivility, bullying, and hazing. Faculty

---

[1] If there is no faculty governance model, then these changes may be made by fiat or decree by a Dean. But when faculty governance is important (or specified in faculty bylaws), these issues (as proposals) generally work their way up through normal internal administrative channels, as they did in this case.

incivility does not occur only between individual faculty members. Clark (2008) earlier noted that student perceptions of faculty incivility toward themselves included faculty members (a) behaving in demeaning and belittling ways, (b) treating students unfairly and subjectively, and (c) pressuring students to conform and comply to unreasonable faculty demands. In academic incivility among faculty, Twale and De Luca (2008), in *Faculty Incivility: The Rise of the Academic Bully Culture and What to Do About It*, a landmark text, write of incivility:

> That is what makes the behavior so insidious, because the meaning behind the interaction could be anything from complete sincerity to sarcasm to flagrant manipulation. It could also be harassment, incivility, passive aggression, or bullying as translated by the receiver. (p. 3)

In other words, the parameters of incivility are in the eye of the receiver and not simply in the eye of the beholder. It is not sufficient if the perpetrator did not mean to be uncivil; if the conduct, speech, or behavior is perceived as such, then it is damaging in its own right. Imber (2010) vehemently disagrees with this approach in his review of Twale and De Luca's book for the journal *Review of Higher Education Writing*:

> [The authors] Yet in repeatedly insisting that "regardless of time, place, or intent, the definition of the situation as civil or uncivil is left up to the victim of the action, not the perpetrator or actor" (p. 6), the book does just that. Any action that someone else does not like, such as rejecting a professor's application for promotion or tenure, is uncivil. Conversely, any action no matter how heinous that does not give offense—perhaps because the victim is self-loathing or masochistic or unaware of the action or its significance—is not uncivil. (p. 6)

Additionally, Imber does not necessarily view that taking the side of the faculty as victim is helpful, as if a faculty member is not doing their work, and it is first discussed, next, confronted, chastised, or even disciplined, that maybe the administrator has done so with cause. He indicated the text ought to be more evidence based, rather than anecdotal.

Twale and De Luca (2010) do conclude that "the only way to eliminate, or at least minimize the impact of, the bully is to recognize the behavior and the perpetrator and address it" (p. 191), and they indicate by doing this the institution is more poised to redirect valuable time and energy to what should occur in higher education: excellent teaching and research.

Also of concern is the ability of nursing faculty to resolve issues of incivility through constructive confrontation or dispute resolution, something we see all too rarely in the nursing profession and in the faculty role. Thomas (2004) wonders whether the "horizontal hostility" in the nursing profession, her phrase for incivility, exists because nurses are predominately women and "trained from birth to be passive-aggressive" (p. 117). Thomas further indicates these behaviors are engrained in nursing students during their nursing education, and it is incumbent on nursing educators to resist this tendency. Role modeling more constructive, assertive behaviors by teaching *and* through mentoring faculty to do the same may be one solution. Chesler (2009), although not a nurse, writes extensively about women's inhumanity to women, and there may be particular parallels to the common acknowledgment that "nurses eat their young"[2] (Brown, 2010).

Faculty-to-faculty incivility can technically be both legal (e.g., rudeness, passive-aggressive behaviors, belittling) and illegal (e.g., defamation, libel, harassment). A defamatory statement is a written or verbal publication of a statement or information that is false and has a tendency to injure a person's reputation. Because defamation is a matter of state law, the elements of a defamatory claim can vary from state to state. In general, to succeed in a defamation case, the plaintiff must prove that a false statement of fact (not a mere opinion) was made that is defamatory in nature and was published to a third party who is not the defendant or plaintiff.

The definition of *harassment* is covered in Chapter 13, Harassment, and although some faculty harassment may not be illegal, if the behavior violates an institutional or human resources department policy, then the faculty member could be disciplined or even terminated.

---

[2] There is a case for ceasing to use the phrase "nurses eat their young" because by using it, it may be itself perpetuated as truth. Maybe the issue should be instead "the incivility of seasoned nurses to novice nurses."

Only a minority of schools have an actual specific faculty code of conduct (see the policy at UC Davis in the "Helpful Resources" section of this chapter). A more common example is faculty codes of conduct covered by general university code of conduct policies (University of Washington, 2019). The University of Kansas (2016) includes nine items under the title Additional Faculty Responsibilities. One item is "Abusive or unprofessional treatment of students, faculty, or other members of the University falls within this category, e.g., see the University policy on consenting relationships. Also proscribed is any form of discrimination, including sexual harassment, as outlined in federal and state law and University policy" (p. 1). It is actually innovative for specific guidelines to be developed that address directly faculty-to-faculty incivility and faculty-to-student incivility—something that is written about less but that remains prevalent even in nursing education (Marchiondo, Marchiondo, & Lasiter, 2010).

DISCUSSION OF CASE STUDY

Recall the first question from Case Study 17.1: Are the six tenured nursing faculty members being uncivil in their submission of this last-minute letter? In this case Associate Dean Fowler was certainly taken aback by the last-minute nature of the approach by these tenured nursing faculty members. Even while acknowledging that there were some valid points in the letter, the complete rejection of the normal procedures for faculty input and voice on matters of curriculum were apparently abandoned with this strategy. Were they really being uncivil or were they simply expressing their opinion on the issue? If Dr. Fowler sanctioned them for this uncivil behavior, would he be violating the faculty members' rights of academic freedom or First Amendment free speech rights as this was a public university?

Concerned that any precipitous action on his part might get the university into legal trouble, Dr. Fowler put in a quick call to an attorney friend in the general counsel's office. The lawyer explained that whereas the university, as a public state university, could not take disciplinary action for free speech that was protected under the First Amendment, the particular speech in question was not protected. The attorney explained that under a 2006 U.S. Supreme Court case, *Garcetti v. Ceballos* (2006), public employees do not have any First Amendment rights when making statements pursuant to their official duties. The attorney felt that because the faculty members were speaking on a matter of internal university operations concerning their own workloads, a court would consider these to be statements pursuant to their official duties. However, the attorney also advised Dr. Fowler that even though he could legally discipline the faculty member, she did not think it was the most prudent course of action given the lack of rules about posting on the blog and its sporadic use for faculty voting. The attorney asked him what he would do if they had posted the letter on the blog just 1 hour before the meeting? Also, wasn't one of the purposes of the meeting to give the faculty member a last chance to debate the proposal before it was voted on?

Further, as tenured faculty members, do they have a greater voice in decision-making as is apparent by the written statement they subsequently submitted: "As tenured faculty we have a responsibility to be leaders in the development of nursing academic policies that affect the whole. We are concerned that as the non-tenured ranks outnumber us, our views, which we contend are indeed valid, may simply be ignored by voting blocks that do not have the best interest of the graduate faculty or particularly the graduate student (master's and doctoral)." Dr. Fowler was immediately reminded of the PhD tenured faculty member who once suggested that she should have first selection over class times for her undergraduate course (over another master's-prepared faculty member) and that she should therefore not have to teach an 8 a.m. class. To Dr. Fowler, this was elitist and he simply responded to the tenured faculty member that this was not how faculty course times were scheduled—taking into consideration doctoral preparation or tenure status—and that he did not view that approach as egalitarian or even fair. Dr. Fowler thought it was irresponsible for these six tenured faculty members to allow 10 days to pass without posting any of their concerns on the blog. He thought they should have posted their concerns and perhaps followed up with a letter; then at least the appearance of being constructive would have been helpful.

The second and third questions in this chapter's case study are: How should Dr. Fowler first respond? What should Dr. Fowler say at the full nursing faculty meeting? Within 10 minutes of receiving the email and complaint, the Dean responded to Dr. Fowler that she thought the last-minute nature of the letter was simply outrageous. The Dean had been following the blog discussion herself but as usual had decided not to post as she did not want to unduly influence the discussion or make other faculty members feel as though they needed to agree with her as Dean. As she was a great believer in faculty governance, she was equally adamant that with faculty governance came great accountability and great responsibility. She knew in the end she herself would have to approve any final proposal, but viewing the posts anonymously at least gave her much insight into the issues surrounding the proposal. She also noted to Dr. Fowler that she had not seen any of the tenured faculty posting on the blog, and asked whether they really were proposing that the tenured faculty members should be the "deciders," as the letter actually seemed to indicate. Dr. Fowler decided not to respond to the protest email (which was probably a good thing—quickly written, terse emails can sometimes cause more harm) and thought the best strategy was to take a deep breath and figure out how best to approach this at the faculty meeting. Fowler, however, reassured the Dean by phone that he would handle it professionally and that he would report to her what took place.

At the full nursing faculty meeting Dr. Fowler made sure every faculty member who entered the room got a copy of the agenda, the previous month's minutes, *and* a copy of the signed letter by the six tenured faculty members. When it was time for that agenda item to be discussed, Dr. Fowler said that some of the tenured faculty members had expressed concerns about the procedures that were being used to vote on the credit allotment for undergraduate and graduate courses and stated to the full congregants that six tenured faculty members had co-authored a letter stating their points. Dr. Fowler had decided that the best strategy was not to be overly confrontational with the four tenured faculty members who attended the mandatory meeting, but calmly ask about the nature of the letter and why they chose not to post these same concerns on the blog. Over the next 45 minutes the four attending tenured faculty members really did not forcefully and publicly defend the letter but one did state it seemed like a foregone conclusion that the change was going to be made. She reiterated that six of them decided to put their view in a more formal letter than in a blog post. Dr. Fowler then asked them to help the rest of the faculty members to better understand their position on the proposal. However, they floundered when trying to defend the letter. One undergraduate faculty member asked one of the tenured faculty members, "What is your solution then to this inequity or do you firmly believe there is no inequity with us teaching almost twice the number of students you do annually?" The tenured faculty in attendance really had no responses, and the room became very silent, but overall there was little discussion because it was apparent it was such a volatile issue.

One of the two tenured faculty members who did not sign this letter (she was uncomfortable signing it and told the six others so) sensed this and decided to intervene as she thought there might be a compromise acceptable to all. She rose up and said, "Although I would have preferred that the issues in the letter had been posted on the blog so we could at least debate them according to our normal procedures, I do agree that there are some valid points in the letter. I said 'some.' I would like to recommend that we table a vote for now, go back to the blog for another 10 days, and that any vote be sent to Faculty Affairs [which had elected members from both tenured or tenure-track and clinical faculty members] for their response because this decision ultimately does affect faculty course load and faculty life. The faculty can then vote up or down the recommendations (however modified) from Faculty Affairs. And of course, we all know the Dean ultimately has to sign off on any of this."

Dr. Fowler immediately stated he thought that was a good idea, and so a vote was taken to follow the new proposed procedures. The vote was 65 in favor, 8 opposed, and 4 abstentions.

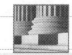 **WHEN TO CONSULT THE UNIVERSITY COUNSEL**

Similar to student violations, a faculty member's contact with the university attorney will generally be through the department chair or other administrator or by a university attorney through human resources. Remember, the job of the university counsel is to represent the institution (this is also counsel's professional and ethical duty as well). The university counsel will not be able to represent an individual faculty member or a group of faculty members who may have a disagreement with institutional policy. If one is from a protected class, then a complaint with the office of equality may be filed if there is bullying, harassment, or discrimination by another faculty member or staff. In extreme circumstances, it may be prudent to consult with a personal attorney if redress within the university is not satisfactory.

FINDINGS AND DISPOSITION

After the conclusion of the meeting, one of the department chairs in attendance informed Dr. Fowler that she thought he handled it well. She said it was definitely a very volatile issue but that he did not let the discussion get out of hand, albeit there was apparent hesitancy by many to speak up. Dr. Fowler hoped his tone was tempered and affirmed that the alternative proposal was fine as this policy was actually both a curriculum and faculty affairs issue and that the dean's signature on any change was required regardless of the proposed course load procedures the faculty wanted to follow. Dr. Fowler did express displeasure with the tenured faculty letter authors, not so much because they wrote the letter (he was quite accustomed to turf battles in academia), but because only four out of six showed up to defend the letter. He affirmed they did have some valid points, but was still perplexed about why they became so quiet upon public questioning by their own peers.[3]

The fourth question is: Should graduate faculty members receive more credit for their courses (as some institutions practice) than for teaching undergraduate courses, or should they receive the same or less credit (as this proposal suggests) for teaching small graduate courses on average? This is a difficult question. It is rather common, although not universal, that faculty members in some colleges and universities receive more credit for teaching graduate courses.[4] More common are faculty expectations that all faculty members will teach both undergraduate and graduate courses and thus there is no need to give graduate courses more credit. Although some traditionalists may say it takes more effort to teach a graduate course or the faculty in graduate courses must have exceptional scholarly credentials, we attest that these perceptions are unproven, however traditional and extremely inegalitarian. At three of these authors' previous institutions, it was standard practice from the Associate Dean's Office that faculty members who had a specific graduate appointment had to have their credentials reviewed by the College's Graduate Council to supervise doctoral students. There is nothing more difficult in nursing education than teaching didactic undergraduate clinical content, especially to a large class and some faculty believe second-degree/accelerated nursing students are more challenging and demanding. In these authors' view, two of whom having taught undergraduate clinical nursing theory and doctoral seminars, we contend doctoral students are not as difficult to teach, and they require using a more collaborative pedagogy.

The fifth question is: Should tenured faculty members have a larger or more influential voice than the non-tenured or non-tenure-track faculty? Our answer, as two tenured nursing faculty members, is a firm no, but others may disagree. Again, while this remains a traditional practice, where, for instance, college or university committees are mostly chaired by tenured faculty, we see this trend changing. Tenured faculty members already receive a host of benefits from being tenured, including a lifetime appointment and always a lower teaching load than non-tenure track (clinical or teaching faculty), and other benefits. Every full-time faculty member has a valuable role to play, and every individual faculty member has made certain choices about their career and has chosen to either emphasize teaching (clinical or classroom) or research or administration. This, therefore, essentially answers the sixth question: How can the contribution of every faculty member, regardless of position and rank, be valued in any respective nursing division or college? It is by constructing effective

---

[3] Or did they consider them "true peers?"

[4] See workload policies at Prairie View A&M University, Prairie View, Texas (2019) where graduate courses receive more credit: Retrieved June 8, 2020 from http://www.pvamu.edu/policies/wp-content/uploads/sites/56/PVAMU-Faculty-Workload-Manual.pdf or the University of Central Missouri (2016) where there is no undergraduate versus graduate course distinction, but whereas large class sizes receive more credit https://www.ucmo.edu/offices/general-counsel/university-policy-library/academic-policies/teaching-workload-guidelines/index.php.

workload policies in which individuals can excel, whether in teaching, research, or administration, without each becoming victim of a strangulating tripartite mission (teaching, scholarship/research, and practice or service) that forces every faculty member to accomplish each equally (including service) and with excellence (Anderson, 2000; Burman, Hart, & McCabe, 2005; Potempa, Redman, & Anderson, 2008). As the first author is a Dean of Nursing, and the second author a former Dean, we agree that:

> No single, simple formula for an equitable faculty workload can be devised for all the academic units. What is fair and works well in Engineering may be inappropriate for the College of Arts and Sciences, and the arrangement thought necessary in the School of Business Administration may be irrelevant for faculty in [Roesch] Library. This is not to say, however, that excessive or inequitably distributed workloads should not be recognized as such. Furthermore, individual faculty members and departments have a right to clarity of expectations. The University must have a system that facilitates accountability in the use of its resources. (University of Dayton, n.d.)

ACADEMIC NURSING ADMINISTRATOR ON FACULTY AND SUBORDINATES ANECDOTAL SCENARIOS

1. A Dean refuses to cancel a faculty meeting for the viewing/funeral of a long-time full-time faculty member and is later overheard by an administrative assistant saying "I have to be strategic about the funerals I attend."
2. An Associate Dean who approved "end of dissertation" accommodation for a program director refuses to give it the following year to an associate director and another full-time faculty member in the department. Having both of them approaching her, she was likely caught off guard being confronted with her actions and questioned, and she resorts to yelling at both of them in the hall.
3. A female department chair suspects her male associate chair is having an affair with one of his male students. While she doesn't want to file a Title IX report based on suspicions or gossip, she resorts to giving her subordinate administrator a bad evaluation. The male administrator in this small program contemplates contesting the evaluation, and begins to feel marginalized and bullied. He contemplates going through the chain of command. But he is fearful of going through the chain of command or going to Human Resources since from his experience Human Resources seems to always support the senior administrator. Fearful of more unchecked reprisals, or possibly the unintended disclosure of his secret behavior (if true), he decides to leave the organization.
4. A School Tenure Committee has convened. For decades anyone on the Committee who supervises any of the faculty being reviewed has rightfully recused themselves for those candidates, although this is not actually specified in the committee bylaws. At the first meeting, a member of the committee, a very senior department chair faculty from a large department in the school, suddenly says she wants to "make a few statements" about the candidates in her department for review which were all highly complimentary. She quickly makes them, stands up, and leaves the room. Startled, the committee members do not know what to do.

With "incivility" often the conceptual umbrella for bullying; mobbing; horizontal, lateral and vertical violence; and relational aggression, these anecdotes also represent clear cases of incivility (Table 17.1). Racial and ethnic slurs and intimidation also include some of these narrower behaviors. What we see in these four anecdotes are cases of incivility.

Anecdote 1: Here the Dean is likely exhibiting aggressive hostile behavior to a group of nursing faculty. It is also a case relational aggression with the insensitive comment made to the subordinate. This is a case of toxic leadership, too (Wilson, 2014). Often, in an organization, according to Brendel and Davis (2017) "All workplaces have an "emotional culture" that shapes how it functions internally and presents itself externally. But top-tier leadership carries the greatest responsibility for shaping this culture" (p. 1). While not described in the anecdote, there may also be horizontal violence as actions of dean were likely covert, where it was also announced that attendance would not be taken. But likely some individuals felt pressured to attend nonetheless.

Table 17.1 Types of Incivility

CONCEPT/SOURCE	DESCRIPTIONS
Workplace bullying/ Emamzadeh (2018)	Situations where an employee repeatedly (more than once or twice) and over a prolonged time period is exposed to harassing behavior from one or more colleagues (including subordinates and leaders) and where the targeted person is unable to defend themselves against this systematic mistreatment.
Workplace mobbing/ Segal (2010)	Mobbing in the workplace is a kind of mass bullying, with collusion or active participation of the management. It is a group campaign of harassment and cruelty, conscious or unconscious, designed to undermine the confidence, impugn the competence, and undercut the effectiveness of certain employees.
Horizontal violence in nursing/Taylor (2016)	Horizontal violence in the workplace has been difficult to define since it has been interchangeably used to refer to lateral violence, bullying, incivility, hazing, mobbing, relational aggression, and disruptive behavior. It is mostly described as hostile, aggressive, and harmful behavior by a nurse or a group of nurses toward a coworker or group of nurses via attitudes, actions, words, and/ or other behaviors. It is mostly covert, hard to discern, or discover or accept— making it difficult to officially complain against.
Lateral violence in nursing/Chu & Evans (2016)	Lateral violence as identified in the nursing workforce is overt aggressive behavior directed by someone toward another person or nurses. This aggression can be verbal or nonverbal; it can have psychological, emotional, and behavioral effects on nurses. The humiliation and putting down of colleagues through rudeness and aggressions eventually demoralize self-confidence and sense of worth. It can lead to negative outcomes in the delivery of quality patient care, increased turnover rate, and cost to the organization. Often, nurses are unwilling to report lateral violence because they consider these events to be part of the job or because they are frightened of retaliation.
Vertical violence/Cantey (2013)	Vertical violence is defined as any act of violence, such as yelling, snide comments, withholding pertinent information, and rude, ignoring, and humiliating behaviors, which occur between two or more persons on different levels of the hierarchical system.
Relational aggression/ Ostrov (2013)	Relational aggression is a type of behavior that is intended to hurt, harm, or injure another person and uses the relationship or the threat of the removal of the relationship as the means of harm. It includes social exclusion, friendship withdrawal threats, giving the silent treatment, and spreading malicious secrets, lies or gossip.

Anecdote 2: In the second anecdote we see incivility alongside workplace favoritism and perhaps discrimination. We cannot rule out lateral violence, as the two nursing faculty may have been hesitant to take their complaints more public and through the common chain of command. They might have also feared reprisal should they do this. We also see vertical violence with the Associate Dean yelling at them.

Anecdote 3: In this anecdote there may be multiple violations and is purposefully derived to demonstrate the complexity of behavior, allegations and actions, both legal and ethical. First, if the junior supervisor is having an affair with a fellow undergraduate student, then this constitutes sexual harassment, a violation of Title IX. Therefore, most colleges, universities, and organizations have explicit policies on Consensual Intimate Relationships.

Second, if the senior supervisor did suspect this behavior, she should have reported it, either to her own supervisor, human resources, in some cases to other "responsible parties" that receive these complaints, or the Title IX officer. However, she is reticent to report this based on suspicions or gossip, and she fears ruining the cohesion of her department or being disparaged by others in the department or school (including students) if it is untrue. Moreover, she could face her own discipline if the evaluation is determined unfounded. Nonetheless, according to Title IX regulations, she is actually required to report this. Second, if her unreported assumptions led to giving him a bad evaluation, this is a violation of workplace policy and he could file an appeal of his evaluation through the chain of command. Third, either the junior administrator felt the chain of command and/or Human Resources had a record of protecting senior administrators, felt fear of reprisal by filing this complaint, including detailing the bullying. Or the junior administrator did violate the law prohibiting intimate consensual relationships between "a faculty member and an undergraduate student" and did not want to report anything through the chain of command or Human Resources at all.

These issues are often difficult to navigate, particularly if they are based on assumptions or gossip, and here we see the dilemma of ethics and the law converge (Cain, 2017). And further, this anecdote does not provide enough information. Was there actual sexual misconduct? If disclosed, could the evaluation complaint also be properly investigated? If not disclosed, could the poor evaluation be determined to emanate from the bullying? We have already discussed what might happen if a report was made and there was no finding of sexual misconduct. If there was evidence of bullying and related to the poor evaluation, how could the Supervisor now report the Title IX complaint, and then possibly be charged with retaliation? Finally, there may be a question, maybe not explicit, that Human Resources may be more aligned to protect the organization (Heathfield, 2019), and neither individual was certain of their own outcome. To escape this complexity, the legal action would be to report the allegation so it could be investigated, no matter the finding, and she would have never resorted to the poor evaluation and bullying instead. This is also the proper ethical action, as the senior administrator followed the law, no matter what others may think. However, she should not be retaliated against in any form by anyone, but the organizational impact of doing the legal and ethical action cannot be divorced from the degree of what others think about what she did.

Anecdote 4: This example is a case of incivility. But perhaps, it raises different issues. First, the lack of specificity in the committee bylaws failed the committee, college, and institution. Bylaws do not receive their proper due, and it has been witnessed by each of these authors how calls to serve on a bylaws committee usually generate little interest. But as evidenced in the case, sensible bylaws that addressed conflicts of interest or prevented a department chair to present her candidates, without other department chairs knowing this had taken place, would have protected the integrity of the committee and its recommendations for tenure and promotion.

Since higher education is a nonprofit, The Association of Corporate Counsels (2014) offers the following recommendations:

1. Understand your state's nonprofit corporation law.
2. Make sure your bylaws are consistent with other regulatory documents.
3. Be sure to address all foreseeable scenarios.
4. Populate your bylaw committee with an accurate cross-section of your organization.
5. Coordinate the actions of your bylaw committee with legal advice.
6. Create bylaws that reflect the appropriate political climate of your organization.
7. Keep your bylaws current.
8. Keep your bylaws flexible.
9. Reserve the details for policies, not bylaws.
10. Ensure that your purposes clause reflects your organization today (this is actually a tax-exemption issue, first and foremost).
11. Closely review the meeting and voting procedures for members and directors.
12. Look at committee composition.
13. Pay attention to the approval process.
14. Do not make your bylaws too difficult to amend.
15. Keep a pulse on the bylaws. (Tenenbaum & Loson, 2014, p. 1)

While all of these do not apply to all committees in a college, a Tenure and Promotion Committee is a high stakes committee, and consultation with the college or university's Office of Legal Counsel is essential.

Bullying seems evident in this anecdote, but technically this behavior would occur more than once. Let's say for example that regardless of the criterion for workplace bullying, this is an example. Likely due to her seniority and position of power, she thought she could get away with the sudden violation, at least, of past committee norms. At a fundamental level it was also a case of lateral violence: It was aggressive behavior and it was going to lead to a negative outcome for the committee with the impact of the supervisor's comment unfairly affecting the decision-making; analogous to a negative outcome in the delivery of quality patient care. Finally, this was an ethical violation, certainly of her profession's ethics and possibly to the university's bylaws that regulated the guidelines of departmental, school, college, and/or university bylaws on Tenure and Promotion Committees. In smaller schools or colleges, there may be no departmental review, but only at one college level. One of these co-authors worked at a small college where at the school level every tenured or tenure-track faculty member voted on all tenure and promotion candidacies. The perilous pitfalls of such a system and opportunities for conflicts of interest are boundless.

Even the leading business literature is replete with articles on bullying, toxic, and unethical bosses and leaders, but as will be discussed later, the nursing literature is not. From the business words here are some recent examples include:

Is Your Boss a True Bully? How to Tell and What to Do About It[5]
What to Do When You Have a Bad Boss[6]
Study Reveals How Damaging a Toxic Boss Really Can Be[7]

In a widely publicized case, in 2012, Ellen Pao, one of a small number of women working in Silicon Valley, filed a lawsuit against her company Kleiner, Perkins, Caulfield & Byers, claiming "allowing her to be sexually harassed by male managers, of punishing and eventually firing her when she complained, and excluding her and other women from business meetings, dinners, and promotion" (Chung, 2015, p. 1). Discrimination, although illegal according to Title VII of the Civil Rights Act, is not so easy to prove, since, in this case, the litigant must prove "intent to discriminate." One rather interesting aspect of this case that Pao (of Asian descent) disclosed was that she was given an "interruption coach" as she allegedly was not deft in the necessary interruption skills [like men in her company] in meetings at the venture capitalist company. The outcome of the lawsuit was that the jury was dead-locked at 6-6 and she lost her case. And while she claimed in her lawsuit asking for $6 million, including loss of potential wages, her next position at the time of the trial was Interim Chief Executive of Reddit (Ferro, 2015). It is a very interesting complex case and had numerous complaints and elements she had to prove.

However, the question remains, while there is now growing literature, even evidence based, on faculty-on-faculty incivility, why is there such a dearth of scholarship on incivility in the academic leader-on-faculty or other subordinate? With so much focus on incivility between and among nursing students and nursing faculty, we have given less attention to the problems with uncivil and unethical leaders and managers in nursing education. The authors of this text hypothesize that it may be risky for some academicians to study this topic. Perhaps a junior faculty member climbing the academic ladder may feel threatened of repercussions, both seen and unseen, that may hamper their careers. Indeed, this issue can be viewed as a sensitive area, and unlike the larger business/corporate world, the network of academic administrators, more visibly Deans, Directors and Chair, but also senior tenured faculty, is much smaller and the network of controversial scholarship often gets more attention. Thus, perhaps tenured, full professors have more freedom to raise and study these issues with less perceived risk. Nonetheless, these authors' view is that the uncivil, particularly the bullying-type behaviors from our leaders/managers in our schools and colleges of nursing may be the most damaging of all since the entire working and teaching environment is threatened.

At a conference session on "Ethical and Legal Issues with Incivility Among Faculty, Students, and Administrators in Nursing Education" led by one of these authors, using anonymous clickers, about 70% of the audience "clicked" that they had been bullied by an academic administrator, and the percent for "bullied by a senior faculty" was even higher (Dreher, 2015). A 2013 study by Beckmann, Canella, and Wantland of 473 nursing academicians "Faculty Perception of Bullying in Schools of Nursing" published in the *Journal of Professional Nursing* reported that: (a) Among 473 nursing

---

[5] Caprino, 2017.

[6] Abajay, 2018.

[7] Morin, 2017.

faculty 36% had personally experienced bullying. (b) Moreover, administrators and senior faculty were more likely than expected to be the perpetrators of bullying.

With regard to senior faculty, Cynthia Clark, PhD, RN, ANEF, FAAN, perhaps the leading expert on civility in nursing education describes the following: "When I politely disagreed with the more senior, tenured professor during a faculty meeting, she didn't say anything then. But it was clear from her nonverbal behavior that she was angry" (2017, p. 1). In this case, the senior faculty later told this nursing professor that she was on the Tenure Committee and she would have to "think about it" [her promotion]. Additionally, there are many cases where even a tenured associate professor knows they must maintain exceptional relationships with the full professors in the respective unit, because they will ultimately vote on their promotion. Further, full professors may feel the need to overlook bullying and unethical behavior by their supervisor, dean, director, or chair if they are approving their sabbaticals and/or international travel for instance. We should note that in Collective Bargaining Agreements these issues may already have agreements. But in any academic environment, there are multiple navigation points in a faculty member's career, and bullying or unprofessional conduct by their leaders may have a detrimental effect on it.

Our view is that if leaders (and senior faculty who should be role models and mentoring junior faculty) are identified as bullies, the environment cannot be perceived as supportive and healthy. These unhealthy environments may have serious consequences related to retaining nursing faculty. Suggestions for improving civility among nursing faculty and academic nursing administrators include the following:

- Examine your own behavior and how you contribute to civility or incivility.
- Don't listen to or tolerate rumors and gossip.
- Encourage other faculty/staff not to jump to conclusions about the intent or motives of other administrators, faculty, or staff.
- Stop the blame game yourself and encourage a solutions orientation to problems.
- Encourage acts of kindness among the entire school team at all levels.
- Go out of your way to say thank you. Set an example for others. Give praise and recognize the efforts of others.
- Look for common ground in dealing with conflict.
- Engage in the practice of forgiveness.
- If you are an administrator, make it safe for faculty and staff to ask questions and discuss problems.

CASE

Ginn v. Stephen F. Austin State University, No. 03-02-00443-CV, 2003 WL 1882264 (Tex. Ct. App. 2003)

In *Ginn v. Stephen F. Austin State University* (2003), Stephen F. Austin State University hired Mr. Gregory Ginn as an associate professor of management in 1989. At the time the university did not have a college-wide smoking policy, and Mr. Ginn determined through his own research that the college was in violation of federal Occupational Safety and Health Administration (OSHA) guidelines for not having a no-smoking policy. On bringing this situation to the attention of university officials, Mr. Ginn was informed that they were technically not in violation of this policy but that they would provide him some access to a smoke-free environment, including moving his office. Over the next 2 years Mr. Ginn continued to complain about the policy. Despite these complaints, his contract was renewed in both 1990 and 1991. In 1992, his contract was not renewed. He responded by suing the university for violation of the Texas Whistleblower Protection Act, claiming that he was fired because he continued his complaints about the smoking policy, including to the university president.

After hearing the evidence, the state court found that he (a) cursed at a student using profane language; (b) referred to a fellow professor by use of an obscene name in one of his classes; (c) engaged in a heated conversation with the same professor when she confronted Mr. Ginn about the name-calling; (d) banged his head against the wall many times in order to stretch his calf while his students were taking exams; and finally, and what the court of appeals ultimately ruled led to his dismissal (e) was charged with assault against his department chair, Mr. Warren Fisher, by shoving him several times while blocking his exit, and finally grabbing Mr. Fisher by the wrists to prevent him from leaving Mr. Ginn's office (Texas Ct. of Appeals, Document, Third District, at Austin, 2003). The court held that these were sufficient to demonstrate that the university had good reasons for not renewing his contract, and ruled against the plaintiff.

Frederick Fagal v. Marywood University, No. 18-2174 (3rd Cir. 2019)

Marywood University terminated Dr. Fagal, a tenured faculty member, after he created and circulated two videos among the Marywood faculty that belittled the university President and mocked the Catholic university as a "fat bureaucratic web and nun casino" and depicted the President and several other university administrators, including one who was Jewish, as Adolf Hitler and SS Nazi officers. Professor Fagal had distributed the videos in response to a dispute he had with the Marywood administrators over flyers he had posted around campus to advertise an event he planned for students.

In his lawsuit Dr. Fagal claimed that Marywood breached its contract with him when it terminated him immediately without following the school's progressive disciplinary policy contained in its faculty handbook which was part of his employment contract. Marywood asserted that the progressive disciplinary policy permitted the school to immediately suspend or terminate faculty for "serious violations of professional responsibility."

After a bench trial, the U.S. District Court denied the breach of contract claim finding that although the policy strongly favored the use of informal process and progressive discipline, it did not require such process for all offending conduct. The U.S. Court of Appeals for the Third Circuit upheld the decision of the District Court finding under the applicable standard of review that the findings of the District Court were not clearly erroneous.

SUMMARY

Is incivility on the rise? It is hard to say, but if there is agreement that there is a rise in incivility in society in general, then it is likely to be happening in academia too. It is very likely that Representative Joe Wilson's yelling out "You lie!" to President Obama during a 2009 speech on the floor of the House of Representatives is at least anecdotal evidence that it is on the rise (Parker, 2009). It is very important that a climate of civility be restored to our institutions of higher learning and that our classrooms actually be places in which safe and civil instruction can take place, and where collegiality among faculty "next door or down the hall" are respectful to each other. It may also be difficult for an individual faculty member to confront a peer who is engaging in some of these behaviors (Knight, 2015). Strong administrative support is essential so that any faculty under obvious attack, and who reports such behavior, believes there is a safe climate to file a complaint. In the following scenario we do not see an example of this: A new high-level administrator is appointed from the outside, hired over an internal candidate (at a lower rank), who coveted the position. In light of this, she harasses this person at every opportunity with insidious, contrarian, dismissive comments whenever this person speaks, and does so with a smile. She even maneuvers her way onto this person's committees, to continue these harassing behaviors. This is obviously an unsafe environment for a new administrator. The concept of collegiality needs to be an ongoing discussion so that faculty members treat each other with respect. Didn't King (Thedarkroome, n.d.) famously say, "Can't we all just get along?" or words to that effect. It may just be that simple. Or maybe not.

ETHICAL CONSIDERATIONS

Civility is a commonly cited virtue. Whether we are considering virtue from an Aristotelian context of achieving *Eudaimonia*, civility, it seems clear, would lead to a good and flourishing life, or in a more modern context like that of MacIntyre (1985), civility is necessary for achieving the internal goods of nursing or college education as a "practice." The first provision of the *American Nurses Association Code of Ethics for Nurses* (2015), while focusing primarily on the nurse–patient relationship, also emphasizes the importance of creating "an ethical environment and culture of civility and kindness, treating colleagues, coworkers, employees, students, and others with dignity and respect" (p. 4). Civility provides for not only a pleasant working environment but also a more safe, efficient, and effective environment. The *1966 American Association of University Professors Statement on Professional Ethics* (2009) indicates the duty to respect both students and colleagues, including respecting others' opinions, acknowledging academic debt to colleagues, striving for objectivity when judging colleagues, and sharing governance responsibilities.

So there no debate that civility is a trait to be sought and to be fostered among nursing faculty. But it is also clear that there is no shortage of problems of incivility within nursing, including in academics. This state of affairs implies a strong duty to continue to foster civility as a virtue among students and rising faculty through role modeling of more experienced faculty. Proactive measures need to be taken in all areas of nursing to turn the tide regarding problems such as these.

CRITICAL ELEMENTS TO CONSIDER

- Victims of bullying or of academic incivility must document these events.
- If attempts to resolve these issues with the offender fail, notify the department chair in writing.
- If the offender is in violation of human resource policies, consider reporting them.
- If the normal chain of command is not working, go to the dean and put a complaint and actions taken in writing.
- For faculty disputes that cannot be resolved at the departmental level, we also suggest making use of the campus Ombudsman or Human Resources.
- A faculty witness to bullying behavior by faculty toward students should make every effort possible to speak to that individual directly. If the violation observed is severe or unethical, then report the activity through normal administrative channels.
- Some universities have ethics hotlines that one can call anonymously.
- Be aware that simply because an activity is reported to a department chair or other administrator, it does not perpetually guarantee the anonymity of the one who reports it.

Helpful Resources

- The Academic Ladder, Academiblog. (2008, February 24). *Mean and Nasty Academics: Bullying, Hazing, and Mobbing*, Retrieved from http://gblog2.academicladder.com/2008/02/mean-and-nasty-academics-bullying.htm
- "UCSF Code of Conduct". Retrieved from https://www.ucsf.edu/sites/default/files/legacy_files/UCSFCOC.pdf
- "UC Davis Administrative Policy: General University Policy for Academic Appointees Section UCD-015, Procedures for Faculty Misconduct Allegations". Retrieved from https://aadocs.ucdavis.edu/policies/apm/ucd-015/ucd-015.pdf

References

Abajay, M. (2018). What to do when you have a bad boss. *Harvard Business Review*. Retrieved from https://hbr.org/2018/09/what-to-do-when-you-have-a-bad-boss

American Association of University Professors. (2009). *Statement on professional ethics*. Retrieved from https://www.aaup.org/report/statement-professional-ethics

American Nurses Association. (2015). *Code of ethics for nurses with interpretive statements*. Silver Spring, MD: Author.

Anderson, C. A. (2000). Current strengths and limitations of doctoral education in nursing: Are we prepared for the future? *Journal of Professional Nursing, 16*(4), 191–200. doi:10.1053/jpnu.2000.7830

Beckman, C. A., Canella, B. L., & Wantland, D. (2013). Faculty perception of bullying in schools of nursing. *Journal of Professional Nursing, 29*(5), 287–294. doi:10.1016/j.profnurs.2012.05.012

Brendel, D. B., & Davis, S. (2017). How leaders can promote psychological safety in the workplace. *Huffington Post*. Retrieved from https://www.huffpost.com/entry/how-leaders-can-promote-psychological-safety-in-the_b_59a55d34e4b03c5da162af6e

Brown, T. (2010, February 11). When the nurse is a bully. *New York Times*. Retrieved from https://well.blogs.nytimes.com/2010/02/11/when-the-nurse-is-a-bully/

Burman, M. E., Hart, A. M., & McCabe, S. M. (2005). Doctor of nursing practice: Opportunity amidst chaos. *American Journal of Critical Care, 14*, 463–464. Retrieved from https://aacnjournals.org/ajcconline/article/14/6/463/398/Doctor-of-Nursing-Practice-Opportunity-Amidst

Cain, A. (2017). What to do when you have a problem at work, and human resources won't help you. *Business Insider*. Retrieved from https://www.businessinsider.com/what-to-do-when-hr-ignores-your-complaints-2017-2

Cantey, S. (2013). Recognizing and stopping the destruction of vertical violence. *American Nurse Today, 8*(2). Retrieved from https://www.myamericannurse.com/recognizing-and-stopping-the-destruction-of-vertical-violence/

Caprino, K. (2017). Is your boss a true bully? How to tell and what to do about it. *Forbes*. Retrieved from https://www.forbes.com/sites/amymorin/2017/01/15/study-reveals-how-damaging-a-toxic-boss-really-can-be/#54baa6426249

Chesler, P. (2009). *Woman's inhumanity to woman*. Chicago, IL: Lawrence Hill Books.

Chu, R. Z., & Evans, M. M. (2016). Lateral violence in nursing. *MedSurg Nursing, 25*(6), S4. Retrieved https://library.amsn.org/amsn/articles/650/view

Chung, R. (2015). The curious case of Ellen Pao and he lessons we can learn from it. *Above the Law*. Retrieved from https://abovethelaw.com/2015/03/the-curious-case-of-ellen-pao-and-the-lesson-we-can-learn-from-it/

Clark, C. (2008). Student perspectives on faculty incivility in nursing education: An application of the concept of rankism. *Nursing Outlook, 56*(1), 4–8. doi:10.1016/j.outlook.2007.08.003

Clark, C. (2017). Seeking civility among faculty, *ASHA, Leader, 12*(22), p. 1, Retrieved from https://leader.pubs.asha.org/doi/full/10.1044/leader.FTR2.22122017.54#.Xt7KeVor-Fg.email

Clark, C. M., & Springer, P. J. (2010). Academic nurse leaders' role in fostering a culture of civility in nursing education. *Journal of Nursing Education, 49*(6), 319–325. doi:10.3928/01484834-20100224-01

Dreher, H. M. (2015). *Ethical and legal issues with incivility among faculty, students, and administrators in nursing education*. Presentation presented to the AACN's Hot Issues Conference, Las Vegas, NV.

Emamzadeh, A. (2018, September 27). Workplace bullying: Causes, effects, and prevention. *Psychology Today*. Retrieved from https://www.psychologytoday.com/us/blog/finding-new-home/201809/workplace-bullying-causes-effects-and-prevention

Ferro, S. (2015). The Ellen Pao trial is not about a woman lacking confidence. *Finance—Yahoo*. Retrieved from https://sg.finance.yahoo.com/news/ellen-pao-trial-not-women-203700600.html

Garcetti v. Ceballos, 126 S.Ct. 1951 (2006).

Ginn v. Stephen F. Austin State University, No. 03-02-00443-CV, 2003 WL 1882264 (Tex. Ct. App. 2003).

Glasgow, M. E. S., Dreher, H. M., Cornelius, H., & Bhattacharya, A. (2009, November). *A final report on the 2009 National Survey of Doctoral Nursing Faculty (both PhD and DNP) in the United States*. Paper presented at the International Conference on Professional Doctorates (ICPD), UK Council for Graduate Education, London, UK.

Heathfield, S. (2019). Reasons why employees hate HR. *The Balance Careers*. Retrieved from https://www.thebalancecareers.com/reasons-why-employees-hate-hr-1917590

Imber, M. (2010). Faculty incivility: The rise of the academic bully culture and what to do about it [Review]. *Review of Higher Education, 33*(2), 293–294. Retrieved from https://muse.jhu.edu/article/365591/pdf

Knight, R. (2015). How to handle difficult conversations at work. *Harvard Business Review*. Retrieved from https://hbr.org/2015/01/how-to-handle-difficult-conversations-at-work

MacIntyre, A. (1985). *After virtue: A study in moral theory* (2nd ed.). London, UK: Duckworth.

Marchiondo, K., Marchiondo, L. A., & Lasiter, S. (2010). Faculty incivility: Effects on program satisfaction of BSN students. *Journal of Nursing Education, 49*(11), 608–614. doi:10.3928/01484834-20100524-05

Morin, A. (2017). Study reveals how damaging a toxic boss really can be. *Forbes*. Retrieved from https://www.forbes.com/sites/amymorin/2017/01/15/study-reveals-how-damaging-a-toxic-boss-really-can-be/#54baa6426249

Ostrov, J. (2013). The development of relational aggression: The role of media exposure. *American Psychological Association.* Retrieved from https://www.apa.org/science/about/psa/2013/07-08/relational-aggression

Parker, K. (2009). Parker: Rise in incivility a threat to concept of civilization. *Chron.com.* Retrieved from https://www.chron.com/opinion/outlook/article/Parker-Rise-in-incivility-a-threat-to-concept-of-1587371.php

Potempa, K. M., Redman, R. W., & Anderson, C. A. (2008). Capacity for the advancement of nursing science: Issues and challenges. *Journal of Professional Nursing, 24*(6), 329–336. doi:10.1016/j.profnurs.2007.10.010

Segal, L. (2010, May 20). The injury of mobbing in the workplace. *Conflict Remedy.* Retrieved from https://conflictremedy.com/the-injury-of-mobbing-in-the-workplace/

Taylor, R. (2016). Nurses' perceptions of horizontal violence. *Global Qualitative Nursing Research, 3.* doi:10.1177/2333393616641002

Tenenbaum, J. S., & Loson, K. J. (2014). The 15 most common non-profit pitfalls: How to avoid the traps. *AAC.* Retrieved from https://www.acc.com/resource-library/15-most-common-nonprofit-bylaw-pitfalls-how-avoid-traps#

Thomas, S. (2004). *Transforming nurses' stress and anger: Steps towards healing* (2nd ed.). New York, NY: Springer Publishing Company.

Thedarkroome. (n.d.). Rodney King Can We All Get Along. *YouTube* [video]. Retrieved from http://www.youtube.com/watch?v=2PbyiOJwNugr

Twale, D. J., & De Luca, B. M. (2008). *Faculty incivility: The rise of the academic bully culture and what to do about it.* Hoboken, NJ: Jossey-Bass.

University of Dayton. (n.d.). *University faculty workload guidelines.* Retrieved from https://www.udayton.edu/provost/_resources/docs/facwrkld.pdf

University of Kansas. (2016). Additional faculty responsibilities. *Faculty Code of Rights, Responsibilities, & Conduct.* Retrieved from https://policy.ku.edu/FacultyCodeKULawrence/faculty-code-of-rights

University of Washington. (2019). Faculty code and governance. *UW Policy Directory.* Retrieved from http://www.washington.edu/admin/rules/policies/FCG/UnivFacCH13.html

Wilson, D. S. (2014). Toxic leadership and the social environments that breed them. *Forbes.* Retrieved from https://www.forbes.com/sites/darwinatwork/2014/01/10/toxic-leaders-and-the-social-environments-that-breed-them/#48f6af05dac5

Wright, M., & Hill, L. (2015). Academic incivility among health sciences faculty. *AAACLE: Journal of the American Association for Adult and Continuing Education, 26*(1), 14–20. doi:10.1177/1045159514558410

Conflict of Interest Issues in the Faculty Role

18

Case Study 18.1
The Love Affair: Dating a Senior Administrator

Your role: You are a Dean for a college of nursing and health sciences.

You are a mid-career academician, having spent 12 years in administration. You have been a dean for 4 years of a large college within a university. You have been asked by the provost to chair a faculty conduct committee convened in the aftermath of a well-publicized case involving another dean colleague, a tenured faculty member in the school, and her husband, a non-tenure track faculty member in the same school at the university. When the dean of the other school began to date a professor in his school, he disclosed the relationship shortly after it commenced. During a period of time before and after this amorous relationship, the professor's husband's performance and teaching evaluations had been in steady decline. The husband-professor has brought a lawsuit against the university claiming that he was wrongfully terminated and subjected to harassment by the dean, who is dating his wife. The provost charges you with organizing the committee and developing a policy addressing romantic relationships between employees of the university staff, faculty, and administrators.

Questions
- How would you proceed with convening a faculty committee?
- What issues would you address?
- How should you best manage the situation from a legal perspective?

CONFLICT OF INTEREST: LEGAL PRINCIPLES AND REVIEW OF THE LITERATURE

In general, a conflict of interest occurs when there is a divergence between a faculty member's private interests and their professional obligations to the university, such that an independent observer might reasonably question whether the faculty member's professional actions or decisions are determined by any considerations other than the best interests of the university (Sugarman, 2005).

In academia, conflicts of interest typically arise in research when scientists or others involved in research have a financial stake in companies sponsoring the research or in companies that may stand to profit from it. The likelihood of such conflicts has increased in recent years, as the percentage of research funding that comes from industry has grown, especially in medicine, biology, chemistry, and engineering. Institutional policies on conflicts of interest have been inconsistent in the academy; many focus on disclosure of conflicts rather than on prohibition of them. Strong policies surrounding such conflicts are needed in the academy.

Another common area ripe for potential conflict of interest is the academic couple, who seem to be pervasive in universities. The term *academic couple* refers to two people who are partners or spouses and work at the same college or university. A potential conflict of interest exists when one or both members of the academic couple hold administrative positions and/or one faculty member in the couple or dyad is not held to the same standard as other faculty because of the position their spouse or partner holds in the university community. The spouse or partner may serve as a senior administrator or generate substantial research dollars or beneficial publicity for the university. To prohibit universities from hiring academic couples would seriously hurt their recruitment of talented faculty, administrators, and researchers (Sugarman, 2005). But allowing discrimination to occur on bases other than merit will contaminate the community, whether the preference (or perceived preference) is given on the basis of sex, race, national origin, or family relationship.

This concern has been expressed at the institutional governance level as well. Nonprofit institutions must file a report each year with the Internal Revenue Service (IRS) that confirms compliance with their charitable tax exemptions. In 2008, the IRS issued a new Form 990 that digs far more deeply into their activities. Among other things, it now asks for disclosures about members of the governing board and about other interested persons—persons or organizations having some kind of close relationship with the nonprofit that might use that relationship to their own benefit, whether through jobs, salary, or contracts, at the risk or disadvantage to the nonprofit. The form seeks disclosures about members of the family, organizations in which the person has a significant financial ownership interest, and members of the family who are employed in those organizations. These disclosures have to be made by every officer and member of the board of directors. They seek not just actual conflicts of interest, but relationships that might be perceived as causing one; and the disclosures are intended to make those relationships transparent, with the objective of forcing the nonprofit to face them and deal with them.

Faculty and administrators should disclose any and all potential conflicts of interest—including familial relationships—and these relationships should be periodically reviewed for any conflict. Members of the same family should not be employed in a situation in which one member of the family works under the administrative supervision of another. Managing interpersonal conflicts and perceptions of favoritism also need to be addressed by administration, as these issues can affect morale and productivity.

DISCUSSION OF CASE STUDY 18.1

What begins as a consensual amorous relationship is fertile ground for a potential sexual harassment claim if things turn sour between the involved parties. Although there are strict policies in place strongly discouraging or prohibiting student–faculty consensual romantic relationships throughout higher education, there remain many institutions that do not have policies addressing faculty–faculty or faculty–administrator relationships (Flaherty, 2015). What begins as a consensual dyad, can rapidly evolve into an unpleasant triad with legal sequelae.

A potential conflict of interest occurs when there is a divergence between private interests and professional obligations to the university such that an independent observer might reasonably question whether the professional actions or decisions are determined by personal financial gain (Kansas Board of Regents, Kansas State University, 2019a; New York University, 2019).

The academic world is replete with legal disputes, many of which never see the light of day because these matters are settled in a board room. There is a dearth of case law on legal issues concerning conflict of interest in the faculty role that is outside of the realm of the scientific research enterprise for several reasons that include the potential expense of court room litigation and the negative publicity to an institution of higher learning. It is often far less expensive to litigate higher education disputes outside of a formal legal proceeding such as a bench or jury trial. As such, there is a limited amount of legal precedent to draw from, further contributing to the likelihood of a remedy through other means such as arbitration, mediation, or an informal settlement hearing or conference.

Conflict of interest issues in academia most often concern the research-related enterprise (42CFR50) or interpersonal relationships. The latter is the focus of this chapter. Interpersonal relationship conflicts of interest may arise within an amorous relationship, hiring of a relative (nepotism), or a sexual harassment claim. All universities have a Human Resources department with written policies relative to each of these potential conflicts of interest. By definition, an *amorous relationship* is one that is a consensual romantic, sexual or dating relationship, not including marriage, domestic partnership, or a civil union relationship. *Nepotism* is understood to mean favoritism granted to relatives or other close relationships not based on merit (Drexel University, 2019, Policy # HR-46) often triggered by hiring of a relative. *Sexual harassment* is a type of harassment (aggressive pressure, intimidation, annoyance) that involves unwelcome sexual advances, requests for sexual favors, disparagement of members of one sex, or other conduct of a sexual nature. Submission to or rejection of such conduct is made either explicitly or implicitly a term or condition of an individual's employment, education, or university activities, programs, or benefits (Kansas Board of Regents, Kansas State University, 2019b).

Sexual harassment claims may be litigated under Title VII of the Civil Rights Act of 1964 "because sexual harassment is a form of discrimination on the basis of sex" (Kaplan, Lee, Hutchens, & Rooksby, 2019, p. 517). Claims against an employer that involve unfair treatment on the basis of sex are most often invoked under Title VII, the most frequently utilized statute in discrimination cases (Kaplan et al., 2019). Conversely, the courts have not looked favorably upon plaintiffs who claim discrimination when a supervisor demonstrates preferential treatment to an employee who is also a paramour because individuals of both sexes are equally disenfranchised by the advantages and benefits received by the paramour. Courts have generally not found Title VII liability under a "paramour favoritism" theory in "isolated instances" of sexual favoritism in the workplace based on consensual romantic relationships. However, favoritism based on coerced sexual conduct may constitute "quid pro quo" sexual harassment under Title VII for other female employees or if favoritism based on granting sexual favors is widespread in the workplace, both male and female employees may be able to establish a "hostile work environment" claim under Title VII. Few courts have ruled in favor of plaintiffs, claiming retaliation due to complaints about paramour favoritism in the workplace. Further, plaintiffs could not have held a reasonable belief that paramour favoritism violated Title VII.

The law does not prohibit a consensual sexual relationship between two adults. However, the sequelae or unintended consequences of such a liaison in the workplace between supervisor and supervisee may potentially trigger a variety of discrimination laws.

 WHEN TO CONSULT THE UNIVERSITY COUNSEL

Consult the **university counsel for advice with a potential or real** conflict of interest.

FINDINGS AND DISPOSITION FOR CASE STUDY 18.1

In Case Study 18.1, the relationship between supervisor and employee allegedly placed another employee at a disadvantage and disfavor with the university. This is an interesting twist to the usual employment discrimination case. The estranged husband's contract was not renewed because his performance evaluations deteriorated as he spent increasing amounts of time at his other job in the tech industry where he was earning a higher income. The estranged husband failed to return to his non-tenure track position at the university after several leaves of absence during which time he was working at his other job. The husband claims "discriminatory treatment by the university due to his entanglement in the dean's love life" (Flaherty, 2015, para. 4). The university's position was that this series of leaves was beyond the permissible normal policy of the university and that the husband chose to pursue his "more lucrative employment" in the tech industry. Ultimately, the Dean decided to step down from his position due to the publicity of the husband's lawsuit against the university that was having an adverse effect on the business and mission of the school. The university, in this instance, did not seek the resignation of the Dean; to the contrary, the university's position was that the Dean correctly followed the university policy of full disclosure and transparency of the amorous relationship with a professor.

Policies should be drafted to address potential scenarios before they occur. Here, a faculty ad hoc committee should be appointed to convene and develop a policy relative to faculty–faculty and faculty–administrator relationships. (A policy addressing faculty–student relationships is most likely already in existence.) The ad hoc policy committee should research other such policies among a variety of universities in the United States. For example, if the committee consists of seven members, each should search 5 to 10 universities for similar policy statements as exemplars. Secondly, the committee should research cases in the literature that could foretell possible conflicts of interest situations to guide anticipatory policy writing. One tenet to follow is that the policy should state that although relationships can develop between individuals, there are certain relationships that by virtue of the status of the individuals present the appearance of impropriety and must be disclosed. Failure to disclose the amorous relationship to the respective supervisors of each individual is grounds for disciplinary action. Before the policy is adopted, it should be reviewed by the university's legal department.

Stanford University (2019) has a policy governing consensual sexual or romantic relationships in the workplace and educational setting. According to university policy, if "such a relationship develops, the person with greater authority must recuse himself or herself from matters involving a romantic partner to ensure 'that he/she does not exercise any supervisory or evaluative function over the other person in the relationship.' Where such recusal is required, the recusing party must also notify a supervisor, department chair, dean or human resources manager, so that person can ensure adequate alternative supervisory or evaluative arrangements are put in place" (Flaherty, 2015, para. 7).

Case Study 18.2
The Faculty Colleague as a Student: Faculty-to-Faculty Conflict of Interest

Your role: You are a non-tenure track clinical professor in a college of nursing teaching a doctor of nursing practice (DNP) course. In your class is a faculty colleague, an assistant teaching/clinical professor who has almost completed her coursework in the DNP program. She has recently been appointed as chairperson of your department and your DNP student is now your direct supervisor to whom you also report. Although the DNP student/department chair has been a very good student in the program, you now feel an obligation to be certain she not only passes your course, but does well. You are concerned about fairness and bias, and apprehensive about the appearance of impropriety that your boss is also your student whose continued employment may be contingent upon successful completion of the doctoral program.

Questions
- How would you distinguish the student from the faculty colleague?
- What action can you take to mitigate a potential conflict of interest?

DISCUSSION OF CASE STUDY 18.2

Conflicts of interest in all levels of education may occur when "your primary responsibility to a student is compromised by competing priorities … [and] could range from unknowingly allowing another priority to affect one's judgment, all the way to outwardly and intentionally violating a policy for personal gain" (Serva, 2019, para. 2). Moreover, a conflict of interest can arise in the nursing faculty role between two faculty members. Conflicts are foreseeable when there is competing interest between an individual and another entity such as: a committee's charge, the department, or a university's strategic plan to balance the budget. Such "conflicts can be financial, political, academic, or commercial" (Anselmi, Dreher, Glasgow, & Donnelly, 2010, p. 214). One scenario is when a faculty colleague is in the classroom as a student pursuing a doctoral degree within the same department, as described herein. The professor and student are professional colleagues outside of the classroom; however, within the classroom there is a hierarchical relationship where the evaluation and grading of the student's work product can have employment consequences if there is poor academic performance. The consequences may translate into compromising the pathway toward continued employment, promotion, and grant opportunities. Moreover, if a disagreement should arise, is the individual a student or an employee? If the individual contests a penalty that has been imposed upon them for an infraction of the school's code of conduct in the student role (Kaplan et al., 2019), what impact does this have upon the individual's employee-faculty role? The occurrence of an infraction or disagreement will trigger the examination and determination of the individual's status of employee-faculty or employee-student.

In this case, measures must be taken to assuage potential conflicts of interest between the dual relationship of employee-faculty and employee-student with good policy that anticipates such incidents (Anselmi et al., 2010). The first measure is to place the employee-student in course sections that are taught by faculty who do not have a supervisory relationship with the student. If this is not possible because there is only one section of the course and there is only one faculty member with content expertise who can teach the class, then action must be taken to eliminate any bias. Students may submit assignments anonymously using an identification number instead of their name. A professional staff person can generate identification numbers to correspond to student names and hold the key for a specific term. Law schools regularly follow this process during midterm and final exams. Furthermore, a second qualified faculty member who does not have a supervisory relationship with the student can evaluate the work product should the employee-student (also known as FAS, faculty as student) receive an unsatisfactory grade. These protocols, in addition to others, can be incorporated into an overall "faculty as student policy" document that is signed by the FAS. The policy should address the avoidance of any appearance of impropriety that the FAS not suffer a positive or negative bias. The policy should state prevention measures, what process will ensue when there is a faculty member in the classroom, action taken to mitigate a conflict of interest, and remedies to resolve conflict when it occurs. Faculty and administrators must disclose actual or perceived conflicts of interest, including familial relationships, and these relationships should be reviewed at regular intervals for any conflict by an objective third party.

The role of university faculty in pedagogy falls along a continuum from caring to professional objectivity. The relationship between faculty and student has been examined and determined that caring intimacy is not in the best interest of the student, faculty, and university (Chory & Offstein, 2016). Cultivating a close relationship with students may result in unintended consequences for the student, faculty, and the university; there are boundaries that must not be crossed. As such, prevention of adverse consequences can be clearly stated in the university and college policy for faculty or employees who take courses at the university. Faculty and employees who are also students should not be treated any differently from other students; in other words, similarly situated persons should be treated the same.

The trend of FAS is increasing, not decreasing; especially in nursing higher education. There is a rising demand for RNs, which translates into a commensurate demand for nursing faculty to educate nursing students (American Association of Colleges of Nursing, 2019). Colleges of nursing are softening their policies to facilitate doctoral education for their faculty "in-house" because it is more efficient and economical. Administrators must be vigilant to keep objective data whenever a potential conflict of interest may arise and adverse consequences must be adjudicated. Clear policy statements will assuage legal challenges.

FINDINGS AND DISPOSITION FOR CASE STUDY 18.2

The non-tenure track clinical professor (who was now supervising her department chair's DNP project) asked to meet with the Dean to discuss her concerns about the situation and its potential impact on her, other students, and faculty. After the discussion, the Dean appointed another supervising professor to oversee the DNP department's chair's DNP project to avoid a conflict of interest. The new supervising professor was a tenured full professor in the PhD program. The Dean followed up with all parties in writing explaining the rationale for the committee change.

RELEVANT LEGAL CASE

DeCintio v. Westchester County Medical Center, 807 F.2d 304 (2nd Cir, 1986)

The plaintiff-appellees in this case were seven male respiratory therapists employed by the defendant-appellant, Westchester Medical Center, who sued claiming that they had been unfairly disqualified from promotion to the position of Assistant Chief Respiratory Therapist in violation of Title VII of the Civil Rights Act of 1664 and the Equal Pay Act. The appellees claimed that the male supervisor of the Respiratory Therapy Department, James Ryan, had initiated a pretextual requirement for promotion to Assistant Chief in order to disqualify the seven male respiratory therapists from promotion and enable the supervisor to hire Ryan's preferred candidate, Jean Guagenti, a female with whom he was engaged in a romantic relationship.

In reversing the decision of the federal district court in favor of the appellees, the Second Circuit held that "voluntary, romantic relationships cannot form the basis of sex discrimination suit under either Title VII or the Equal Pay Act."

The Appeals Court found that the dispositive issue in this action is whether, under Title VII of the Civil Rights Act of 1964 ... the phrase "discrimination on the basis of sex" encompasses disparate treatment premised not on one's gender, but rather on a romantic relationship between an employer and a person preferentially hired. The meaning of "sex," for Title VII purposes, thereby would be expanded to include "sexual liaisons" and "sexual attractions." The Court said such an overbroad definition was "wholly unwarranted." The Court reasoned:

> Even assuming that appellees' allegations are true and that the district court's findings are correct, appellees have not set forth a cognizable Title VII claim for sex discrimination. Appellees allege, and the district court found, that Ryan and Guagenti were engaged in a romantic partnership; that Ryan established a special requirement for the Assistant Chief position solely as a pretext to enable him to cause Guagenti to be hired; that appellees were precluded from applying for the position due to the special requirement; and that Guagenti was hired on the recommendation of Ryan. Ryan's conduct, although unfair, simply did not violate Title VII. Appellees were not prejudiced because of their status as males; rather, they were discriminated against because Ryan preferred his paramour. Appellees faced exactly the same predicament as that faced by any woman applicant for the promotion: No one but Guagenti could be considered for the appointment because of Guagenti's special relationship to Ryan. That relationship forms the basis of appellees' sex discrimination claims. Appellees' proffered interpretation of Title VII prohibitions against sex discrimination would involve the EEOC and federal courts in the policing of intimate relationships. Such a course, founded on a distortion of the meaning of the word "sex" in the context of Title VII, is both impracticable and unwarranted.

Subsequently in 1990, the EEOC revised its position on paramour favoritism and issued new guidance which followed the 2nd Circuit's holding in the *DeCintio* case that "isolated instances" of sexual favoritism are not prohibited under Title VII. This EEOC guidance is still in effect today.

SUMMARY

Faculty members (like all university employees) are counseled to report potential or real conflicts of interest. It must be noted that legal proceedings cannot always capture the interpersonal conflicts, motives, and nuances that exist in the work environment. Legal cases are decided on facts provable by admissible evidence, and the legal casebooks are filled with decisions that were wrongly decided because the real evidence never got to the judge or jury. Administrators must be careful to keep focused on objective data when making adverse employee actions, and must figure out ways to deal with the subjective, personal, and political issues that can also greatly affect the performance of individuals and units.

ETHICAL CONSIDERATIONS

The appearance of impropriety can erode faculty and students' confidence in the academy. Faculty and students expect fairness and equity in the academy. If relationships exist that give an individual preferential treatment or the appearance of preferential treatment, an ethical dilemma can arise. Equally important, faculty and students need to feel safe in a university—that their work is judged on its merits and not less than or more than due to a special relationship. Administrators need to be aware of conflicts of interest and intervene appropriately when one exists to promote an ethical environment.

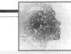

BEST PRACTICE EXEMPLARS

Academic administrators may be well served to develop a collaborative arrangement with another university to create a faculty tuition exchange program. Faculty members could obtain their doctoral degree at no or limited cost at another university and avoid internal conflicts of interest that may occur if faculty members obtain a degree at their place of employment (e.g., Duquesne University and St. Louis University Schools of Nursing).

Prevention Tips

Faculty and administrators should disclose any and all potential conflicts of interest—including familial relationships—and these relationships should be periodically reviewed for any conflict by an objective body.

CRITICAL ELEMENTS TO CONSIDER

- Refer to the university's conflict of interest policy.
- Report any potential conflicts to your supervisor and those noted in the conflict of interest policy.
- If you are an administrator, treat all direct reports equitably, regardless of "special" relationships.
- Refrain from participating in any employment, salary, or other important decision regarding an immediate family member or person with whom you are in a personal relationship.
- To avoid a perception of conflict of interest, members of the same family may not be employed in a situation where one member of the family works under the administrative supervision of another.
- Document performance issues in a formal and timely fashion—do not wait until there are numerous performance concerns that result in negative employment decisions.

References

American Association of Colleges of Nursing. (2019). *Fact sheet: Nursing shortage*. Retrieved from https://www.aacnnursing.org/Portals/42/News/Factsheets/Nursing-Shortage-Factsheet.pdf

Anselmi, K. K., Dreher, H. M., Glasgow, M. E. S., & Donnelly, G. (2010). Faculty colleagues in your classroom as doctoral students: Is there a conflict of interest? *Nurse Educator*, *35*(5), 213–219. doi:10.1097/NNE.0b013e3181ed83c7.

Chory, R. M. & Offstein E. H. (2016). "Your professor will know you as a person": Evaluating and rethinking the relational boundaries between faculty and students. *Journal of Management Education*, *41*(1), 9–38. doi:10.1177/1052562916647986

Code of Federal Regulations, *Title 42, Volume 1*, Part 50, 180–183 (42CFR50).

Drexel University. (2019). *CPO-2 conflict of interest and commitment*. Retrieved from https://drexel.edu/cpo/policies/cpo-2/

Flaherty, C. (2015, September 16). Dating the dean. *Inside Higher Ed*. Retrieved from https://www.insidehighered.com/news/2015/09/16/when-it-comes-dating-other-faculty-members-or-supervisors-proceed-caution

Kaplan, W. A., Lee, B. A., Hutchens, N. H., & Rooksby, J. H. (2019). *The law of higher education: A comprehensive guide to legal implications of administrative decision-making* (6th ed.). San Francisco, CA: John Wiley & Sons.

Kansas Board of Regents, Kansas State University. (2019a). *Conflict of interest policies*. Retrieved from https://www.k-state.edu/provost/universityhb/fhxs.html

Kansas Board of Regents, Kansas State University. (2019b). *Policy prohibiting discrimination, harassment, sexual violence, domestic and dating violence, and stalking, and procedure for reviewing complaints*. Retrieved from https://www.k-state.edu/policies/ppm/3000/3010.html#define

New York University. (2019). *Academic conflict of interest and conflict of commitment*. Retrieved from https://www.nyu.edu/about/policies-guidelines-compliance/policies-and-guidelines/academic-conflict-of-interest-and-conflict-of-commitment.html

Serva, C. (2019). Conflicts of interest in education. In *Praxis school psychologist: Practice and study guide*. Retrieved from https://study.com/academy/lesson/conflict-of-interest-in-education.html

Stanford University. (2019). *1.7.2 Consensual sexual or romantic relationships in the workplace and educational setting*. Retrieved from https://adminguide.stanford.edu/chapter-1/subchapter-7/policy-1-7-2

Sugarman, S. D. (2005). Conflict of interest in the role of the university professor. *Theoretical Inquiries in Law*, *6*, 255–275.

Title VII of the Civil Rights Act of 1964, 42 U.S.C. §§ 2000e *et seq*.

Disability Issues for the Student

Case Studies
Physical and Learning Disabilities

Your role: You are Dr. Callahan, the BSN program coordinator in a college's nursing department.

This chapter offers analyses of several scenarios regarding undergraduate nursing students with disabilities who make requests for academic accommodations to faculty and academic program administrators. Although these cases initially appear unique, close examination of the underlying principles and related case law reveals common themes that emerge as a basis for discussion of programmatic issues and considerations related to the education of nursing students with disabilities.

Case Study 19.1

During the first clinical rotation in a fundamentals nursing course, Lisa Bowman informs her clinical instructor, Professor Lowell, that she (Lisa) is unable to participate in physical care activities of adults because of a previously undisclosed physical limitation that does not allow her to lift more than 10 pounds. Ms. Bowman declares that she is protected from discrimination in her student role and states that she has a qualified disability. She further states that her intent is to work in a neonatal intensive care unit after graduation and threatens legal action if prevented from continued progression in the nursing program.

Case Study 19.2

Janet Golden was admitted to the nursing program and scheduled to begin classes in less than 1 month. She presented to the Dean's office and requested a meeting to discuss concerns related to some newly identified medical issues that could potentially impact her success in nursing clinical coursework. During that meeting, Janet explained that she was newly diagnosed with multiple sclerosis. At the time of diagnosis, Janet's only deficit was a numbness and loss of feeling in her fingertips, but the possibility and unpredictability of progression was extremely overwhelming. She was obviously distraught and concerned that her medical condition would prevent her from becoming a nurse.

The Dean offered emotional support and articulated the program's commitment to helping Janet achieve her goal, but also explained that due to the unpredictable nature and management of the disease, exacerbation of symptoms could result in the need for accommodations beyond the scope of programmatic/university resources. Should such a situation occur, a temporary leave or medical withdrawal from the nursing program would be warranted. Janet was advised to contact the office of disability services and encouraged to be proactive in identifying needed accommodations that would enable her to meet clinical and academic standards of the program. She was also encouraged to contact student counseling services for assistance in dealing with the emotional and physical upset of her recent medical diagnosis

Unfortunately, within the first weeks of the semester, the student returned to the Dean's office in tears explaining that, due to the loss of sensation in her fingertips, she was having difficulties taking peripheral pulses and that her clinical faculty member suggested she would not likely pass the course if she were unable to master this basic clinical skill. In collaboration with the clinical instructor, it was determined that a reasonable accommodation would be for the student to use a handheld Doppler as an assistive device for obtaining the needed clinical information in patient assessments. Although the initial discourse between student and faculty was unfortunate, the incident afforded the opportunity for mutual understanding, open communication, and support. Janet encountered no further difficulties mastering foundational clinical skills.

 Case Study 19.3

Debra Gormley, a nursing student midway through the nursing program, was denied employment as a nurse extern for a cooperative education experience in a telemetry unit at a local hospital because of her disclosure of a hearing deficit. Hospital officials cite concerns related to patient safety because Ms. Gormley will not be able to hear cardiac monitor alarms. The student wears bilateral hearing aids and is able to converse reasonably well in face-to-face situations. Ms. Gormley has been approved for accommodations from the university's office of disability services. The accommodations consist of note-taking support in class and use of an amplified stethoscope in the clinical setting. She has met all academic and clinical requirements to date. However, Ms. Gormley acknowledges significant auditory processing problems in large groups or with multidirectional auditory stimuli. The prognosis is that her auditory capacity will continue to decline and she will become totally deaf within an unspecified time frame. Ms. Gormley approaches the BSN program coordinator, Dr. Callahan, and questions how the recent denial of employment and associated functional limitations will influence both her continued progression in the nursing program and her career aspirations of becoming an RN.

 Case Study 19.4

Jacob Patel, a nursing student, enrolled in a nonprofits and healthcare course, given his minor in health services administration. He provided to the faculty member an Accommodation Verification Letter, which allowed for time and a half for any in-class assessment. He

participated very little in the in-person class. Unsolicited he told the faculty member he had a serious chronic disease, and would miss only two classes for a procedure. There were five assessments, including a group assessment in the course. The faculty member gave a very generous grade to this student for his class participation. When the student learned that he would get an A minus for the course, he challenged the faculty member on the fairness of not getting more credit for class participation; presumably, this could tip the final grade to an A. The student complained to both the instructor and department chair that he was penalized due to his illness, which made him anxious and ostensibly not able to participate fully in class.

 Case Study 19.5

David Issacs, a 21-year-old student with attention deficit hyperactivity disorder (ADHD) who was previously unsuccessful in a fast-paced second-degree accelerated nursing curriculum, was granted admission to your BSN program on the premise that he would be able to meet program outcome standards given that the coursework would be spread over a longer time period. However, David did not proactively initiate the request for academic accommodations with the office of disability services confident that no such supports would be required in a slower paced academic environment. After scoring poorly on the first two tests, David informed his instructor that he had ADHD and demanded that he be afforded extra time and reduced distraction environment for testing. David seemed surprised and annoyed that he was directed to the office of disability services for assistance. However, due to the urgent nature of the request, he was granted temporary (one term) academic accommodations by the office of disability services. Doing so gave him time to complete the necessary processes and procedures associated with assessment and evaluation of the nature and extent of formal accommodations needed on an ongoing basis. An instructor who had significant experience in supporting students with ADHD also offered support and suggestions directed at helping him improve his academic performance.

Unfortunately, even with accommodations in place and intense faculty support, David's academic difficulties continued. He was disruptive in class and often belligerent with professors when they would attempt to provide clarification and direction related to assignments. He also struggled in adapting to the dynamic nature of the clinical setting and had great difficulty with critical thinking and clinical judgment in both care activities and interactions with faculty, staff, and patients. In efforts to support student success, David was encouraged, on multiple occasions, to utilize the full array of academic supports available from both the nursing program and the university but declined to do so. He refused to accept personal accountability for shortcomings consistently blaming others for his academic and clinical issues or claiming discriminatory bias. When David's academic and clinical deficiencies culminated in dismissal from the nursing program, his parents initiated legal action.

Questions
- In each of these cases, do you believe there is a valid disability claim by the student?
- How would you resolve each case individually if you were the academic nursing administrator charged with making a final determination?

DISABILITY ISSUES FOR THE STUDENT: LEGAL PRINCIPLES AND REVIEW OF THE LITERATURE

As the majority of disability issues in higher education pertain to students, the impact of disability law on students are thoroughly addressed in this chapter. Legal protection for students with disabilities was initially established by section 504 of the Rehabilitation Act of 1973 but was limited in its applicability to institutions that received federal funds. This protection was extended to all educational institutions by Title II and Title III of the Americans with Disabilities Act (ADA) of 1990. Moreover, in 2008, President George W. Bush signed a major amendment to the ADA making it less onerous for individuals to prove that they had a disability within the meaning of the ADA (U.S. Equal Employment Opportunity Commission, 2008). In addition, equivalent state laws will prohibit discrimination against students due to disability. These acts require universities to make reasonable and necessary modifications to rules, policies, and practices to prevent discrimination against students on the basis of disability (Cope, 2005).

Because of these legislative mandates, advances in technology, and educational supports, the number of students with disabilities who are seeking higher education has tripled in the past 25 years. Data from the National Center for Educational Statistics [NCES] show that 11% of undergraduates in both 2007 to 2008 and 2011 to 2012 reported having a disability. In 2011 to 2012, the percentage of undergraduates who reported having a disability was 11% for both males and females (NCES, 2019). The NCES report indicates that the most common disabilities in higher education are psychiatric disorders, learning disabilities, and ADHD.

This trend is also evident in educational programs for health professionals, but the proportion of students enrolled in these programs who report some type of disability is significantly lower than it is in the general undergraduate population. It is unclear whether this disparity is a result of selective admission policies, technical standards, or educational requirements characteristic of health-related disciplines (Newsham, 2008). In a recent study of nursing faculty knowledge and expertise in dealing with disabled nursing students, responses to the types of student disabilities encountered in classroom/clinical settings revealed that 63 of 88 (72%) respondents currently or previously taught students with disabilities. Further breakdown of faculty experiences with students presenting with varied types of disabilities revealed that 60% had encountered students with learning disabilities; 28% had encountered students with ADHD; 25% had encountered students with physical disabilities; 18% had encountered students with significant hearing impairment; and 13% had encountered students with visual impairment (Sowers & Smith, 2004).

In 2014, a roundtable was organized by the U.S. Department of Labor's [USDOL] Office of Disability Employment Policy, in collaboration with the National Organization of Nurses with Disabilities and co-sponsored by the Department's Employment and Training Administration and the U.S. Health Resources and Services Administration. The roundtable discussed the health professions' disability trends, best practices, and made a "call to action" for how those with a disability could play a role in meeting health professions' growing workforce needs (USDOL Office of Disability Employment Policy, 2014). This same year, a requirement from the Office of Federal Contract Compliance Programs mandated that healthcare organizations with federal contracts demonstrate that their nursing workforce be comprised of at least 7% of qualified individuals with disabilities (USDOL Office of Federal Contract Compliance Programs, 2014).

Learning disabilities and attention deficit disorders are a heterogeneous group of medical conditions manifested by significant difficulties in acquisition and use of listening, speaking, reading, reasoning, or mathematical skills. They often present as comorbidities with similar clinical presentations. These disorders are intrinsic to the individual and presumed to be caused by central nervous system dysfunction (Rosenbraugh, 2000). Although physical disabilities are more distinct in etiology and varied in presenting symptoms, there are often similarities in the categories of accommodations needed in the educational setting. Consequently, for purposes of discussion, this chapter focuses on addressing the needs of students with physical disabilities generically.

Nursing, as a profession, maintains a strong advocacy role for individuals with special needs; however, the education of nursing students with disabilities poses unique challenges. Nursing faculty, similar to their counterparts in other professional health disciplines, often exhibit personal bias related to student capabilities, a lack of information, and a lack of confidence in dealing with student disabilities. Clinically focused professional education programs such as nursing are faced with the challenges of simultaneously supporting student learning within the context of public safety, meeting mandated program outcome standards, and ensuring student competency to pass licensure requirements.

Nursing educators have a vested interest in student success, and tend to respond favorably to student requests for assistance in meeting learning objectives. However, granting informal student requests for special considerations related to performance assessments, assignments, or clinical rotations on an ad hoc basis may inadvertently create inequities for other students, delay student access to needed formal academic intervention/supports, and pose legal challenges of discrimination. Limited knowledge about disability issues often contributes to indecision and inconsistency on the part of faculty when approached by students requesting special considerations related to assignments/examinations and/or formal academic accommodations. There is general consensus that educators and administrators alike need to develop a better understanding of the rights of and responsibilities of students and programs within the context of quality in educational curricula and the provision of high-quality healthcare services to the public (Newsham, 2008; Sowers & Smith, 2004; Stacey & Carroll, 2000).

Meloy and Gambescia (2014, p. 142) remind faculty about the "unique distinction between *consideration*, the multiplicity of day-to-day decisions faculty make when students experience changing and extenuating circumstances but not related to documented disability, and *accommodation*, that is, those actions faculty are required to take after an official designation is made by an office of disability services." They admit that nursing faculty by nature approach student issues in a caring manner but need to balance academic considerations with risk of pitfalls, perceived or real, in giving students preferential treatment. They warn that enabling students to rely on their good nature for consideration may delay or mask much needed academic support including official accommodation by the office of disability services. Repetitive requests for special considerations from any student should raise concerns and consideration for referral to student counseling and/or the Office of Disability.

Legal protection for students with disabilities in higher education is addressed in federal laws specifically in section 504 of the 1973 Rehabilitation Act (29 U.S.C. § 794) and Title II of the 1990 ADA (42 U.S.C. § 12132). These somewhat overlapping laws aim to protect the rights of disabled individuals, those individuals who have a physical or mental disability that "substantially limits" one or more of their major life activities. In academic settings, learning is viewed as a major life activity (Helms, Jorgensen, & Anderson, 2006). These laws require universities to make reasonable and necessary modifications to rules, policies, or practices to prevent discrimination against qualified students based on disability. The ADA also requires that institutions designate a compliance officer (and disability staff as needed) to address ADA compliance issues, qualify students with disabilities, and identify appropriate academic adjustments as indicated (Cope, 2005).

Although these two federal regulations do not specifically address higher education, subsequent administrative rules and case law provide insight and guidance related to a nursing program's obligation to the student, its educational mission, preparation for licensure, and eventual employment of the student as an RN. Courts are understandably particularly interested in cases involving the health professions because of the direct effect on the health and safety of patients. Initially, few suits from students came forward. However, legal experts in this area suspect that more cases will arise given the dramatic increase in accommodation given in the high schools making more students with disabilities eligible, the increase in activity from disability advocacy groups, and the interest from policy makers to expand those eligible for accommodations (Rothstein, 2000).

Three foundational terms must be defined to understand these laws. A *qualified disability* is a physical or mental impairment that substantially limits one or more major life activities of an individual compared to the conditions, manner, or duration under which these activities can be performed by the general public or comparable student group. *Otherwise qualified* in postsecondary educational settings means that a student with a disability is one who is able to meet a program's admission, academic, and technical standards either with or without accommodation *in spite of* the limitations imposed by the disability. *Reasonable accommodations* are the program/activity adjustments that enable an otherwise qualified individual fair opportunity to achieve outcome standards.

---

[1] Just a reminder that due process for private universities is not required. What private universities follow is something close to due process but is technically not called due process.

[2] See Gambescia, S. F., & Donnelly, G. D. (2017). Managing and monitoring student "issues" in higher education. *Journal of Allied Health, 44,* 183–187, and Anselmi, K., Glasgow, M. E., & Gambescia, S. F. (2014). Using a student conduct committee to foster professional accountability. *Journal of Professional Nursing, 30*(6); 481–485. doi:10.1016/j.profnurs.2014.04.002

Adjustments are not intended to create unfair advantage or require significant adjustments to program/activity—do not result in lowering program/activity standards—and are not intended to cause undue burden to the sponsoring entity.

Several principles guide the fair and reasonable implementation of accommodating students during the continuum of their enrollment to graduation in an academic nursing program. These include the following:

1. Formal notification by the student of perceived or qualified disability
2. Disability verification/qualification by designated disability personnel
3. Integrity of educational program and academic standards
4. Determination of reasonable accommodations
5. Notification and implementation of accommodation
6. Established procedures for complaints and appeals[1,2]

It should be noted that the students entering postsecondary education face a substantially different dynamic in terms of guaranteed access to support services. Special education legislation governing primary and secondary schools provides extensive due process rights for disabled students and their families. At the postsecondary level, the burden of responsibility shifts from the institution to the individual necessitating that students assume ownership and accountability for initiating needed academic supports. Consequently, it is the student's responsibility to formally notify an institution, either through the program administrators or the office of disability services, to self-identify the existence of disability (perceived or qualified), and to request consideration of formal academic accommodations. However, in a recent survey of California Nursing Programs, Betz, Smith, and Bui (2012) identified that 72% reported that they have encountered students who do not self-disclose their disability status or proactively request accommodations. If the student fails to make such notification to an institution, program administrators and faculty cannot be held responsible for untoward student outcomes, requests for retroactive accommodations, or related allegations of disability discrimination. Once the student requests disability status, the case should be handled in a confidential, expeditious, and comprehensive manner.

Assuming a student appropriately reports a disability, the student must then provide supporting documentation from appropriate/qualified medical or educational professionals to establish a qualified disability. However, the existence of documentation of physical or learning limitations, in and of itself, may not be sufficient to qualify the student for academic accommodations because the associated impairment must substantially limit major life activities. In addition, disabling conditions that can be mitigated or ameliorated with medications or corrective devices may negate requests for disability accommodation. In instances in which supporting documentation is not available (or deemed inadequate) to support a claim of disability, the cost of all related testing and professional evaluative measures to document the existence of a qualified disability are the responsibility of the student. The institution and its representatives bear no accountability for the provision or procurement of these services. Qualified disability status (and related accommodations) cannot be granted unless all verification requirements are met in accordance with the law.

Accommodations/academic supports are intended to minimize the impact of a qualified disability and enable the student to participate fully in the educational process. These adjustments are not intended to fundamentally alter the education and training program in an academic setting, create excessive burden to the sponsoring organization, or create an unfair advantage with regard to other students in learning experiences and evaluative measures. However, courts have asked that institutions bear the higher burden than the individual because they are better situated to do so (Rothstein, 2000).

Once reasonable accommodations are determined by the office of disability services, the student is given an academic verification letter (AVL), or equivalent documentation, outlining the specific nature of the accommodation and related considerations. It is extremely important that faculty do not grant any academic adjustments in any way without the AVL. Granting accommodations in the absence of this documentation establishes precedence that the academic unit acknowledges the student as disabled. As a result, the individual is automatically qualified to receive similar academic supports/considerations in the future, thereby circumventing the evaluation/verification processes inherent in disability legislation. Once established, institutions have limited recourse for cessation of academic accommodations, even if it is felt that they are no longer warranted (Newsham, 2008). It is the institution's responsibility to ensure that accommodations are implemented in a consistent and equitable manner and that equivalent backup supports are available in the event that usual accommodation mechanisms fail. Both students and faculty (who are charged with implementing accommodations) should also have access to formal appeal mechanisms should the designated accommodations be viewed as inadequate or unreasonable.

Academic accommodations are not intended to lower program outcome standards in any way. It is important for both faculty and students to understand the important distinction that all students, even those with qualified disabilities and academic accommodations, are held to the same academic standards and program outcome requirements. Correspondingly, technical standards/essential functions are established for the continuum of students' participation in the nursing program from admission, to graduation and practice as an RN. These standards typically range from the very general, such as sense functioning and locomotion, to motor ability, observational ability, communication ability, conceptual and quantitative ability, sociobehavioral ability, and ability to handle stress (Evans, 2005). Individuals who are unable to meet such technical standards, with or without reasonable accommodations, are not permitted to complete the nursing program and will be counseled to pursue alternative careers. In circumstances in which achievement of technical standards or course/program outcomes is deemed unsatisfactory, the student should be afforded access to formalized appeal procedures.

DISCUSSION OF CASES, FINDINGS AND DISPOSITION, AND RELEVANT LEGAL CASES

Unlike previous chapters, this one explores several different cases exemplifying the complexity of the issues at hand and the individual nature of student-specific circumstances. Therefore, the discussion of each case, the resulting findings and disposition, and relevant legal citation will be integrated in one section. Case Studies 19.1 and 19.2 provide examples of the myriad of instances where students present with physical disabilities. In Case Study 19.1, Lisa Bowman, a fundamentals nursing student, stated that she was unable to lift more than 10 pounds. Despite Ms. Bowman's claim of protection under ADA legislation, she did not disclose her physical limitation, nor did she proactively seek the office of disability services with request for accommodation on admission to the nursing program or in advance of her clinical rotations. She, like many others, assumed that the mere existence of a severe physical limitation would place her in a protected class and afford special consideration with regard to meeting clinical requirements and technical standards inherent to the nursing curriculum.

Ms. Bowman's case was referred to the office of disabilities services for evaluation and recommendation. Although the medical documentation of her physical limitations met the criteria of substantially limiting her performance of manual tasks, the nature of her disability made it impossible for her to meet programmatic technical standards associated with motor ability and patient care activities for individuals across the life span. In addition, it was determined that her physical condition would place her at significant risk for personal harm and she did not have the physical stamina to meet the demands of physical exertion required for safe performance in the clinical setting. There were also no medications or ameliorating devices that would permit her to meet these requirements. It was noted that students who have disabilities for which there are no reasonable accommodations do not meet the criteria of being reasonably qualified for admission to or continued progression in a nursing education program. In addition, internships and clinical requirements are considered essential components of nursing curricula. Dismissal from the nursing program was upheld on the basis that Ms. Bowman's requested accommodations would necessitate significant alteration to the undergraduate nursing curriculum and related program requirements and necessitate significant alterations/limitations in student clinical learning activities beyond the scope of available resources.

In Case Study 19.2, Janet Golden was proactive in identifying her disability and the need for accommodations. The student was informed that diagnosis of her condition, in and of itself, would not necessarily preclude completion of the nursing program. The Dean emphasized the existence of a supportive environment and a commitment to provide the student with needed resources on an ongoing basis and referred the student to appropriate support services. It was also appropriate that the Dean responded honestly about the uncertainty of the student's medical prognosis and did not provide assurances that could well be beyond her control.

This case also exemplifies the need for faculty education and examination of bias regarding nursing students with physical disabilities. Ashcroft et al. (2008) assert that faculty members' approach to nursing students with disabilities is often a result of their personal view of disability. In this instance, the faculty member's initial response to the student's condition was likely grounded in the medical model of disability, in which disability is viewed as an abnormality or deficiency needing correction, thereby precipitating safety concerns and the belief that students with a disability cannot be successful in nursing education (Marks & McCulloh, 2016). Aaberg (2012) examined the implicit attitudes of 132 nurse educators toward disabled individuals, which revealed a strong preference for able-bodied individuals. There is clearly a need for increased education and exploration of implicit bias by nursing faculty; however, a collaborative approach to resolution of the issue at hand (including consultation with the office of disabilities) and facilitation of an open dialogue between the student and the instructor resulted in enhanced mutual understanding, facilitated a shift in perspective on the part of the faculty member, and included the student as an active partner in identification of needed academic supports. Unfortunately, due to the unpredictable nature of the student's illness, it is impossible to predict the nature of "reasonable accommodations" and what performance standards will be met in the future.

RELEVANT LEGAL CASES

Doherty v. Southern College of Optometry, 862 F.2d 570, 575 (6th Cir. 1988), cert. denied, 493 U.S. 810, 110 S.Ct. 53, 107 L.Ed.2d 22 (1989)

Courts have been clear that health professions education programs can require the full complement of standards and practice. For example, in *Doherty v. Southern College of Optometry*, an optometric student was not otherwise qualified because his neurological disorder inhibited him from using necessary clinical tools of the profession. The court also ruled that reasonable accommodation does not include waiving an essential component of the educational program.

Shin v. University of Maryland Medical System Corp., 369 F. App'x. 472 (4th Cir. 2010)

In the case of *Shin v. University of Maryland Medical System Corp.* (2010), a medical intern with mental and behavioral disabilities associated with attention deficit disorder (a low working memory and impairment in visual–spatial reasoning) was not deemed an otherwise qualified person under the ADA because he was unable to meet program requirements. The courts upheld that the nature and extent of needed accommodations would require extensive restructuring of the academic program and modifications in academic/clinical standards resulting in undue burden for the academic entity.

Southeastern Community College v. Davis, 442 U.S. 397 (1979)

In Case Study 19.3, Debra Gormley was a nursing student midway through her nursing program but with significant hearing impairment. The seminal case of a student with disabilities in the nursing context is the U.S. Supreme Court case of *Southeastern Community College v. Davis* (1979). The court determined that a nursing college's denial of enrollment to a deaf applicant was not a violation of section 504 of the Rehabilitation Act of 1973, in which accommodation to perform essential functions of work would require major accommodations by, and lowering the standards of, the nursing program (e.g., taking only academic classes and not participating in the clinical portion of the nursing program). However, subsequent cases have clarified the original ruling explaining that programs could be expected to make reasonable accommodations such as those made available to this student to date.

In this case, Ms. Gormley continued to meet all academic and clinical requirements of the nursing program, but there was ongoing concern that her academic performance on examinations was negatively affected by the continued progression of her hearing deficits. She had been provided a stenographer to take notes during class sessions as an auxiliary aid to enhance learning. It is well established that students with sensory impairments may require an intermediary to facilitate communication in areas and activities outside the classroom. However, the use of these intermediaries is highly controversial in the clinical healthcare arena. Privacy concerns related to patient confidentiality and potential violation of the Health Information Portability Accountability Act (HIPAA) of 1996 are inherent to inclusion of an independent third party in the client–caregiver relationship. It is also difficult to determine to what degree the intermediary simply transfers information or influences the nature of the communication and student judgment (Hafferty & Gibson, 2003). Cost and availability of providing such services outside the classroom raise considerations of undue financial burden on the part of the program; however, the burden of proof in this situation rests largely with the academic entity and the overall financial resources of the university or college, not the individual student's program, will be considered by courts in determining whether an accommodation might be unreasonable because it imposes an undue financial burden on the institution (Newsham, 2008).

The denial of Ms. Gormley for employment for a university and program-sponsored cooperative education requirement highlights the fact that while on clinical rotations and cooperative work-related activities, students are invited guests of the host facility and subject to their decisions regarding patient care delivery in their respective institutions. The nursing program maintained that it would continue to assist Ms. Gormley in finding quality clinical educational experiences and alternative clinical sites that would provide opportunities for her to increase knowledge and skills in fulfillment of her degree requirements. However, it was beyond the academic program's purview to demand that healthcare facilities honor the range of accommodations provided to students in the academic environment. If Ms. Gormley's disability worsens to the extent that her academic/clinical performance is significantly compromised, safety issues emerge, or reasonable accommodations are no longer feasible, her continued progression in the nursing program would need to be reevaluated. Ms. Gormley was also advised that, although there is established precedent that individuals with significant hearing impairment have successfully transitioned to clinical practice roles as RNs, there is no guarantee that the extent of accommodations available in postsecondary education programs will be deemed reasonable by potential employers. Consequently, she was counseled that her employment options in the future, although available, may be limited by the nature of her disability.

In Case Study 19.4, you see how students may confound an actual accommodation with the other expectations of a course and try to expand an instructor's consideration to an accommodation. As mentioned above, Meloy and Gambescia (2014) explain the important distinction between giving students consideration with that of a formal and legal accommodation. The instructor actually gave some consideration to the student, with a serious illness, in giving a boost to the class participation grade. In fact, the instructor allowed the student to substitute part of one assignment, given the student's ostensible anxiety. The students were required to interview an executive director of a community nonprofit in the area to learn about the major skills and competencies needed to run a nonprofit health organization. The instructor allowed this student to review leadership competencies of health service administrators, rather than interview (in person or by phone) an executive of a nonprofit health group.

Regarding the class participation grade, the student made claim to unfair treatment given his chronic illness, but the official accommodation letter said nothing about relieving the student from class participation. The student was not satisfied with the instructor's explanation, and took his case to the chair of the department. The chair agreed that there was no official relief of the student from class participation and explained to the student that the instructor was "quite considerate" of his circumstance. The chair did explain to the instructor that while she made a reasonable and student-friendly consideration for the one assignment, a consult with experts from the office of disabilities may have been helpful and consequently avoided a slippery slope expectation from a student with a disability accommodation. Meloy and Gambescia (2014) warn:

> Faculty working without some thoughtful consult will have a hard time determining where to draw the line for *academic considerations*. Each request seems to be different as the students' issues seem to involve such varied extenuating circumstances. The variance is uncanny. This creates a slippery slope for inadvertently encouraging students who seek academic considerations, and the faculty member's litmus test becomes more liberal. (p. 140)

In Case Study 19.5, nursing student David Issacs had ADHD. He successfully completed all academic and clinical requirements during the first semester with temporary accommodations (extended time and reduced distraction environment for testing) in place. However, he did not complete the qualifications process within the initially agreed-on time line and did not contact the office of disability services for an extension of academic supports. Mr. Issacs verbally notified course faculty of his diagnosis of ADHD, but did not follow through with faculty recommendations to contact the disability services despite being reminded of academic policies prohibiting special considerations in the absence of official verification of qualification for academic accommodation. During the second semester of classes, Mr. Issacs once again elected to take exams without the accommodations of extended time or a distraction-free environment that were in place previously, citing that he did not want to take advantage of the system. He subsequently failed two of four exams and was in jeopardy of course failure and significant delay in progression of his nursing studies. He appealed both failing grades and demanded the opportunity to retake the failed exams citing that his previous accommodations served as an acknowledgment of disability by the nursing program and that prior accommodations should have automatically been extended.

Mr. Issacs then contacted the office of disability services and requested additional time to complete the disability certification process. He was granted an additional 3-month extension of temporary accommodations, but was notified that retroactive application of academic supports was not possible and that he had no basis for appeal in that regard. Correspondingly, the nursing program permitted Mr. Issacs to continue in the nursing program, but with the clear stipulation that (with or without academic accommodations in place) he must meet all established academic and clinical requirements or face dismissal from the nursing program.

This case highlights several important considerations associated with students who request disability accommodations. Although the diagnosis of ADHD was medically documented, the diagnosis alone is insufficient to qualify the student as disabled. In addition, responsibility to complete the certification process or request extension of time to do so rests solely with the student.

The faculty member's response to the student's verbal notification of a diagnosis of ADHD and denial of accommodations in the absence of an official AVL, consistent with program and university policies, was appropriate. A faculty member is technically an agent of the university. Consequently, had the faculty member granted academic accommodations without formal documentation of same, it would have resulted in the student being regarded as disabled. In this instance, it would be virtually impossible to discontinue related accommodations, whether or not they were justified, in the future (Thomas, 2000).

The case of Mr. Issacs also exemplifies the requirement that student disability (perceived or qualified) does not exempt an individual from academic policies and technical standards. It is well established in case law that students with disabilities (with or without related accommodations) must demonstrate that they are otherwise qualified to meet all programmatic requirements or are subject to denial of continued academic progression and dismissal (*Hash v. University of Kentucky*, 2004; *Rosenberger v. Rector and Visitors of the University* of Virginia, 2005).

It should also be noted that, at 21 years of age, Mr. Issacs is a millennial. David's inattentiveness to rules, regulations, deadlines, and instructions is consistent with behaviors typically found with millennial students (Coomes & DeBard, 2004). His lack of accountability for actions/outcomes is likely a result of his parents being heavily involved in all aspects of his life and "taking care" of anything they perceive needing attention. While the request for disability accommodations in this age group is not different from previous cohorts, the often-intense approach to disability issues on the part of millennials and their parents can be extremely challenging for educators and administrators (Rothstein, 2008). Although the parents did seek legal counsel, the Dean had accumulated substantial documentation over time highlighting efforts in support of Mr. Issacs's success in the nursing program and it was determined that there was no basis for legal recourse to his dismissal.

Powell v. National Board of Medical Examiners, 34 F.3d 79 (2nd Cir. 2004)

Another case from the University of Connecticut (*Powell v. National Board of Medical Examiners*, 2004) describes a situation in which a student diagnosed with dyslexia, attention deficit disorder, anxiety, and depression was dismissed from medical school after failing to meet academic standards despite being afforded multiple opportunities to do so. The court held that she never proved that she was a qualified individual with a disability. As a result, the court found that the university did not discriminate against the student in any way. The court further acknowledged that by granting the student multiple opportunities to meet academic standards, the university went above and beyond usual standards to support her educational endeavors. The temporary academic accommodations granted to the nursing student in this case scenario (in support of the student completing the necessary verifying processes to qualify her ADHD as a disability) would likely be viewed in a similar manner.

 WHEN TO CONSULT THE UNIVERSITY COUNSEL

As mentioned earlier in this chapter, the need to support students with disabilities has intensified in both its nature and extent, and university officials should expect that students will seek legal representation. Therefore, it is important for academic administrators in nursing programs to first be familiar with the representative from the general counsel office who will handle such cases; know how to access this individual for a consult; and be proactive in the educational process and information exchange. In most universities, the director of the office of disability services will have more frequent contact in handling students with disability concerns than will the academic administrators. However, as emphasized in this chapter, nursing program administrators need to ensure that legal counsel is briefed on how a clinical education program differs from other academic programs in handling student progression and overall clearance for licensure examination. It would be important to meet with general counsel staff prior to the rise of a problem to explain the types of issues anticipated. Updated student handbooks should be on file in the general counsel office with more in-depth discussion about competencies and technical standards. General counsel should also periodically review admission standards as they relate to students' ability to *fully participate* in didactic and clinical components of the program.

General counsel should be able to review correspondence sent to these students, especially if there may not be agreement between the office of disability services director and the nursing program administrators. Dismissal letters should, without a doubt, be reviewed by counsel. Communiqués that significantly alter the student's degree plan or time to degree completion should be reviewed by counsel. Rulings and decisions on official complaints (not necessarily grievances) are worth reviews by counsel. Decisions on rulings that the student may believe their disability confounded the less than expected score or grade on an assessment is worth a review by general counsel. Nursing program administrators should not be hesitant about contacting general counsel on these matters.

Considerations of Students With Disabilities in Nursing Education

Sharby and Roush (2009) suggest that the process of supporting students with disabilities begins long before the student submits an accommodation verification letter endorsed by the office of disability services to a faculty member. It is important that academic administrators and nursing faculty develop a systematic process to anticipate, review, and respond to student requests for accommodation. A discussion of considerations in nursing education must address the specific needs and challenges of students with disabilities from both a legal and conceptual viewpoint.

Clear Articulation of Admission Policies, Pedagogical Requirements, Academic Policies, and Technical Standards

The first step in addressing the needs of nursing students with disabilities involves a detailed review of existing university/program admission criteria for compliance with current legal mandates. Preadmission inquiry concerning whether a prospective applicant has a disability is not permissible under the law. However, questions related to substance abuse and criminal convictions are permissible because of the direct relationship with clinical nursing practice, professional licensure requirements, and the student interface with vulnerable patient populations during clinical rotations (Thomas, 2000).

The use of testing, evaluation of preexisting course work, or other criteria that may influence the admission decision is permissible only if applied equitably to prospective students and if the criteria have been deemed valid and reliable predictors of student success in the nursing program. It is also important to note that when standardized testing is used as a major criterion in the admission decision process, these tests must reflect the applicant's aptitude or achievement level rather than sensory, manual, or verbal skills (Thomas, 2000). It is common for third-party testing administrators to note if the tests were taken in nonconforming conditions (testing accommodations provided). Preadmission test scores with such a notation should not be relied on as a sole predictor for admission or rejection of a candidate's application, and should be viewed within the context of other universally applied admission criteria, including prior academic performance, background, and life experiences.

Technical standards deemed fundamental for admission and successful student progression/ graduation in the nursing program must also be clearly defined and must be defensible as essential elements of the curriculum. These essential requirements are generally classified in terms of (a) the ability to observe and communicate; (b) physical capacity and motor skills; (c) cognitive skills and intellectual capacity; (d) decision-making skills; and (e) behavioral, social, and professional attributes (Helms, Jorgensen, & Andersen, 2010). Once established, the technical standards should be included in student recruitment and application materials, posted in program websites, and published in student handbooks. This information should also be readily available to both theory and clinical faculty so that the standards are applied in a consistent manner. Refer to the *Drexel University Technical Standard Policy* located at https://drexel.edu/cnhp/academics/ departments/nursing-undergraduate/technical-standards-nursing/ for a detailed example.

Courts have consistently demonstrated great respect for faculty professional judgment and expertise with regard to establishment and implementation of technical standards in professional education programs when reviewing disability discrimination cases. However, it is also necessary for program administrators to ensure timely and ongoing review of these standards to verify conformance with current standards of practice, fair and equitable application of principles, and ongoing compliance with disability law. It is essential that academic administrators take a systematic, disciplined approach to these reviews and seek consultation from legal counsel as needed.

Centralized/Integrated Student Disability Services Functions

The ADA also requires institutions to designate a compliance officer to oversee compliance issues, student disability qualification processes, and accommodation determinations and to serve as a subject matter expert for consultation with faculty and program administrators. This function can be operationalized in a variety of ways. Small, stand-alone nursing programs may choose to designate a faculty member and committee supported by outside consultants and legal counsel. Nursing programs associated with most colleges and universities have the benefit of institutional legal counsel and a formal department dedicated to disability services.

Academic adjustments in nursing and other healthcare education programs may be similar to other academic programs in many instances, but often differ substantially in clinical education activities. As noted previously, the office of disability, legal counsel, and their respective staffs are content experts in disability law and generally accepted academic accommodations, but they often lack the professional insight and expertise to adapt generic academic adjustments to clinical course work and related clinical experiences. Close collaboration among nursing program administrators, faculty, university academic support services, and office of disability is needed to address the specific nuances and challenges of addressing discipline-specific nuances and clinical agency requirements for the development and implementation of accommodations in the clinical setting.

Consideration of accommodations in the clinical setting must take into consideration policies and procedures of the host clinical facility and availability of associated resources that may present associated challenges of feasibility or undue burden. Until now, it has not been uncommon for nursing programs to establish policy that academic accommodations do not transfer to the clinical arena because of patient safety concerns and the inability of the university to mandate policies and procedures of clinical affiliates. However, ongoing advances in technology and the availability of sophisticated assistive devices for students with disabilities continue to stretch the limits of possibility in developing creative, unobtrusive, and economically feasible support for students with disabilities in clinical settings. Consequently, it is imperative that the office of disability, program administrators, nursing faculty, and representatives from clinical affiliate sites work together in consideration of student requests for accommodation and evaluation of program standards and related organizational policies/procedures.

Support From Key Stakeholders

Although the law and institution-specific policies serve as the foundation for the determination of applicable accommodations, inherent complexities in nursing education necessitate active involvement and support from key stakeholders.

Nursing Faculty

Nurse educators have the responsibility of ensuring that disabled students have equal access to the nursing profession. The most significant factors affecting disabled student access and academic success in nursing education programs are the perceptions and attitudes of faculty (Ashcroft et al., 2008; Dupler, Allen, Maheady, Fleming, & Allen, 2012; Sowers & Smith, 2004). Unfortunately, for nursing students with disabilities, there is often a disproportionate preoccupation with safety concerns compared to the general nursing student population. However, there is no documented evidence to support those concerns. There have also been no reported instances of students or nurses with qualified disabilities causing harm or substandard care.

Another misconception often voiced by faculty is concern that accommodating students with disabilities will have a negative impact on program outcome standards. These concerns reveal a misunderstanding of intent and requirements of the law, which is to an otherwise qualified individual fair opportunity to achieve outcome standards. Accommodations are not intended to create unfair advantage or require significant adjustments that would substantially alter the nature of the activity.

A study by Sowers and Smith (2004) focusing on faculty perceptions about nursing students with disabilities revealed that nursing faculty viewed students with learning disabilities less favorably than those with physical disabilities. The researchers were also surprised to find that given the emphasis on technical standards in nursing education, respondents were less negative than expected regarding the ability of wheelchair-bound individuals to complete a nursing program and practice as nurses. They suggest that possible contributing factors to these findings include prior experience with wheelchair-bound professional colleagues; minimal faculty effort associated with accommodations associated with physical infirmities that can be implemented with minimum disruption to faculty routines; a lack of understanding of the need for accommodations associated with hidden disabilities; and the need to exert substantial effort in modifying teaching practices to meet the needs of students with learning disabilities (Sowers & Smith, 2004). There is general agreement regarding a significant need for faculty orientation and ongoing education related to potential for students with disabilities to complete an academic nursing program; strategies to promote student success; implementation of needed accommodations; and associated legal mandates (Ashcroft et al., 2008; Konur, 2002; Sowers & Smith, 2004).

Clinical Affiliates

Agencies contracted as clinical sites for nursing student experiences with direct patient care have the dual responsibility of fulfilling these contractual obligations to nursing education programs and the provision of quality healthcare. These entities are faced with several regulatory requirements (e.g., accreditation standards, licensure requirements, health information privacy laws, patient-quality benchmarks) and liability concerns. Although they may be philosophically supportive of nursing education, their primary focus is the "business" of healthcare. Nevertheless, they are also subject to compliance with disability statutes.

Understandably, perceived potential liability issues and patient perceptions become important considerations in granting access to a disabled student (who is essentially a guest in the host facility). It is incumbent on nursing faculty and academic administrators to provide education and needed supports to alleviate affiliate clinical agency concerns. It may also be beneficial for the program administrator to take advantage of established relationships with key individuals in clinical agencies when soliciting cooperation and support for student accommodations when appropriate in the clinical setting such as introducing the use of adaptive devices and suggesting possible modifications to policies/procedures that will enhance student learning and the provision of safe, effective nursing care. Once the feasibility of such accommodations is established, it is likely that other clinical affiliates will be more receptive to requests for needed clinical accommodations in their respective organizations.

Students

For those who have had little exposure to individuals with disabilities, it may be difficult to understand the associated challenges faced by peers with physical or learning disabilities. Students may sense faculty concern about the ability of disabled students to meet clinical and academic standards. Nondisabled students may have apprehensions that sharing the learning environment with individuals who need extra support may negatively affect their own personal learning objectives and outcomes. Open dialogue, experiential learning, and faculty support will provide opportunity for students to reframe paradigms, work collaboratively with individuals with disabilities (in both personal and professional roles), and provide nursing care from a more holistic framework that will enhance the learning experience for all.

Embrace the Use of Technology and Evolving Pedagogy

Rapid advances in technology and assistive devices and evolving pedagogy continue to open new worlds of possibilities for assimilation and achievement for individuals with disabilities thought impossible not long ago (Dorman, 1998; Glasgow, Dunphy, & Mainous, 2010; Leigh, 2008). In addition to increased sophistication of adaptive and assistive devices, these technological supports are also becoming more affordable and accessible to the general public.

Corresponding advances in special education and the move from teacher-dominated to learner-focused pedagogies, which enable students with diverse learning needs to process information more efficiently and effectively, enhance student acquisition of knowledge and skills. Simulated patient care experiences and virtual learning environments enable nursing students to practice clinical skills, develop clinical judgment, and demonstrate mastery of essential professional competencies (Azzopardi et al., 2013; Glasgow et al., 2010; Leigh, 2008). Although the advances in technology have benefited the entire nursing student population, these scientific and technological breakthroughs have had a profound effect on minimizing or eliminating barriers for nursing students with physical and learning disabilities in both the classroom and clinical arena (Ashcraft et al., 2008; Broadbent, Dorow, & Fisch, 2006; Busby, Gammel, & Jeffcoat, 2002; Coombs, 2002; Evans, 2005; Preece et al., 2007; Sowers & Smith, 2004; Tee et al., 2010; Tincani, 2004). Consultation with colleagues in other nursing programs and other health-related disciplines will provide insight into innovative teaching strategies, evaluative measures, physical adaptation devices, learning aids, and technological supports that would enable disabled nursing students to meet program outcome standards both in the classroom and at the point of care.

Create a Supportive Environment

It is generally accepted that a supportive educational environment is conducive to learning and achieving program outcomes for all students. Information for the range of academic and clinical support services available, including the office of disability services, should be made available to students in advance of matriculation into the nursing program, at general orientation sessions, and on an ongoing basis. Because students with disabilities may be hesitant to disclose limitations for fear of negative consequences, it is essential that an attitude of acceptance and support permeate all aspects of the educational experience. There are many and varied strategies and accommodations that provide students with learning and other disabilities an equal opportunity to be successful in didactic and clinical settings. An open, supportive environment will encourage students with disabilities to feel more comfortable in openly discussing their learning needs and accessing available supports. Some examples of how this can be accomplished include the following:

1. Inclusion of an introductory course (or equivalent) focusing on the transition to college which includes information related to time management, organizational skills, study strategies, stress management and personalized introductions of staff from student support services available through the university
2. Inclusion of the office of disability services in course syllabi
3. Implementation of a non-faculty adviser role that serves as a student advocate and liaison for addressing student issues and concerns in a nonjudgmental manner
4. Ongoing monitoring of student progress in course work with established early warning mechanisms to facilitate recognition and activation of needed support systems
5. Development of nursing-specific academic and clinical support functions that complement course content (practice labs, content review, remediation activities, test-taking skills, etc.) that accommodate the need for additional time and practice associated with mastery of course content and proficiency in clinical skills
6. Education of administrators, faculty, and staff regarding disability law, and information regarding accommodation and access
7. Provision of sensitivity training workshops and understanding of disability as a cultural competency throughout all aspects of the nursing curriculum
8. Encouragement of student input and maintenance of ongoing dialogue regarding needed educational supports
9. Provision of timely responses and comprehensive ongoing follow-ups for inquiries and issues associated with disability services
10. Development of case-by-case evaluation, complaint, and appeal procedures for student disability issues
11. Establishment of ongoing review, update, and widespread dissemination of practices and policies associated with student disability services

Evolving Trends

As a result of greater acceptance of individuals with disabilities in society, many nursing educators are questioning the long-standing emphasis on physical attributes associated with technical standards for admission and progression in nursing programs. Marks (2007), Aaberg (2012), Neal-Boylan and Smith (2015), Neal-Boylan and Miller (2016), and Matt, Maheady, and Fleming (2015), assert that nursing students with disabilities will foster a new set of knowledge, skills, and abilities in the nursing profession and challenges that technical standards and essential standards in nursing curricula need to be redefined accordingly. They also suggest that students with disabilities have the potential to improve nursing care and advance culturally relevant care as a result of their unique understanding of disability issues. There is also a growing number of nursing faculty and professionals who argue that relying exclusively on a list of physical attributes and technical skills that tend to dominate the nursing profession undermines the profession's desire to move beyond the perception of nurses as skilled laborers (Sowers & Smith, 2004). The National Council of State Boards of Nursing (2018) reports that advances in technology, the rapidly evolving healthcare system, and new care delivery models have and will continue to expand professional nursing roles and practice settings resulting in a shift from hospital-based employment to community-based and ambulatory settings necessitating new approaches in nursing education. Carroll (2004) suggests that the technical standards model in nursing should be replaced by a creative access model that is outcomes based and acknowledges that more than one process can be used to achieve desired outcomes. This model focuses on the availability of accommodations, not the type and severity of the associated disability. Arndt (2004) proposes that because delegation, direction, and supervision of certain tasks are essential components of professional nursing practice, it should also be considered as a possible accommodation for nursing students with physical disabilities in the clinical setting. She further asserts that "every nurse needs to be caring, deliver that care with integrity, effectively interact with others and able to think critically. Not every nurse needs to be able to lift 25 lbs., climb stairs, or be able to start an intravenous solution" (Arndt, 2004, p. 205). (Had that philosophical underpinning existed in Case 1, it is likely that the outcome of Case 1 would differ substantially.)

Evans (2005) presents a compelling example of a paraplegic student who successfully completed a baccalaureate nursing program and successfully transitioned to practice as an RN. She outlines curricular and procedural adaptations that permitted the student to meet both academic and clinical program standards and enabled faculty to think in new ways about clinical competencies and innovative teaching strategies. Faculty deemed that when the student learned the concepts underlying a psychomotor skill and demonstrated her knowledge through verbalization, simulation using a manikin, and theoretical testing, she had fulfilled her academic obligations similar to nondisabled students who learn the same concepts but never had the opportunity to practice on a live patient in the clinical setting (Evans, 2005).

Matt (2008) studied the experience of nurses with disabilities working in a hospital setting. Findings revealed that although navigation issues were identified as problematic without accommodations, self-advocacy, personal innovation, and support from administrators/colleagues provided the foundational elements of success in an acute care setting.

Azzopardi et al. (2013) report results of a critical analysis of the effectiveness of using low-, medium-, and high-fidelity simulation activities to support undergraduate nursing students with disabilities. Findings suggest that simulation can be a useful tool in the determination of reasonable accommodations that meet legislative requirements, embrace the advancement of learning technologies in nursing education, and assist in the identification of supports tailored to individual student needs. They further assert that simulation offers nursing students with disability the opportunity for deeper learning and enhancement of preparation for clinical practice (Azzopardi et. al., 2013).

The works of Aaberg (2012), Neal-Boylan and Smith (2016), Neal-Boylan and Miller (2017), Matt et al. (2015), and Allen and Marks (2017) represent an increasing consensus among nurse educators calling for revision of historic technical requirements grounded in outmoded practice settings and nursing roles. The requirements should reflect the principles of contemporary nursing practice and the evolving role of professional nurses in today's rapidly changing healthcare environment.

In revisiting these important concepts, nursing educators are challenged to move away from a task-oriented perspective and the mind-set that disabled students need special treatment, and focus instead on the range of strategies and technologies that will enable these students to exercise their full range of abilities in meeting essential functions inherent in professional nursing practice. The dialogue and debate will undoubtedly continue; however, ongoing communication and collaboration will serve as a foundation for curricular innovation now and in the future.

SUMMARY

Federal laws require universities to make reasonable and necessary modifications to rules, policies, and practices to prevent discrimination against students on the basis of disability. As a result of these legislative mandates, advances in technology, educational supports at all levels of schooling, and the work of advocacy groups for students with disabilities, more and more students with disabilities are seeking postsecondary degrees. Nursing, as a profession, maintains a strong advocacy role for individuals with special needs; however, the education of nursing students with disabilities poses unique challenges. Clinically focused professional education programs such as nursing are faced with the dichotomous challenge of supporting student learning within the context of public safety, mandated program outcome standards, and licensure requirements. Despite the significant body of literature on postsecondary students with disabilities, there is a paucity of literature related to students with disabilities in nursing and the health professions compared with other disciplines (Sharby & Roush,

2009). There is also no definitive agreement regarding the nature and extent of accommodations and related academic supports in meeting the needs of nursing students with disabilities with regard to program outcome standards at this time. Courts are, understandably, particularly interested in cases involving the health professions because of the direct effect on the health and safety of patients.

In your role as an academic nursing administrator to support faculty and students in the teaching and learning process, you also have a legal and moral responsibility to protect your school from claims of discrimination on the basis of disability. However, the complex and varied roles of the nurse educator and academic administrator also necessitate that you transcend legal mandates and embrace the associated ethical and professional responsibilities to students, faculty, clinical affiliates, and the public for the education of nursing professionals who provide high-quality, culturally sensitive nursing care. This chapter offered analyses of several scenarios regarding undergraduate nursing students who present requests for academic accommodations (perceived or officially verified) to faculty and academic program administrators and pointed out significant considerations in the management of these issues. Additionally, it pointed out the crossover and subsequent complications that may occur between academic considerations and actual disability accommodations (Meloy & Gambescia, 2014). In both types, faculty naturally will be supportive but need to be aware when they are invoking a consideration versus when they are exercising formal and legal accommodations.

Bohne (2004) suggests consideration of two essential questions that provide the foundation for personal reflection and academic leadership in policy development, curricular evolution, and programmatic accommodations/supports for nursing students with disabilities: (a) "If people with disabilities can use their skills to execute the nursing process to achieve desired nursing outcomes in a nursing role, do these individuals have a right to pursue a career in nursing?" *and* (b) "... beyond the letter of the law, does the nursing profession have a professional responsibility to support them to doing so?" (p. 202)

As an academic administrator of a nursing program, you are positioned in a key leadership role to challenge traditional paradigms and proactively assist faculty in exploring curricular innovation and academic/clinical supports, which will support disabled nursing students in achieving program outcome standards as they transition to professional nursing roles. An emphasis on faculty education that addresses continually evolving disability related laws, and the unique challenges and opportunities for creating academic supports while supporting academic rigor is essential. May (2014) asserts that these goals are not mutually exclusive and emphasizes transforming mind-sets and traditional approaches to nursing education requires commitment and recognition of the value and contributions of students with disabilities. The voice of nursing students with disabilities and their counterparts in professional nursing practice is also a critical component in the success of such initiatives.

The disposition of cases in this chapter is based on the technical standards model prevalent in nursing education today. As a result of ongoing advances in technology, changing societal perceptions, new conceptual models of nursing education, and the evolution of increasingly diverse professional opportunities, similar cases may have very different outcomes in the future. The principles and practices presented in this chapter also provide a framework for compliance with legal mandates, evaluating and implementing academic accommodations, and understanding the needs of students with physical and learning disabilities in contemporary nursing education programs.

Qualified individuals with physical and learning disabilities have the potential to improve nursing care and advance culturally relevant care with their unique understanding of related obstacles and challenges. Consequently, it is also critical that academic administrators in nursing education build upon the status quo and assume a proactive role in reexamining existing admission criteria; redefining technical standards and essential competencies; exploring creative teaching and evaluation strategies; and participating in the ongoing evolution of best practices and professional standards for individuals with disabilities in nursing education and practice, now and in the future.

ETHICAL CONSIDERATIONS

There are several ethical considerations when addressing students with disabilities in nursing education programs. Underlying most of these is a fundamental conflict between justice and beneficence. On the one hand, we have a duty to provide equal educational access to students with disabilities. On the other hand, we have a duty to produce competent professionals. It may seem at times that meeting one of these obligations makes it difficult or impossible to meet the other. One concern is the direct effect of the nursing student's disability on the health and safety of patients. Essentially, does the disability and its required accommodation cause any harm to patient care? Do the potential harms outweigh our duty to provide education for such students? One also needs to consider whether the patient has perceived confidence and competence in the caregiver. One does need to ask, should the patient, who is already sick and vulnerable, experience an increase in stress as a result of a nurse with a disability? The other concern is the amount of fiscal or human resources required to assist an individual student in a nursing program of study versus offering the financial or human resources to many students. For example, is it ethical to spend $800,000 in accommodation costs from a limited pool of resources for one student to be a nurse or should the student pursue another health career that does not require extensive accommodations? Can we determine, in economic terms, how far our duty to provide equal access to education extends? From a perspective of virtue, we also must consider the possible bias, including unconscious bias, of faculty and administration toward students with disabilities. Are our evaluations of these cases affected by a lack of understanding and empathy for persons with disabilities? How do we go about improving ourselves and other faculty to remove these possible vices from our reactions and thinking? The last consideration is one of fairness—does the accommodation provide an unfair advantage to the student with a disability or fundamentally alter the program of study. There are also different considerations with respect to accommodations in different nursing programs—ideally, there should be technical standards for each degree. The technical standards are different for an undergraduate clinical degree versus a nonclinical MSN or PhD for example. A student may very well be blind and enrolled as a PhD student but would not meet with technical standards for a pre-license BSN program. Another view would be, are we ethically bound to admit students who may not be able to perform the regular duties of a professional nurse? There are many ethical considerations to reflect upon when contemplating a student with a disability's impact on fiscal and human resources, patient safety, and patient emotional well-being. These ethical considerations need to be viewed in the context of the current legislation on students with disabilities in higher education.

 CRITICAL ELEMENTS TO CONSIDER

- Examine admission and progression policies for conformance with disability laws; consult legal counsel as needed.
- Maintain working knowledge of regulatory changes, case law, and professional standards, and licensure regulations affecting nursing education and practice.
- Provide early and ongoing student access to comprehensive disability services and individualized case analysis and disposition.
- Review technical standards and essential competencies with regard to trends in nursing education and professional practice.
- Expand conceptualization of disability beyond the focus of physical limitations and disorders.
- Provide education sessions for faculty related to evolving trends and advancements in addressing students with physical and learning disabilities.
- Develop collaborative relationships for determination and implementation of student academic and clinical accommodations; ensure that accommodations are not made without formal verification.
- Keep abreast of evolving advances in technology and educational practices that will assist disabled individuals in achieving programmatic outcomes.
- Participate in ongoing dialogue regarding evolving trends and best practices in addressing the needs of nursing students with disabilities within the context of quality in educational curricula and the provision of high-quality healthcare services to the public.

Helpful Resources

- U.S. Department of Education, "Students With Disabilities Preparing for Postsecondary Education: Know Your Rights and Responsibilities": http://www2.ed.gov/about/offices/list/ocr/transition.html
- "10 Tips for College Students With Disabilities": https://www.npr.org/templates/story/story.php?storyId=94728312
- College Funding for Students With Disabilities: https://www.washington.edu/doit/college-funding-students-disabilities
- Colleges With Programs for Learning Disabled Students: http://www.college-scholarships.com/learning_disabilities.htm

A BEST PRACTICE EXEMPLAR

As the convergence of academic standards, ADA accommodations, and accountability within higher education presents itself to nursing education professionals, it is critical to consider the time frame and method of communicating a student's academic accommodation (or AVL) to the appropriate parties. This has special considerations in the context of the nursing field, as multiple parties may be involved in making an academic accommodation happen once the request has been approved by a disability services office: student services professionals, academic advisers, clinical coordinators, testing coordinators, or technology professionals, to name a few. The notification process is often varied, depending on the size and operation of a given university or college.

A best practice is the utilization of a course management or online scheduling system, with the capability of creating a student success network for the student, based on their attributes and academic program. For example, a nursing student with a disability, that plays a varsity sport, and plans to study abroad, would have the following people in their success network: academic adviser, disability services staff, athletic adviser, faculty members, international programs staff, residence life staff, and their clinical coordinator. These networks can be custom built based on student interaction and program attributes. Once the network is established, the professionals in the network can communicate in a private and secure way to meet the needs of a student. A hallmark of these systems is the ability to instantly communicate and "flag" students to each other. A professor can report that a student did poorly on an exam, or an adviser can indicate that a student has not turned in an appropriate registration form, and flag that student. From this, a notification is automatically sent to the members of the network. The flag would remain until cleared by the appropriate parties.

Using this network, disability services professionals can upload a student's academic accommodation letter instantly, and send out a confidential system-wide message to the appropriate members of the student's success network. One of the most helpful features of this system is the ability to look at a student profile and immediately determine when a request was granted, when faculty members were notified, when flags were raised and cleared, and other important pieces of information. This is of immense use, as academic accommodations are never retroactive under the ADA. As the numbers of students with disabilities are increasing in academic programs all over the country, methods such as this offer an efficient way to serve students with disabilities in a timely and personalized manner.

AN EXAMPLE OF TECHNICAL STANDARDS

An individual must be able to independently, with or without reasonable accommodation, meet the following technical standards of general abilities and those specifically of (a) observation; (b) communication; (c) motor; (d) intellectual, conceptual, and quantitative abilities;

(e) essential behavioral and social attributes; and (f) ability to manage stressful situations. Individuals unable to meet these technical standards, with or without reasonable accommodation, will not be able to complete the program and are counseled to pursue alternate careers.

General Abilities: The student is expected to possess functional use of the senses of vision, touch, hearing, and smell so that data received by the senses may be integrated, analyzed, and synthesized in a consistent and accurate manner. A student must also possess the ability to perceive pain, pressure, temperature, position, vibration, and movement that are important to the student's ability to gather significant information needed to effectively evaluate patients. A student must be able to respond promptly to urgent situations that may occur during clinical training activities and must not hinder the ability of other members of the healthcare team to provide prompt treatment and care to patients.

Observational Ability: The student must have sufficient capacity to make accurate visual observations and interpret them in the context of laboratory studies, medication administration, and patient care activities. In addition, the student must be able to document these observations and maintain accurate records.

Communication Ability: The student must communicate effectively both verbally and nonverbally to elicit information and to translate that information to others. Each student must have the ability to read, write, comprehend, and speak the English language to facilitate communication with patients, their family members, and other professionals in healthcare settings. In addition, the student must be able to maintain accurate patient records, present information in a professional, logical manner and provide patient counseling and instruction to effectively care for patients and their families. The student must possess verbal and written communication skills that permit effective communication with instructors and students in both the classroom and clinical settings.

Motor Ability: The student must be able to perform gross and fine motor movements with sufficient coordination needed to perform complete physical examinations utilizing the techniques of inspection, palpation, percussion, auscultation, and other diagnostic maneuvers. A student must develop the psychomotor skills reasonably needed to perform or assist with procedures, treatments, administration of medication, management and operation of diagnostic and therapeutic medical equipment, and such maneuvers to assist with patient care activities such as lifting, wheel chair guidance, and mobility. The student must have sufficient levels of neuromuscular control and eye-to-hand coordination as well as possess the physical and mental stamina to meet the demands associated with extended periods of sitting, standing, moving, and physical exertion required for satisfactory and safe performance in the clinical and classroom settings including performing CPR, if necessary. The student must possess the ability of manual dexterity that would be required for certain activities, such as drawing up solutions in a syringe.

Intellectual, Conceptual, and Quantitative Abilities: The student must be able to develop and refine problem-solving skills that are crucial to practice as a nurse. Problem-solving involves the abilities to measure, calculate, reason, analyze, and synthesize objective and subjective data, and to make decisions, often in a time urgent environment, that reflect consistent and thoughtful deliberation and sound clinical judgment. Each student must demonstrate mastery of these skills and possess the ability to incorporate new information from peers, teachers, and the nursing and medical literature to formulate sound judgment in patient assessment, intervention, evaluation, teaching, and setting short- and long-term goals.

Behavioral and Social Attributes: Compassion, integrity, motivation, effective interpersonal skills, and concern for others are personal attributes required of those in the nursing programs. Personal comfort and acceptance of the role of a nurse functioning under supervision of a clinical instructor or preceptor is essential for a nursing student. The student must possess the skills required for full utilization of the student's intellectual abilities; the exercise of good judgment; the prompt completion of all responsibilities in the classroom and clinical settings; and the development of mature, sensitive, and effective relationships with patients and other members of the healthcare team. Each student must be able to exercise stable, sound judgment and to complete assessment and interventional activities. The ability to establish rapport and maintain sensitive, interpersonal relationships with individuals, families, and groups from a variety of social, emotional, cultural and intellectual backgrounds are critical for practice as a nurse. The student must be able to adapt to changing environments; display flexibility; accept and integrate constructive criticism given in the classroom and clinical settings; effectively interact in the clinical setting with other members of the healthcare team; and learn to function cooperatively and efficiently in the face of uncertainties inherent in clinical practice.

Ability to Manage Stressful Situations: The student must be able to adapt to and function effectively to stressful situations in both the classroom and clinical settings, including emergency situations. The student will encounter multiple stressors while in the nursing programs. These stressors may be (but are not limited to) personal, patient care/family, faculty/peer, and or program-related.

Source: Drexel University. (2019). *Technical standards for nursing.* Retrieved from https://drexel.edu/cnhp/academics/departments/nursing-undergraduate/technical-standards-nursing.

References

Aaberg, V. A. (2012). A path to greater inclusivity through understanding implicit attitudes toward disability. *The Journal of Nursing Education, 51*(9), 505–510. doi:10.3928/01484834-20120706-02

Anselmi, K., Glasgow, M. E., & Gambescia, S. F. (2014). Using a student conduct committee to foster professional accountability. *Journal of Professional Nursing, 30*(6), 481–485. doi:10.1016/j.profnurs.2014.04.002

Arndt, M. E. (2004). Educating nursing students with disabilities: One nurse educator's journey from questions to clarity. *Journal of Nursing Education, 43*(50), 204. doi:10.3928/01484834-20040501-09

Ashcroft, T., Cheronomas, W., Davis, P., Dean, R. A., Seguire, M., Shapiro, C. R., & Swiderski, L. M. (2008). Nursing students with disabilities: One faculty's journey. *International journal of Nursing Education Scholarship, 5*(1), 1–26. doi:10.2202/1548-923X.1424

Azzopardi, T., Johnson, A., Phillips, K., Dickson, C., Hengstberger-Simms, C., Goldsmith, M., & Allan, T. (2013). Simulation as a learning strategy: Supporting undergraduate nursing students with disabilities. *Journal of Clinical Nursing, 23*, 402–409. doi:10.1111/jocn.12049

Betz, C. L., Smith, K. A., & Bui, K. (2012). A survey of California nursing programs: Admission and accommodation policies for students with disabilities. *Journal of Nursing Education, 51*(12), 676–684. doi:10.3928/01484834-20121112-01

Bohne, J. J. (2004). Valuing differences among nursing students. *Journal of Nursing Education, 43*(5), 202–203. doi:10.3928/01484834-20040501-06

Broadbent, G., Dorow, L. G., & Fisch, L. A. (2006). College syllabi: Providing support for students with disabilities. *Educational Forum, 71*, 71–80. doi:10.1080/00131720608984569

Busby, R. R., Gammel, H. L., & Jeffcoat, N. K. (2002). Grades, graduation and orientation: A longitudinal study of how new student programs relate to grade point averages and graduation. *Journal of College Orientation and Transition, 10*(1), 45–50. doi:10.1080/00131720608984569

Carroll, S. M. (2004). Inclusion of people with physical disabilities in nursing education. *Journal of Nursing Education, 43*(5), 207–212. doi:10.3928/01484834-20040501-07

Coombs, N. (2002). FIPSE: Empowering students with disabilities. *Change, 34*(5), 42–48. doi:10.1080/00091383.2002.10544035

Coomes, M. D., & DeBard, R. (Eds.). (2004). *Serving the millennial generation* (New directions for student services, No. 106). San Francisco, CA: Jossey-Bass.

Cope, D. (2005). The courts, the ADA, and the academy. *Academic Questions, 19*(1), 37–47. doi:10.1080/00091383.2002.10544035

Doherty v. Southern College of Optometry, 862 F.2d 570, 575 (6th Cir. 1988), cert. denied, 493 U.S. 810, 110 S.Ct. 53, 107 L.Ed.2d 22 (1989).

Dorman, S. M. (1998). Assistive technology benefits for students with disabilities. *Journal of School Health, 68*(3), 120–123. doi:10.1080/00091383.2002.10544035

Drexel University. (2019). *Technical standards for nursing.* Retrieved from https://drexel.edu/cnhp/academics/departments/nursing-undergraduate/technical-standards-nursing

Dupler, A. E., Allen, C., Maheady, D., Fleming, S., & Allen, M. (2012). Leveling the playing field for nursing students with disabilities: Implications of amendments to the Americans with Disabilities Act. *Journal of Nursing Education, 51*(3), 140–144. doi:10.1080/00091383.2002.10544035

Evans, B. C. (2005). Nursing education for students with disabilities: Our students, our teachers. In *Annual review of nursing education* (Vol. 3, pp. 3–22). New York, NY: Springer Publishing Company.

Gambescia, S. F. & Donnelly, G. D. (2017). Managing and monitoring student "issues" in higher education. *Journal of Allied Health, 44*, 183–187.

Glasgow, M. E., Dunphy, L. M., & Mainous, R. O. (2010). Innovative nursing educational curriculum for the 21st century. *NLN Educational Perspectives, 31*(6), 355–357.

Hafferty, F. W., & Gibson, G. G. (2003). Learning disabilities, professionalism, and the practice of medical education. *Academic Medicine, 78*, 189–201. doi:10.1097/00001888-200302000-00014

Hash v. University of Kentucky, 138 S.W.3d 123 (Ky.Ct. App. 2004).

Helms, L., Jorgensen, J., & Anderson, M. A. (2006). Disability law and nursing education: An update. *Journal of Professional Nursing, 22*(30), 190–196. doi:10.1016/j.profnurs.2006.03.005

Konur, O. (2002). Access to nursing education by disabled students: Rights and duties of nursing programs. *Nurse Education Today, 22*, 364–374. doi:10.1054/nedt.2001.0723

Leigh, G. T. (2008). High-fidelity patient simulation and nursing student's self-efficacy: A review of the literature. *International Journal of Nursing Education Scholarship, 5*(1), 37. doi:10.2202/1548-923X.1613

Marks, B. (2007). Cultural competence revisited: Nursing students with disabilities. *Journal of Nursing Education, 46*(2), 70–74. doi:10.1054/nedt.2001.0723

Marks, B., & McCulloh, K. (2016). *Success for Students and Nurses With Disabilities: A Call to Action for Nurse Educators. Nurse Educator 41*(1), 9–12. doi:10.1097/NNE.0000000000000212

Matt, S. (2008). Nurses with disabilities: Self-reported experiences as hospital employees. *Qualitative Health Research, 18*, 1524–1535.

Matt, S. B., Maheady, D., & Fleming, S. E. (2015). Educating nursing students with disabilities: Replacing essential functions with technical standards for program entry criteria. *Journal of Post-secondary Education and Disability, 28*(4), 461–468.

May, K. A. (2014). Nursing faculty knowledge of the Americans with Disabilities Act. *Nurse Educator, 19*(5), 241–245. doi:10.1097/NNE.0000000000000058

Meloy, F., & Gambescia, S. F. (2014, May/June). Guidelines for response to student requests for academic considerations: Support vs. enabling. *Nurse Educator, 39*(3), 138–142. doi:10.1097/NNE.0000000000000037

National Center for Educational Statistics. (2019). *Students with disabilities.* Washington, DC: U.S. Department of Education. Retrieved from https://nces.ed.gov/fastfacts/display.asp?id=60

National Council of State Boards of Nursing. (2018). The nursing regulatory environment in 2018: Issues and challenges. *Journal of Nursing Regulation, 9*(1), 52–65. doi:10.1016/S2155-8256(18)30055-3

Neal-Boylan, L., & Miller, M. (2017). Treat me like everyone else: The experience of nurses who had disabilities while in school. *Nurse Educator, 42*(4), 176–180. doi:10.1097/NNE.0000000000000348

Neal-Boylan, L., & Smith, D. (2016). Nursing students with physical disabilities: Dispelling myths and correcting misconceptions. *Nurse Educator, 41*, 13–18. doi:10.1097/NNE.0000000000000191

Newsham, K. (2008). Disability law and health care education. *Journal of Allied Health, 37*(2), 110–115.

Powell v. National Board of Medical Examiners, 34 F.3d 79 (2nd Cir. 2004).

Preece, J., Roberts, N., Beecher, M., Rash, P., Shwalb, D., & Martinelli, E. (2007). Academic advisors and students with disabilities: A national survey of advisors' experiences and needs. *NACADA Journal, 27*(1), 57–72. doi:10.1097/NNE.0000000000000348

Rosenberger v. Rector and Visitors of the University of Virginia, 145 Fed. Appx. 7 (4th Cir. 2005).

Rosenbraugh, C. J. (2000). Learning disabilities and medical schools. *Medical Education, 34*, 994–1000. doi:10.1046/j.1365-2923.2000.00689.x

Rothstein, L. (2008). Millennials and disability law: Revisiting Southeastern Community College v. Davis. *Journal of College and University Law, 34*(1), 169–202. Retrieved from https://papers.ssrn.com/sol3/papers.cfm?abstract_id=1266333

Rothstein, L. F. (2000). The Americans with Disabilities Act: A ten-year retrospective: Higher education and the future of disability policy. *Alabama Law Review, 52,* 241.

Sharby, N., & Roush, S. (2009). Analytical decision-making model for addressing the needs of allied health students with disabilities. *Journal of Allied Health, 38*(1), 54–62.

Shin v. University of Maryland Medical System Corp., 369 F. App'x. 472 (4th Cir. 2010).

Southeastern Community College v. Davis, 442 U.S. 397 (1979).

Sowers, J., & Smith, M. R. (2004). Nursing faculty members' perceptions, knowledge, and concerns about students with disabilities. *Journal of Nursing Education, 43*(5), 213–218. doi:10.3928/01484834-20040501-03

Stacey, M., & Carroll, S. M. (2004). Inclusion of people with physical disabilities in nursing education. *Journal of Nursing Education, 43*(5), 207–212. doi:10.3928/01484834-20040501-07

Tee, T. R., Owens, K., Plowright, S., Ramnath, P., Rourke, S., James, C., & Bayliss, J. (2010). Being reasonable: Supporting disabled students in practice. *Nurse Education in Practice, 10,* 216–221. doi:10.1016/j.nepr.2009.11.006

Thomas, S. B. (2000). College students and disability law. *Journal of Special Education, 33*(4), 248–257. doi:10.1177/002246690003300408

Tincani, M. (2004). Improving outcomes for college students with disabilities. *College Teaching, 52*(4), 128–132. doi:10.3200/CTCH.52.4.128-133

U.S. Department of Labor, Office of Disability Employment Policy. (2014). *Health care professionals with disabilities career trends, best practices and call-to-action policy roundtable.* Washington, DC: Author.

U.S. Department of Labor, Office of Federal Contract Compliance Programs. (2014). *Regulations implementing section 503 of the Rehabilitation Act.* Retrieved from https://www.dol.gov/ofccp/regs/compliance/section503.htm

U.S. Equal Opportunity Commission. (2008). *The Americans with Disabilities Act Amendments Act of 2008.* Retrieved from https://www.eeoc.gov/laws/statutes/adaaa_info.cfm

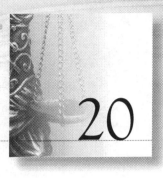

When Academic Nursing Policies Are Ignored, Not Enforced, or Overruled?

Case Study 20.1
Academic Policy: Interference or Overruled

Your role: You are Dr. Clark, a new dean for the School of Nursing.

As dean, you are responsible for the academic outcomes in the School of Nursing. You and the faculty implemented a standardized testing protocol in the curriculum in response to low NCLEX-RN® scores. Faculty worked with a standardized testing company to develop custom final exams in all major clinical courses in addition to an exit exam. Ten percent (16 students) of the seniors failed the exit exam after two attempts and are thus failing the capstone course. You receive a call from the university president because one of the students who failed is the daughter of his close friend. The president, an English professor, begins to interrogate you about the standardized tests and failure rate. He tells you he does not support standardized tests.

Case Study 20.2
Academic Policy: Not Enforced

Your role: You are Dr. Boyle, a nursing faculty member in the second degree BSN program. Jane O'Rourke, a second degree student, fails the Fundamentals of Nursing clinical rotation for poor skills acquisition. Jane cannot perform basic skills in a safe manner. You wonder how she passed the lab portion of the course since there is a skills competency testing for every basic skill. Students need to pass the core basic skills in order to begin clinical rotations. In your opinion, Jane clearly did not pass the skills testing based on her performance.

Case Study 20.3
Academic Policy: Ignored

Your role: You are Dr. Simon, Chair of the BSN program in a small liberal arts college. The program has experienced a major dip in NCLEX-RN scores. A faculty task force developed the "no rounding policy" that was voted on unanimously by the BSN faculty. You have also received a fair amount of appeals recently where students are claiming that some faculty are rounding test scores to help students pass despite the no rounding policy while others are not, which is problematic from a fairness perspective. Your university places a lot of weight on student evaluations and you suspect that faculty do not want to be the bad guy or girl and are also equally concerned about the student evaluations of their teaching for promotion purposes.

Questions
- When academic policies are ignored, not enforced, or overruled, what are the underlying reasons?
- What are the legal and ethical implications when academic policies are not followed?

HOW TO DEVELOP AND ENFORCE ACADEMIC POLICIES: REVIEW OF THE LITERATURE

Academic policies reflect the values of the faculty and institution. Policies and procedures are an essential part of any university or academic program. Together, policies and procedures provide a road map for day-to-day operations or guidelines to be followed in certain circumstances. They ensure compliance with laws and regulations, give guidance for decision-making, and streamline internal processes. Consistency in practices is also important for students and faculty as individuals. They know the expectations and what they can expect from various individuals (such as faculty, chairs, or deans). When faculty follow policies and procedures, there is also a decrease in the risk of liability. Students become more upset and possibly litigious when they suspect that they are not being treated fairly. Faculty also object to not being treated in an equitable manner (Gasior, 2019).

Keep in mind that the failure to follow promulgated policies and procedures can also subject the institution to breach of contract claims from aggrieved students. Although courts characterize the student–university relationship as contractual in nature, since contract law is often an area of state law interpretation, you will find that state courts have applied different legal analysis and theories when considering student breach of contract claims (Kaplin, Lee, Hutchens, & Rooksby, 2019). As a result, the student–university contract theory continues to evolve in judicial opinions. Consultation with institutional counsel is advisable to ensure you are following the most current law in your jurisdiction.

In general, steps should be followed when developing or revising an academic policy so that it is fair, transparent, and clear. The general question needs to be asked, "What is the problem we are trying to solve?" In other words, will a policy help address the issue at hand and assist faculty or students with guidance or compliance in a certain situation?

In addition, including disclaimers or reservation of rights provisions in program handbooks, policies, and syllabi will help protect from breach of contract claims. A sample provision might read as follows:

> The School of Nursing reserves the right to make changes in this handbook at any time without prior notice. The School provides the information herein solely for the convenience of the reader and, to the extent permissible by law, expressly disclaims any liability which may otherwise be incurred.

The Maine Supreme Court ruled in *Millen v. Colby College*, 874 A.2d 397 (Me. 2005) that the preceding statement was sufficient under Maine law to find that a student handbook was not legally binding on the college and rejected the plaintiff's breach of contract claim.

Steps in Policy Development or Revision

- Determine the need for a policy.
  - ◈ Form a working group with subject matter experts to determine the need for the policy or revision.
  - ◈ Designate a policy owner.
- Develop and draft policy.
  - ◈ Policies should be developed by knowledgeable stakeholders.
  - ◈ Review near final draft for brevity, clarity, consistency, and readability.
  - ◈ Listen to critics.
  - ◈ Think about procedural aspects.
    - ◯ Policy and procedures should be separated into two distinct documents.
    - ◯ Procedures/processes should not be overly burdensome.
- Dissemination and change management.
  - ◈ Distribute near final draft to stakeholders for review and feedback with a deadline the policy will be submitted for approval.
  - ◈ Failure to follow academic policies must have consequences for the students and faculty.
- Maintain and monitor.
  - ◈ Make policies accessible (online and searchable by term).
  - ◈ Integrate policy information into the faculty and student orientation.
  - ◈ Encourage accountability.
  - ◈ Regularly review policies and procedures on an annual or biannual basis.
  - ◈ Consider reasons why stakeholders may not follow policy and attempt to educate. (University of California Santa Cruz, 2019)

DISCUSSION OF CASE STUDIES

Case Study 20.1—Academic Policy: Interference or Overruled

"Many nursing schools have adopted the practice of using standardized exit examination testing to provide an indication of student preparedness for NCLEX-RN. Policymaking is a cyclical, evolving process based on program needs. Program guidelines are tailored to the individual philosophy of the institution" (Stonecypher, Young, Langford, Symes, & Wilson, 2015, p. 189). Success on the NCLEX-RN is important to students who are ready to engage in the professional nursing role, and nursing programs need to demonstrate adequate student educational preparation as evidenced by the percentage of students passing the first time when taking the licensure examination (Stonecypher et al., 2015). There are often misunderstandings related to the integration of standardized testing in nursing programs. The use of a single exit exam in the absence of a comprehensive approach to standardized testing is not recommended. Also, when schools of nursing do not provide remediation or create a clear communication plan to help students, the students or their parents often contact the State Board of Nursing looking for answers or some type of recourse (Spector & Alexander, 2006).

> Boards of nursing have made several recommendations to prevent this type of scenario from occurring. A comprehensive assessment program throughout the curriculum, with adequate remediation resources, is the foundation for preparing students to pass the NCLEX-RN. The objective of using standardized assessment examinations is to identify students who have gaps in their nursing knowledge so remediation can occur sooner, rather than later. Care must be taken to ensure that the exit examination selected is psychometrically sound. Standardized examinations that are integrated throughout the program provide valuable feedback for students, as well as program administrators and faculty. Students become accustomed to taking standardized examinations, their strengths and learning needs can be assessed, and intervention can be provided throughout the program. (Spector & Alexander, 2006, p. 291)

It is not surprising that the university president lacks a deep understanding about the comprehensive approach that Dean Clark and her faculty have implemented in response to low NCLEX-RN scores. Dean Clark communicated this major change and rationale to Provost Young but he apparently did not communicate this change to President Jordan. At this juncture, Dean Clark should communicate the president's dissatisfaction with her supervisor, Provost Young, and provide research on standardized testing in nursing, the school's comprehensive approach to standardized testing, and the grades and attendance records of the 16 students to both the provost and president, in addition to the school's NCLEX-RN first-time pass rates for several years and the implications of NCLEX-RN failure to the student and school. Dean Clark should also communicate that "Standardized examinations can also provide faculty with information not only about how their students are doing, but also about how the students compare to other students in nursing programs across the country" (Spector & Alexander, 2006, p. 291).

 BEST PRACTICE EXEMPLAR

Many of the students who have difficulty passing a school's exit examination also had trouble in their clinical experiences and coursework. Students and parents may still contact the university President or Provost and their respective state boards of nursing regarding a standardized exit exam even if a solid comprehensive standardized exam approach has been established by the school. Deans, chairs, or directors should be prepared to respond to these challenges.

In summary, cumulative testing is well supported in the educational research literature as a valuable learning tool (Karpicke, 2012; Soderstrom & Bjork, 2014; Weimer, 2014). Sometimes, even when academic nursing administrators and faculty have the best intentions and have thoughtfully developed an evidence-based academic nursing policy, they may experience interference from senior administration or pushback from students and parents. In these cases, the Dean and faculty should remain calm and provide the necessary evidence on the subject. The President, in theory, should not interfere with academic nursing policies that are evidence-based or advocate on behalf of his friend's child.

Students and parents should be reminded of the implications for failing NCLEX-RN. For students who repeat the NCLEX-RN because of first-time or subsequent failures, their pass rates drop significantly (National Council of State Boards of Nursing, 2017). For the student, a first-time NCLEX-RN failure is associated with consequences. There is the loss of time the student is required to prepare for retaking the test. There is potential loss of employment if already employed and continued employment is based on passing the exam. In relation to this failure, there is loss of compensation for not being able to obtain an RN position or loss of income due to losing one's position for failing the NCLEX-RN. There are also potential psychosocial consequences, such as being embarrassed among peers and losing professional status (Glasgow, Dreher, & Schreiber, 2019).

Case Study 20.2—Academic Policy: Not Enforced

We can have the best strategies to improve academic and clinical education quality, but if we do not have the culture to support them, they will fail. Traditionally, healthcare's culture has held individuals accountable for all errors or mistakes that happen to patients under their care—no matter the reason. A just culture recognizes that individual practitioners should not be held accountable for system failings over which they have no control. A just culture also recognizes many errors represent predictable interactions between human operators and the systems in which they work (Dekker, 2008). A just culture also has zero tolerance for reckless behavior. Reckless behavior is behavioral choice to consciously disregard a substantial and unjustifiable risk.

Reckless Behaviors in Nursing Education
- Lack of preparation
- Failing to seek remediation when advised to do so

- Disregard clinical policies or safe practice
- Failing to raise or report a safety concern
- Speak or act disrespectfully toward another person
- Engage in or tolerate abusive, "bullying" behaviors
- Look up or discuss private information about patients outside of specified patient assignment/responsibilities
- Attend clinical, while impaired by any substance or condition that compromises one's ability to function safely
- Reporting false-positive information to faculty to gain favor (Barnsteiner & Disch, 2012, 2017)

In Case Study 20.2, if Dr. Boyle is correct that the student, Jane, was passed and deemed satisfactory on core basic skills competency even though she was not competent, it is reckless behavior on behalf of the lab faculty member. Dr. Boyle can report her concerns to her chair *without assigning any blame to the lab faculty*. At this point, Dr. Boyle does not have any objective evidence that Jane was passed without demonstrating competence or that the lab faculty did not test Jane. Since Dr. Boyle does not supervise the lab faculty, she should allow her chair, Dr. Thompson, to investigate the situation. Dr. Thompson should impose a sanction/penalty if it is found that lab faculty did not engage in basic core skills competency testing. To improve the quality and safety of patient care, we must pay attention to what happens in academic settings. Like clinicians, nursing faculty and students must be actively involved in learning about safety science (Barnsteiner & Disch, 2017).

BEST PRACTICE EXEMPLAR

Nursing faculty and academic administrators should discern why academic policies are not enforced. Education on "Just Culture" should occur with students, faculty, and staff.

Case Study 20.3:—Academic Policy: Ignored

In Case Study 20.3, Dr. Simon had conducted an internal review and determined that faculty awarded points to students who were close to passing. After recognizing this issue, she formed a Nursing Grading Task Force for faculty to review rounding policies. She did so because she recognized that it was unfair or "unjust" to give failing students additional points while other students with higher grades did not receive this benefit. She also recognized that students who minimally passed the course had academic difficulty in future classes because they had not synthesized the content. The Nursing Grading Task Force developed the policy below:

> Students must achieve an average grade of ≥77% (a grade of C) on all exams to pass the course.
> Final grade calculation: Grades will be calculated for each exam and made visible to students. At the end of the semester, exam grades will be averaged, and that score will not be rounded. Per mathematical rules, for example: a score of 76.499 will be recorded as 76, and a score of 76.99 will be recorded as 77.

Dr. Simon was perplexed that faculty enthusiastically endorsed the policy in the meeting but were not following it in practice. She was aware of the heavy influence of student evaluations of faculty teaching.

FINDINGS AND DISPOSITION

Case Study 20.1 Academic Policy: Interference or Overruled

Dr. Clark effectively convinced the President of the value of standardized testing in nursing education. She had demonstrated a significant increase in NCLEX-RN scores for the BSN program after implementing a comprehensive approach to standardized testing with associated remediation. President Jordan admitted that he was having a bad day and responded to his close friend's emotional outburst concerning his daughter's test score.

Case Study 20.2—Academic Policy: Not Enforced

Dr. Boyle's supervisor, Dr. Thompson, investigated the testing issue concerning the student, Jane O'Rourke. Professor Lewis, the lab faculty member responsible for testing Jane on core basic skills, admitted that she felt sorry for Jane and passed her even though against her better judgment she should have not done so. Professor Lewis explained that Jane was a single parent who had financial troubles and significant school loans, and that she thought she was helping her. Professor Lewis recognized that in hindsight, she was wrong. Dr. Thompson offered several workshops on "Just Culture" and formed a Task Force for faculty to integrate just culture into the curriculum. Professor Lewis received a written warning and was mandated to attend a conference on Just Culture. She was reminded of the importance of following policies.

Case Study 20.3—Academic Policy: Ignored

Dr. Simon was distressed that faculty ignored the rounding policy. It was creating a lot of problems for her and was not fair and equitable to all students if the policy was not followed and some students were awarded additional points while others were not. Dr. Simon convened a faculty meeting to discuss the issue. After listening to faculty, it was clear that the policy was overly restrictive and faculty could not defend it. Dr. Simon convened another Nursing Grading Task Force to review the policy and make recommendations. The task force put forth a new policy:

> Students must achieve an average grade of ≥77% on all exams to pass the course. Final grade calculation: Grades will be calculated for each exam and made visible to students. At the end of the semester, exam grades will be averaged, and that score will be rounded, if necessary, as described below. Rounding will not be applied to individual exams in a course. Per mathematical rules, rounding to the nearest whole number is only affected by the digit immediately to the right of the decimal point. For example: a score of 76.499 will be recorded as 76, and a score of 76.50 will be recorded as 77.

Faculty unanimously approved this new policy. Dr. Simon organized a faculty development workshop related to legal and ethical academic decision-making.

RELEVANT LEGAL CASES

Davis v. University of North Carolina at Greensboro, and Raleigh School of Nurse Anesthesia, US District Court for the Middle District of North Carolina, 1:2019cv00661 [Filed July 2, 2019]

In state and federal lawsuits filed in July 2019, Autumn Davis, nurse anesthesia student, alleges that she was sexually harassed by a supervisor while performing clinical work as part of University of North Carolina Greensboro program. When she complained, she says, administrators subjected her to a hostile, retaliatory environment that "victimized and damaged her," including mocking her physical disability. Ultimately, the lawsuits allege, she was drummed out of the program a month before graduation—and to facilitate her removal, the complaints suggest, administrators may have falsified or destroyed medical records. Davis's federal lawsuit, filed on July 2, 2019 in the U.S. Middle District of North Carolina, names as defendants UNCG, the UNC Board of Governors, and the Raleigh School of Nurse Anesthesia, a nonprofit associated with UNCG. It alleges that the nursing program has a "history of turning a blind eye towards sexual harassment and engaging in unlawful retaliation" toward female students who complain.

The adherence to sexual harassment policies and the university's response (UNC Greensboro and Raleigh School of Nursing Anesthesia) is at the center of this lawsuit.

Ottgen v. Clover Park Technical College, 928 P2d. 1119 (Wash.Ct.App., 1996)

In this case, a Washington state appellate court held that oral statements made by an instructor in a real estate appraisal program were not contractually binding on the college. The faculty member had verbally promised several students that they would get on-the-job appraisal experience along with their class lectures. When the appraisal experiences did not occur, several students sued the college for breach of contract and under the state's consumer fraud statute. Materials published by the college about the program discussed the classroom-based instruction only and did not mention the on-the-job appraisal component promised by the faculty member. The court ruled the only contract between the institution and students based on the written materials published about the program was for classroom-based instruction and the failure to provide the appraisal experience was not a breach of contract or in violation of consumer fraud statutes.

SUMMARY

The underlying reasons why academic policies are ignored, not enforced, or overruled are often not clearly understood. In many cases, faculty do not follow policies due to self-interest (influence on their teaching evaluations, time and energy involved in failing a student, or sympathy for student rather than a focus on safe patient care). Administrators or senior executives sometimes do not appreciate academic nursing policies because of lack of knowledge and/or competing demands with donors or associates (valuing associates' or donors' wishes over nursing faculty policies) or are unsupportive because they do not want additional conflict or work. In the end, nonadherence to sound and just academic policies is an ethical and legal matter. Following an evidence-based continuous quality improvement model and just culture principles can potentially positively impact student outcomes and graduate new nurses who are prepared for today's complex healthcare environment (Barnsteiner & Disch, 2017; Serembus, 2016). Failure to follow academic nursing policy that has the goal of safe patient care has significant adverse implications.

ETHICAL CONSIDERATIONS

Policies should be developed and followed to protect students, patients, and faculty. Whether a policy focuses on student conduct, incivility, or clinical evaluation, accountability and consequences for policy violations must be an integral part of nursing education throughout the world to ensure quality and safety and mitigate the adverse effects of nursing errors. The American Nurses Association (ANA) Code and ANA Standards also indicate patients (by increasing patient safety) are the beneficiary of ethical conduct among and between nurses and nursing students. The culture of civility, professional responsibility, patient safety, and ethics must be introduced in the nursing school and reinforced for both students and faculty (Anselmi, Glasgow, & Gambescia, 2014). Too many times, competing interests adversely impact academic policy enforcement and/or ethical conduct.

As noted earlier, policies are an essential part of any institution. Policy allows for smooth and efficient functioning and achievement of inherent institutional goals. Policies should be fair, transparent, and clear. Yet, with all this in mind, we should avoid fetishizing policy. Ideally, policies cohere with the mission of the institution and central ethical values. Yet, this may not always be the case. Policy, like law, differentiates from ethics in sometimes focusing on expedience. Clear and general standards are necessary but may not foresee every significant circumstance. Thus, policies, like law and like a professional code of ethics, should always be open to critique to ensure the best, most ethical standards are maintained. We see this in Case Study 20.3 when a necessary change in policy was recognized. And when a change is necessary, a fair, reflective, and well-defined system should be in place to do so. Also, we must avoid the temptation to abuse a "reservation of right" provision in order to justify just any action. Rather, such disclaimers should be used as intended, to ensure fair and ethical action when published policy might fall short.

CRITICAL ELEMENTS TO CONSIDER

- Offer Faculty Development Sessions on "Just Culture."
- Consult the university attorney when developing or revising academic policies to ensure they are fair, transparent, and consistent with laws and regulations.
- Involve all stakeholders on policy development and review.
- Consult your State Board of Nursing to determine if there are advisory policies in place related to exit standardized testing.

References

Anselmi, K. K., Glasgow, M. E. S., & Gambescia, S. (2014). Using a student conduct committee to foster professional accountability. *Journal of Professional Nursing, 30*(6), 481–485. doi:10.1016/j.profnurs.2014.04.002

Barnsteiner, J., & Disch, J. (2012). A just culture for nurses and nursing students. *Nursing Clinics of North America, 47*(3), 407–416. doi:10.1016/j.cnur.2012.05.005

Barnsteiner, J., & Disch, J. (2017). Creating a fair and just culture in schools of nursing. *American Journal of Nursing, 117*(11), 42–48. doi:10.1097/01.NAJ.0000526747.84173.97

Dekker, S. (2008). *Just culture: Balancing safety and accountability*. Burlington, VT: Ashgate Publishing.

Gasior, M. (2019) *Following policies and procedures and why it's important: Ideas for making sure your staff knows how to follow procedures*. Retrieved from https://www.powerdms.com/blog/what-is-a-policy-vs-a-procedure/

Glasgow, M. E. S., Dreher, H. M., & Schreiber, J. (2019). Standardized testing in nursing education: Preparing students for NCLEX-RN® and practice. *Journal of Professional Nursing, 35*, 440–446. doi:10.1016/j.profnurs.2019.04.012

Kaplin, W. A., Lee, B. A., Hutchens, N. H., & Rooksby, J. H. (2019). *The law of higher education: A comprehensive guide to legal implications of administrative decision making* (6th ed.). San Francisco, CA: John Wiley.

Karpicke, J. D. (2012). Retrieval-based learning: Active retrieval promotes meaningful learning. *Current Directions in Psychological Science, 21*(3), 157–163. doi:10.1177/0963721412443552

Millen v. Colby College, 874 A.2d 397 (Me. 2005)

National Council of State Boards of Nursing. (2017). *2017 Number of candidates taking NCLEX examination and percent passing, by type of candidate*. Retrieved from https://floridasnursing.gov/forms/nclex-pass-rates-2017.pdf

Serembus, J. (2016). Improving NCLEX first-time pass rates: A comprehensive program approach. *Journal of Nursing Regulation, 6*(4), 38–44. doi:10.1016/S2155-8256(16)31002-X

Soderstrom, N. C., & Bjork, R. A. (2014). Testing facilitates the regulation of subsequent study time. *Journal of Memory and Language, 73*, 99–115. doi:10.1016/j.jml.2014.03.003

Spector, N., & Alexander, M. A. (2006). Exit exams from a regulatory perspective. *Journal of Nursing Education, 45*(8), 291–292. doi:10.3928/01484834-20060801-01

Stonecypher, K., Young, A., Langford, R., Symes, L., & Wilson, P. (2015). Faculty experiences developing and implementing policies for exit exam testing. *Nurse Educator, 40*(4), 189–193. doi:10.1097/NNE.0000000000000152

University of California Santa Cruz. (2019). *Administrative policy*. Retrieved from https://policy.ucsc.edu/resources/index.html

Weimer, M. (2014). *Do cumulative exams motivate students? Faculty focus*. Retrieved from http://www.facultyfocus.com/articles/teaching-and-learning/cumulative-exams-motivate-students/

Individual Rights and Public Safety: Addressing Conduct and Mental Health Issues Among Students

Case Study 21.1
Conduct and Mental Health Issues

Your role: You are the Associate Dean, Dr. Patrick Monahan.

James Thompson is a 20-year-old nursing student in his junior year in the BSN program. There have been multiple episodes where James ignores faculty directives in class and clinical and is argumentative when instructed to comply, believing he is correct. He has been counseled both verbally and in writing by the faculty involved and you, the Associate Dean. James is very charming until his requests are not met and then he becomes very argumentative and aggressive. Recently, James was argumentative with a faculty member, Dr. King, about his final exam grade and refused to leave her class during a test review. Due to his size and behavior, the faculty member, Dr. King, felt very threatened and was "essentially rescued" when students entered the class for a remediation session. James was also placed on clinical warning and subsequently received a clinical failure in his Adult Health II course for poor clinical preparation, failure to communicate with patients in a therapeutic manner, failure to demonstrate empathy with patients, demonstrating inappropriate emotional responses to patient situations, and failure to follow faculty directives.

James appealed the clinical failure. The clinical faculty member denied the appeal. The School of Nursing Academic Standing Committee reviewed James' clinical evaluation in Adult Health II and concurred with the clinical failure recommendation. You send a letter to James with the Committee's recommendation as per the protocol. You also ask to meet with James as you have concerns about his behavior. When you meet with James, you note that he is very unstable. He is initially very amiable and overly solicitous; however, when James realizes that you support the clinical failure, he becomes very angry with you. He informs you how smart he is and how this is a big misunderstanding. He glares at you and tells you that you think you are so smart but he is smarter. He also invades your interpersonal space and points his finger at your chest, poking you and then smiles. You have to insist that he leave your office. You have concerns about his mental health/stability and potentially your and others' safety.

Questions
- Whom should you consult?
- Is the student a safety risk?
- What is your best course of action?

LEGAL PRINCIPLES AND REVIEW OF THE LITERATURE

There is no doubt that higher education in general, and course work in clinical care in particular, is stressful. Students have always had difficulty in responding to the stress, and faculty have dealt with that issue for years. However, mental health crises appear to have exploded on college and university campuses around the country. Nearly one third of newly admitted college students report a history of mental illness or experiencing psychological problems (Marsh & Wilcoxon, 2015). According the American College Health Association National College Health Assessment (2015), 30% to 45% of students ($n = 93,034$) reported having mental health problems over the last 12 months (Gallagher, 2014). Problematic student behavior or psychopathology falls along a continuum that can range from disruptive and disturbing to openly threatening and dangerous (Kirsch, Doerfler, & Truong, 2015).

One likely cause of this is the evolution of our culture. The 1960s and 1970s exposed a generation to the right to express themselves as individuals and to act out, and those students are today's administrators and faculty. Another likely cause is the law: Lawsuits and lawyers (and the fear of both) and the ease with which claims can be asserted (and costs imposed) have caused college administrators to accept and retain students longer than they had been willing to do so in years past. These forces have combined in two landmark federal laws—the Rehabilitation Act of 1973 and the Americans with Disabilities Act (ADA) of 1990—which together afford students a better chance of entering and remaining in college by protecting their rights as persons with psychiatric (or physical) disabilities (Bowe, 1992). Section 504 of the Rehabilitation Act was the first to require all postsecondary institutions receiving federal aid (i.e., virtually all colleges and universities) to make their programs accessible to students with mental health issues (Meunier & Wolf, 2006).

A third likely cause is the prevalence of psychopharmacologic therapy/medications. The numbers of students who are able to function in an academic setting despite anxiety disorders, mood disorders, depression, psychiatric illness, and other such issues have grown as treatments that are more effective and medications have been developed and made available (Kaplan & Reed, 2004). More and more students have been diagnosed and treated successfully in high school, leading to greater opportunity for students with mental health issues to enter college. These issues may or may not be disclosed to the university.

 BEST PRACTICE EXEMPLAR

A university may or may not want to know about a student's mental or physical health issues. Unlike high school, a university is not obligated to take care of students. Conversely, if the college knows about a student's problems (and medications), it can react appropriately when the student begins to demonstrate those problems. Such knowledge may become problematic, however. If the college asks for and has this knowledge, it might be considered to have created a "special relationship" with the student, and might be held liable for failing to step in and act to prevent harm to the student or others. This is often called *parens patriae*. Many universities do not want to assume this responsibility voluntarily, and have disclaimed such responsibility.

An additional factor contributing to students' dealing with mental illness on campus involves the timing of psychiatric illness presentation. Psychiatric illnesses are most often diagnosed in young adulthood and may very well be triggered by stressful situations germane to college life. Some of the stressors that contribute to the development of mental health problems in college students include living in a new place, sharing a confined space, peer pressure, greater academic demands, and less structure (Cook, 2007; Eisenberg, Hunt, & Speer, 2013). College students are faced with these multiple changes during this transition, not to mention the physical absence of parents and decreased structure in their lives in general. Nursing majors not only must cope with the general pressure associated with college life, but they also have additional stress associated with clinical education and the hospital environment. Although policies may exist for students in crisis on academic campuses, there is a shortage of literature related to the undergraduate nursing student in the clinical area with severe exacerbation of his or her mental illness.

Although many students with a psychiatric disability will register with the office of disability services, there are still others who choose not to disclose a disability, especially students with a mental illness or psychiatric disability who are concerned about stigma and believe that they will not be treated confidentially or fairly. When any of these nursing students starts to experience psychiatric symptoms and exhibits distress in the classroom and/or the clinical area, a different type of problem solving is required, one that takes on a more complex set of stakeholder considerations. In these cases, faculty may not be clear about how to manage a student emergency situation. It is useful for a university to have an emergency student protocol in place to assist faculty in supporting students when they begin to act out seemingly unreasonably or suggest that they may be acting in imminent danger to themselves. It is important that faculty members are aware of distress signals, methods of immediate intervention, and sources for help for students.

The situation is made more complex by the rights that college students have to privacy. The Family Education Rights and Privacy Act (FERPA; 20 U.S.C. § 1232g; 34 CFR Part 99) is a federal law that protects the privacy of student education records. The law applies to all schools that receive funds under an applicable program of the U.S. Department of Education. In essence, it requires schools to keep confidential—from anyone at the college unless they have a need to know, and even from parents—the student's education records unless the student consents to the disclosure of their education record or the disclosure is permitted by FERPA without the student's consent. FERPA defines "education records" as records that are "directly related to a student" and "maintained by an educational agency or institution or by a party acting for the agency or institution" (34 CFR § 99.3). This is a broad definition and can include complaints about behavior, allegations of misconduct, and event punishments imposed by student judicial bodies. For this reason, it is sometimes not easy for a member of the faculty or administration to decide whom they can talk to or what they can say. However, FERPA permits disclosure of education records without student consent to "school officials" whom the institution has determined to have legitimate educational interests. The institution's FERPA policy will define who is a school official and what constitutes a legitimate educational interest, but the U.S. Department of Education's model policy provides institutions with wide latitude: "[a] school official has a legitimate educational interest if the official needs to review an education record in order to fulfill his or her professional responsibilities of the school." This broad definition, if included in your institution's FERPA policy, will permit the faculty member to discuss concerns about a student to a supervisor or other support personnel at the institution (such as personnel in student life, academic administration, disability services, public safety, counseling center and legal) without violating FERPA. There are also other exceptions under FERPA that may permit disclosure outside the institution to appropriate parties such as parents if the disclosure is made "in connection with a health or safety emergency" (34 CFR § 99.31(a)(10)) (U.S. Department of Education, 2019).

A nursing faculty member or administrator who has concerns about a student's behavior or conduct, but is worried that disclosing these concerns, either within or outside the institution, may potentially violate FERPA, should immediately contact their institutional legal counsel for guidance because the sharing of information within the institution is critical for appropriate management of these very serious situations.

Threatening or Violent Behavior

A threatening or violent event requires the combination of a person with some (high or low) predisposing potential for violent behavior, a situation with elements that create some risk of violent events, and usually a triggering event (Reiss & Roth, 1993; Salzer, 2012). Under the law, people have the right to be free of the threat of violence, and this is protected by both the criminal law and the civil law of torts (see Chapter 2, Legal Issues Commonly Encountered by Faculty and Academic Administrators). A person commits an assault if they put someone else in reasonable fear of being harmed, and the actor intended either to do the act that causes the fear or to cause the fear itself. Words alone are not enough, but they are if they are coupled with an act that suggests the ability to carry out the threat.

Virtually all student codes of conduct prohibit students from acts of violence, and the sanctions for violation are severe. But codes will never deter emotion. In 2002, a nursing student shot three nursing instructors to death at the University of Arizona and then killed himself ("Gunman in Arizona," 2002). On Friday, February 12, 2010, University of Alabama Huntsville Professor Amy Bishop opened fire at a faculty meeting, killing three colleagues and wounding three others. Allegations emerged that a denial of tenure for Bishop played a role in the shootings (Bartlett & Wilson, 2010). The tragedies at University North Carolina-Charlotte, Virginia Tech, and Northern Illinois University have focused enormous attention on mental health issues and violence among college-aged students. In 2019, a shooter on the University of North Carolina at Charlotte campus killed two and injured four on the last day of classes. The alleged gunman, Trystan Andrew Terrell, opened the front door and smiled before firing his weapon at random, showing no other reaction. Mr. Terrell had withdrawn from the university earlier in the semester (Helsel & Fichtel, 2019). In two separate attacks in 2007 in Blacksburg, Virginia, 32 Virginia Tech students and faculty were killed before the gunman, who was a senior English major, killed himself, resulting in what has become not just the deadliest school shooting, but also the deadliest shooting rampage by a single gunman in all of U.S. history. This shooting resulted in many universities reviewing and revising their student mental health policies, in addition to the establishment of a campus emergency alert system if an active shooter is on the campus. Less than a year later, in February 2008, on the campus of Northern Illinois University, a 27-year-old former graduate sociology student shot 22 victims and killed 6 (including himself; "6 Shot Dead," 2008). Less than 2 years after the mass shootings devastated the campus, Virginia Tech was shaken by yet another horribly violent crime. Graduate student Xin Yang had befriended doctoral candidate Haiyang Zhu because of their shared ethnicity; Yang had just come from China 2 weeks earlier. The two were having coffee in a campus restaurant, giving no indication to witnesses that either was upset. Suddenly Zhu attacked Yang, stabbing her multiple times and then decapitating her in front of horrified students. Latina Williams, a 23-year-old nursing student at Louisiana Technical College killed two classmates and herself in a second floor classroom in 2008. In 2012 at Oikos University in Oakland, California, a former nursing student, One Goh returned to a nursing class and told his former classmates, "Get in line…. I'm going to kill you all." He then fired indiscriminately around the room, killing seven people and injuring three (Lee, 2014). As these tragic events indicate, faculty and administrators have good reason to be concerned for their safety.

DECISIONS TO ALERT PUBLIC AUTHORITIES

The shooting of U.S. Representative Gabrielle Giffords in January 2011 highlights another aspect of this situation: potential harm to the public after the university has dealt with the problem internally. The alleged shooter, Jared Lee Loughner, had exhibited behavior at Pima Community College that was so erratic that it caused his suspension and ban from campus. The college had revised its student code of conduct to better identify potentially violent students after the Virginia Tech massacre in

2007, when a student fatally shot 32 teachers and students before killing himself; however, the responses and remedies ended at the geographic borders of the campus.

College officials confirmed that Loughner attended the school from the summer of 2005 through the fall of 2010. They said he was suspended for violating the college's code of conduct after five disruptions in classrooms and libraries on two different campuses and after the discovery of a YouTube video that Loughner had posted in which he claimed that the college was illegal under the U.S. Constitution. On September 29, 2010, two college police officers delivered a letter of suspension to Loughner at the house where he lived with his parents. After meeting with administrators on October 4, the college sent a second letter on October 7, indicating Loughner could return to campus only if he resolved his violations and obtained "mental health clearance indicating, in the opinion of a mental health professional, his presence at the College does not present a danger to himself or others," according to a statement issued by the college.

Under Arizona law, anyone can call the county or regional health authorities with concerns about a person's mental health, and authorities are required to send out mobile units to assess the person's condition. The person who files a request for commitment must list the names of two witnesses who can attest to the subject's behavior, although they do not have to sign the document themselves. Unlike the laws in other states that allow involuntary commitment only if people pose a danger to themselves or others, or if they are profoundly disabled by their mental illness to the point of being unable to take care of themselves, Arizona apparently allows for involuntary commitment if someone is deteriorating from a mental illness and could benefit from treatment.

Laws such as these do not themselves impose obligations on individuals perceiving the mental health problem, but they do allow the observer to share the information officially and in a way that is privileged, protecting them from liability for having made a slanderous statement against a person or having violated their privacy. Under Arizona law, any one of Loughner's classmates or teachers at Pima Community College who were concerned about his behavior could have contacted local officials and asked that he be evaluated for mental illness and potentially committed for psychiatric treatment. However, none did. It remains to be seen whether any of the victims of the shootings will attempt to impose legal liability upon the college for having failed to notify the public authorities (Szabo & Lloyd, 2011).

The Higher Education Security Act requires universities to report the previous year's crime statistics to the entire campus community (Siegel, 1994). The university must also report whether any of the crimes were motivated by race, gender, sexual orientation, religion, ethnicity, or disability, otherwise known as hate crimes. This will tell consumers (potential and current students, faculty and staff) how safe the area is, but it is nothing more than historical fact. "What is perhaps most troubling about campus crime is that the majority of the incidents, excluding theft but including rape and other sexual assaults, are impulsive acts committed by students themselves, according to nationwide studies conducted by Towson State University's Campus Violence Prevention Center." Because universities are often regarded as protected environments, incidents of violence are particularly shocking for the college campus and extended community. "There are many types of campus violence—including rape, assault, fighting, hazing, dating violence, sexual harassment, hate and bias related violence, stalking, rioting, disorderly conduct, property crime, and suicide" (Langford, 2004, p. 2). Today, students learn about campus crime statistics and ways to ensure their safety in university orientation and other programs.

In response to acts and threats of violence, "user-friendly" harassment policies and complaint procedures are now common on university campuses. To minimize events of (and potential liability for) harassment, colleges and universities should make their anti-harassment policies and procedures clear; publish and disseminate them as widely as possible; make sure there are hotlines in place to which reports can safely and effectively be made; and provide training to potential complaint handlers and faculty, staff, and students (Alger, 1998).

IDENTIFYING BEST PRACTICES IN NURSING EDUCATION

Faculty and administration need to be cognizant of triggering events that would cause a student with a propensity for violence to become violent. A violent event requires the combination of a person with some (high or low) predisposing potential for violent behavior, a situation with elements that create some risk of violent events, and usually a triggering event (Reiss & Roth, 1993). Increased vigilance and preventive measures during times of high stress—such as during midterm and final examinations—are recommended. For nursing faculty, the award of a clinical warning notice or grade of clinical failure would also constitute a triggering event. During these times, faculty are cautioned to take preventive measures, such as alerting one's supervisor that a student will be receiving a failing grade. The faculty member should meet with the student during a high-traffic time when many faculty and staff members will be outside the conference room or office. The member should notify faculty and staff that they will be meeting with a student to deliver bad news. If the faculty member suspects that the student may become violent, they should notify security to be on standby as a precautionary measure. The university should also teach faculty how to identify behaviors that are consistent with harassment or potential violence, and it should emphasize its zero tolerance for workplace harassment and violence (Equal Employment Opportunity Commission [EEOC], 2010). Faculty and students should also be educated to report concerning behavior such as severe depression, anger outbursts, and fascination with weapons to university public safety officials. Equally important, complainants should be treated with respect and compassion, provided anonymity when possible, and given protection from retaliation or further harm (Box 21.1).

After a university receives notice of the harassing conduct, it has a duty under Title IX to take some action to prevent the further harassment or harm of the student or students (Kaplin, Lee, Hutchens, & Rooksby, 2019). Student-to-student harassment is also the most common form of sexual harassment on campus. College-wide prevention programs, and procedures by which there can be prompt and direct intervention, are critical in addressing and minimizing harassment and violence. Harassment policies need to be widely publicized, as do the universities' methods for reporting and responding to incidents of harassment.

Clinical Education Implications

A student may not recognize that they are not well enough to participate in a clinical rotation providing care for sick, vulnerable patients and could refuse to take a temporary leave from the clinical experience. At the same time, university officials may be reluctant to remove the student

---

Box 21.1
Faculty Recommendations on Managing a Student With Mental Health Issues

1. Recognize signs of psychological/behavioral distress and/or substance abuse.
2. Talk with the student privately about your concerns arising from the student's recent behavior or conduct. Share your observations and assess the urgency of the situation. *During this discussion, the faculty member should focus on describing the behavior or conduct that is causing concern, rather than the suspected causes of that behavior or conduct (i.e., psychiatric illness). Even where strongly indicated, the faculty member should avoid diagnosis of psychological illness until the student mentions it.*
3. Determine if the situation requires immediate intervention. *The most basic criteria are whether the student is an immediate danger to self or others. If this is the case, the faculty member needs to contact security or public safety representatives immediately. It is imperative that the student receive appropriate evaluation and subsequent treatment.*
4. Do not isolate yourself when dealing with a student with a serious mental health issue. Consult with academic nursing administrators and staff at the university's counseling center and legal department.

Source: Adapted from Ashcroft, T., Chernomas, W., Davis, P., Dean, R., Seguire, M., Shapiro, C., & Swiderski, L. M. (2008). Nursing students with disabilities: One faculty's journey. *International Journal of Nursing Education Scholarship, 5*(1), 1–26. doi:10.2202/1548-923X.1424

from their clinical rotation, as they may be fearful that they are violating the student's rights or unnecessarily harming their educational progress. Clinical faculty teaching students with emerging mental health problems have other, competing obligations including addressing needs of other students, maintaining patient safety, and maintaining collaborative relationships with nursing leadership and staff at clinical agencies. In managing such at-risk student situations, faculty, nursing administrators, and institutional officials will want to act in a manner that does not violate the legal rights of the individual student and give rise to potential legal liability. To accomplish this, the institution can conduct a direct threat review prior to initiation of any involuntary leave or suspension. The objective of this review is to assess whether the student poses a direct threat to themselves or to others, and whether the institution could or could not provide a reasonable accommodation that would reduce or eliminate that threat. As part of this assessment, the institution determines whether there is a high probability of substantial harm and not just a slightly increased, speculative, or remote risk. The institution will need to conduct an individualized and objective assessment about whether the student can continue to participate in the institution's programs safely, based on a reasonable medical judgment relying on the most current medical knowledge or the best objective evidence. The assessment should determine the nature, duration, and severity of the risk, the probability that the potential threatening injury will actually occur, and whether reasonable modifications of policies, practices, or procedures will sufficiently mitigate the risk (Kucirka, 2017; Lee & Abbey, 2008).

In the event that the student refuses to take a temporary leave from the clinical experience while having a mental health crisis, a university can convene a threat assessment task force with university officials made up of representatives of mental health counseling, public safety, student life, legal counsel, and nursing academic administration to evaluate the situation and the student's fitness for clinical educational responsibilities at this time and to consider whether an involuntary leave or temporary suspension from specific educational activities is appropriate based on an individualized assessment of the situation. Proper documentation that this assessment process was followed will help the institution defend itself in the event of legal challenge.

Using a Best Practice Framework

In Case Study 21.1, it is important that the faculty member speak in a low tone, be empathetic to the student, and call the student by name. You can discuss how difficult the program is, how many students have difficulty in the third term as adult health is challenging, and how often students suffering from stress and other mental health issues can be helped by seeking assistance from student counseling. You can promise to review his case again with the Dean *if you are feeling threatened at the time*, in an attempt to have the student leave your office.

It is always best if faculty members have their offices arranged in a manner so that their chair is close to the door. With this arrangement, the faculty member can exit the office quickly if necessary. It is best if faculty members do not stay in their offices late at night or early in the morning, when the campus is isolated. If it is necessary to work late, then the faculty member should lock the office door and alert public safety or security that they are alone in the office.

Faculty should be particularly vigilant after giving students bad news. If possible, faculty office buildings should be locked during the evening hours. In this case, you need to report the student to the student conduct committee and the office of public safety for uncivil and threatening behavior. It is difficult to predict if Mr. Thompson will resort to physical violence; however, his recent behavior is of great concern and warrants further investigation and action.

An emergency student protocol guide is also warranted in guiding the nursing faculty on the proper procedures in the event of a violent or potentially violent incident involving students or other personnel. These protocols serve as a resource in assisting faculty during interventions with students who may be in imminent danger to themselves or others. The need for management protocols for nursing students in crisis must be underscored.

A threat assessment task force, as previously discussed in this chapter, will consider the student's fitness for educational responsibilities at this time and whether an involuntary leave or temporary suspension from specific educational activities is appropriate based on an individualized assessment of the situation. Proper documentation that this assessment process was followed will help the institution defend itself in the event of legal challenge. In the event of a violent act, the police would be notified and take appropriate *action*. If the alleged perpetrator and victim are still on campus, as in *Kelly v. Yale University* (2003), the university is obligated to provide academic or residential accommodations to prevent possible future harassment or harm.

DISCUSSION OF CASE STUDY

The authors have specifically selected a case where the student presents with concerning mental health behaviors and the faculty member is very uncomfortable or even fearful. Nursing faculty should trust the inherent "gift" of their gut instinct and recognize various warning signs and precursors to violence, and take appropriate precautions (de Becker, 1998). Faculty can surely understand this student's distress, and they will want to be supportive. What makes the situation reach a higher level of concern is the student's anger, labile mood, and physical contact with the Associate Dean and prior incident of refusing to leave a classroom when requested to do so by another faculty member. Thus, the response is clear: Faculty must immediately consult public safety and the Dean with respect to convening a threat assessment task force. A psychiatric evaluation (for the student's good) and to the university's office of student life (for the good of all students and the health of the academic community) should be recommended. All campus personnel who play a part in this student's campus experience should be notified of the faculty member's self-initiated descriptions of safety concerns. The situation is hopefully successfully addressed with outpatient anger management and other psychiatric treatment and possibly medication and counseling. However, as long as the student is exhibiting threatening behaviors, the administration needs to ensure the safety of students and patients. The student's clinical experiences should be suspended until such time as a mental health professional confirms that the student can safely return to the clinical arena and assume patient care responsibilities or the university makes a final determination on the student's academic status based on the Code of Conduct. It is also essential to maintain (and continuously update) a detailed timeline of events as they transpire and to compile a complete file of all related materials and correspondence, including updates as they occur from the various officials consulted. "What is the next action step?" is a crucial question to be asked both when sharing initial concerns and providing updates to the situation. A communication or intervention plan must be established, approved, and implemented, and it must be commonly understood.

WHEN TO CONSULT THE UNIVERSITY COUNSEL

Consult the university counsel related to policy development and implementation related to students with mental health issues.

Consult the university counsel if you believe FERPA or other privacy laws prevent you from fully disclosing information or knowledge you have about a student to other school personnel or to others outside the school.

FINDINGS AND DISPOSITION

The Dean requested that the Threat Assessment Taskforce meet to evaluate James's behavior to determine whether he is a safety concern to the university campus given he had refused to leave a classroom and made physical contact with the Associate Dean. The Chair of the Threat Assessment Taskforce consulted with a number of campus entities, including representatives from the following: campus police, student affairs, counseling staff, central academic affairs, and legal counsel since it is not uncommon for a disruptive student to be "on the radar" of the personnel of more than one entity—based upon prior, seemingly isolated interactions—without always rising to the threshold of a safety concern. Based on the investigation, patterns of inappropriate behaviors may emerge, aiding further in substantiating a rationale for decisive and swift intervention. This is particularly important when the student's behaviors are veiled, implied threats rather than overtly menacing, physical actions or verbal statements. In this case, James did make physical contact with the Associate Dean Monahan (poking him in the chest) and refused to leave a classroom, not allowing the faculty member, Dr. King, to exit the classroom. Resident's Life had a complaint concerning a roommate dispute on file suggesting James has an anger management issue. James was required to attend counseling.

Before the Threat Assessment Taskforce Committee could convene, James sent some concerning emails to Associate Dean Monahan stating, "You think you are so clever, I would be careful if I were you." And "I am not going to let this go." The Threat Assessment Taskforce met late that week and recommended suspension (involuntary leave) and temporary removal from campus to the Vice President of Student Life. The Vice President of Student Life placed James on an involuntary leave and banned him from campus pending a psychiatric evaluation. His threatening emails were reported to the University and local police. The university victim advocate and police reached out to Associate Dean Monahan to discuss personal safety strategies due to the disturbing emails. The Threat Assessment Taskforce also recommended that James's case be sent to the Office of Student Conduct after the recommendation of the psychiatric evaluation is sent to the Vice President of Student Life.

Prevention Tips

- *Offer faculty development sessions on signs of psychological distress, and appropriate support resources for students.*
- *Educate faculty about the emergency protocol for students exhibiting severe psychological distress.*
- *Remind students on a routine basis to consult university counseling services during high-stress periods (midterm and final exams, etc.).*

Safety Tips

- *Deliver bad news to students during normal office hours in a private office located in a high-traffic area.*
- *Do not keep concerns related to student harassment to yourself. Alert your supervisor and public safety.*
- *Alert security ahead of time if you suspect that a student, faculty, or staff member may be violent when you deliver bad news.*
- *Alert security when you are working late, then lock your office and take necessary safety precautions.*
- *Educate faculty, students, and staff about the need to report concerning behavior to public safety.*
- *Educate and promote bystander intervention (Langford, 2004).*
- *Convey clear expectations for conduct among students, faculty, and staff (Langford, 2004).*
- *Create and disseminate comprehensive policies and procedures addressing behavior— strong enforcement of violent behavior sends a clear message about intolerance for violent behavior (Langford, 2004).*
- *Provide a range of support services for students, including mental health services, crisis management, and comprehensive services for victims (Langford, 2004).*
- *Offer campus safety classes in orientation and offer campus escort service.*

RELEVANT LEGAL CASES

Chang v. Purdue University, 985 N.E.2d 35 (Ind. Ct. App. 2013)

The law clearly shapes university policies that are related to student conduct issues whether or not associated with mental illness. Recent complaints of student harassment and violence on college campuses give academic administrators and their legal counsel pause as they are charged with keeping students safe at their respective universities. Universities are usually challenged on one of the following legal theories: duty to protect, duty to prevent, and permitting or allowing the cause (Smith & Fleming, 2007). In *Chang v. Purdue University* (2013), Judy Chang, an undergraduate nursing student was dismissed for unprofessional conduct that jeopardized the health and/or safety of classmates. Students and faculty reported hateful speech, argumentative behavior, agitation, and intent to push a pregnant student down the stairs. The nursing department committee determined that there was sufficient evidence of faculty and student complaints to support dismissal. The decision was based on the pattern of action of verbal abuse that involved an expressed or implied threat to a person's safety. Ms. Chang appealed her dismissal through the internal [University] process based on lack of due process and discrimination but was denied. Chang filed a lawsuit based on a violation of her 14th Amendment rights and a breach of the implied contract between Purdue University and herself with respect to the Purdue University adherence to due process policies, and against the faculty in their individual capacities under a theory of tortious interference with contract pertaining to Chang's contract with Purdue University. The court affirmed the university's decision. Because the university's decision to dismiss the student was not arbitrary or made in bad faith, the university did not breach its contract with the student. The student's due process rights were not infringed because she had the opportunity to appeal the decision. The student's tortious interference claims failed because she did not comply with state statutory notice requirements.

Regents of the University of California, et al. v. the Superior Court of Los Angeles County (Cal. 2018)

Katherine Rosen was a student at UCLA who sued the university and several employees after she was stabbed by another student, Damon Thompson, without warning during a chemistry lab. She claimed the school was negligent in failing to protect her from Thompson's foreseeable violent conduct.

Thompson had been admitted to UCLA in 2008. Beginning in the first term, the school received several reports involving his auditory hallucinations and suicidal thoughts. He admitted to thinking about harming others but did not identify any specific victims or plans. Thompson was treated by UCLA counseling and psychological services and by third-party providers who diagnosed possible schizophrenia and major depressive disorder. However, he did not comply with medical treatment options recommended to him. While in his dorm room he claimed he heard voices coming through the wall calling him an idiot. In February 2009, campus police responded to another complaint that he heard clicking noises above his room that sounded like a gun and that other residents were planning to shoot him. After a search found no weapons, police took him to a local emergency department for an evaluation. He entered and withdrew from treatment during the March to April 2019 period. He was banned from University housing in June 2009 after shoving another resident he accused of making too much noise. His case was brought to the University's Consultation and Response Team for review and monitoring. During the summer of 2009, Thompson complained to two faculty about insults and harassment he claimed to be experiencing in his chemistry lab. After the fall 2009 semester began, he emailed a faculty member complaining that disruptive behavior of other students was interfering with his experiments. On September 30, 2019, he met with two separate counselors at UCLA and both their evaluations noted guarded attitude, slowed speech, delusional thought process and impaired insight. Two different teaching assistants reported to the chemistry lab professor in early October that Thompson was accusing students of verbally harassing him and that Katherine Rosen, who worked right next to Thompson in the lab, was one of the students calling him stupid. These reports were forwarded to the University Consultation and Response Team. Although potential options were discussed among the team and concern was expressed that urgent outreach may be needed, no actions were taken or warnings issued.

While doing classwork in the chemistry lab on October 8, Thompson suddenly and without warning or provocation attacked Rosen from behind with a kitchen knife while she was placing items into a lab drawer. Although taken to the hospital with life-threatening injuries to her chest and neck, Rosen fortunately survived the attack. Thompson was arrested by campus police in the laboratory and charged with attempted murder. He pleaded not guilty by reason of insanity.

Rosen's suit against UCLA and several UCLA employees alleged a single count of negligence and argued that the school had a special relationship with her as a student and, therefore, a duty to take reasonable measures to protect her from reasonably foreseeable criminal conduct. Rosen alleged that the school breached this duty because it was aware of Thompson's dangerous "propensities" but failed to warn or protect her or control Thompson's foreseeable violent conduct. One of the grounds on which UCLA filed for summary judgment in the case was that colleges and universities had no duty to protect adult students from criminal acts. The trial court denied this ground and UCLA appealed the ruling to the state's Court of Appeals. A divided panel of the Court of Appeals held that UCLA had no duty to protect Rosen based on her status as a student or business invitee. Rosen then appealed to the state's highest court, the California Supreme Court.

The California Supreme Court reversed the Court of Appeals and held that "universities have a special relationship with their students and a duty to protect them from foreseeable violence during curricular activities." The Court elaborated that under certain circumstance the "duty to protect" could be fulfilled by giving adequate warning to the students at risk. The Court remanded the case back to the lower court to determine if UCLA failed to exercise reasonable care under the circumstances of the case.

In its legal analysis, the California Supreme Court noted that there is generally no duty to protect others from conduct of third parties. However, there are exceptions to this general rule if the defendant has a "special relationship" with the plaintiff.

The Court determined that a "special relationship" existed between UCLA and Rosen because (a) college and university students are comparatively vulnerable and dependent on the college for a safe environment; (b) colleges and universities have a superior ability to provide for that safety in activities they sponsor or facilities they control; and (c) the relationship is bounded by the student's enrollment status.

SUMMARY

Nursing faculty members may respond to a student having a mental health crisis by acting in accordance with their professional nursing training and attempt to help the student. This is the wrong response, because it will impose much higher obligations and duties as a result of the special relationship doing so creates. Nursing faculty should immediately contact the university counseling center, as should faculty members from other academic disciplines. Just as nursing faculty would call 911 as they provided CPR or other lifesaving emergency techniques in an emergency situation, they should also ensure the safety of the student in a psychological emergency and seek qualified psychiatric care for the student. Case law clearly cautions faculty about switching their role to care provider (establishing a special relationship). It is in the student's and clinical faculty's best interest for the clinical faculty member to refer a student rather than attempt to counsel the student on their own, as this could be considered a special relationship. In nonemergency situations, faculty should also refer students to the university counseling center, as would be expected of faculty members from other academic disciplines. Psychiatric and mental health nursing faculty members are especially cautioned not to establish a special relationship with students (Cook, 2007; Lane & Corcoran, 2016).

In an effort to manage students in crisis effectively, universities need to develop protocols on emergency situations to guide faculty. Protocols serve as a resource in assisting faculty during interventions with students who may be in imminent danger to themselves or others (see the Emergency Student Protocol Guide in Appendix 21.1). The need for management protocols for nursing students in crisis, particularly those with suspected severe mental health issues or psychiatric disabilities, cannot be understated. Academic nursing programs need to be cognizant of the safety of the student and the patients that student might treat, while respecting the student's own rights and the law (e.g., the ADA). Furthermore, faculty encounter problems in the clinical setting when a student has not disclosed a mental health problem; therefore, it is important for the faculty member to consult the counseling center, academic administrator, office of disability, and legal counsel for advice.

An analysis of how colleges and universities have responded in the aftermath of the horrific shootings at Virginia Tech was reported at the 2008 Annual Forum of the Association of Institutional Research (The Midwestern Higher Education Compact, 2008). According to a media report published by *insidehighered.com*, data indicate that many colleges have significantly altered their campus safety procedures, especially how students are notified of possible danger and how procedures are implemented to deal with students who display signs of trouble. However, these same reports indicate that campus leaders resisted "wholesale changes to their admissions or other policies that might have been seen as severely restricting the campus culture or trampling on individual rights." Over 50% of the respondents disclosed that "they had considered installing metal detectors at entrances to classroom buildings," while approximately 30% disclosed that they had considered including questions to admissions applications that asked potential students about receiving previous psychiatric treatment (p. 1). Finally, and perhaps sadly, one coauthor of the report stated, "It's interesting what they talked about and *didn't* do" (p. 1). Dealing with students exhibiting mental health problems needs to be proactive, professional, and cognizant of both the student's and patient's well-being.

Unfortunately, there are not always red flags (e.g., harassment, anger management issues) to predict violent behavior; therefore, a comprehensive university approach that combines education, sound code of conduct policies, vigilance, and clear reporting mechanisms are in the best interest of the college community. Harassment and other violent behavior compromise the sense of community to which most universities aspire (Kaplin et al., 2019). Faculty, students, and staff all desire a safe campus environment. Individuals want to go about their daily lives without fear of physical, emotional, or psychological harm. Personal safety is a basic human need that must be upheld; therefore, violence prevention and safety promotion should be seen as a broader mission of all universities (Bickel & Lake, 1999; Roark, 1993).

 CRITICAL ELEMENTS TO CONSIDER

Faculty should consider these essential recommendations on how to manage a student with a mental health issue effectively:

- Recognize signs of behavioral distress, such as deterioration of clinical performance or attendance, lack of energy, disruptive behavior, confused thoughts or speech, anxiety, mood changes/swings, weight change, and loss of contact with reality. This should be documented in the student's file.
- Speak with the student privately about your concerns, share your observations, and make an assessment of the urgency of the situation. This should be documented in the student's file.
- Determine if the situation requires immediate intervention. The most basic criterion is whether the student is a danger to themselves or to others. If the student is perceived to be a danger, then the faculty member must contact security or public safety representatives immediately. It is imperative that the student receive a psychiatric evaluation and subsequent treatment. Do not isolate yourself when dealing with a student with a serious mental health issue: Consult with staff at the university's counseling center and legal counsel.

- Universities can support their faculty members—and, more specifically, their nursing faculty members—by making sure that they have the policies and procedures in place to manage emergency situations that involve the rights of the person with a disability, the care and safety of patients, the care and safety of the student at risk, and the safety of other students involved.
- Faculty development sessions should be offered to new faculty members to acquaint them with behaviors that warrant concern as well as the appropriate action to take in these situations, with periodic reinforcement of this information to ensure awareness and accessibility of these possibilities. Written guidelines should be prepared and made easily accessible to all faculty, instructing them what to do, and when.
- Consult the university attorney. (*Note:* University administrators and legal counsel are not clinicians and may not fully appreciate the specific safety implications of an accommodation respective to the clinical arena.)
- Consult with the student counseling office.
- Know university policies and procedures as well as the appropriate state laws. The university's interpretation of FERPA and its emergency exceptions should be emphasized.
- Initiate an emergency protocol for any reference to harm self or others or extreme emotional distress.
- Focus on the academic performance and conduct of the student only, and do not diagnose the student.
- Contact the director or dean or department chair regarding the distressed student.
- Do not provide an accommodation without official accommodation from the office of disability.
- Be familiar with the nursing program's technical standards.
- Implement preventive strategies such as emails related to student counseling services during times of high stress such as midterms and finals.
- Offer faculty development sessions to faculty related to best practices in addressing students with mental health issues and psychiatric disabilities; particularly warning signs that warrant attention.

ETHICAL CONSIDERATIONS

Nursing faculty members also have an ethical duty to protect the student in distress and the public. The *American Nurses Association's Code of Ethics for Nurses* does not clearly and specifically address issues such as this. However, the general concerns can be seen as covered by interpretive statements 3.5 and 3.6, which address questionable practice and impaired practice. These statements develop the duties of nurses to protect vulnerable patients but also the possibility that nursing practice could lead to harm instead of well-being in certain circumstances. Thus, with students who may have potentially harmful (to themselves or others) mental health issues, the faculty can analogously be perceived as having a duty to protect the student as well as the public. The majority of clinical experiences are outside the college and in hospitals, and other clinical settings. As such, nursing programs, students, and faculty are subject to the procedures and policies of that institution. Today, distance learning adds yet another dimension to addressing anyone with mental health issues and the environment where student learning is taking place. In particular, the nursing student with mental health problems may be at a clinical site that is quite a distance from the student's respective college in today's distance learning environment. In this situation, the faculty member should alert the administration of the student's concerning behavior immediately. Similarly, the university administration has an ethical obligation to protect the Associate Dean and faculty members and other students by sometimes requiring students to take an involuntary leave from the university and banning the student from campus depending on the severity of the behavior. The counseling office should assist the student in obtaining the needed mental healthcare.

References

6 shot dead, including gunman, at Northern Illinois University. (2008, February 14). *CNN*. Retrieved from http://www.cnn.com/2008/US/02/14/university.shooting/

American College Health Association. (2015). *American College Health Association National College Health Assessment II: Spring 2015 Reference Group Executive Summary*. Linthicum, MD: ACHA.

Ashcroft, T., Chernomas, W., Davis, P., Dean, R., Seguire, M., Shapiro, C., & Swiderski, L. M. (2008). Nursing students with disabilities: One faculty's journey. *International Journal of Nursing Education Scholarship*, 5(1), 1–26. doi:10.2202/1548-923X.1424

Bartlett, T., & Wilson, R. (2010, June 17). Amy Bishop is indicted in 1986 shooting death of her brother. *The Chronicle of Higher Education*. Retrieved from http://chronicle.com/article/Amy-Bishop-Is-Indicted-in-1986/65970/

Bickel, R.D., & Lake, P.F. (1999). *The Rights and Responsibilities of the Modern University: Who Assumes the Risks of College Life*. Durham, NC: Academic Press.

Bowe, F. (1992). *Adults with disabilities: A portrait*. Washington, DC: President's Committee on Employment of People With Disabilities.

Chang v. Purdue University, 985 N.E.2d 35 (Ind. Ct. App. 2013).

Cook, L. J. (2007). Striving to help college students with mental health issues. *Journal of Psychosocial Nursing*, 45(4), 40–44. doi:10.3928/02793695-20070401-09

de Becker, G. (2008). *The gift of fear: Survival signals that protect us from violence*. New York, NY: Dell Publishing.

Drexel University. (2019). *Student handbook*. Philadelphia, PA: Drexel University College of Nursing & Health Professions, 2018–2019.

Eisenberg, D., Hunt, J., & Speer, N. (2013). Mental health in American colleges and universities: Variation across student subgroups and across campuses. *Journal of Nervous and Mental Disease*, 201, 60–67. doi:10.1097/NMD.0b013e31827ab077

Equal Employment Opportunity Commission. (2020). *Harassment*. Retrieved from https://www.eeoc.gov/harassment

Gallagher, R. P. (2014). *National Survey of Counseling Center Directors*. Alexandria, VA: International Association of Counseling Services.

Gunman in Arizona wrote of plan to kill. (2002, October 22). *The New York Times*. Retrieved from https://www.nytimes.com/2002/10/31/us/gunman-in-arizona-wrote-of-plan-to-kill.html

Helsel, P., & Fichtel, C. (2019, April 30). University of North Carolina at Charlotte shooting kills 2, injures 4. *ABC News*. Retrieved from https://www.nbcnews.com/news/us-news/least-2-dead-2-injured-after-report-shooting-university-north-n1000436

Kaplan, B., & Reed, M. (2004, March). College student mental health: Plan designs, utilization, trends and costs. *Student Health Spectrum*. p. 31–33.

Kaplin, W. A., Lee, B. A., Hutchens, N. H., & Rooksby, J. H. (2019). *The law of higher education: A comprehensive guide to legal implications of administrative decision making* (6th ed.). San Francisco, CA: John Wiley & Sons.

Kelly v. Yale University, WL 1563424, 2003 U.S. Dist. LEXIS 4543 (D. Conn. 2003).

Kirsch, D. J., Doerfler, L. A., & Truong, D. (2015). Mental health issues among college students: Who gets referred for psychopharmacology evaluation? *Journal of American College Health*, 63, 50–56. doi:10.1080/07448481.2014.960423

Kucirka, B. G. (2017). Navigating the faculty–student relationship: Interacting with nursing students with mental health issues, *Journal of the American Psychiatric Nurses Association*, 23(6), 393–403. doi:10.1177/1078390317705451

Lane, A. M., & Corcoran, L. (2016). Educator or counselor? Navigating uncertain boundaries in the clinical environment. *Journal of Nursing Education*, 55(4), 189–195. doi:10.3928/01484834-20160316-02

Langford, L. (2004). *Preventing violence and promoting safety in higher education settings: Overview of a comprehensive approach*. Newton, MA: U.S. Department of Education, Higher Education Center for Alcohol and Other Drug Abuse and Violence Prevention.

Lee, B. A., & Abbey, G. E. (2008). College and university students with mental disabilities: Legal and policy issues. *The Journal of College and University Law, 34*(2), 349–391.

Lee, H. K. (2014, September 17). Details of Oikos University massacre tell of terror in Oakland. SFGate. Retrieved from https://www.sfgate.com/crime/article/Oakland-school-massacre-Jury-told-of-5 -minutes-5760283.php#photo-2769726

Marsh, C. N., & Wilcoxon, S. A. (2015). Underutilization of mental health services among college students: An examination of system-related barriers. *Journal of College Student Psychotherapy, 29*, 227–243. doi:10.1080 /87568225.2015.1045783

Meunier, L. H., & Wolf, C. R. (2006). Mental health issues on college campuses. *NYSBA Health Law Journal, 11*(2), 42–52. Retrieved from https://nysba.org/

The Midwestern Higher Education Compact. (2008, May). The Ripple Effect of Virginia Tech: Assessing the Nationwide Impact on Campus Safety and Security Policy and Practice Retrieved from https://files.eric .ed.gov/fulltext/ED502232.pdf

Roark, M.L. (1993). Conceptualizing campus violence: Definitions, underlying factors, and effects. *Journal of Student Psychotherapy, 8*(1/2), 1-27.

Salzer, M. S. (2012). A comparative study of campus experiences of college students with mental illnesses versus a general college sample. *Journal of American College Health, 60*, 1–7. doi:10.1080/07448481.2011.5 52537

Siegel, D. (1994). What is behind the growth of violence on college campuses? The United States of Violence. *USA Today*. Retrieved from https://www.questia.com/magazine/1G1-15282515/ what-is-behind-the-growth-of-violence-on-college-campuses

Smith, R., & Fleming, D. (2007). Student suicide and colleges' liability. *Chronicle of Higher Education, 53*, B24–B26. Retrieved from http://chronicle.com/

Szabo, L., & Lloyd, J. (2011, January 13). Loughner could have been committed under Arizona law. *USA Today*. Retrieved from https://www.questia.com/magazine/1G1-15282515/ what-is-behind-the-growth-of-violence-on-college-campuses

U.S. Department of Education. (2019). FERPA general guidance for parents. Retrieved from https://www2 .ed.gov/policy/gen/guid/fpco/ferpa/parents.html

Appendix

21.1

Sample Emergency Student Protocol Guide

A GUIDE FOR FACULTY

Students entering the University are called upon to manage special challenges of academic life. In addition to learning, students need to integrate into a large and diverse student population. Many nursing students encounter a range of academic, personal, and social stress during their educational experience. While many students cope successfully with the demands of their educational endeavors and the interpersonal experiences that go along with it, others have difficulties that can become overpowering and unmanageable. The inability to cope effectively with emotional stress poses a serious threat to a student's overall functioning. This guideline will be helpful in assisting faculty during interventions with students who may be in imminent danger to themselves or others.

What Can Faculty Do?

If you observe behavior changes indicating behavioral distress (deterioration of clinical performance or attendance, lack of energy, disruptive behavior, confused thoughts or speech, anxiety, mood changes/swings, dramatic weight change, loss of contact with reality, mood altering substance use), you should:

1. Talk to the student privately about your concerns and share your observations.
2. Make an assessment of the urgency of the situation.
3. Listen to the student and respond reflectively.
4. Refer student to the **Student Counseling Center**. (Provide the student with Student Counseling Center's information.)
5. If warranted, ask the student directly if they are considering harming themselves.
6. Discuss your concerns with the course coordinator at the first indication of a problem. Together you will decide on the next steps. The course coordinator will notify the program director.
7. If you are in the clinical setting and the student's condition requires immediate intervention, inform the staff nurse and unit supervisor that you will be leaving the floor and going with the student to the Emergency Department for an assessment. Immediately notify the course coordinator and director of the nursing program.
8. Once the student is stable or another faculty representative is available to stay with the student, return to the unit. Do not share specifics with the other students. However, it may be helpful to inform them that their colleague was under stress and has been seen by a medical professional.

9. It is helpful to spend some time at the beginning of the semester (before or after the first exam) and again at the end of the semester mentioning the potential or actual stress of the program and taking the "pulse" of the class to assess how students are doing.
10. It is also useful to maintain careful awareness of students during critical flashpoints whereby their failure in the course would prevent/limit progression in the program. Examples of these times are after midterm and final exams.
11. If you are teaching in the classroom and, if the situation permits, speak with the student after class as outlined in Points 1 and 2. If the student is very distressed or disruptive and the student's condition requires immediate intervention, ask another student in the class to get help from the nearby university office if feasible. The student should be assessed by one of the following: (a) the Counseling Center or (b) the Emergency Department.
12. After the student has been assisted to the appropriate center, follow Point 8.

EMERGENCY/INCIDENTS IN YOUR OFFICE OR HOME SETTING

If a Student Presents in Distress at Your Office Between the Hours of 8:30 a.m. and 5:00 p.m.

Monday through Friday:

- Encourage the student to call the Student Counseling Center. Let the student know that counseling services are free and confidential. If the student prefers to see someone off campus, referral information can be provided. Mental health services may be available through the student's health insurance.
- Walk the student over to the Student Counseling Center.
- If the student declines, document your interaction and place it in the student's file.
- Notify both the Program Director and the Student Counseling Center concerning the situation.

If Self-Harm or Harm to Others Appears Imminent to the Student (Threats in Your Office) and the Student Counseling Center Is Not Open:

- Call Campus Security, notifying them of the location and nature of the threat.
- Escort the student to the Emergency Department (if possible) or if the student refuses call 911.
- If the student's anger/loss of control seems to be escalating, and you feel yourself to be in danger, ask the student to leave your office and contact Campus Security.

If You Receive a Distressing Phone Call at Home (Student May Be at Distant Location)

- Ascertain student's address/location.

Source: Drexel University. (2019). Student Handbook. Philedlphia, PA: Drexel University College of Nursing and Health Professions, 2018-2019.

- Listen to student's voice; assess the danger student is in (workable plan to harm himself).
- Convey your concern, your own limited potential to help in this situation, and your intention to call for help.
- Students living on campus: Call Campus Housing Student Residents and call University Student Counseling Center
- Students living off campus: *Call 911 for emergency assistance.* Call will be routed to appropriate emergency jurisdiction.
- Notify Director or Department Chair of appropriate Nursing Program and Student Counseling Center concerning the situation.

22

Substance Misuse: Assessment and Confrontation in Nursing Education

Case Study 22.1

Your role: You are the Director of a BSN Second Degree Nursing Program.

Amy Burke is a 25-year-old female who has a bachelor's degree in psychology and decided to enroll in a BSN Second Degree Program, a 1-year program where she can obtain a Bachelor of Science in Nursing degree. She is married and has a 2-year-old daughter. Although her husband was initially supportive of her decision to return to school, his support is variable and she often describes her life as overwhelming—going to school full time, caring for her child, and intensive studying. Although she was active in her church, she did not get much support or satisfaction from her work there. Her faculty members and fellow students have often noticed that she comes to school tired and distracted. However, recently, she has been "overactive" demonstrating high levels of energy. As she progressed in the program, her energy levels were replaced with periods of irritability and especially during her clinical rotations, she would frequently disappear from the unit for short periods without notifying staff. Some staff have noticed significant changes in the size of her pupils—sometimes they are very dilated; other times they are pinpoint. When approached by her faculty member, she reports only that her behaviors are a result of marital and family discord and she apologizes. When her faculty members point out that her behavior seems to be more inappropriate in her treatment of patients and staff, she displays anger. Ultimately, her faculty member reports her behaviors to the school and, since both the school and the hospital are designated as Drug Free Workplaces, following the federal guidelines, the school mandates a urine specimen for a drug screen. She initially refused, becoming inappropriately angry and stating her rights are being violated. She is told that if she refuses, she will be placed on leave from the school. Ultimately, she agrees and an observed urine specimen is collected and, following chain of custody procedures, it is sent to an outside laboratory for evaluation. The results indicate the presence of cocaine, opiate, and benzodiazepine metabolites. In conference with school officials, Amy discloses that as a result of her anxiety and depression, her primary care physician (PCP) prescribed Xanax. She almost immediately began to misuse the prescription and eventually her PCP told her she was being "cut off" from more prescriptions. She eventually began buying the drug from the street. A well-intentioned friend gave her a few oxycodone tablets to "calm her down." However, again, she liked the feeling these drugs caused and she also added opioids to her "shopping list." Eventually, her friends and family noticed her sedated sensorium and her supplier told her that cocaine would reverse the sedation. She got some cocaine and noticed how much energy it gave her—the very thing she needed to help her through the day. However, because of the "ups and downs" the various drugs caused, she was constantly medicating herself with all three drugs—benzodiazepines, opioids, and cocaine—trying to find the proper "cocktail" to help get her through the day. She agreed that her use was out of control.

Questions

- What is the best course of action when a student's behavior is suspicious of substance misuse/abuse?
- Who should the Director of the BSN Second Degree Nursing Program consult?
- What is best practice with respect to this case?

SUBSTANCE MISUSE: LEGAL PRINCIPLES AND REVIEW OF THE LITERATURE

The use, misuse, and abuse of psychoactive substances continues to pose major threats to the health of the nation in general and specifically to nurses, nursing students, and other healthcare practitioners. Alcohol and other drug abuse must be identified swiftly in the college/university and healthcare setting in order to protect patients and to provide for the safe withdrawal management of the impaired nurse/student. However, it is important to note that substance abuse causes, complicates, or coexists with other health problems that lead to hospitalization and signs of substance abuse may be masked by more obvious symptoms of the admitting diagnosis.

The phrase "substance use disorder" refers to the full range of complaints from abuse to a dependency or an addiction to alcohol or drugs. The term "addiction" refers to the compulsive use of chemicals (drugs or alcohol) and the inability to stop using them despite all the problems caused by their use. A person with an addiction is unable to stop drinking or taking drugs despite serious health, economic, vocational, legal, spiritual, and social consequences. The American Nurses Association (ANA) estimates that 6% to 8% of nurses use alcohol or drugs to an extent that is sufficient to impair professional performance (National Council of State Boards of Nursing [NCSBN], 2011).

So, what does a person who is addicted to a psychoactive substance look like? Addiction affects people from all walks of life. We have identified pedestal professionals—those licensed to work with patients in the healthcare system. The unfortunate reality is that substance abuse is the number one public health problem in the United States in this time of the "opioid epidemic"; there is greater morbidity and mortality occurring as a result of the use and abuse of alcohol, tobacco, illicit and prescribed psychoactive drugs than any other single preventable cause of illness and death in the United States (Gordis, 2009). General signs/symptoms of substance use problems include: excessive use of days off and sick time, absences without notice, improbable excuses for absences or late work, long trips to bathroom, and disappearance from clinical or lab site, and so forth. One also needs to be vigilant for diversion of medications at the worksite. This can include coming to work on days off and volunteering for overtime. Of course, colleagues misinterpret these behaviors as dedication and the diversion can continue without concern. Other signs include incorrect narcotic counts, consistent volunteering to administer medications, and "forgetting" to get witnesses to verify the wasting of unused medications. Substance abuse is an issue that must be managed in nursing education for the safety of patients, students, and the profession. "Clear policies show a commitment to professional standards by academic administrators and faculty and specify what occurs when standards are violated" (Monroe, 2009, p. 276). Substance abuse policies should address the policy and procedures related to any unlawful use, manufacture, distribution, or possession of controlled or illegal substances or alcohol, as substance abuse may significantly affect the ability of students to administer safe care to patients entrusted to them in a clinical healthcare setting. The development of such a policy should include nursing faculty, academic administrators, substance abuse experts, legal counsel, and consultation from clinical affiliates and the state board of nursing.

Every state is given the power to regulate professionals within their jurisdiction whereby rules and regulations are implemented and enforced as they are related to the practice of nursing (Dunn, 2005). Boards of nursing are the administrative agencies that were created by statute to regulate nursing with an explicit duty to protect the public from unsafe nursing practice. These statutes are referred to as Practice Acts, and among other purposes define the qualifications of nurses, define the practice of nursing and scope of practice and establish disciplinary procedures. The boards of nursing have no inherent authority and have only those powers granted by the statute. They cannot conflict with existing law or go beyond the delegated rulemaking authority. The board's rulemaking function operationalizes the general statutory framework and sets standards for the profession. In this way, nurses/students are provided with information related to misconduct, unprofessional conduct, and incompetence or being unfit to practice. Although jurisdictions vary as to whether all or some of the regulations are included in their Nurse Practice Act, they generally provide the authority for a board to develop a nondisciplinary alternative program for nurses with a substance use disorder. The board will also act whenever it receives information alleging that a nurse has engaged in some form of misconduct. Each state's board of nursing has its own outline for the complaint process, which must be followed. A nurse/student with a substance use disorder, and the presence of impairment and diversion are potential areas of concern and boards of nursing must have rules to address these concerns. Related causes for disciplinary action by boards of nursing may include:

- Drug diversion
- A positive drug screen for which there is no lawful prescription
- Addiction to a controlled substance
- Violation of a state or federal narcotics or controlled substances act
- Criminal convictions
- Illegal use of a drug or controlled substance
- Impairment from use of a drug or controlled substance (either physically, mentally, or both)

Some of the important laws that have implications for how boards of nursing manage substance use disorders include the following.

The *Rehabilitation Act of 1973* defines "disability" as any record of, or current, physical or mental impairment that substantially limits one or more major life activities. The Act protects those with disabilities from discriminatory employment practices in the federal sector, including programs that receive federal financial assistance. Under the Act, individuals who are *recovering* from alcohol abuse (as evidenced by active treatment in a rehabilitation program or successful completion of such a program) may be deemed as having a disability and are thus protected under the Act. Individuals who are *recovering* from abuse of an illegal substance (as evidenced by active treatment in a rehabilitation program or successful completion of such a program) may also be deemed as having a disability, and are protected under the Act. In both cases, employers must provide reasonable accommodations in the workplace for those individuals, unless doing so would cause undue hardship. Reasonable accommodations may include such things as limited access to controlled substances, stable shift assignments, or no overtime (NCSBN, 2011). Individuals who are currently engaged in illegal drug use are not deemed as having a disability and are not protected under the Act. In such cases, employment can be denied or terminated. Likewise, despite the designation of having a "disability," if employment of an individual is determined to be a threat to patients' or the employees safety, or if there is diversion, theft of property, or violation of an established conduct code, employment can be terminated. The Americans with Disabilities Act of 1990 (ADA) prohibits discrimination on the basis of a disability by an employer, unrelated to receiving federal funds. Similar to the Rehabilitation Act, illegal use of drugs or alcohol is not included within ADA's definitions of a disability. An employee may receive protection by the ADA if the employee has successfully completed a drug rehabilitation program and is no longer engaging in the illegal use of drugs. The Health Insurance Portability and

Accountability Act of 1996 (HIPAA) protects any and all information that could reasonably be used to identify an individual and requires that disclosures be limited to the information necessary to carry out the purpose of the disclosure.

As already stated, the organization and structure of the disciplinary process varies among states. For example, in some states, the board of nursing makes the final administrative determination concerning discipline, with review available only in court. In other states, the board does not make the final administrative decision on discipline, and it is an administrative hearings commission or larger public agency, of which the board of nursing is one component, that makes the final determination subject to judicial review. In some states, an administrative hearings commission may make the findings of fact, but the nursing board makes the final determination as to violation and penalty. Some state licensing acts limit access to judicial review. At any rate, nurses, students, and nursing faculty should be aware of their state's statutes regarding procedural requirements for disciplinary actions. Undergraduate students (who do not hold an RN license) will generally not be subject to the board's disciplinary action; however, any past drug charges may impede the student from obtaining an RN license.

DISCUSSION OF CASE STUDY

Given the serious allegations, the faculty member consults with the assistant dean for clinical compliance, who is responsible for clinical health clearance and safety. Concurring in the concern, the assistant dean calls Ms. Burke to a meeting in her office and from there escorts her to the office for student and employee health for a drug test. A urine and hair analysis are obtained in accordance with the college's substance abuse policy for student majors that include a clinical component in the curriculum. You also suspend Ms. Burke from her clinical rotation pending an investigation and drug screen results.

Once a problem of alcohol or other drug misuse has been identified, documentation of all findings (including behavioral changes and impairing behavior) must be completed. Additionally, the faculty member should note any physical and psychological signs of withdrawal as well as any drug-seeking behavior. Most, if not all, state boards of nursing mandate the reporting of a nurse, to either the board itself or a state-sponsored peer assistance agency. For those fearing retaliation, when the nursing faculty has a duty imposed by law to disclose confidential information about a student who is misusing drugs, and the disclosure is made in compliance with such law, the nursing faculty is protected from liability. It is important to check with the respective state board of nursing for specific guidelines. Additionally, as in Case Study 22.1, since the student, Amy Burke, is *not yet licensed*, the academic program/college/university must have clear guidelines as to how to handle cases of substance use/abuse including referral for treatment. DiClemente (2003) recommends, when interacting with the nursing student, to use an empathic, nonjudgmental, nonconfrontational style. Nursing students with an untreated addiction can jeopardize patient safety because of impaired judgment, slower reaction time, diverting prescribed drugs from patients for their own use, neglect of patients, and making a variety of other errors (Dunn, 2005). Many states have Peer Nurse Assistance Programs for nursing students, which are discussed later in this chapter.

Clinical rotations occur at independent hospitals, healthcare facilities, and organizations that are affiliated with academic nursing programs. Under the law, employers are allowed to investigate the fitness of applicants for jobs and to continue doing so after they have become employed, as long as they have provided notice to the employee of their requirements and those requirements have a reasonable relationship to the job being performed. The application for employment (or even volunteering) at a clinical site may require a fairly rigorous investigation of the applicant's past because of the sensitive nature of the services being performed, the personal disclosures made by and vulnerability of the patients, and the accessibility of drugs. The investigation can include, among other things, a criminal background check, child abuse check, FBI fingerprinting, drug test, and a check for immunizations prior to the start of the clinical practicum rotations. Students participating in clinical practica are subject to rigorous background checks before entering a clinical facility.

Participation in clinical practicum rotations is a required part of the curriculum for most nursing students. Students need to comply with the university's drug and alcohol policies as outlined in the student handbook. Clinical affiliates generally do not permit students with a positive drug screen into their facilities. In Case Study 22.1, a student may be unable to complete the nursing program, as the clinical sites may be unwilling to allow the student a clinical placement unless the student has completed a Peer Nurse Assistance Program and has demonstrated sobriety for a required length of time. The ramifications are even greater than just the one job: RN-BSN and graduate nursing programs (where students hold an RN license) may be required to report any positive results of background checks and drug screens to the board of nursing in the state where the student is licensed. It is also likely that university procedures require that students with a positive drug screen for illegal substances also be referred to the office of student conduct (or similar judicial office) for review and adjudication.

University policies may prohibit employees from working while they are taking certain kinds of prescription drugs. They may also impose sanctions for conduct involving substance abuse, even if it occurs after hours and off premises.

Substance abuse policies and procedures should also include methods for assessing substance abuse problems, intervention, and student follow-up (Clark, 1999), in addition to specifying the range of sanctions that can be imposed. Because nursing students are trusted with caring for patients, a nursing program may impose a harsher penalty for a drug violation than would otherwise be imposed by the university.

Nursing majors are at high risk for developing substance abuse problems. Clark (1999) noted that many impaired professional nurses were addicted as students. Students who abuse drugs typically will exhibit a pattern of objective, observable behaviors that eventually compromise patient safety and clinical standards of performance. Such behaviors include irritability, excessive absenteeism, tardiness, red eyes, hand tremors, leaving clinical area frequently, unsafe clinical performance, and impaired judgment (Dunn, 2005).

It is imperative that colleges and schools of nursing develop fair, comprehensive policies and procedures regarding this important issue. Policies need to offer assistance to the student in distress while at the same time safeguarding the needs of patients. Although most nursing academic administrators recognize that substance abuse is an illness requiring early intervention, academic administrators also need to comply with state boards of nursing, university policies, and clinical affiliation requirements.

For similar reasons, policies need to be developed for students who have separated from the school or college because of substance abuse issues and who wish to return; to do so, they must comply with the requirements of these regulatory bodies and affiliates. Such polices typically specify that students may be eligible to reenter the nursing program in certain circumstances if they can demonstrate satisfactory evidence of successful completion of treatment and documentation of 24 months of sustained recovery. Factors that have been identified as helpful for reentry into practice include 12-step program participation, random drug screens, and sponsorship on a peer-assisted support group. The student must also provide medical clearance from the appropriate individual coordinating the therapeutic intervention and evidence of current, active nursing licensure if enrolled in a post-licensure program. A nursing student in active recovery from substance abuse will be monitored closely, particularly in clinical practice. Frequent evaluations will be mandated and stipulated in the contract delineating the contingencies of programmatic return.

Nursing faculty and academic administrators need to be humanistic in their approach to impaired students while removing them quickly from the clinical practice site. It is the goal of schools of nursing to ensure patient safety while promoting the student's well-being (Monroe, 2009).

 WHEN TO CONSULT THE UNIVERSITY COUNSEL

Consult the university counsel when you need:

- To seek advice related to verbal/written communication with student
- To interpret the state board of nursing reporting law(s)
- To seek advice related to temporary suspension
- To review documentation

FINDINGS AND DISPOSITION

The director of BSN Second Degree Nursing Program first confirmed that Amy Burke's urine drug screen was positive for cocaine, opiate, and benzodiazepine metabolites. The director then scheduled a meeting with Ms. Burke and the Dean. Because the use of illicit drugs is a crime, the Director sought advice from university counsel. In accordance with counsel's advice, the director began by warning Ms. Burke that using cocaine, opiate, and benzodiazepine was a serious violation of the university's code of conduct; that anything she said would be written down and reported; that it was all right if she chose not to answer any questions, but that her refusal to answer would be included in her file; and that the director would refer the matter to the office of student conduct following the meeting. At the meeting, Ms. Burke admitted to having a problem and states that she took the drugs to get through the day. You encourage her to seek treatment and she begins to cry and admits that she has a problem and wants help. She states, "I have a 2-year old daughter, I do not want to live like this anymore." As a result of the meeting, Ms. Burke agrees to enter to the Peer Nurse Assistance Program in your state. You contact the Peer Nurse Assistance Program to arrange Ms. Burke's initial evaluation. You also report the matter to the nursing student conduct committee for review, noting that Ms. Burke is entering the Peer Nurse Assistance Program. Ms. Burke takes a medical leave from the BSN Second Degree Nursing Program and the drug violation is placed in her academic record. Her reentry will be contingent upon her compliance with the Peer Nurse Assistance Program contract. She is expected to be out of school for the remainder of the school year.

The ANA estimates that 6% to 8% of nurses use drugs or alcohol to an extent that it impairs professional performance (Brent, 2019). One way the stigma of substance misuse is perpetuated is through the reluctance that nurses have toward confronting another nurse or student when the disease is suspected or even known (McKenna, 2005). Nurses/students/faculty members need to be aware of their own stereotypes and evaluate themselves for any generalizations, images, and misconceptions they may hold about addiction. For example, one study discovered that male nurses with a substance use disorder issue often go unnoticed because they do not fit the stereotypical image of someone who has a substance use disorder (Dittman, 2008).

Nursing faculty members who suspect a substance use disorder in students need to be provided with guidelines and a clear process for reporting their concerns in a discreet and nonthreatening manner. If guidelines are not provided, the nursing faculty member may inadvertently cover up for the person instead, which can contribute to additional dangers for the affected student as well as for patients. Data indicate that the likelihood of successful treatment outcomes is higher when treatment is implemented earlier in the addiction process (Martin, Schaffer, & Campbell, 1999).

For students who hold a license, a license to practice nursing carries with it the ability to earn a living, which means the license is a form of property and cannot be taken away without giving the nurse due process of the law, as granted by the 14th Amendment of the U.S. Constitution. The concept of due process at its most basic involves giving the nurse a notice of the charges and an opportunity to be heard by an impartial tribunal. The degree of process that is due in any given situation is a balancing of the property interest and risk of error in depriving someone of that interest (*Barry v. Barchi*, 1979). That being said, many states allow the regulatory agency authority to take immediate action against the license, which would render it inactive or suspended, and then to follow up with a hearing on the issues. Unfortunately, following this procedure is not without complications. The process is very resource intensive due to the right of the nurse to have a prompt hearing and the need of the nurse's counsel to obtain evidence, prepare motions, and prepare witnesses in a short amount of time. This process is not without criticism since the nature of the emergency action supersedes due process. Proponents of the regulatory process would argue that patient safety takes precedence over the nurse's right to a license.

ALTERNATIVE TO DISCIPLINE PROGRAMS

Since the 1970s, non-disciplinary programs, which offer an alternative to traditional discipline, have been used by a growing number of boards of nursing. The requirements for participation by nurses in an alternative program require the nurse to sign a contract for participation in the program and/

or have a board order. The nurse is also required to undergo drug testing, workplace monitoring, and to take part in counseling—group and/or individual. Utilizing an alternative program allows the nurse to remain active in nursing, after treatment and demonstrated sobriety, while being monitored. In this way, by continuing to work or go to school, they contribute to their financial status or future, further supporting recovery. Such programs are often referred to as Peer Assistance Programs since they help nurses remain substance-free and active in the workforce (Fogger & McGuinness, 2009). Although each state has its own contractual requirements, they have common requirements such as a written contract, drug screening protocol, evaluation criteria for treatment and treatment providers, including total abstinence from mood-altering drugs and alcohol, participation in educational programs, and therapeutic modalities. Student nurses who are not yet licensed are also able to participate in Peer Assistance Programs in some states, thereby staying in school with subsequent monitoring and contractual obligations (Cotter & Glasgow, 2012). In the states having alternative programs (a rehabilitation option in lieu of discipline), confidential reporting to the programs absolves the colleague from reporting to the nursing regulatory board (American Association of Nurse Anesthetists, 2019).

When investigating alleged illicit use of controlled substances or drug diversion, the faculty member should consult their supervisor or legal counsel, and identify and follow university policies/protocols. Faculty should consider the following recommendations:

- Note changes in observed performance. Documentation of problematic performance should be objectively stated to avoid any potential liability issues with wrongful accusations.
- Identify and maintain documents that contain information about possible impairment or diversion of drugs.
- Ensure that all related documents are kept confidential but are easily accessible to appropriate university, hospital, and law enforcement officials.
- Any documented observations should be objective and fact based rather than opinions or conclusions. (For instance, document behaviors such as gait, mood swings, outbursts, and observations such as appearance, speech, pupil size, etc.). Remember, the observed symptoms could be attributed to conditions other than substance misuse.
- Include any incident reports and witness statements and ensure that they are fact based.
- If the nursing student admits to diverting, obtain the statement in writing. Have a witness present. (Sometimes, the student may state they were unwillingly pressured to make such a statement which is later recanted.)
- Obtain information from the student as to what drugs were diverted or used, during what time period, and the process followed in getting, using, and recovering from the substance.
- The student, upon identifying impairing behavior, should be referred for a urine drug screen and Breathalyzer for alcohol, pursuant to the university's policy.
- Ensure that patient and staff safety are not be compromised.
- Prevention or early identification of illicit use of controlled substances is most important.

Monitoring Tips That Are Warning Signs of Potential Diversion

- *Medication administration reports show that a single nurse administers more PRN medications than other nurses.*
- *When the medication administration is documented as given, the patient is not on the unit.*
- *Although the medication was signed out on the narcotics log, there is no documentation that it was actually administered in the medication administration record or nurses' notes.*
- *There is regular and frequent documentation of the nurse/student administering medications to other nurses' patients.*
- *Discarding of unused controlled substances is regularly documented without the signature of a witness, or it appears that the witness signature is forged.*

> ▪ *Patients regularly report that pain medication was not effective when the identified nurse/ student documents administering the medication.*
>
> ▪ *Controlled substances are signed out for patients that have no record of an order for the medication.*

RELEVANT LEGAL CASES

Mississippi State Board of Nursing v. John Wilson, No. 91-CA-0054, 624 So.2d 485 (Miss. 1993)

Woodis v. Westark Community College, 160 F.3d 435 (8th Cir. 1998)

In the case of *Mississippi State Board of Nursing v. John Wilson* (1993), John Wilson was an RN who was employed as a nursing supervisor in the chemical dependency unit at the Mississippi State Hospital. Following the introduction of considerable evidence at hearings, the state board concluded that he was guilty of three violations of using habit-forming drugs—primarily cocaine—and issued a final order revoking his license. Mr. Wilson appealed this decision to the local court (the Hinds County Chancery Court). After a trial, the court found that Mr. Wilson did have a history of drug use, but that the incidents were isolated, being separated by periods of 3 to 8 years. Because this did not constitute continuous use of habit-forming drugs, the court reversed the finding of the board that Wilson was addicted to or dependent on habit-forming drugs. For that reason, the court held that his license should not have been revoked and reversed the decision of the state board. The state board then filed an appeal, and the Mississippi Supreme Court upheld its original decision, reversing the trial court and sending the case back to the state board to implement its original decision.

In *Woodis v. Westark Community College* (1998), Rosia Woodis was enrolled as a nursing student and pursuing a degree as an LPN. In her third semester in the program, the police arrested Ms. Woodis for attempting to obtain a controlled substance using a fraudulent prescription. Upon receiving notice of the arrest and the charges against the student, Dr. Sandi Sanders, the community college's vice president of student affairs, promptly suspended Ms. Woodis pending the outcome of the police investigation. Dr. Sanders sent a letter to Ms. Woodis advising her of this decision and of her due process rights as set forth in the Westark student handbook. Ms. Woodis appealed the decision to a five-member disciplinary appeals committee, which not only upheld the suspension but, hearing the evidence behind the arrest, concluded that Ms. Woodis had violated the school's code of conduct and imposed the sanction of expulsion. Ms. Woodis appealed those decisions to the court. In upholding the expulsion decision, the court held that the disciplinary committee had properly found that the student had violated the school's code of conduct and that the student's rights to due process had not been violated.

Although the courts ruled differently in each of these cases, both *Woodis v. Westark Community College* (1998) and *Mississippi State Board of Nursing v. John Wilson* (1993) reveal that specific policies regarding drug use and abuse are invaluable when acting on suspicion or reports of student substance abuse. For example, the Westark student handbook's specific descriptions of the conduct that was not allowed and the process that would be followed during a drug and police investigation left the courts satisfied that the student's interests were protected while the university was conducting its investigation. The problem for the Mississippi State Board of Nursing's substance abuse policy was that it was not entirely clear: Had it been specific in stating that the board could revoke a nurse's license solely based on illegal drug use (as opposed to addiction or regular use), then there probably would not have been a disagreement between the trial court and the supreme court, and the trial court would have been more likely to affirm the decision of the board based on clear warning given in the policy. In other words, the question of whether the appellee was addicted to the drug would not have made a difference in their decision. These cases illustrate the need for colleges and universities to have a policy for drug use, testing, and monitoring that is clear, and a process for investigating allegations of violations that moves quickly toward a resolution while protecting the rights of all involved.

Prevention Tips

To help prevent substance abuse in students, educate students about the risk of chemical dependency among healthcare providers and the risk that it causes not just to patients, but also to society at large. Enhance their ability to recognize impaired healthcare professionals, and reinforce the importance of reporting and the significance of appropriate intervention. Make sure that students have the contact information for people who can help them or their colleagues if substance abuse becomes an issue. It is also important to remind students of the school's substance abuse policy and to show them where they can locate a copy of it.

SUMMARY

When a student or nurse is suspected of substance abuse, it is suggested that faculty or fellow nurses and peers confront the student or nurse by taking the individual aside and privately addressing their concern about the behavior. The faculty member should also consult an administrator to receive assistance and support (Banerjee, 2006). Except in extreme situations, it is likely that an appropriate response is for the individual and the university to enter into an agreement by which the individual agrees immediately to cease the improper conduct and begin addictions treatment with the goal to return to work/school and maintain client safety (O'Hagan, 2005). The academic institution will have to render a decision regarding the student's eligibility to continue in the program—at the time, after a suspension, or never. The student should be allowed to continue in school based on conditions consistent with the institution's drug and alcohol policy. Although a report of the transgression may be required at the time of the conduct, the state board of nursing will not become involved until the student graduates and a decision is needed about whether to issue an initial registered professional nursing license. If a student participates in a Peer Nurse Assistance program under the auspices of the board of nursing and complies with prescribed treatment, the board will generally view this participation favorably and permit licensure. What is certain is that faculty and students require education about this very important issue. Academic institutions need drug and alcohol use and screening and monitoring policies firmly in place to deal effectively with this persistent social problem.

ETHICAL CONSIDERATIONS

In considering ethical policies regarding substance misuse, all stakeholders need to be taken into account. These stakeholders include, of course, patients and future patients who may be at risk of malpractice due to substance abuse by a nurse or nursing student. The nursing duty to protect the health and safety of patients is not only in conflict with substance abuse by nurses but obligates nursing education programs to screen for and provide education about these problems. The nursing program or department itself may be seen also as a stakeholder as a nursing student on a clinical rotation with a substance problem could reflect poorly upon the program. And the nurse or nursing student is also a stakeholder. The disease model of addiction is continuing to eclipse the moral model. This perception further emphasizes the obligation to treat the affected professional with care, respect, and dignity. The disease may be one that places innocents at risk, but it is still one for which a chance of recovery should be offered, rather than abandoning the affected when they become inconvenient.

Healthcare professionals—especially nurses and nursing students—have specific and unique workplace risk factors that may increase their risk for the development of a substance use disorder. These include access, attitude, stress, and lack of education about a substance use disorder. They share many other risk factors with the general population that also contribute to their susceptibility to developing a substance use disorder. Nurses with an addiction rarely self-report for fear of losing their jobs, licenses, and livelihoods (Copp, 2009). Students are afraid that they will be dismissed from school and lose their chance of becoming a nurse. Aside from seriously affecting the physical and psychological integrity of the user, substance abuse may significantly affect the ability of students to administer safe care to the patients who are entrusted to them in a clinical healthcare setting. For these reasons, it is important that academic nursing programs have policies and procedures related to the detection of drug and alcohol use and that they authorize the testing and monitoring of students. This is particularly important for those who are involved in patient-care activities. Such policies should inform students who are enrolled in a major that includes a clinical healthcare component.

Creating an environment that encourages reporting is most important for reducing the stigma, maintaining transparency, rehabilitating the student, and protecting the public. In utilizing a nonpunitive monitoring program, most nurses and students will agree to undergo treatment and monitoring to save their licenses and/or to stay in school. However, the fact that alternative programs are not punitive does not mean individual accountability is ignored. Nursing students who enroll in an alternative program are accountable to themselves, their program monitor, their counselors and other nurses, and their clinical site supervisors/faculty members, and are held responsible for abiding by the contract they signed upon entering the program. Relapse is yet another important issue to consider as the risk of relapse doubles in people with comorbid psychiatric disorders such as depression and anxiety (Schellekens, deJong, Buitelaar, & Verkes, 2015). There is also an increase in the prevalence of substance use disorders among nurses working in medical–surgical units, long-term care facilities, and outpatient centers for reasons less understood (Mumba, 2016). Addiction is a disease and alternative approaches to discipline with required treatment are humane and ethical. Peer Nurse Assistance Programs ensure that nurses or nursing students with addictive and/or other psychiatric disorders receive needed care that enables them to return to practice and prevent disciplinary action and loss of licensure. In severe cases where a patient is harmed due to a student's substance use, disciplinary action may be warranted and just. Spirituality can also provide a sense of meaning to life, ability to cope with stressful situations, and interpersonal connectedness (Monod et al., 2011), all of which are important to successful recovery from chemical dependency and the prevention of relapse.

CRITICAL ELEMENTS TO CONSIDER

- Assess students for signs of substance abuse.
- Offer faculty development programs on substance abuse.
- Maintain student confidentiality.
- Follow your institution's substance abuse policy.
- Consult legal counsel for advice.
- Consult the dean of students for assistance and support.
- Document faculty report of suspicion of drug/alcohol use.

Include the following information in documentation:

- Date, time, and location of incident
- Behavioral, visual, olfactory, or auditory observations
- Whether the student admitted to use of drugs/alcohol
- Whether drugs/alcohol were discovered on the student
- Witnesses to the student's behavior
- Whether the student agreed to drug/alcohol testing
- Results of drug/alcohol test (if completed)
- Consult the state board of nursing for reporting advice
- Consult the university attorney and the dean of students
- Offer education sessions on substance abuse to students during orientation and throughout the student experience
- Offer faculty development sessions on substance abuse among students
- Develop clear, comprehensive policies related to student substance abuse with multiple stakeholders (faculty, dean of students, substance abuse experts, legal counsel, clinical affiliates, and state board of nursing consultation)
- Include the substance abuse policy in the student handbook

- Provide a list of support groups for students if they suspect substance abuse in their peers
- Designate a faculty member to become a peer assistance advisor or faculty advocate who is current and knowledgeable about substance abuse as well as serves as a liaison between professional assistance programs and the school (Monroe, 2009)
- Adhere to all policies and affiliation agreement requirements
- Provide due process to students. Suspend the student from clinical activities until allegations of substance abuse are cleared
- Keep all information related to the student's substance abuse confidential
- Consult individual state board of nursing related to reporting requirements for RNs
- Develop a reentry policy for those students who are separated from the university for substance abuse

Helpful Resources

- The International Nurses Society on Addictions (IntNSA): www.intnsa.org
- The American Association of Nurse Anesthetists Health and Wellness Peer Assistance (AANA): https://www.aana.com/practice/health-and-wellness-peer-assistance
- National Council of State Boards of Nursing. (2011). *Substance use disorder in nursing: A resource manual and guidelines for alternative and disciplinary monitoring programs.* Chicago, IL: Author.

References

American Association of Nurse Anesthetists. (2019). *Health and wellness: Peer assistance.* Retrieved from https://www.aana.com/practice/health-and-wellness-peer-assistance

Barry v. Barchi, 443 U.S. 55 (1979).

Banerjee, L. (2006). Ask a practice advisor: Substance abuse and chemical dependency by nurse. *SRNA Bulletin.* Regina, SK: Saskatchewan Registered Nurses Association.

Brent, N. (2019). When a BON disciplinary process is based on substance misuse disorder. *American Nurse Today, 14*(3), 14–16. Retrieved from https://www.myamericannurse.com/bon-disciplinary-substance-use-disorder-part-1/

Clark, C. (1999). Substance abuse among nursing students: Establishing a comprehensive policy and procedure for faculty intervention. *Nurse Educator, 24*(2), 16–19.

Copp, M. A. B. (2009). *Drug addiction among nurses: Confronting a quiet epidemic.* Retrieved from http://www.nursingworldnigeria.com/2015/02/drug-addiction-among-nurses-confronting-a-quiet-epidemic/

Cotter, V., & Glasgow, M. E. S. (2012). Student drug testing in nursing education. *Journal of Professional Nursing, 28*(3), 186–189. doi:10.1016/j.profnurs.2011.11.017

DiClemente, C. C. (2003). *Addiction and change: How addictions develop and addicted people recover.* New York, NY: Guilford Press.

Dittman, P. W. (2008). Male nurses and substance use disorder masterminding the nursing environment. *Nursing Administration Quarterly, 32*(4), 324–330. doi:10.1097/01.NAQ.0000336731.64878.66

Dunn, D. (2005). Substance abuse among nurses: Defining the issue. *AORN Journal, 82*(4), 573–596. doi:10.1016/S0001-2092(06)60028-8

Duquesne University. (2019). *Bachelor of Science in Nursing 2019-2020 academic year student handbook.* Retrieved from https://duq.edu/assets/Documents/nursing/Handbooks/Undergradaute%20student%20handbook-2019-2020.pdf

Fogger, S.A. & McGuinness, T. (2009). Alabama's nurse monitoring programs: The nurse's experience of being monitored. *Journal of Addictions Nursing, 20*, 142–149. doi:10.1080/10884600903078928

Gordis, E. (2009). *Epidemiology* (4th ed.). Philadelphia, PA: Saunders Elsevier.

Martin, A. C., Schaffer, S. D., & Campbell, R. (1999). Managing alcohol-related problems in the primary care setting. *Nurse Practitioner, 24*(8), 14. doi:10.1097/00006205-199908000-00002

McKenna, G. A. (2005). Diagnosis and treatment of substance use disorder in professionals. *Hawaii Dental Journal, 36*(4), 13–15.

Mississippi State Board of Nursing v. John Wilson, No. 91-CA-0054, 624 So.2d 485 (Miss. 1993).

Monod, S., Brennan, M., Rochat, E., Martin, E., Rochat, S., & Bula, C. J. (2011). Instruments measuring spirituality in clinical research: A systematic review. *Journal of General Internal Medicine, 26,* 1345–1357. doi:10.1007/s11606-011-1769-7

Monroe, T. (2009). Addressing substance abuse among nursing students: Development of a prototype alternative-to-dismissal policy. *Journal of Nursing Education, 48*(5), 272–278. doi:10.3928/01484834-20090416-06

Mumba, M. N. (2016). A retrospective descriptive study of chemically impaired nurses in Texas. *Proquest Dissertations and Theses Global.* Retrieved from http://www.proquest.com/products-services/pqdtglobal.html

National Council of State Boards of Nursing. (2011). *Substance use disorder in nursing: A resource manual and guidelines for alternative and disciplinary monitoring programs.* Chicago, IL: Author.

O'Hagan, R. (2005). Consensual complaint resolution agreement: Dealing with an addiction/chemical dependency. *SRNA Bulletin.* Regina, SK: Saskatchewan Registered Nurses Association.

Schellekens, A. F. A., deJong, C. A. J., Buitelaar, J. K., & Verkes, R. J. (2015). Co-morbid anxiety disorders predict early relapse after inpatient alcohol treatment. *European Psychiatry, 30*(1), 128–136. doi:10.1016/j.eurpsy.2013.08.006

Woodis v. Westark Community College, 160 F.3d 435 (8th Cir.) (1998).

Appendix 22.1

Sample Substance Abuse Policy

The School of Nursing has a vested interest in the health and welfare of its students. Moreover, it has a responsibility in ensuring that students enrolled in the pre-licensure nursing program are eligible to secure a license upon successful completion of the program and all students licensed and enrolled in graduate program are able to maintain their licensure. Furthermore, the School has a duty and obligation to protect the public health and safety.

The School recognizes that a substance use disorder is a medically recognized condition as defined by the *Diagnostic and Statistical Manual for Mental Disorders (DSM) 5th edition* that poses a risk for substantive harm to affected individuals, their contacts, and the general public. Therefore, the School will refer individuals who are identified as being at risk for a substance use disorder for professional assessment and, when so indicated, follow-up treatment.

The University and the School of Nursing are committed to providing compassionate and proactive assistance for students with substance abuse issues and their families and to afford students, who are not legally restricted and are no longer chemically impaired, the opportunity to continue their education without stigma or penalty, and to protecting society from harm that impaired students could cause.

INDICATIONS FOR REFERRAL FOR EVALUATION

Students subject to referral for a professional assessment include, but are not limited to, any or all of the following conditions:

- A positive finding on a criminal background check that suggests a potential active substance use disorder. Please note that the withdrawal or dismissal of legal charges or a "not guilty" disposition is separate and distinct from the presence of a substance use disorder and does not relieve the student from complying with referral for assessment when so warranted.
- Referral from the University Office of Student Conduct
- Positive drug screen
- Being identified as the subject of a drug-related criminal investigation
- Reliable information from independent sources
- Evidence of drug tampering or misappropriation
- Accidents or illnesses caused by impairment related to substance use
- Impairment or intoxication in the clinical and/or didactic setting
- Following a clinical-related injury or illness
- Observation of poor judgment or careless acts which caused or had the potential to cause patient injury, jeopardize the safety of self or others, or resulted in damage to equipment
- Suspicion of a substance use disorder based on behavioral cues as reported by faculty, staff, experiential preceptors, employers, peers, and/or other stakeholders

- Odor of drugs or alcohol on a student
- Physical symptoms (including but not limited to behavior such as slurred speech, decreased motor coordination, difficulty maintaining balance, etc.)
- Possession of an illegal substance
- Self-referral

DRUG AND/OR ALCOHOL TESTING

The School reserves the right to order a drug/alcohol screen for cause, such as a student who unexpectedly has a major deterioration in academic performance or who demonstrates bizarre, erratic, or unprofessional behavior. Drug screens are also performed as a condition of participating in the clinical education component of the curriculum.

If a didactic or clinical faculty member suspects possible substance abuse by a student who is in class or in a clinical setting, they will report the suspicious behavior to the Faculty of Record and the Assistant Dean of Student Affairs immediately.

Once notification occurs that a student is suspected of violating the substance abuse policy, the student will be instructed to report to the designated testing laboratory. The cost of any drug or alcohol testing will be assumed by the nursing program. The Chair of the Undergraduate program has the authority to temporarily suspend the student from the clinical practicum pending the final results of any tests.

REFERRAL FOR EVALUATION: PENNSYLVANIA NURSING PEER ASSISTANCE PROGRAM

Students who are enrolled in the pre-licensure (traditional or second degree) program, and those students enrolled in any of the Program at the School of Nursing who hold a nursing license in the state of Pennsylvania, will be referred to the Pennsylvania Nurse Peer Assistance Program (PNAP) for further assessment. PNAP is an organization sanctioned by the Pennsylvania State Board of Nursing whose purpose is to aid individuals who may need treatment, protect the ability of individuals to secure and maintain a nursing license, and ensure the public health and safety. Its recommendations are supported by the School and the University.

In the event of a positive diagnostic impression by an independent drug and alcohol counselor as identified by PNAP, continuation of the student in the pre-licensure program, or post-licensure program if licensed in Pennsylvania, will be contingent upon compliance with any treatment recommendations endorsed by PNAP. Where so indicated, such students will also be required to engage in a monitoring contract administered by PNAP. Those individuals who are enrolled in any of the post-licensure nursing program and who hold a nursing license in a state other than Pennsylvania will be referred to the appropriate state board or peer assistance program.

PROCEDURE FOR VIOLATION OF SUBSTANCE USE/ABUSE POLICY

1. Students identified as in need of assessment of a possible substance use disorder (via faculty staff report or any other mechanism described previously) will be required to schedule an appointment to meet with the Assistant Dean for Student Affairs and a designated member of the School of Nursing staff or administration within three university days of notification.
2. If it is determined that a referral for a professional assessment is indicated, the student must contact PNAP within three university days for an initial intake and referral to a qualified drug and alcohol counselor as selected by PNAP.
3. When referral for assessment is indicated by PNAP, the Assistant Dean for Student Affairs and the Director of the PNAP program must be notified by the student, within five university days, of the scheduled date of the assessment.
4. Signed releases must be executed within five university days from referral to PNAP, allowing designated individuals to send and receive confidential information regarding the student referral, treatment, and progress, as applicable.

5. Professional assessments must be conducted within 10 university days of notification of the scheduled appointment.

6. Students who are recommended for treatment will be required to enter into a monitoring contract with PNAP. Designated individuals from the School, including the Assistant Dean for Student Affairs and the Dean, will be signatories to the contract. Enrollment in the PNAP program will continue for the duration of the student's enrollment in the nursing program, but not less than a period of 3 years. When applicable, students progressing into the profession after graduation, who have not yet completed the contracted time period in the PNAP program, will continue to be enrolled in the PNAP program under contract, until they have completed the minimum monitoring requirement.

7. Refusal to contact PNAP, submit to an assessment, enter into a monitoring contract, or comply with treatment recommendations, when so indicated, may result in notification to the Pennsylvania State Board of Nursing and dismissal from the nursing program.

8. A negative diagnostic impression or completion of previous treatment recommendations does not preclude a subsequent referral in the event of a new event, additional evidence, or continuation of a suspect behavioral pattern.

9. Costs for external assessments, treatment program, monitoring program, and any related fees are the responsibility of the student.

10. All records related to referrals, assessments, and monitoring of substance use disorders will be kept confidential.

The School will not support the matriculation and/or continued enrollment of anyone found guilty of

- Illegal possession of controlled substances with the intent to divert or distribute
- A felony

Final decisions for continuance in all nursing Program rest with the Assistant Dean for Student Affairs. Written appeals can be made to the Dean within 10 university days of notification of the dismissal from the program. Failure or refusal to comply with any aspect of the substance abuse policy is grounds for disciplinary sanction, including dismissal from the program. Examples of noncompliance include, but are not limited to, refusal to submit to immediate drug and alcohol testing, tampering or alteration of specimens, attempts to submit the samples of another person as the student's own, and failure to appropriately complete associated program or testing laboratory documents.

Note: Please consult Legal Counsel before adopting or revising this policy for your school.

Source: Duquesne University. (2019). *Bachelor of Science in Nursing 2019-2020 academic year student handbook.* Retrieved from https://duq.edu/assets/Documents/nursing/Handbooks/Undergradaute%20student%20handbook-2019-2020.pdf

23

Medical Marijuana and Nursing Students: An Evolving Higher Education Quandary

 Case Study 23.1
Medical Marijuana

Your role: You are Dr. Calumet, Associate Dean for Pre-licensure Nursing Programs

Emily Zoe is a new student in your university's second-degree, direct entry clinical nurse leader program, which grants both eligibility for registered nurse licensure and a master's degree with eligibility for clinical nurse leader certification. This program admits individuals who already have bachelor's degrees in other fields; students take nursing courses immediately in their first term and begin the clinical sequence in their second term. Emily, who previously earned a bachelor's degree in sociology at another university, has just started her first term in the program. She makes an appointment to speak with you about preclinical clearance screening. At your university, as at most others, all nursing students must undergo a criminal background check and a nine-panel urine toxicology screen that includes cocaine, opiates, amphetamines, tetrahydrocannabinol (THC), benzodiazepines, barbiturates, methadone, and other drugs prior to beginning any course with a patient care clinical experience.

During the meeting, Emily tells you that she has questions about the drug screening process. She discloses that she has rheumatoid arthritis and has struggled since her diagnosis 3 years previously to manage the condition and the chronic pain associated with her condition, all under the care of her rheumatologist. She has discussed her condition with the university's disability services office and has not requested accommodations. However, she also discloses to you that, because her pain management regime has not adequately controlled her chronic pain, her rheumatologist has strongly recommended that she begin a trial of medical marijuana, legal in your state and available through a certified dispensary. Both she and her provider feel strongly that this change in the pain management regimen is needed for her to feel well enough to complete the nursing program. She asks you how the decision to go ahead with a trial of medical marijuana might affect her standing as a nursing student in light of drug screening.

Questions
- What are the major considerations for the university and the program?
- What legal constraints are at play?
- How can the rights of the student be balanced, or even addressed, in the context of federal law that restricts the university's approach to students who use medical marijuana?

REVIEW OF THE LITERATURE AND LEGAL PRINCIPLES

State-Level Landscape of the Therapeutic Use of Marijuana

Since 1996, when California became the first U.S. state to legalize the use of marijuana for therapeutic purposes (National Conference of State Legislatures [NCSL], 2019), perspectives on its recreational and therapeutic uses have been evolving. In 2016, according to the Substance Abuse and Mental Health Services Administration (SAMHSA, 2017), approximately 24 million people, close to 9% of those aged 12 and older, reported using any form of marijuana in the past month. Many states in the United States have considered decriminalization of recreational use of marijuana, with varied outcomes by the respective state legislatures. Fourteen states currently have some legalized form of nonmedical use by adults (NCSL, 2019).

According to the National Conference of State Legislatures, as of summer 2019, 33 states, along with the District of Columbia and several U.S. territories, have enacted legislation that creates a comprehensive program in their state or territory for the use of one, some, and/or many forms of medical marijuana. Some state laws provide only for referral by licensed and certified providers and/or require access to licensed dispensaries for patients; some others are less restrictive. Thirteen other states have laws that permit, in some cases, limited use of products that are low in THC, considered the psychoactive ingredient in marijuana affecting cognition and sensorium, without criminal penalty (National Institute on Drug Abuse, 2019). A metabolite of THC, 9-carboxy-THC, is the constituent that is recognized in urine immunoassay drug screening (Centers for Disease Control and Prevention [CDC], 1983). Cannabidiol (CBD) is another cannabinoid in marijuana that, although not psychoactive, can have sensory-cognitive as well as therapeutic effects (Mead, 2017).

Federal Law and Guidance

Title 21, Code of Federal Regulations, includes the federal Controlled Substances Act (CSA). The CSA categorizes marijuana as a Schedule I controlled substance. This category refers to substances considered to have high-abuse risk, no defined medical use, and a lack of safety under medical supervision; only highly restricted research uses, approved by the federal government, are permitted (U.S. Department of Justice, Drug Enforcement Agency [DOJDEA], n.d.; Title 21 U.S.C.). Cannabis, or marijuana, as defined in federal law, also includes its components, derivatives, and extracts including THC and CBD; stalks, fiber, and seeds are exempted from the definition of marijuana. Hemp, a different variety of the plant, is low in THC and is not currently a controlled substance (DOJDEA, 2016). The term "medical marijuana" is not defined legally in federal statute, but reflects various provider and state regulatory perspectives on the use of marijuana, its derivatives and extracts, for therapeutic (medically related) purposes, based on specific state laws (Mead, 2017). Substances currently used for medical/therapeutic purposes include an array of products and formulations, many of which are THC based, although any formulation may contain different proportions of THC and/or CBD as specified by state laws. However, many CBD formulations also contain THC; the percentage of THC permitted in CBD products varies greatly by state statute, up to 5%. Individuals taking a CBD formulation can test positive on urine screens for THC that are completed by commercial laboratories (Quest Diagnostics, 2019).

The Drug-Free Schools and Communities Act Amendments of 1989 (Public Law 101-226) specifies that higher education institutions must certify to the federal Secretary of Education that the college or university has a program to prevent illegal drug and alcohol use by students and employees. This is required in order to retain eligibility for federal funds or federal financial assistance, including federally funded or guaranteed loans. The law additionally specifies that such programs include the imposition of sanctions for the use of illegal substances including drugs and alcohol, in accordance with local, state, and federal laws, up to and including such sanctions as suspension, expulsion, or referral for prosecution by law enforcement.

As marijuana is federally categorized as a Schedule I substance, despite decriminalization/medical marijuana legislation across a range of states, colleges and universities in these states hesitate to change their adjudication approaches to marijuana use by students. Specifically, concerns about loss of eligibility for federal funds continue to result in disharmony between colleges' procedures, sanctioning marijuana use on campus in line with both the CSA and the Drug-Free Schools and Communities Act Amendments, and the respective state laws decriminalizing adult or therapeutic uses (Bauer-Wolf, 2017). Therefore, higher education institutions are likely to sanction students when there is evidence of use of marijuana or other substances that are classified illegal by federal law. There is no waiver provision in the CSA or any other federal regulation or law for the use of medical marijuana, despite state laws that have decriminalized its use. According to Davidson (2015), "An institution that knowingly permits possession, use, or distribution of marijuana is at risk of losing, and even having to repay federal funding, although few, if any institutions have been required to do so." Issues regarding the location of use of legal marijuana have been raised, with some colleges and universities creating specific policies addressing off-campus versus on-campus use of medical marijuana and establishing procedures to allow off-campus living arrangements for students who require this therapy, while still prohibiting use on campus or at college-sponsored events (Tufts University, 2014; Williams College, n.d.).

Nursing Regulatory Guidelines

Little literature was located at the time of this writing regarding the use of medical marijuana by healthcare providers or by students, particularly students in the health sciences. The National Council of State Boards of Nursing (NCSBN) has promulgated extensive guidance related to the preparation of students and clinicians for care of people using medical marijuana (NCSBN Medical Marijuana Guidelines Committee, 2018). In 2018, the NCSBN also published *NCSBN Guidelines for the Boards of Nursing for Complaints Involving Marijuana*, which provides general guidance regarding three major types of complaints related to marijuana:

1. Licensed nurses with positive urine tests for THC;
2. Advanced Practice Nurse certification of patients for a state's medical marijuana program;
3. Improper administration by a licensed individual that breaches state law. (NCSBN, 2018, p. 11)

With regard to nurses' use of marijuana in states where such action is legal, such as those states with comprehensive medical marijuana programs, the NCSBN (2018, p. 13) noted:

> The federal government's position on prosecuting the use of cannabis that is legal under applicable jurisdiction law has been set out in U.S. Department of Justice position papers. In 2009, the U.S. Attorney General took a position that discourages federal prosecutors from prosecuting people who distribute or use cannabis for medical purposes in compliance with applicable jurisdiction law; further similar guidance was given in 2011, 2013 and 2014. In January 2018, the U.S. Office of the Attorney General rescinded the previous nationwide guidance specific to marijuana enforcement. The 2018 memorandum provides that federal prosecutors follow the well-established principles in deciding which cases to prosecute, namely the prosecution is to weigh all relevant considerations including priorities set by the attorneys general, seriousness of the crime, deterrent effect of criminal prosecution and cumulative impact of particular crimes on the community.

In light of these considerations, the NCSBN encouraged state nursing boards to be specifically mindful of their respective state laws regarding marijuana use, well-informed regarding laboratory testing data, capabilities, standards, and limitations of such testing, and to consider its mission to protect the public while applying appropriate levels of "regulatory force … to achieve the desired result" in light of risks to the public and the need for appropriate disciplinary measures (NCSBN,

2018, p. 14). No guidance with regard to students is provided. However, higher education institutions are subject to the previously described constraints of the Drug-Free Act Amendments of 1989, while state boards of nursing are not.

DISCUSSION OF THE CASE STUDY

Before meeting with the student, Dr. Calumet closely reviews the state statutes regarding the use of medical marijuana; procedures used by the laboratory to identify, validate, and report positive urine test findings; university policies regarding drug use by students; and policies related to both clinical behaviors and the mandatory drug screening, both of which are documented in both the nursing student handbook and the university catalog. In light of federal law, this university imposes sanctions on students when there is evidence of drug use on campus and at any university-sponsored event; students who meet these criteria, using any drugs defined by federal law as illegal, are referred to the community standards committee, comprised of faculty, students, and academic administrators. Evidence of drug use results in the sanction of withdrawal from the respective program of study. Students who have been through this adjudication process must show evidence of treatment, including documentation of drug abstinence, before reapplying for admission to the university.

The university's legal counsel advises Dr. Calumet to follow the established procedure, documented in the nursing program student handbook, for handling drug screens that are positive for illegal substances. The procedure used for management of positive urine screen results is one that is common to most laboratories that perform such drug screening. Students who are aware of prescribed substances that may cause positive results on the test are instructed by the laboratory to self-report prior to submitting to the screening and to submit documentation that such substances are legally prescribed by an authorized clinician. Any positive result on the test is subsequently reviewed by the laboratory's medical review officer (MRO), a qualified physician with expertise in this area. The student with the positive result is contacted by the MRO with a request for further information. If a documented prescription for the substance is provided to the MRO, the result is reported as negative. However, in light of the university's compliance with the Drug-Free Schools and Communities Act Amendments of 1989 and the CSA, all screens that document THC are reported as positive, without consideration of whether or not there is a medical marijuana referral[1] that follows the medical marijuana program law in the state where the university is located. According to the established nursing program policy, a student with a positive drug screen is referred by the associate dean to the community standards committee. The university's community standards committee is responsible to determine the sanction, but the standard sanction for a positive drug screen is withdrawal of the student from the nursing program.

First and foremost, Dr. Calumet's discussion with Emily is based in caring, concern for her as an individual, empathy, and respect for her autonomy. As an advocate for students, Dr. Calumet's goal is to ensure that Emily has accurate information about the policies that affect her status as a student, so that she can make informed decisions about her academic progress. In consideration of the "letter of the law," which is clearly addressed through the university's policy, Dr. Calumet informs Emily about the procedure used when a drug screen is positive. She discusses the university policy, grounded in federal law. The current policy indicates that when there is evidence of use of illegal substances, including positive results of a urine drug screen despite any conditions qualifying the student for the medical marijuana program, the student involved would indeed be referred to the university's community standards committee. The committee is responsible for recommending the appropriate sanction.

Should Emily and her healthcare provider determine that therapeutic treatment with a form of marijuana is indicated during the nursing program, her use of the substance would be documentable through the preclinical urine screening process. Depending on the formulation of the drug, if her urine test were found to be positive for THC, Emily would be referred to the community standards committee. Dr. Calumet also refers Emily to the policies outlined in the nursing program handbook regarding behaviors reflecting impaired judgment in clinical experiences. She additionally refers Emily to information regarding criteria for licensure on the state board of nursing website.

---

[1] Comprehensive state programs involve certification by an approved clinician that patients have conditions that qualify them for medical marijuana, rather than prescription of the substance.

BEST PRACTICE EXEMPLAR

Universities are subject to the federal CSA. Marijuana is classified as a Schedule I drug according to the CSA. The use, possession, cultivation, or sale of marijuana violates federal policy. This prohibits the university from allowing any form of marijuana use on campus. Additionally, federal grants are subject to university compliance with the federal Drug-Free Schools and Communities Act and the federal Drug-Free Workplace Act.

FINDINGS AND DISPOSITION

Several weeks later, Emily reveals to Dr. Calumet that she had an extensive discussion with her medical provider to strategize for improved management of her condition. She shares that she has decided to forego treatment with medical marijuana for the immediate future, but may return to speak with the Associate Dean if her circumstances change. Dr. Calumet encourages Emily to stay in touch and to consider reaching out again to the university's disability services.

Prevention Tips

Technical standards should address student's reaction time and clinical judgment such as: A student must also possess the ability to perceive pain, pressure, temperature, position, vibration, and movement that are important to the student's ability to gather significant information needed to effectively evaluate patients. A student must be able to respond **promptly** *to urgent situations that may occur during clinical training activities and must not hinder the ability of other members of the healthcare team to provide prompt treatment and care to patients.* **Students cannot take substances that have the potential to slow their reaction time in providing prompt treatment and care to patients.**

Please refer to Technical Standards in Chapter 19, Disability Issues for the Student.

RELEVANT LEGAL CASES

Coats v. Dish Network, LLC, COA 62, ¶ 23, 303 P.3d 147, 152 (2013)

Currently, case law reflects employment, not higher education issues related to medical marijuana. Payne and Mort (2018) published a comprehensive overview of relevant court decisions that highlight employers' rights to rescind employment offers or to terminate employment in circumstances where marijuana is involved. Payne and Mort outline several recent decisions, including the case of *Coats v. Dish Network* (2013), where the plaintiff was an individual with a severe physical disability who was a legally registered medical marijuana user in Colorado, a state with a comprehensive medical marijuana program. Mr. Coats used medical marijuana in the evenings to assist in sleep and worked during day hours for his employer in a telephone call customer service center. Despite good evaluations and no complaints of impaired job performance, the employer required urine drug tests of all employees. Mr. Coats was fired from his job after the results of the urine screen were positive for marijuana; he then sued the employer, using the rationale that the termination from his position was in violation of a Colorado statute protecting employees who engage in legally permitted activities during nonwork hours. The argument used was that Mr. Coats's use of marijuana was legal in the state. The court found for the defendant, his employer; this decision was upheld at the state court of appeals and state supreme court levels. Payne and Mort also cite several medical marijuana use cases based in claims of disability discrimination: *Noffsinger v. SSC Niantic Operating Company LLC* (2018; Connecticut courts); *Barbuto v. Advantage Sales and Marketing LLC* (2017; Massachusetts courts). In these, the users' rights to treatment with the drug and to retain employment were upheld to larger or lesser degrees. However, other cases alleging disability discrimination in Washington and California did not result in the same outcomes. The authors suggest that the intersection of disability law with states' marijuana laws is an evolving area of legal decision-making that is not settled; these types of cases may eventually establish a framework for future understanding of disability discrimination or similar claims related to student or employee use of medical marijuana. No cases related to student use of medical marijuana could be located at the time of this writing.

SUMMARY

Despite a rapidly changing state-level context for legal use of marijuana and the extensive growth of comprehensive medical marijuana programs across 33 states and several U.S. territories, marijuana remains classified as a Schedule I, illegal substance, defined as having no therapeutic use. Higher education regulation, as outlined in the Drug-Free Schools and Communities Act Amendments of 1989, places those institutions of higher education located in states that legalized marijuana at risk of losing eligibility for an array of federal funds, should their policies regarding marijuana be harmonized with state rather than federal law. Since marijuana has psychoactive effects, use of medical marijuana by healthcare providers is a controversial issue that the NCSBN has attempted to address in a general sense in its guidance to state boards of nursing. However, this guidance does not extend to students currently in academic nursing programs, which remain subject to the higher education law restrictions. The interplay of these creates unavoidable ethical and personal rights considerations that nursing education leaders will need to sort through. Navigating these in an evolving legal landscape is challenging for even the most law-savvy nurse educator.

ETHICAL CONSIDERATIONS

Due to the relatively recent but accelerating acceptance of marijuana as a form of therapy, there is little guidance to be found in the ethics literature or the published statements of professional organizations like the American Nurses Association (ANA) on a question like the one posed by this case. The ANA has a statement on "Substance Use Among Nurses and Nursing Students" (ANA, 2016), but the focus of this statement is the response to nurses and students with substance use disorders. A nurse or nursing student using marijuana or some other cannabinoid form in a legal and medically prescribed manner would not be fairly described as having a substance use disorder. In 2016 the ANA published a statement titled, "Therapeutic Use of Marijuana and Related Cannabinoids" (ANA Center for Ethics and Human Rights, 2016). This document does not address the rather narrow (but inevitable) question of medical marijuana use by nursing students, but it does advocate quite strongly for the reclassification of marijuana from a Schedule I controlled substance to a Schedule II controlled substance in order to facilitate further research on its therapeutic potential. This position clearly expresses the ANA's belief, at least potential if not actual (as the statement also notes the mixed evidence of limited anecdotal and controlled studies), in the clinical and ethical appropriateness of the drug. More recently, the ANA has published "The Ethical Responsibility to Manage Pain and the Suffering It Causes" (ANA Ethics Advisory Board, 2018). This document focuses largely on the difficult balance between adequate treatment of pain and concern for opioid addiction. But the perhaps interesting and relevant part of the article for our question here is the strong emphasis found in the document on the obligation to relieve pain. Given this emphasis and the context of the other noted documents, one can only conclude at least the potential acceptance of medical marijuana use by nurses and nursing students. Nurses (and nursing students) are also sometimes patients. And, as nurses noting Provision 5 of the ANA Code or patients, they too deserve respect and appropriate treatment. At the same time, one cannot ignore the possibility of altered mental states caused by this drug to impair practice. However, marijuana is not the only prescribed pharmaceutical that may cause an altered mental state. So, for any of these some balance must be found between the right to treatment/respect for autonomy on one side and the safety of patients on the other.

In this particular circumstance, the student's concern could be resolved with changes to her medical management plan. However simple this solution appeared to be for Emily's immediate future, there are multiple unresolved concerns of an ethical nature for academic nursing programs, related to the disposition of students requiring treatment with a therapy that is legal by state legislation, but illegal by federal law and higher education regulation.

- Is sanctioning of health professions students who have legitimate therapeutic needs for medical marijuana a discriminatory practice?
- Do the restrictions on college student use of medical marijuana infringe on personal rights?
- How are student rights balanced with any nursing program's implicit obligation to ensure that a student's presence is not a risk to the public? Considering the recognized absence of concordance between urine THC levels and cognitive/sensory impairment (NCSBN, 2018), is drug screening for THC an effective public protection strategy to be used with nursing students?
- Is coercion occurring when students are faced with the choice between abandoning their preferred medical treatment and continuing their treatment with resultant sanctions?

Until such time as there are changes in federal law governing controlled substances or in the umbrella higher education regulations that are described by the Drug-Free Schools and Communities Act Amendments, these considerations will leave the disposition of nursing students being treated with medical marijuana in the ethical and procedural "gray area." Nursing program leadership who face this dilemma in the immediate future will need to have proactive discussions with legal counsel regarding students' rights and risks to the university with regard to federal fund eligibility, clear guidelines for handling evidence of marijuana use grounded in university policies, and sound understanding of state and federal laws to direct thinking and decision-making about nursing students being treated with medical marijuana. If medical marijuana slows the student's reaction time or clouds the student's judgment, the nursing academic administrator will need to consider patient safety first and foremost and inform the student that they cannot participate in clinical education activities while taking medical marijuana. There is no doubt that more studies and guidance are needed.

CRITICAL ELEMENTS TO CONSIDER

- Know the state law regarding use of marijuana for recreational and therapeutic purposes, in order to understand how students may be treated with medical marijuana.
- Ensure that there are clear policies about the handling of impairment of judgment or behavior outlined in the program handbook or college catalogue.
- Consult with university's legal counsel, especially in situations where a student discloses the use of medical marijuana.
- If urine screening is part of the clinical compliance policy, be familiar with the laboratory's disposition of THC-positive results; ensure that there is a clearly written explanation of the management of any positive results disseminated to students.
- Follow the current university or college policies regarding drug use in students.

References

American Nurses Association. (2016, October). *Substance use among nurses and nursing students*. Retrieved from https://www.nursingworld.org/practice-policy/nursing-excellence/official-position-statements/id/substance-use-among-nurses-and-nursing-students/

ANA Center for Ethics and Human Rights. (2016). *Therapeutic use of marijuana and other cannabinoids*. Retrieved from https://www.nursingworld.org/~49a8c8/globalassets/practiceandpolicy/ethics/therapeutic-use-of-marijuana-and-related-cannabinoids-position-statement.pdf

ANA Ethics Advisory Board. (2018). *The ethical responsibility to manage pain and the suffering it causes*. Retrieved from http://ojin.nursingworld.org/MainMenuCategories/ANAMarketplace/ANAPeriodicals/OJIN/Columns/ANA-Position-Statements/ANA-Position-Ethical-Responsibility-Manage-Pain.html

Barbuto v. Advantage Sales & Marketing, LLC, 477 Mass. 456 (2017).

Bauer-Wolf, J. (2017). Despite more open marijuana laws, colleges still banning it. Inside Higher Ed. Retrieved from https://www.insidehighered.com/news/2017/12/19/despite-more-open-marijuanalaws-colleges-still-banning-it

Centers for Disease Control and Prevention. (1983). Urine testing for detection of marijuana: An advisory. *Morbidity and Mortality Weekly Report, 32*(36), 469–471. Retrieved from https://www.cdc.gov/mmwr/preview/mmwrhtml/00000138.htm

Coats v. Dish Network, LLC, COA 62, ¶ 23, 303 P.3d 147, 152 (2013).

Davidson, E. S. (2015). *Marijuana and the drug free schools and campuses*. Illinois Higher Education Center. Retrieved from https://www.eiu.edu/ihec/Marijuana%20and%20DFSCA.pdf

Drug-Free Schools and Communities Act Amendments of 1989, P. L. No. 101-226, 103 Stat. 1928 (1989). Retrieved from https://www.govinfo.gov/content/pkg/STATUTE-103/pdf/STATUTE-103-Pg1928.pdf

Duquesne University. (2019). *Bachelor of Science in Nursing 2019–2020 academic year student handbook*. Retrieved from https://duq.edu/assets/Documents/nursing/Handbooks/Undergradaute%20student%20handbook-2019-2020.pdf

Mead, A. (2017). The legal status of cannabis (marijuana) and cannabidiol (CBD) under U.S. law. *Epilepsy and Behavior, 70*, 288–291. doi:10.1016/j.yebeh.2016.11.021

National Conference of State Legislatures. (2019). *State medical marijuana laws*. Retrieved from http://www.ncsl.org/research/health/state-medical-marijuana-laws.aspx

National Council of State Boards of Nursing Medical Marijuana Guidelines Committee. (2018, July). The NCSBN national nursing guidelines for medical Marijuana. *Journal of Nursing Regulation, 9*(2), S6–S52. Retrieved from https://www.ncsbn.org/The_NCSBN_National_Nursing_Guidelines_for_Medical_Marijuana_JNR_July_2018.pdf

National Institute on Drug Abuse. (2019). *Marijuana: How does marijuana produce its effects?* Retrieved from https://www.drugabuse.gov/publications/research-reports/marijuana/how-does-marijuana-produce-its-effects

Noffsinger, Plaintiff, v. SSC Niantic Operating Company LLC. d/b/a Bride Brook Nursing & Rehabilitation Center, Defendant, No. 3:16-cv-01938 (D. Conn. 2018).

Payne, S. E., & Mort, G. A. (2018). Medical marijuana in the workplace: A current look at cannabis law. *New York State Bar Association Journal*. Retrieved from https://nysba.org/NYSBA/Meetings%20Department/Section%20Meetings/Labor/LABRFA19/Workshop%20A%20Materials.pdf

Quest Diagnostics. (2019). Drug testing for marijuana. Retrieved from https://www.questdiagnostics.com/home/companies/employer/drug-screening/drugs-tested/marijuana/

Substance Abuse and Mental Health Services Administration. (2017). *Key substance use and mental health indicators in the United States: Results from the 2016 National Survey on Drug Use and Health* (HHS Publication No. SMA 17-5044, NSDUH Series H-52). Rockville, MD: Center for Behavioral Health Statistics and Quality, Substance Abuse and Mental Health Services Administration. Retrieved from https://www.samhsa.gov/data/

Tufts University. (2014). *Tufts University medical marijuana policy*. Retrieved from https://legal.tufts.edu/tufts-university-medical-marijuana-policy/

U.S. Department of Justice, Drug Enforcement Agency. (2016). *Marijuana: Clarification of new code (7350) for marijuana extract*. Retrieved from https://www.deadiversion.usdoj.gov/schedules/marijuana/m_extract_7350.html

U.S. Department of Justice, Drug Enforcement Agency. (n.d.). *Controlled substance schedules*. Retrieved from https://www.deadiversion.usdoj.gov/schedules/index.html

Williams College. (n.d.). *Marijuana policy FAQ*. Retrieved from https://president.williams.edu/writings-and-remarks/college-policy-regarding-marijuana/

Appendix

23.1

Excerpt Sample Policy

1. Medical Marijuana Policy: Pennsylvania law allows for the controlled use of medical marijuana in the Commonwealth. The university, however, is subject to the federal Controlled Substances Act (CSA). Marijuana is classified as a Schedule I drug according to the CSA. The use, possession, cultivation, or sale of marijuana violates federal policy. This prohibits the university from allowing any form of marijuana use on campus. Additionally, federal grants are subject to university compliance with the federal Drug-Free Schools and Communities Act and the federal Drug-Free Workplace Act.

2. Students in Preprofessional Programs: Students are reminded that nursing, health science, pharmacy, and certain other preprofessional programs maintain separate or additional requirements relating to the use of controlled substances, and therefore, students in preprofessional programs who are legal medical marijuana users under Pennsylvania law must consult with their respective chairs for additional guidance and requirements. Please refer to the Substance Abuse Policy in the *BSN Handbook*.

EXCERPT FROM TECHNICAL STANDARDS

A student must be able to respond *promptly* to urgent situations that may occur during clinical training activities and must not hinder the ability of other members of the healthcare team to provide prompt treatment and care to patients. *Students are not permitted to take substances that have the potential to slow their reaction time in providing prompt treatment and care to patients.*

Note: Please consult Legal Counsel before adopting or revising this policy for your school.

Source: Adapted from Duquesne University. (2019). *Bachelor of Science in Nursing 2019–2020 academic year student handbook.* Retrieved from https://duq.edu/assets/Documents/nursing/Handbooks/Undergradaute%20student%20handbook-2019-2020.pdf

IV

SPECIFIC CLINICAL
EDUCATION ISSUES

Clinical Probation and Failure

Case Study 24.1
Remediation of a Nursing Student Failing to Meet Clinical Objectives

Your role: As the clinical faculty in a pediatric nursing rotation, you are responsible for teaching, supervising, coaching, and evaluating eight nursing students who are in their third clinical rotation.

One of your students, Rona Joyce "RJ" Jacobson, is not progressing as expected. In particular, RJ is not meeting clinical objectives related to comprehensive patient assessment and to the safe performance of previously learned technical skills. You feel that RJ is highly likely to fail the clinical rotation unless she shows immediate improvement.

The students have been through a Fundamentals of Nursing and an Adult Health/Medical–Surgical clinical rotation at other hospitals. Their current clinical placement, with you, is on an acute care general pediatric unit. It is the fourth week of an 8-week clinical rotation. During week 1, students had an orientation to the rotation, clinical objectives, expectations, and clinical unit, and then obtained a health history and provided basic nursing care to a pediatric patient and family. The following 3 weeks involved progressively more complex daily clinical objectives, including, but not limited to, comprehensive assessment; maintaining safety; providing comprehensive care; and administering medications, treatments, fluids, and other prescribed or independent interventions for an infant or child and family members, consistent with pediatric nursing standards.

Questions

- What should the faculty member consider when developing a clinical evaluation plan?
- What policies should the faculty member consult with respect to this situation?
- What behaviors should the faculty member document related to the student's clinical performance?

IDENTIFYING BEST PRACTICES IN NURSING EDUCATION

Clinical Evaluation Plan

The foundation for management of a student who is struggling to meet clinical objectives is established through the overall clinical evaluation plan. Evaluation of clinical performance may be compared to the tracking of a moving target, subject to multiple variables and changes in the patient care situation.

> Evaluation of student learning and mastery of clinical learning objectives or clinical performance criteria can be very challenging in the patient care setting. Students need to demonstrate understanding of information, develop particular competencies, and demonstrate the development of critical thinking, decision-making, clinical judgment, and technical skills in an unstable, rapidly evolving patient care environment. They need to learn skills to distinguish what works from what does not work in a rapid-fire setting where the context of patient care is not static and where patient care needs and expectations can change in an instant. (Gardner & Suplee, 2010, p. 105)

As Ironside, McNelis, and Ebright (2014) attest, clinical nursing education is a time-intensive and resource-intensive aspect of contemporary nursing education. We would add that the evaluation of those clinical experiences is necessary and critical. Clinical evaluation validates that the student's practice is safe, sound, and validly represents the progression of learning what professional nursing is and how it is practiced for optimal patient outcomes. Clinical evaluation, and thus management of failure to meet clinical objectives, begins with a full understanding, by the clinical faculty,[1] of the end of program learning objectives (clinical objectives) for the clinical experience, along with a clear understanding of the benchmarks, daily objectives, or progression objectives that gauge students' progress toward these objectives. In addition, the instructor should keep in mind the need for students to learn and practice before being evaluated. Providing adequate time for development of skills and judgment is important. Evaluation also includes the clinical faculty's assessment, which involves subjectivity (Brown, Neudorf, Poitras, & Rodger, 2007). However, this challenge can be addressed by attention to the connection between performance behaviors and explicit clinical objectives or competency standards.

The clinical evaluation plan includes formative and summative evaluation.[2] Students as well as faculty benefit from concrete daily performance objectives that are clearly related to the overall clinical objectives for the rotation and unbiased, iterative feedback, including daily feedback, to each student about clinical performance along with opportunities for improvement. Instructors should keep documentation of each student's progress via weekly summaries and incident-specific anecdotal notes (Gardner & Suplee, 2010).

Communicating Clinical Performance Issues

Student evaluation of performance is a high-stakes process that can have financial, academic, legal, and personal consequences for the student. Discovering that he or she is at risk for or has failed objectives in the clinical setting can be devastating for students. However, communicating failure to students can be difficult for clinical faculty and requires them to justify and document objective data to support their decision. It is therefore important to ensure that clinical evaluation is free from bias, based on behaviors linked to clear clinical objectives, and that communication of expectations for clinical performance and the results of evaluation are explicit and in writing so that student and faculty have a shared understanding of the issues and the process for correction, if needed. Rapport with the student, coupled with effective communication of clinical performance, is also crucial for student progression and preservation of the student's sense of efficacy and self-worth (Benor & Leviyov, 1997; McGregor, 2007).

---

[1] For the purposes of this chapter, we will use the title "Clinical Faculty" as a proxy title for both Clinical Faculty, Clinical Adjunct Faculty, and Faculty. It is recognized that while most clinical instruction is now performed by Clinical Adjunct Faculty, some instruction remains taught by full-time (or part-time) Faculty who may not identify as a Clinical Faculty.

[2] Formative evaluation is done progressively during a clinical semester, where mastery learning principles are principally followed. A summative evaluation generally takes place at episodic endpoints, perhaps a midterm or final clinical evaluation.

Faculty should be familiar with and adhere to the academic and clinical policies of their academic institution. They should consult with experienced colleagues, such as the respective course or program director or dean, to assist in accurately assessing clinical performance problems, documenting and communicating clearly and objectively, ensuring explicit and timely notice of problems, making recommendations for improvement to the student, and adhering to the established policies and regulations as well as laws. Information presented here represents general concepts related to clinical evaluation of nursing students. Clinical faculty should consult with their program's academic administrators and legal counsel for guidance and advice related to any student issues and problems.

The first step that must take place at the beginning of any clinical experience is to ensure that the clinical objectives for each clinical encounter are clearly communicated in writing as well as verbally to all students. The clinical faculty should discuss the meaning of each objective and provide examples of related behaviors, and thus establish shared understanding of clinical expectations between student and teacher. Some nursing programs may have a template for clinical orientation and discussion of expectations, but if not, all expectations should be in writing so that students have a reference point from the beginning of the clinical rotation. At the point of clinical concern, assess the nature of the clinical performance issue. Safety issues require immediate intervention and/or immediate failure.[3] Expectations related to safe clinical practice, as well as consequences for breaching safe practice guidelines, such as removal from the clinical setting and/or clinical failure, must also be communicated clearly and in specific detail to students in writing, prior to beginning a clinical rotation.[4] A student who is grossly unsafe in the clinical area, who needs continual supervision to provide safe nursing care, or who does not recognize their deficits or limitations may be one who cannot continue in the rotation because patients are placed at significant risk for injury. In this case, immediate, detailed, and written documentation of student behaviors related to clinical objectives; immediate communication with the academic administrator; and careful, frank communication, both verbally and in writing, with the student will need to take place. Other issues related to clinical objectives, such as lack of preparation, poor skills performance, care planning, or organization, among others, may allow for a more prolonged remediation and opportunity to demonstrate improvement. In any case, attention to students' rights to academic due process along with a perspective focused on student learning, performance improvement, and the likelihood of success are needed. Students' clinical performance issues should be discussed directly and immediately with them, and documented in writing, so that opportunities for improvement can be provided and students are fully aware of their problems and the resources available to help them improve. Be sure to obtain a student signature and date for all communication related to clinical performance. All of these actions must take place within a context of respect for the student, confidentiality and privacy, timely notification with adequate time allowed for remediation, and adherence to regulatory guidelines including academic policies as well as the Family Educational Rights and Privacy Act (FERPA), the Health Insurance Portability and Accountability Act (HIPAA), the Americans with Disabilities Act (ADA), and other regulations.

Clinical Probation and Remediation

Once an assessment has been completed, place the performance in the context of clinical learning objectives by tying it specifically to one or more clinical objectives. It is essential to document in writing any serious concerns that need follow-up or improvement and explicitly communicate these to the student. If the clinical issue is one that can be improved with practice, review, further study, or clarification, a remediation plan is appropriate. Most nursing programs will have a template or form for documentation of clinical issues, but the template or form should include a description of the behaviors of concern linked to clinical objectives from the formal clinical evaluation tool, a clear outline of the steps the student must take to improve clinical performance, behavioral criteria

---

[3] That is giving medication to the wrong patient.

[4] It is not uncommon in clinical instruction to send a student home who is not prepared for the care of their patient(s) the morning/day of clinical.

for evaluation of improvement, a time line for improvement, the date by which improvement must be shown, and consequences should remediation not take place or improvement in clinical performance does not occur (Gallant, McDonald, & Higuchi, 2006). The focus of the remediation plan should be to support student learning and mastery of competency. However, it is important that students are fully informed of their rights. Student rights include, but are not limited to: due process of rights outlined in the program or university policy; student requirements, expectations, and responsibilities; and the risk of clinical failure or other consequences. Depending on the severity of the problem and the program policies, written documentation may take the form of a clinical memo, warning, or learning contract.

Schedule an immediate, private meeting with the student. Sensitively, but explicitly, outline the concerns, clinical objectives, and remediation requirements. Although privacy and confidentiality are essential, so is safety of both faculty and student. Students receiving this type of feedback about their performance may become upset, defensive, disruptive, angry, or may dispute the instructor's feedback and threaten legal or other actions. A private session should not continue if the instructor feels unsafe in any way. The instructor should tell the student that the meeting has ended and will be rescheduled, seek assistance and consultation from the academic administrator, and involve the health system or academic unit's security department, if indicated. Student's legal challenges to poor grades, including those related to clinical evaluation, have not been upheld when the following actions have taken place: Students are informed in writing of expectations; students are treated equally and fairly with respect to expectations, assignments, evaluation, and grading with lack of absence of arbitrary or capricious action by the instructor; students have been given written feedback and afforded opportunities for improvement; students are informed about progress or lack of progress in a timely manner; and the instructor has followed, with documentation, established program and university policies which include attention to due process rights.

In giving feedback about clinical performance standards or the need for improvement, be timely and specific, and clearly outline the specific area of concern and the steps to be taken to improve. Provide an opportunity for the student to voice their perspective, explanations, and questions. Ask the student to describe the problem and requirements for improvement in their own words. Further, document all of these, including date and time. The student and instructor should both sign the form or memo. Copies of the signed documentation should be provided to the student and remediation faculty, learning laboratory staff, or other individuals who would be legitimately involved with the student's performance and improvement plan in accordance with program policies and FERPA regulation if appropriate. The remediation plan should be clearly outlined so that the student has a full understanding of the steps to take and the time line involved. Feedback for unsatisfactory clinical performance should be provided in writing and discussed with the student (Figure 24.1).

Outcomes of Remediation

Follow-up to the remediation plan should include close communication between the clinical faculty, laboratory or instructional faculty involved with the student (if any), and the student themselves. Once the student has completed the prescribed remediation, they should provide documentation to the clinical faculty. The student should be provided opportunities to demonstrate mastery of the specific objectives, which include formative and summative evaluation. As noted earlier, formative evaluations are used throughout the student's clinical rotation to assess progress and include informal strategies such as discussion and observation of student participation (Billings & Halstead, 2015). Summative evaluations are conducted at the end of the course and are conducted to assess the student's achievement (Billings & Halstead, 2015). If the student fails to complete the required remediation within the prescribed time line, or does not meet the respective clinical objectives, the consequences may include a clinical failure. The consequence of failing to meet clinical objectives should be clearly outlined in writing to all students prior to the beginning of any clinical rotation or experience. Daily formative feedback to students during each clinical experience across the clinical rotation will ensure that all students are aware of their progress toward achievement of the clinical objectives, including at a minimum a written midpoint or mid rotation evaluation. A final written summative evaluation is given at the conclusion of the clinical rotation. Feedback for unsatisfactory

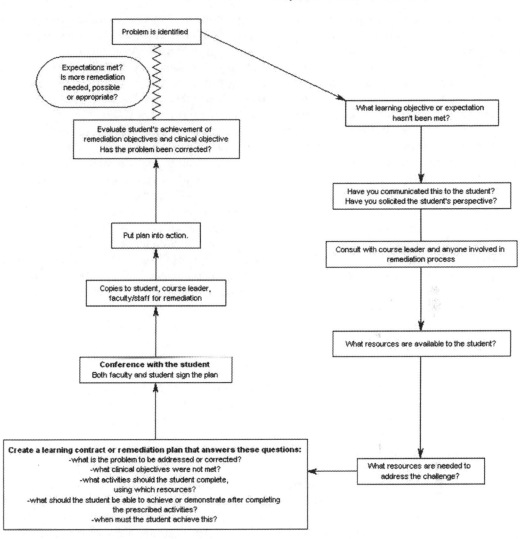

Figure 24.1 Remediation model.
Source: Gardner, M. R., & Suplee, P.D. (2010). *Handbook of clinical teaching in nursing and health sciences.* Sudbury, MA: Elsevier. Used with permission by Elsevier.

clinical performance should be provided in writing and discussed with the student. Clear and full documentation of the instructor's communication of the clinical performance problem, the process of evaluation, the opportunities for remediation, and behavioral data supporting the judgment of the instructor that the student did not meet objectives after remediation are essential. A discussion and review of the documentation with the course leader and/or academic program director, depending on program policies, should occur as soon as possible, respecting program and academic policies as well as FERPA regulations related to communication of student information.

WHEN THE STUDENT FAILS CLINICAL

Once the decision to issue a failing clinical grade to a student has been made, the clinical faculty should schedule a conference with the student to discuss the failure. A clear, explicit, but empathetic and sensitive approach is needed. To acknowledge emotional difficulties that students may have when confronting a clinical failure, it may be helpful to remember common strategies for breaking bad news: providing privacy; speaking objectively using data, not labels; acknowledging effort; gauging comprehension of and response to the information; and supporting a realistic perspective about the situation (Gardner & Suplee, 2010; Vaderkieft, 2001; Walsh, Girgis, & Sanson-Fisher, 1998). The clinical faculty should be familiar with the crisis management policies of the program or university, as well as academic and counseling resources available for students. The clinical evaluation form and clinical objectives, along with observed behavior (rather than subjective) data, should be the basis for the discussion. Document the discussion, date and time, and the student's response and have the student sign the written evaluation, but it cannot be coerced. The student may elect the immediate opportunity to respond to the evaluation in writing, may state the response will be made later, or the student may refuse to sign it at all. The student should be informed that the signatures do not necessarily indicate agreement with the feedback, only that the information has been received. Should the student refuse to sign the evaluation form, document the student's refusal, response to the discussion, the date and time, and seek consultation from the academic administrator. While these are the ordinary steps of the formality of the expected process of communicating a clinical failure, human behavior often does not follow prescribed administration processes. That is why appeals and lawsuits can be the final outcome of a clinical failure in any health professions discipline (Westrick, 2007).[5] Fiona Dobson (2019) of Open University has an excellent module that addresses the issues of clinical failure, especially how to mentor the underperforming student, giving the student feedback, and failing the student. We suggest this module would be very helpful to clinical faculty.

CASE STUDY

Verbal feedback was given to RJ about specific problems during the third week of the clinical rotation and this was documented in the instructor's anecdotal notes. During the fourth week, the instructor noted ongoing problems. The instructor completed a clinical memo (based on the program's policy and template) that summarized data about the student's performance, and related the data directly to clinical objectives about assessment skills and about safe performance of technical nursing skills. The clinical memo included a learning contract outlining remediation requirements to be completed in the campus clinical skills learning laboratory, a timeline for remediation, criteria by which the student would be reevaluated, and the potential consequence—clinical failure—should improvement not been seen. After developing the memo, the instructor reviewed the memo, remediation plan, and approach to the student with the program director in accordance with FERPA guidelines specific to the communication of educational information, and scheduled a private conference with RJ. During the conference, instructor and student reviewed and discussed the progress and performance and reviewed the memo in detail. The student's perspective was elicited. RJ initially emphatically denied that there were clinical performance problems. After listening to RJ's perspective, the instructor brought the student's attention to the behaviors documented on the clinical memo, emphasizing remediation as an opportunity to improve performance but realistically identifying risks for clinical failure. RJ reluctantly agreed that remediation and additional practice were needed. RJ was asked to sign the clinical memo and copies of the signed clinical memo were sent to the learning laboratory faculty.

RJ completed the prescribed remediation within the prescribed time frame and was provided additional opportunities to demonstrate competency in clinical skills. Despite additional practice and remediation, the student was unable to meet the clinical objectives for the rotation. Ongoing feedback was provided to the student. A detailed evaluation of student performance, tethered to clinical objectives, was written and all of the documentation was reviewed with the nursing program administrator. The clinical faculty then scheduled a conference with the student and reviewed the clinical evaluation point by point. RJ signed the evaluation form and was offered the opportunity to respond in writing to the evaluation. The student was directed to the university handbook outlining due process procedures (e.g., student academic grievance procedure) and was encouraged to consult with her faculty adviser and with the program director. The clinical faculty offered support and a reminder that no-cost student counseling services were available. RJ had the

---

[5] *Jillian Marlowe v. Keene State College, University System of New Hampshire, Rebecca Lytle, and Thomas W. Connelly, Jr.* (2016).

academic standing to repeat this course and successfully repeated the course and clinical rotation the following semester.

SUMMARY

It is our experience that there are many factors that impact and can lead to a clinical failure. Additionally, we have seen students fail a didactic or clinical course, repeat it successfully and pass the NCLEX® the first time. In other words, a grade of clinical failure may not be completely determinative to a student finishing their degree (maybe not on time) and successfully beginning their nursing career. Nursing professors Diekelmann and McGregor (2003) seem to agree (see Table 24.1). A proactive approach, including a clearly defined plan for student evaluation, is the starting point for effective evaluation and remediation. Clear and explicit communication of student progress toward clinical objectives, along with documentation based on observed behaviors, will support realistic,

Table 24.1 Common Steps to Clinical Failure[a]

STEPS	REMEDIATION	IMMEDIATE OUTCOME	LONG-TERM OUTCOME
Grave incident which can take many forms (incompetent clinical practice)	No opportunity	Clinical failure	Could result in dismissal from nursing program
Illegal or unprofessional conduct	Would be individually evaluated	Clinical probation of clinical failure	Could result in dismissal from nursing program and possibly the College/University
1. Incident requiring a verbal warning, but is documented by clinical faculty	If warranted, remediation is required; if not skill based, student will be counseled	Student supported and given opportunities to demonstrate progress in the clinical agency; reminded of evaluation policy	None
2. Incident recurs or another incident occurs; a written warning is made and jointly signed by student and faculty	Remediation is required; satisfactory remediation must be demonstrated before student can return to clinical	Student is again supported and given opportunities to demonstrate progress in the clinical agency; reminded that next infraction will result in Clinical Probation, placing the student at risk for Clinical Failure; a Team Meeting is held with relevant faculty to develop a plan of action for the underperforming student to prevent Clinical Probation; the plan is shared with student; student asked to sign statement; policy should indicate the student has not failed, but must sign this contract agreeing to remediation plan; the student can ask for modifications or extra resources and these requests will be considered, but not guaranteed	Risk for Clinical Probation

(continued)

Table 24.1 Common Steps to Clinical Failure (*continued*)

STEPS	REMEDIATION	IMMEDIATE OUTCOME	LONG-TERM OUTCOME
3. Student has a third infraction	Remediation is required; satisfactory remediation must be demonstrated before student can return to clinical; a second faculty must sign off on the remediation plan before the student can return to clinical	Student placed on Clinical Probation: School policy on Clinical Probation should be enacted; student informed of risk of clinical failure; student signs statement understanding status; last plan for remediation filed and signed	Risk of clinical failure
4. Final infraction		Clinical failure; often clinical is linked to the didactic course and thus resulting in a course failure; there should be a policy on what final grade is awarded should the student fail clinical	Clinical failure. Depending on previous course failures, student may or not progress; may be dismissed from program if course failure or progression policy is violated
5. Readmission policy		More schools are developing readmission policies. Both nursing authors of this text have seen very successful readmissions and performance, but not always. The policy must be outlined in detail	

ᵃ From our experience, this table outlines the simplest and most student due process procedure for documenting clinical failure (outside of an incident leading to immediate clinical failure). All clinical evaluation policies should be in the student handbook and on the syllabus. The policy should be orally reinforced at the beginning of class or/and the beginning of clinical.

unbiased appraisals of clinical achievement. When adequate progress toward achievement of clinical objectives is not apparent, a clear, explicit, written plan for improvement, tied to the clinical objectives of the rotation, should be designed, discussed with the student, and implemented. Once adequate opportunities for improvement, if appropriate, are provided, further appraisal of student achievement of objectives should occur before a failing grade is levied.

ETHICAL CONSIDERATIONS

According to the American Association of University Professors (2002), one of the fundamental purposes of a university is to "develop experts for various branches of the public service" (p. 182). This purpose implies an ethical duty of a university and its faculty to ensure that the students they produce and place their imprimatur upon are adequately prepared, and they in fact are the experts they are meant to be. This duty then implies derivative duties regarding the setting of uniform standards, benchmarks, and metrics for determining students who achieve these. From the perspective of nursing ethics, the *American Nurses Association's Code of Ethics* (ANA, 2012) explicitly identifies an obligation of educators to "ensure that basic competence and commitment to professional standards exist prior to entry into practice" (p. 11). These similar conceptualizations of moral duties for education can be seen as largely utilitarian. The greatest good is served by competent professionals, though there is a character issue at play here as well. Faculty members of a university act within a particular role, one which in part defines their identity. Faculty to meet these standards for student preparation fail also to achieve the *telos* (end, purpose, or goal) of that role. So, though they may have the titles associated with education and university faculty, they do not truly fulfill the role as it is defined.

At the same time a duty to respect students exists. This is a very broad principle which means many things. In this context we have to recognize that reasons for failure can be multivariate and not patently evident. To respect students in these types of situations would include the consideration of factors beyond one's control and thus the opportunity for remediation. Some degree of compassion can be at play here as well, acknowledging the reality and struggle of this other person beyond our full understanding. In addition, there should be a uniform due process in place to ensure fair treatment in like cases across the board. Failure to provide consideration and due process in these forms amounts to treating the student as a disposable resource rather than a person with dignity and inherent value. Considering these two duties, some balance must be achieved between the utilitarian duty to provide adequately prepared professionals and the obligation to respect the dignity of students. Still, there must be a limit in providing further opportunities for failing students, which needs to be clearly stated as part of their due process and a professional assessment of student performance. Assuming there is no limit to meet neither duty, unreasonably lowering expectations for a student that unquestionably is less able to establish the required competency and safety in nursing care, may be ultimately deserving of clinical failure outright at some point.

CRITICAL ELEMENTS TO CONSIDER

Critical elements of the process include the following:
- Clearly defined performance objectives
- Clearly outlined expectations and possible consequences for not meeting expectations
  - Discussion and written communication to ensure shared understanding of clinical objectives and expectations
  - Formative feedback after each clinical experience, tied to daily and overall clinical objectives
  - Documentation of student progress using weekly as well as incident-specific instructor notes
  - Opportunity for improvement with a clearly outlined plan, time line, and criteria for remediation
- Feedback on outcomes of remediation
- Clear, objective, detailed documentation of facts and behaviors
- Empathetic but clear communication
- Attention to program and university policies and procedures, in line with higher education regulations and laws

References

American Association of University Professors (AUUP). (2002). *1915 AAUP general declaration of principles.* Appendix B in N. W. Hamilton, *Academic ethics: Problems and materials on professional conduct and shared governance.* Westport, CT: Praeger Publishers.

American Nurses Association. (2015). *Code of ethics for nurses with interpretive statements.* Silver Spring, MD: Author.

Benor, D. E., & Leviyof, I. (1997). The development of students' perceptions of effective teaching: The ideal, best, and poorest clinical teacher in nursing. *Journal of Nursing Education, 36*(5), 206–211. doi:10.3928/0148-4834-19970501-05

Billings, D. M., & Halstead, J. A. (2015). From teaching to learning: Theoretical foundations. In *Teaching in nursing: A guide for faculty* (p. 205). St. Louis, MO: Elsevier Health Sciences.

Brown, Y, Neudorf, K., Poitras, C., & Roger, K. (2007). Unsafe clinical performance calls for a systematic approach. *Canadian Nurse, 103*(3), 29–32. Retrieved from https://www.researchgate.net/publication/6410931_Unsafe_student_clinical_performance_calls_for_a_systematic_approach

Diekelmann, N., & McGregor, A. (2003). Students who fail clinical courses: Keeping open a future of new possibilities. *Journal of Nursing Education, 42*(10), 433–436. doi:10.3928/01484834-20120427-01

Dobson, F. (2019). Supporting the failing student. Open University. Retrieved from https://www.open.edu/openlearn/ocw/mod/oucontent/view.php?id=20107&printable=1

Gallant, M., McDonald, J., & Higuchi, K. S. (2006). A remediation process for nursing students at risk. *Nurse Educator, 31*(5), 223–227. doi:10.1097/00006223-200609000-00010

Gardner, M. R., & Suplee, P. D. (2010). *Handbook of clinical teaching in nursing and health sciences.* Sudbury, MA: Jones & Bartlett.

Ironside, P. M., McNelis, A. M., & Ebright, E. (2014). Clinical education in nursing: Rethinking learning in practice settings. *Nursing Outlook, 62*(3), 185–191. doi:10.1016/j.outlook.2013.12.004

Jillian Marlowe v. Keene State College, University System of New Hampshire, Rebecca Lytle, and Thomas W. Connelly, Jr. No. 4:16-CV-40054-TSH (D. Mass. 2016).

McGregor, A. (2007). Academic success, clinical failure: Struggling practices of a failing student. *Journal of Nursing Education, 46*(11), 504–511. doi:10.3928/01484834-20071101-05

Vandekieft, G. K. (2001). Breaking bad news. *American Family Physician, 64*(12), 1975–1978. Retrieved from https://www.aafp.org

Walsh, R. A., Girgis, A., & Sanson-Fisher, R. W. (1998). Breaking bad news 2: What evidence is available to guide clinicians? *Behavioral Medicine, 24*(2), 61–72. doi:10.1080/08964289809596382

Westrick, S. J. (2007). Legal challenges to academic decisions. *Journal of Nursing Law, 11*(2), 104–107. Retrieved from https://search.proquest.com/openview/72b48cb8d9833767dc56d067de6118b5/1?pq-origsite=gscholar&cbl=34122

The Testing Environment

25

 Case Study 25.1

Your Role: You are Dr. Juanita Johnson, Chair of the Undergraduate Programs.

Alejandra Lopez is a second-degree nursing student in your BSN program, taking her final capstone course. She requests to take her final, third attempt of the HESI exam in her hometown of El Paso, Texas because her mother is terminally ill. You grant her request and make arrangements for Alejandra to take her third attempt at a testing center. You receive notice from the testing company that Alejandra obtained a score of 839; however, Alejandra vehemently denies taking the exam in El Paso, where you arranged the test. You write Alejandra the following letter and refer her to the School of Nursing Student Conduct Committee.

Dear Ms. Lopez:

During the fall 2019 semester you did not achieve a minimum score of 900 on a standardized HESI exit examination after two attempts in order to pass your capstone course. You received a grade of "D" on your first and second HESI exam attempts. Based on the Senior Capstone syllabus, you have three attempts to achieve a score of 900 to successfully pass the class. You requested that, in lieu of taking the exam on campus, you be allowed to take the HESI exit examination at a testing center or university in El Paso, Texas, because your mother is very ill and you need to go home to care for her. As Chair of the BSN Program, I granted approval for you to take the test for a third time in Texas and notified you of that decision so that you could register for the test near your mother's home.

The School of Nursing was notified that you achieved a score of 839 on your third attempt on the HESI exit examination on December 6, 2019. This grade did not meet the minimum required score of 900 which means you are required to retake NURS 411: Senior Capstone again.

Since that time, you have stated that you did not take the HESI exit examination on December 6, 2019 in Texas at the Testing Center. There is sufficient evidence that you indeed took the test as scheduled. Therefore, I am proceeding with the academic integrity policy violation and am referring you to the School of Nursing Student Conduct Committee.

Sincerely,
Dr. Juanita Johnson

Questions
- What information do you need to gather from the testing center?
- What are the exam security procedures at a national testing center?
- What information should the School of Nursing Student Conduct Committee consider in their deliberations?

Testing Site Requirements Considerations:
- Student needs two forms of photo identification at the testing site, one being the university identification to test.
- Student needs to sign an "agreement to test" form, which includes academic integrity procedures (clean desk, no phones or papers in testing area) and knowledge that the testing environment includes digital video recording of a student taking the exam.
- Student needs a secure password from the professionally developed standardized testing company to take the exam at the testing site.
- Student signs an agreement to send her exam results to the university.

The School of Nursing Student Conduct Committee reviewed the testing procedures at the testing center, the signed agreements and disclosures by the student, and digital video recording of the testing environment compared to the student's photo identification and agreed that the student did indeed take the exam. The student was dismissed for making false statements and violating the American Nurses Associations's [ANA] Code of Ethics and Academic Integrity Policy. Alejandra appealed to the Dean and admitted to lying after receiving the School of Nursing Student Conduct Committee's decision stating she was under a lot of stress and did not have the money to retake the course. The Dean, although empathetic to Alejandra's personal circumstances, upheld the committee's decision to dismiss the student.

 ## Case Study 25.2

Your role: You are a new Dean arriving mid-spring and during your first summer you have a cheating scandal.

The summer is nearly here and seven students who failed Fundamentals in the spring semester (they all passed Health Assessment and Pharmacology and all their other courses) are requesting that a repeat Fundamentals class be offered in the Summer, albeit in a 10-week format, not the regular 15 weeks. As a new Dean, you do want to display that you are supportive of students. From your previous experience as a faculty member or administrator at four other institutions, you don't recall someone retaking Fundamentals and then moving successfully through the program and passing NCLEX, particularly the first time. But of course, you do not absolutely know this. You do realize this is a new demographic of student than you have previously taught,[1] very often heavily dependent on financial aid, a high degree of other economic, social, and family/work obligations that can all interfere with time-on-task for class preparation, and who see an RN license as a ticket to the middle class (Preston,

---

[1] We discourage the use of the word "disadvantaged" or "high risk" here, but we struggle like many to find more respectful, alternative words. Commonly, the word "disadvantaged" is not used with Caucasian college students, but instead from one source, as "low-participation neighborhoods" where few students go to college in the U.K. (British Broadcasting Corporation, 2019). One college has the following statement in their grants to supplant such labels: "this grant is directed toward students who have not had a seamless transition from high school to college." Yes, that is long, but less derisive. It is similar to the change of word from "disabled" to "differently abled." We do need to find a word to replace "disadvantaged" or "underprivileged" and "high-risk." Is the use of "dis" or "under" an appropriate way to begin to describe an individual?

2018). You do have reservation about letting these students repeat the class in an intensive format, but you agree to offer the class. The class begins at an early point in the summer, and the Clinical Lab Coordinator who served as a test administrator and proctor for the exam, urgently notifies you and the faculty member teaching the course that *all the exams and Scantron sheets* have been stolen from her office drawer where she put them before she would later score them. The drawer was not locked, but she had no recollection that any student would know where she would keep the tests. You, the faculty, and instructor were not only flabbergasted, but incredulous that a student would be so brazen to attempt and pull off this theft. You as new Dean are also completely disappointed that one or more students in this small class of seven students would act so unethically. You are more than extremely disappointed.

Questions

- What should be the Dean's first action?
- Does the Dean initially ask the Instructor to investigate or get involved immediately?
- What will be the process to determine who, or if more than one, person was involved?
- If the individual is not identified, what is the next step that should be taken?
- What is the broader context of this event and should its occurrence be kept quiet or used as a teaching case in some format to other faculty?
- Or how about a teaching case to other students and in what format?

Academic Integrity Considerations:

- While it is probably unlikely the entire class was involved, this cannot be excluded if no one comes forward.
- If there is punishment, will it be fair to those who may have not cheated?
- Was there a student-testing-protocol in place and was it followed?
- Was there a faculty-administration-testing protocol that was standard practice for any faculty administering an exam, and was it followed?
- This occurred at a religious-affiliated institution. Is there any additional context, implications, or actions that should be taken, or should the remedies be the same as a public institution?

The students were asked to confidentially come forward and identify the person or persons involved. The class was assured the person making the complaint would not be identified. The students were first asked in class by the Instructor and subsequently in an email by the Dean. In this case, no student came forward. The Dean, Instructor, and Lab Coordinator who administered the test then caucused and decided to deliver a completely different exam. This remedy has often met with outcries of "this is not fair" when some students claim they did not cheat and are being punished for it. However, a cheating scandal like this is usually treated this way. Sometimes if grades are calculated and there is evidence of widespread cheating, a new exam is administered, and patterns of "grades significantly decreasing" from the first test can give the faculty some assumption that these substantial grade declines point to cheating, but even these are difficult to prove. The retest did not indicate any certain testing pattern. But the Dean decided this had to be addressed in some format to other students.

At the first Fall Student Nursing Association-sponsored "Meeting with the Dean" (to a mostly packed theater), the Dean made her usual greeting to the new students, and welcomed back the returning students. Various items were covered as typical in welcoming the students back to a new academic year. At the end, the Dean decided she wanted to share with them an incident that had happened "in the last academic year"—trying to avoid specific attention on seven summer students. She briefly outlined the most salient point of the incident. She reaffirmed each student's compliance with the Mission of the College, the Nursing School Code of Conduct, and the College's Code of Conduct. She made specific references to what cheating means in the education of nurses and the practice of professional nursing. She ended by telling the packed auditorium, that "a student who will cheat on a test is the kind of person who will cheat a patient." Maybe the nurse will "cheat" a patient if no one is looking, not clean up the patient properly, ignore a less communicative patient, get impatient with a difficult patient, get lazy and not keep up with the latest clinical literature, make derogative comments about a patient to someone, and other issues. The Dean then elevated the students with what great promise they were going to make for the profession, that one incident by no means reflects on them all, and finally implores them to keep the ethical conduct as a student and future nurse "close to their heart." Then she took general questions from students as was her practice, and no one (probably not unexpected) asked a question about the incident.

THE COMPLEX TESTING ENVIRONMENT

Today's testing environment is complex and ever evolving. While not all schools have moved past Scantron scored tests, most have, and tests are now administered on desktop computers, either on tests prepared by publishing companies[2] or now increasingly commonly, faculty-made tests administered through secure software[3]—and often now Cloud based. The purpose of this chapter is to provide an overview of (a) some guidance on test protocols or students which are different from (b) test administration policies for faculty; also included are (c) a short primer on basic psychometrics in test scoring and (d) a background on use of the Standardized Patient (SP) Testing[4]; (e) an overview of some of the current controversies in test taking; and (f) finally a very lengthy legal case study. This chapter will not focus on any type of low- to high-fidelity simulation testing, as that is a new, largely untested area—the actual validity and reliability of scoring/testing students on actual simulations. Simulation is widely used in nursing education and is increasingly determined to improve student learning outcomes in some large cohort studies.[5] This chapter will also not focus on the future NGN NCLEX Testing Model which is the focus of Chapter 26, Changing the NCLEX-RN* to the Clinical Judgment Measurement Model: Educational, Legal, and Ethical Implications.

Test-Taking Protocols for Students

As part of any nursing program handbook for both students and faculty are procedures for test taking by students and test administration by faculty. Some of the essential procedures for students ensure they fully understand how a test is taken. Some tests may be quizzes, exams, final exams, or "high-stakes" exams that are nationally normed exams. But even the name "high-stakes" is an improper description of these type of tests. This is addressed in the last section of this chapter. Students must be aware of any "missed test" policy consequences for cheating, plagiarism, or any form of academic dishonesty and other important testing information. Following is a sample student test taking policy that one nursing program uses:

UNDERGRADUATE HANDBOOK

ADA Accommodations

Students requesting academic accommodations must register with the Office of Disability Services. This request must be made each term while the student is enrolled at the University. University policies surrounding academic accommodations can be found here: www.duq.edu/

---

[2] We are not very supportive of publisher-made tests for major classroom texts, except perhaps quizzes. Publisher or text examinations do not undergo the rigor of validity and reliability of nationally normed tests like HESI (https://evolve.elsevier.com/education/hesi) and ATI offers (https://atitesting.com).

[3] ExamSoft is the leading vendor for secure classroom testing on student laptops and notebook computers in the classroom. Other competitors to ExamSoft are at this link www.g2.com/products/examsoft/competitors/alternatives

[4] The nursing authors of this text were leaders in implementing the first standardized patient education requirement in undergraduate nursing.

[5] A large meta-analysis of various levels of fidelity in nursing education simulation by Kim, Park, and Shin (2016) indicated that there were large effects on the psychomotor domain in educational simulation; however, the effects were not specifically related to a specific type of fidelity.

life-at-duquesne/student-services/disability-services/academic-accommodations. Students requesting accommodations and services at the University need to present a current accommodation verification letter (AVL) to faculty before accommodations can be made. AVLs are issued by the University Office of Disability Services.

Test Proctoring Protocol

Faculty has the responsibility and obligation to provide a secure testing environment that ensures fairness for all students and supports academic honesty and integrity. Faculty must be empowered to manage the testing area assigned for the test, the students' behaviors, and materials used to take or administer the test. The following are some *best practice guidelines* for proctoring student test taking in undergraduate nursing:

Test Materials

1. Faculty may use methods of varying either content and/or physical makeup of a test to create such variance that may have prophylactic value against student cheating.
2. Faculty may use varying methods of test distribution and collection to authenticate the test taker.
3. Students must return all test materials to the proctor or designee before retrieving any personal materials.
4. Faculty can invoke various methods of establishing unique identifiers to validate students' work as authentic.

Student Seating

1. Faculty reserves the right to arrange seats in the testing area.
2. Faculty reserves the right to assign students their seats for test taking.
3. Faculty reserves the right to move students during a test, if he/she suspects that academic integrity has been compromised. When a faculty member asks that a student move his/her seating during a test, this should not be construed as an accusation that the student(s) was cheating.

Students' Belongings and Test Aids

1. Faculty will identify what test aids are to be used for both test taking execution, (e.g., pencil, computer) and content support (e.g., calculator). Use of any unauthorized aid will result in a zero for the test, and/or an Academic Integrity Violation.
2. The University makes every reasonable effort to provide an environment conducive to testing. However, the university cannot guarantee a distraction-free testing environment. Students are permitted to use foam or rubber earplugs during testing. Audio devices of any kind are not permitted as substitutions for earplugs. It is the responsibility of the student to bring earplugs to the testing environment.
3. Students must place all personal belongings in a designated area established by the proctor and not to access these belongings until all test materials have been turned into the proctor, unless explicit permission has been given by the proctor. Any unauthorized access of personal belongings will result in a zero for the test and/or an Academic Integrity Violation.
4. All electronic equipment taken into the testing area must be silenced and placed in the front of the room (this could include timepieces if such timepiece is distracting). Students are not permitted to wear any type of smart device during an exam. Devices include but are not limited to Bluetooth Ear Buds, smart watch or other wearable smart device.
5. Faculty reserves the right to ask students to remove nonessential clothing (e.g., hat or scarf) if he/she suspects that it compromises academic honesty, and to place such item(s) in the front of the room.

Test Ending Protocol

1. When the proctor signals that test time is over, students must cease writing of any kind (or typing/clicking if using an electronic testing device). If a student continues marking a test, the student could receive a zero and/or an Academic Integrity Violation.

2. Faculty can invoke various methods of establishing unique identifiers to validate students' work as authentic.

Dealing With Transgressions

1. If the faculty proctor suspects that there has been a violation of academic honesty by a student or group of students, he/she reserves the right to act in ways that confirm or negate such acts. These acts may include, among others:
   a. Ask a student to move his/her seat or move to another seating area.
   b. Ask a student to focus his/her eyes on test materials.
   c. Ask a student to produce a "cheating source," especially if concealed.
   d. Ask a student(s) to stop taking a test; collect the test materials.
2. If a student alerts the faculty proctor that another student or group of students are cheating, the faculty member may act in ways that confirm or negate such acts and are delineated above.

   Such acts should not immediately be construed that the student(s) is in fact cheating, but that the faculty member must undertake the appropriate due diligence to ensure academic honesty during test taking.
3. Under no circumstances are students to take a photograph of their exam materials during the examination or during the review of the examination with their cell phone, iPad, or any other electronic device.

Sanctions

Faculty who find students in violation of clear directives related to ensuring the academic integrity of the test taking environment and test taking procedures will result in an academic integrity action and/or an Academic Integrity Violation.

Testing Issues

Any issue of concern related to testing conditions must be brought to the immediate attention of the test proctor at the time of the test. The student must notify the course faculty of the issue of concern within 24 hours of the testing experience. The university cannot guarantee a distraction-free environment, but every effort will be made to provide a testing environment conducive to test taking.

Review of Testing Items

Students are permitted to review quizzes, midterm, and final exams. The method for review is determined by the individual course faculty. Requests to review test items must be made within 2 weeks of posting of the grade. Requests made after this time may not be considered. Students are not permitted to duplicate or take a photograph of the examination materials during the review. Students are able to review the rationales after completing the examination for non-Exit HESI Examinations. For HESI exams given in 8-week courses, students taking a HESI during term one will review their rationales for their HESI exam at the end of the full semester.

Examinations and Quizzes

Students are required to take all examinations and quizzes on the scheduled date. In the extreme, extenuating event that a makeup exam is required, the faculty member will determine the date, time, location, and format of the makeup exam. If a student misses both the regularly scheduled exam and the makeup exam, the student will earn a grade of zero for that exam. The student should be aware that as the number of students taking the makeup exam is typically very small, no statistical inferences can be drawn, and therefore, no numerical adjustment will be applied. Additionally, if a student who is not feeling well elects to sit for an exam, the student's exam effort cannot be rescinded. Furthermore, once the exam containing the exam questions is accepted by the student, the exam effort is considered to have begun. Vacations and social events are not considered to be excused absences. Students are advised not to make any personal or travel plans, including job interviews until all course requirements have been met.

Failure to contact a faculty member prior to a student's absence for an examination or quiz (without a documented emergency) is considered a no call, no show and a grade of 0 will be given for the examination or quiz.

Test Taking Administration Protocols for Faculty

In a review of several random faculty handbooks across the country, only in one did this author find faculty test administration instructions. Perhaps these instructions are documented elsewhere. Perhaps they are often dispensed by word of mouth. Procedures must be documented so that test construction, test administration, psychometric review, and student review of their tests are all carried out in a consistent and fair way. The advances in testing software have also introduced new procedures that must be followed by the student and faculty administering the exam. It is also important that faculty understand the screens the students are seeing, not just the side of the software for the instructor. An example in one nursing program that uses ExamSoft has a policy that all students must download their exam at 10 p.m. the night before the exam (the exam is downloaded to inaccessible cloud that is encrypted) so that when they come into the room the next day for testing the student can immediately log into their exam. Students who wait to do this right before class or during class may experience difficulties in access, potentially distract the professor/proctor to help them, and delay the class (or just themselves) from beginning the exam on time. Also, the professor is assured the night before that all students have accessed the exam and that it can begin on time, hopefully in an uncomplicated way. This is just an example of how changes in test taking may require more detailed test administration policies. Below is an example of a faculty test administration policy provided by the first author of this text.[6]

Testing Policies

FACULTY HANDBOOK

Exam Proctoring and Scheduling Makeup Exams for Excused Absences
Faculty members are expected to proctor examinations scheduled in their assigned courses and be available to answer student questions during the testing session. At least two proctors should be present to proctor an exam. All faculty members are requested to assist other faculty in proctoring exams to provide assistance, as needed, in the testing room. Faculty is responsible for scheduling and monitoring private testing for students who missed scheduled exams due to special approved circumstances (i.e., illness, unplanned events, athletics, family deaths, etc.) and should offer a different but equivalent exam in those instances.

Faculty needing private or special testing arrangements for students (with written permission from the Office of Freshmen Development and Student Affairs) should contact the School of Nursing Testing Coordinator (see Scheduling Special Testing Accommodations for Students policy).

Scheduling Special Testing Accommodations for Students
Faculty needing special testing accommodations for students enrolled in assigned courses and presented with written permission from the Office of Disability Services should schedule such arrangements at least 2 weeks in advance with the School of Nursing Testing Coordinator. This does not include makeup exams unless the student has special needs as previously mentioned.

Faculty Responsibilities: Provide the Testing Coordinator with the following *at least 2 weeks prior* to the first exam of the semester that will be administered in your class:

1. List of dates and times of all exams/quizzes that will be administered during the semester. This form will be emailed to you from the Testing Coordinator.
2. Inform the selected students that all testing accommodation info will be sent to them via email from the Testing Coordinator. They are to report to the testing room at least 10 minutes prior to the start of each exam.

The Testing Coordinator will develop a special testing schedule for the entire semester and share with GAs who will sign up to proctor various exams. Each week, the Testing Coordinator will email students their special testing schedule and will Cc the appropriate instructors. At least

---

[6] Used with permission by Duquesne University School of Nursing.

three business days before each scheduled exam, submit the online ExamSoft request form with accurate information. On the day of the exam, 15 minutes prior to the start time, the proctor will secure the exam code packet from the Testing Coordinator and go to the testing room and administer the exam. Following the exam, the proctor will return the packet to the Testing Coordinator.

Exam Item Analysis Results

Faculty members must review the item analysis report following each scheduled course examination and notify the appropriate Program Chair if the exam's mean or median score falls below 80; more than 15% of the class scored below a passing grade (C+); or more than 25% of the class attained an A grade.[7]

A Short Primer on Basic/Essential Psychometrics

In a chapter on the Testing Environment it would still be helpful to review some of the principles of psychometrics and test item construction. These are extremely critical aspects of evaluation, and when they are not followed and used consistently, and when faculty do not regularly update their test banks and improve the reliability of their questions, then faculty are simply not doing their job. They are actually negligent.

There are two types of tests, one of which is **norm referenced** (typically classroom tests where student performance is measured relative to other test takers). Our classroom tests (objective multiple-choice tests, not essay), HESIs and NCLEX are all norm-referenced tests. **Criterion-referenced** tests are employed solely to determine whether a student has mastered specific content or behaviors. Our clinical evaluation and our Skills Check-off Competencies that are used are examples of criterion-referenced tests.

All tests administered must have an acceptable level of **validity** and **reliability**. This may not be important for a history exam, but it is critically important for nursing exams where the student potentially passes or fails a course based on the results of one or more exams, and whose scores carry a risk to progression or expulsion. On a small quiz, reliability and validity may be less important, but for a major exam, midterm, or final—this is an expectation. Moreover, because students must eventually postgraduation take NCLEX or NP Certification Exams, they must be exposed to reliable and valid measures of their mastery of necessary content while they are in school.

Validity

Validity is the degree to which test items measure what they are supposed to measure. *Question: Does this test measure neurological nursing care or not (or something else)?* **Content validity** is essential for norm- and criterion-referenced exams. To establish content validity, you need (a) the use of a test blue print and (b) test items reviewed/judged by content experts—with minimum acceptable = 80% agreement among "expert judges." This means an ideal **test blue print for students** indicates how many questions on specific content will be on the exam. For example, you spent 2 hours on Neuro, 2 hours on Cardiac, and 30 minutes on Hematology. On a 60-item test, you cannot administer a test with 20 items on Neuro, 20 items on Cardiac, and 20 items on Hematology. The test would not be a valid measure of the time allocated to that content. In this case, for a 40-item test, you would only include 6 or 7 questions on Hematology and 16 or 17 questions each on Neuro and Cardiac. **A test blue print for faculty** (and not typically shared with students) would include not only the number of questions per content area, but a distribution of questions deliberately selected among their emphasis on knowledge (the lowest), comprehension, application, and analysis (the highest level of Bloom's Taxonomy for which test items can generally be devised). Constructing items at the synthesis/evaluation level are nearly impossible for a pen-and-pencil test, including NCLEX. As students move through an undergraduate program, the emphasis should be less and less on knowledge and progressively more from the comprehension, application, and analysis level. Senior tests should

---

practically have no knowledge questions but have application and analysis-based questions for which knowledge must be first demonstrated in the individual test question before the full question can be analyzed. For example, a nephrology content question at the analysis level would first require the student to know ranges (both high, low, normal, and abnormal) for BUN and creatinine before being able to fully analyze and answer the rest of the question which outlines the case of the question. One example of a junior level 60 item exam might include 20% knowledge, 30% comprehension, and 50% application test items. Your secure test bank must have your individual questions tagged or categorized to accomplish this. For individual test items, at minimum you should have your test reviewed by another expert for both content and test construction evaluation. An individual faculty member administering any objective test (undergraduate or graduate) should never administer a test that "only their eyes" have seen. The expert peer feedback is critical.

Reliability

Reliability is the accuracy or precision of measuring what you are trying to measure. *Question: Does this test measure student performance on mastery of neurological nursing care content at an acceptable and consistent level or not?* The primary measure of reliability that we can ascertain is Kuder-Richardson KR-20 and KR-21—whereas KR-21 somewhat underestimates reliability compared to KR-20, but is sufficient for our measures. We must run KR-20/21 on all our major exams and .70 or greater is good for a classroom test (and the higher, the better!). A score of .60 to .69 is acceptable but somewhat low (in this case, items that are too easy or too difficult, the "rigor of test items," need to be revised before they are used again). "Rigor of test items" will be discussed in the following. Below .60 indicates the test needs revision and must be seriously analyzed before final grades for that test are posted. A test with less than .50 KR-20/21 is really not reliable and should not be used as a "high-stakes test." Individual tests with a reliability less than .50 should be seriously evaluated and scores adjusted. In program the test evaluation policy is that any test with a reliability less than between .60 and .70 has to be reviewed with another faculty member. A test, and a proposed "fix" to the test, must be reviewed by a three-member faculty team. Here is a website where it is easy to calculate your KR-21. You just need to insert your test mean, standard deviation, and number of test items: www.cedu.niu.edu/~walker/calculators/kr.asp

With ExamSoft or Scantron Performance Series and others test taking software, these are the essential psychometrics:

- **% Correct** (this number will give you an indirect measure of the rigor or *level of difficulty* of each test item); 100% correct means the individual test item/question did not discriminate, was too easy, and if this is a Foundations of Nursing exam a couple of these might be acceptable (a few early "success questions" are acceptable), but for a senior exam, test items that have no discrimination are just not helpful to the student or valuable information to us as faculty. Conversely, a test item that no one gets correct has the same effect on student and faculty evaluation. Your percent correct should range between 30% and 80%. Above 80% indicates the item was too easy and below 30% indicates the item was too hard. In each of these cases, examine the distractors and modify them to improve the test item for use the next time. Upon revision, ExamSoft will identify this as a new question.
- **Point biserial statistic** is the Item to Total Score Correlation (Discrimination Level). This is the primary statistic you should use to determine whether a question should be "kept" or "thrown out." The Point Biserial Correlation should be +.20 or greater. A negative correlation is bad and may indicate that your "best students on this test" missed the question too often and "weak students on this test" got it correct too often (here, the most common explanation is the "weak students on this test" simply guessed the correct answer). Examine all questions with a point biserial correlation of less than .20 and make a decision whether more than one answer ought to be accepted or whether the entire test question needs to be eliminated.
- **Response frequency** (# who answered A, B, C, D). "E" should not be used since NCLEX and HESI give four options). Moreover, on HESI and NCLEX at least 30% of questions are "Select all that apply," so students should be exposed to these types of questions at the very beginning.

- **Unused distractors** (you should not have distractors that no one uses or selects). If so, this means your distractor was not a good one and did not "distract" at least some (more than one!) student. Example: Test A had 64% of all possible options NOT selected by any student. That means that 64 of 108 distractors did not distract at all. This would seriously decrease the rigor of this test. Test B: 100% of students got 31 test questions correct. Again, this means 31 items had zero discrimination and also likely affected the rigor of the test. Again, when you analyze your test and see these occurrences (distractors unused or items where not a single distractor was used—you need to modify these questions in your individual secure test banks so this does not happen again). This is the kind of "test" quality improvement that must be done.

- Finally, a few points about the writing of test questions. This is an important skill and new faculty who have not had coursework or experience in test construction will need continuous faculty development in this area. You should not use fake names or real names. There should be no "Mr. Smith is…." You should write: "The patient is…." or "The client is…." Second, you should not use age, gender, ethnicity, or race of the patient or client in the stem (the body of the question) or as options (the four different possible answers) *unless it is relevant to the answer.*

- **The most critical problems to avoid with stems include:**
  - Do not use "You"—it is "The Nurse or the Registered Nurse…."
  - Do not use negative stems— "Which of the following should you not do…."
  - No grammatical errors

- **The most critical problems to avoid with the four options include:**
  - Avoid nonparallel construction (you cannot have three options where the nurse "performs" an action and one option where the nurse "observes"). There are literally hundreds of improper uses of nonparallel construction. In parallel logic, each item should be similar.
  - Avoid options of unequal length (cannot have one option with 4 words and one with 11)
  - Avoid bias of placement of options; ideally 25% of your correct options should be balanced between a, b, c, and d and you should avoid multiple patterns (e.g., four straight answers of "a" followed by a b, d, then three items with "c").

Writing good test items is difficult and test items must be constantly updated in order to properly evaluate student performance. Last, every effort must be made to make sure test banks remain absolutely secure.

The Standardized Patient in Nursing Education and Scoring

It was a very radical idea when Drexel nursing students first went to the Drexel University College of Medicine for an standardized patient (SP) experience in 2002. The students were videotaped performing a history and basic health assessment on patient actors, with numerous nursing faculty behind one-way mirrors, observing student–patient interactions, and taking prodigious notes. This was the beginning of perhaps the first premier SP nursing simulation program in the United States, now named the Center for Interdisciplinary Clinical Simulation and Practice (CICSP) at Drexel University in Philadelphia and now includes low- to high-fidelity simulation too.

The history of the first SP dates to 1963 when Dr. Howard S. Barrows, a neurologist and medical educator at the University of Southern California, "trained" the first "patient actor" to portray a paraplegic patient with multiple sclerosis (Howard University Health Sciences Clinical Skills Center, n.d.). For many people, their first exposure to "what is a standardized patient?" comes in the ninth and last season of *Seinfeld* in 1998. In this episode, Kramer plays a patient with gonorrhea to an attending and a group of physicians-in-training. He then gets upset when he is asked to come back and repeat his stellar performance, fearing being "typecast!"

While use of Standardized Patient Health Simulation is now required in medical education (including use in the United States Medical Licensing Examination), it is used to varying degrees across other health and healthcare professions education. It is now common in many graduate nursing programs, but its use in undergraduate nursing education has been limited (Andrea & Kotowski, 2017). The Objective Structured Clinical Examination (OSCE), developed for use in any healthcare discipline, can be incredibly diverse. Cases can focus on substance abuse and ethical issues; have cultural implications; and span an incredible array of medical, health-related issues. The depth and breadth of an OSCE is constrained only by the expertise and creativity as developed by the writing and testing team. In one example, a medical student worked with a female SP actor who was portraying a Muslim patient trying to control her hypoglycemia as she fasted for Ramadan. The student was from a small Missouri town and had never heard of this Muslim holy period. Afterward, including with feedback from the SP, he stated "I couldn't tell you how amazing this was … it helped calm my fears; it helped me learn how to say things [and avoid hurting patients' feelings]" (Brinn, 2017).

In baccalaureate nursing education, SPs are reportedly used with fundamentals of nursing students, health assessment, mental health nursing, and often to facilitate development of effective communication skills. An excellent example of the use of SPs with BS nursing students describes a theater major playing an SP actor, with nursing students portraying the role of the nurse, and another the patient's friend (Sideras et al., 2013). The moulage of teaching cases, from simply having a faculty member create an OSCE and observing students performing the scenario to the formal use of trained SPs who are examined in formal labs, encompasses the pedagogy of the SP. But like other forms of simulation, we need better validity studies and scoring instruments to demonstrate these teaching strategies are truly educational and foster learning. Further, with the rapid implementation of simulation particularly in nursing education (for a variety of issues, including competition for clinical sites) within some 900 to 1,000 nursing programs in the United States and its territories that prepare RNs, there are disparities in resources with which to offer a Comprehensive Simulation Program (CSP). Sideras et al. (2013) also emphasized that "While simulation is a burgeoning strategy to augment and complement clinical practice education, full implementation requires a broader scope than dependence on manikin-based simulation alone" (p. 421).

In 2002, there was no literature on the validity and reliability of scoring an SP, and certainly not for nursing students. How would we create a scoring system that could be psychometrically credible to the faculty and students. The faculty team discussed at length some scoring models (please refer to Appendix 25.1). Before further discussion here, it is noted that in a 2017 multi-study (Park et al., 2017) of SP scoring medical schools, where SP testing is far more prevalent than undergraduate nursing, (but could certainly be used as a template for Advanced Practice or Doctoral Advance Practice Nursing students). It is interesting to note that there still remains a lot of creative models to arrive at a satisfactory evaluation system and scoring that is deemed acceptable by the associated faculty. This is an example of a Team Meeting where validity was extensively reviewed for another text SP administration.

In our first scoring model, we relied 50% on the trained SP scores that were computerized. One common OSCE used was a case where an RN who was admitting a patient to a medical unit was tasked to perform the typical patient history and physical that the professional RN (not an advanced practice nurse) would perform. After the SP exam, the SP would sit at a computer in the room and rate the student on a series of questions as (a) Did the nursing student use effective communication skills to me? (b) Did the student demonstrate compassion and care during communication? (c) Did the student nurse exhibit professional behavior? The other 50% came from the score sheet that scored whether the student performed the "skill" or not. Not all skills were scored, especially ones all students might always perform and this would not discriminate in scoring. For instance, "taking a blood pressure" would likely be performed by all students so it would not be scored. But the student may have skipped or improperly performed an abdominal exam, so that skill would be scored as absent. In our first years, we watched students perform the exams behind the one-way mirror and scored them. Later, with digital tapes, the scoring could be performed remotely. We then first calculated all students' raw scores to determine a mean and standardized deviation. Next, we converted standardized scores into Z-scores.[8] A Z-score is the number of standard deviations a particular value is from the mean. Using Z-scores, we closely examined the lowest quartile of scores, the lowest 25% Z-scores. We looked for a logical cut point, not a specific statistical

---

[8] Note that these calculations were performed independently of knowing individual student names, to maintain the integrity of the scoring.

Z-score as cut point. We also looked at outliers. Generally, in a class of 65 students there might be around five failures. They then had to review their videotape (after 2 years we were converted to fully digital), do a self-review, receive remediation, and prepare for a retake examination. Passing a standardized examination was one of the final grade components used to pass their last course and graduate. Finally, it should be noted in that very first class of undergraduate nursing students, the SPs had only ever worked with medical students; at the end of the semester they stated that the nursing students had better communication skills than the medical students. This finding has been confirmed in a study by Rezaei and Mehrabani (2014) where 80 physicians examined 93 real and 90 SPs and 12% of the "patients" were not satisfied with the physician's communication skills. The medical students, however, had more confidence in their physical examination skills. Not that the nursing students were less knowledgeable, but that they were not assertive enough during the exam. In other words, the nursing students didn't want to hurt the patient (e.g., an abdominal palpation) or were overly concerned about their privacy (e.g., were hesitant to lift up the patient's gown and expose them). Overall, the faculty were very proud these very pioneering nursing students.

RELEVANT LEGAL CASE (AND COMMENTARY BY AUTHOR)

Jonathan Dorfman, Plaintiff and Appellant, v. University of California, San Diego et al., Super. Ct. No. 37-2012-00101760- CU-WM-CTL (2015)

This is a case of a student at the University of San Diego, California heard by the California Supreme Court and Court of Appeals. A student (Dorfman) was accused of cheating on a math exam and his professor filed Academic Misconduct charges against him based on a statistical analysis of his exam. He was dismissed twice before winning on Appeal over 5 years later.

On July 4, 2011, the Dean of the College Dorfman attended notified him that his CHEM 6B Instructor, Professor John Crowell, had accused him of academic misconduct by cheating on his chemistry exam. The exam was administered on March 25, 2011, but the student was not notified of the charges until after the semester.

The testing protocol was that four versions of the exam (A, B, C, and D) were administered to 618 students (there were multiple sections of the same course). Each student had a Scantron score sheet to score the exam and an exam booklet. The score sheet had the version of the exam in pencil and in pen ink on the back of the exam booklet. The students were instructed to place their name on each item. The exam was administered in four separate classrooms (probably large lecture halls). There were proctors in each classroom and they were instructed to put a summary of the Test Taking Procedures on the blackboard. The instructions written included instructions to compare the penciled version of their exam to the pen ink version and notify the proctor if they were different. In large capital letters on the blackboard was written "DO NOT ALTER YOUR SCANTRON." Crowell also stated that it was his practice at the beginning of each exam to go from to room to room reminding students to notify the Proctor if the two item numbers did not match.

After the semester ended, Crowell discovered that Dorfman and four other students had changed the version of their exam on the score sheet. Crowell determined that Dorfman likely changed his penciled version from D to A. On June 19, 2011, Crowell submitted a report to the university's Academic Integrity Coordinator, Tricia Gallant. UCSD's "Instructions for Prevention and Processing Incidents of Academic Honesty" identified that it was up to instructors/faculty to prevent academic misconduct, and that students who witnessed academic misconduct were required to report it to the faculty or the appropriate administrator.

Dorfman admitted his score sheet and exam booklet did not match, he did not notify the proctor, and made the change himself. He admitted he had to change rooms to take his exam since the others were full. He did not recall seeing the instructions on the blackboard, nor hearing about the instructions that he should notify a proctor because his items did not match. He was not accused of cheating by any other student nor any proctor. Because Crowell let all students take their exam booklet home, he had no direct knowledge of the discrepancy. Dorfman reported he did not have his exam booklet anymore since he had moved and thrown it in the trash.

The University Proceedings

Because Dorfman was already on probation for a prior incident of academic misconduct, he faced expulsion. He denied wrongdoing and requested all of Crowell's documentation which he was provided. On July 25, 2011, he filed for a hearing before the Academic Integrity Review Board (AIRB) to dispute the charge.

He was notified that he would receive a briefing packet 5 days before his hearing. He hired an attorney, Robert P. Ottilie (heretofore identified as "Counsel"), and on July 25, 2011, Dorfman requested a hearing before the AIRB to dispute the charge. Counsel also requested a seating chart and test forms of other students who sat near Dorfman. Counsel asked if there was additional documentation but got no answer. On the fifth day before the hearing it was first learned that Dorfman was accused of copying another student's exam. Additionally, Crowell charged that 24 of 26 answers on his exam matched another student, identified as "Student X,"[9] and that of the 24 items, eight wrong answers and 16 correct answers matched. Student X had Version A of the exam, the same version Dorfman admitted changing his score sheet to. He also reported moving after the semester and throwing the exam booklet away. Two days before the hearing Crowell reported that he had consulted with an expert outside the University and was told it would be a one in billion chance the matched score sheet could be random. Immediately Dorfman and Counsel demanded that Gallant identify Student X, but they were informed the identity of Student X was not relevant to the discussion. After the hearing, the AIRB ruled that Dorfman had violated UCSD's Policy on Integrity of Scholarship. This Council was charged to rule on the punishment and Dorfman contended: (a) Altering his version of the exam was not a violation of academic misconduct, (b) there was insufficient evidence that he copied another student's exam, (c) he was denied due process in various ways, (d) he was not alerted until after the semester, and (e) the University would not identify Student X, and the testimony of a consultant was inappropriate. They ruled to expel him. As per UCSD policy, he was permitted to petition the Council of Provosts. Here he claimed: Gallant worked with Crowell to procure the consultant, thus was assisting against him, failure to provide data only 2 days before the hearing, not 5 as per the procedure, thus precluding Dorfman from obtaining his own expert. In this case, the Council of Provosts suspended the actions of the Council of Deans, until there could be a new AIRB hearing.

The Second University Hearing

In the second AIRB hearing Counsel to Dorfman again sought the identity of Student X. Then a letter was sent to the Office of Student Conduct requesting the following three motions: (a) exclude reference to Student X's score sheet; (b) dismiss and replace the new presiding hearing officer, his own Dean, Patti Mahaffey, as she was already involved in his case and would introduce bias into his hearing as she was on the Council of Deans which had already ruled against him, presenting a conflict of interest; and (c) exclude all mention of the four other students alleged to have cheated. The Office of Student Conduct denied the appeal to remove Dean Mahaffey as it was an expectation of the Dean of any student's respective College to contribute to the discussions surrounding the student's case. With permission of Dorfman and Counsel she would contact Student X to see if the student wanted to provide a written statement or participate in the review, and agree to drop mention of the other students. But Counsel disagreed with contacting Student X as they had earlier claimed contact with the consultant improper and this contact would also fall into that category, both in their view against the Academic Integrity Policy. They were concerned that Mahaffey might get information from Student X that they might not share with Dorfman. Instead Counsel requested Mahaffey "make an evidentiary ruling and exclude reference to the Student X [S]cantron evidence..." (p. 9), which was denied. The second AIRB took place on April 27, 2012. Crowell testified that even if the consultant's estimations were excluded, the statistical analysis did not support coincidence. There was no evidence offered of the seating arrangement of Student X. Dorfman refuted he copied from

---

[9] Student X would never be identified in any University or Court proceedings, nor was evidence ever presented that Student X was aware of the incident.

anyone and disclosed that 40 other students had matching answers to 23, 24, and 25 questions, and some were in different rooms. On May 2, the AIRB ruled Dorfman had changed his scorecard from version D to A, that his exam matched only one other exam on 24 of 26 test items, and that Dorfman offered no explanation for this. They ruled that it was more likely than not that he had engaged in Academic Misconduct. The following day the Council of Deans affirmed the decision. Another appeal to the Council of Provosts included repeated claims of another claim of lack of due process from the failure to identify Student X, the delay in notifying Dorfman of the charge until after the semester, and insufficient evidence to support findings. On June 6, 2012, the appeal was rejected.

Legal Proceedings

On August 12, 2012, Dorman filed a petition of writ against UCSD and the Board of Regents of California in state court. The plaintiff claimed due process violations and insufficient evidence by AIRB findings. On February 10, 2014, after a full briefing and hearing, the Court issued a writ of mandate concluding the AIRB evidentiary findings did not support the ultimate finding that the student had cheated on the exam. Writing, the Court stated the AIRB failed to provide evidence that the matching of the two exams could not have been a statistical anomaly. The Court rejected the claim that the student had no due process. The Court set aside the AIRB's decision and ordered a rehearing at the option of the Regents. The Board of Regents chose to commence another AIRB. Dorfman elected to challenge any rehearing but was overruled. On appeal, after another briefing and rehearing, the Trial Court granted the Regents reconsideration and reversed its ruling setting aside its decision that AIRB's decision was unfounded, leading to the ultimate dismissal of Dorfman from UCSD.

CASE STUDY

On appeal, Dorfman argued that his right to a fair trial was impacted by excluding Student X as a witness, allowing Mahaffey to be the presiding officer at the second AIRB hearing, and that Crowell did not provide sufficient evidence to support the findings by the AIRB. The Appeals Court ruled, "We agree with Dorfman that the university's refusal to provide him with the identity of Student X violated the Regents' and UCSD's own policies mandating certain minimum procedural protections in disciplinary proceedings" (pp. 12–13). Their ruling stated that Dorfman could not amount an adequate defense not knowing the identity of Student X and the ability to refute the charges of copying Student X's exam. Dorfman may have presented exculpatory evidence if it were disclosed where Student X sat. The Court ruled on this point alone the University's ruling should be dismissed. Additionally, Crowell did not provide a seating chart, let students take their exam booklet home, or enforce his policy that students submit their exam with the names of students sitting beside them. There was no evidence presented that the proctors wrote this information on the blackboard as they were instructed to "summarize" the procedures for taking the exam, mentioned earlier in this discussion in the Case Study. The University's assertions were based entirely on a statistical analysis and not on the identity of Student X. Since there was no evidence that the two students were cooperating, "evidence that Student X was not seated where Dorfman could see his or her exam could establish the matching answers were that rare coincidence. Without any ability to determine where Student X sat, Dorfman's defense was unfairly crippled" (p. 17). The University stated their policy of not identifying any student who was not a direct witness or had direct information of the allegation was designed to protect the student from reprisal. The UCSD was criticized for this narrow interpretation of their Policy on Integrity of Scholarship, but they claimed by not identifying Student X, there was sufficient evidence to find Dorfman guilty of misconduct. However, UCSD Counsel did admit this information could have been "dispositive" (p. 18). Finally, the University argued if this were his first violation of the academic integrity policy, he would only be facing probation, not expulsion. Dorfman's Counsel did admit that while first requesting Student X be contacted, they later withdrew this request for Mahaffey to contact Student X. This change of position was based on Mahaffey previously working with Crowell on getting a consultant's report, their fear of what information might be garnered, and fear the full disclosure of this meeting might not be shared with Dorfman. Counsel claimed this was ex parte communication and could not be used under the Academic Integrity Policy. This final claim would ultimately be determinative in the outcome of the appeal.

The finding of the Appeals Court was that this communication was ex parte, and that even if the request was made and later retracted, Dorfman was not acquiescing his rights to due process under the Fifth and Fourteenth Amendments to the Constitution. Dorfman made three motions to the Office of Student Conduct: First requesting disclosure of Student X and if not, second, then requesting removal of Student X's score sheet from the second AIRB hearing, and, third, basically a prohibition of Mahaffey to contact Student X for reasons previously mentioned.[10] The Appeals Court ruled on a technical point that the motions and determinations, made formal and informal to Dorfman, were outside the sections of the procedures of the academic integrity policy; that requesting, then declining Mahaffey contact Student X did not preclude Dorfman from not waiving his right to due process by the University's refusal to identify Student X. The Court wrote, "Courts will not presume acquiescence in the loss of a fundamental constitutional right …; rather, we must indulge in every reasonable presumption against the waiver of such a right" (p. 19). In October 2016, around 5-1/2 years after this incident occurred, Dorfman's writ of mandate was reversed. UCSD was required to retract the dismissal, and the Court ruled the case could be returned UCSD, and if the student later enrolled, the University could pursue actions that were consistent with this ruling. On November 8, 2016, Dorfman had a hearing to request the University pay his legal fees of $200,000. It was stated by Counsel that they believed UCSD knew who Student X was and if they had kept information from the Plaintiff that they found not helpful to their case, they would refer the incident back to the California Board of Regents (Warth, 2016). There is no evidence that the student returned to the College nor any other details of the hearing or its disposition.

The *Dorfman v. University of California* case illustrates the importance of following applicable institutional policies and procedures when dealing with issues of student academic misconduct. In addition, unlike cases where dismissal is based on academic grounds, legal courts will not be as deferential to the judgment of the faculty in cases where the student is being dismissed because of cheating and will be more willing to scrutinize the underlying facts and evidence supporting the institution's decision.

Some Current Controversies in Nursing Education

From our view, there are no major controversies today in testing in nursing education. Probably the most public issue surrounds the use of what has been called "High-Stakes" testing that occurs in a nursing program, particularly as an exit point for graduation. The tests are almost always nationally normed tests like HESI and ATI, which are used widely throughout the country because they have a long track record of high validity and reliability. We contend the use of the term "High-Stakes" for these exams as technically false and we suggest the nursing community find a more appropriate term. The SAT, GRE, MCAT, LSAT and others like it are all high-stakes. The student first takes the test, and the student fails it or doesn't achieve a certain score required by the school or program they are applying to, they likely will not be admitted. NCLEX is a "high-stakes" exam, but it has even higher stakes then the exams just mentioned. The student has already graduated from a nursing program, but if they fail the exam (the student truly only passes or fails), they are not allowed to obtain a license and cannot practice. Other tests like NCLEX include the test for Pharmacists (NAPLEX), Medicine (USMLE, Steps 1–3), Dentistry (ADEX CIF—The Patient Centered Curriculum Integrated Format), Registered Dietician (CDR), and others. We are not going to weigh in whether NCLEX or ATI is more predictive of passing NCLEX, but HESI has now over 25 years of high success of predicting passing NCLEX and high validity and reliability (Morrison, Adamson, Nibert, & Hsia, 2005; Vessey & Brunnert, 2019). Vessey and Brunnert (2019) present data on the HESI exam with a KR20 of 0.90 on almost 80,000 examinees. Dreher, Glasgow, and Schreiber (2019) argue that HESI and ATI are not high-stakes tests because they can find no evidence of any nursing program that uses a single

---

[10] Mahaffey previously offered to contact the student to see if there was any willingness to participate in the hearing or provide a written testimony, but Counsel declined for fears of Mahaffey collaborating with Student X as she had done previously with Crowell.

administration of an exit exam as a requirement for graduation. Any program that allows more than one attempt on an exit exam to achieve the score an autonomous faculty decide is the passing rate is not a high-stakes exam. It is something else. On any issue, there are opponents of these types of exams (Hunsiker & Chitwood, 2017; Sosa & Sethares, 2015), but opposition has not diminished their use. We are even aware of an Associate Degree program in Texas that had very poor, sustained NCLEX scores and resorted to 100% standardized tests throughout their program, and their scores reportedly improved significantly (personal communication, March 17, 2017). We concur that the use of high-stakes testing (as our revised definition indicates) is used through education, from K-12 through higher education. And some arguments about potential cultural bias are valid. But their use in nursing education, particularly when the NGN NCLEX is implemented, will have higher levels of difficulty and require more valid and reliable tests and simulations than current NCLEX testing. When implemented exit exams will increase in rigor and likely increase their prevalence. We list in the following some potential areas of future debate in testing in nursing education:

1. Are we moving toward too much simulation in nursing? At one recent conference attended by both nursing authors, we were amazed how sparse the poster sessions were on evidenced-based nursing practice, ethics, or studies in nursing education that did not deal with simulation. Practically every poster was on simulation, almost exclusively high-fidelity simulation.
2. Will new faculty without experience or graduate courses in test construction, evaluation, including psychometrics, be able to properly develop their skills?
3. Will faculty move rapidly to adjust their testing procedures for the NGN NCLEX?
4. Will someone conduct a study of whether teacher-made tests are more valid and reliable than nationally norm-referenced tests that programs use as exit exam tests (High-Stakes Tests)? Maybe the resolution of this question might alleviate some of the remaining anti-standardized test sentiment.
5. Will NGN be successful? What will happen if NCLEX scores across the United States plummet?

ETHICAL CONSIDERATIONS

A primary purpose of universities and other tertiary educational institutions is to educate students in order to produce experts in various areas of public service (American Association of University Professors, 2002). From the perspective of a nursing program, this translates to a duty to educate competent nurses. "Nurse educators," reads the *American Nurses Association's Code of Ethics* (2015), "… must ensure that basic competence and commitment to professional standards exist prior to entry into practice" (p. 11). Testing is one of our educational system's prime mechanisms for ensuring competency of students. This implies then an obligation to ensure that tests utilized indeed ensure the acquisition of knowledge and skill, that is, validity and reliability. And even the most valid and reliable exams are rendered useless without ensuring academic honesty. So, some standards and policies to protect the integrity of testing are also morally obligatory. It is not possible to prevent all possibility of academic dishonesty, but reasonable steps to ensure integrity need to be taken, and policies and procedures to follow when they are not need to be in place.

Even having all the preceding in place does not guarantee no problems or difficult conflicts will arise. At times, for example, issues of epistemic uncertainty, as in the main case of this chapter will complicate decision-making. In that case at least one, maybe more, maybe all students involved cheated. But the determination of who and how many cheated does not seem forthcoming. In such a case, some degree of unfair treatment of innocent students is almost inevitable. This potential for injustice needs to be weighed against the potential for unprepared or mal-prepared graduates. The potential for injustice toward the innocent needs to be reduced as much as possible, but the duty of preparing competent professionals must also be met. In the case we see an attempt to balance these, though with some degree of unavoidable unfairness almost certainly being visited upon innocent students. There is no perfect answer, so conflicting duties need to be met as far as possible with recognition that some unfortunate compromise must be made.

The Dorfman case also demonstrates concerns of epistemic uncertainty, as the charge of cheating is largely based upon uncertain inferences. But further, the case demonstrates another concern of fairness and justice. Rigorous consistency of policy and procedure must be maintained. Possible inconsistencies in the testing procedures may have contributed to this conflict. And later charges of inconsistent application of policy in responding to the case only furthered and deepened the conflict. Policy, procedure, and due process all have the tinge of vacuous bureaucracy. And they can devolve into such when they become treated as ends in themselves or they are otherwise followed without attention to their proper ends. When attended to properly, these instruments can ensure fair and just treatment. When applied inconsistently, or without just warrant in cases of exceptions, injustice toward students will ensue.

SUMMARY

The testing environment has become extremely complex. Nursing faculty have a duty to develop and administer psychometrically sound examinations in an environment that values academic integrity. The delivery of valid and reliable examinations in a testing environment that adheres to testing protocols is necessary and prudent for the credibility of the nursing profession. To achieve an optimal testing environment, faculty will require significant development on test construction and training on item analysis to write and evaluate test items. Knowledge of testing and measurement coupled with a strong ethical compass are important for a trustworthy testing environment and educational system.

CRITICAL ELEMENTS TO CONSIDER

- The integrity of the testing process must be guaranteed.
- Cheating in any form destroys the integrity of this process.
- Detailed processes for faculty administration of tests and students taking tests must be clear, documented some place, and reinforced.
- All forms of testing policies must be continuously reviewed.
- The use of psychometrics to ensure that tests are reliable and valid is required.
- The confidence students have in the validity of their tests may reinforce that there are positive outcomes from the learning.
- Program, school, college, and university policies on academic conduct must be announced, written, reinforced, and enforced.
- Adherence to these policies is essential as cases of academic misconduct are processed through the various offices of enforcement.
- Members of the faculty need guidelines on how to deal with academic misconduct.
- Offices and institutional members that handle and manage these cases may need to understand some basic legal procedures.
- The concept of due process is critical to those who are accused of misconduct.

Helpful Resources

- Marilyn Oermann and Kathleen Gaberson: *Evaluation and Testing in Nursing Education*, Fifth Edition (2016).
- William A. Kaplin, Barbara A. Lee, Neal H. Hutchens, Jacob H. Rooksby. *The Law of Higher Education: Student Version,* 6th Edition (2020).
- The American Association of Nurse Attorneys: https://www.taana.org/
- NYC Standardized Patient Program: https://www.nycsprep.com/standardized-patients-sp
- Association of Standardized Patient Education: https://www.aspeducators.org/

References

AAUP. (1915). APPENDIX I 1915 Declaration of Principles on Academic Freedom and Academic Tenure, Retrieved from https://www.aaup.org/NR/rdonlyres/A6520A9D-0A9A-47B3-B550-C006B 5B224E7/0/1915Declaration.pdf

American Nurses Association. (2015). *Code of ethics for nurses with interpretive statements*. Silver Spring, MD: Author.

Andrea, J., & Kotowski, P. (2017). Using standardized patients in an undergraduate nursing health assessment class. *Clinical Simulation in Nursing, 13*(7), 309–313. doi:10.1016/j.ecns.2017.05.003

Brinn, D. W. (2017, November 28). Standardized patients teach skills and empathy. *Association of Medical Colleges, AACM News*. Retrieved from https://news.aamc.org/medical-education/article/ standardized-patients-teach-skills-and-empathy/

British Broadcasting Corporation. (2019). Half of universities have fewer than 5% poor white students. *Education News*. Retrieved from https://www.educationviews.org/half-of-universities-have-fewer-than -5-poor-white-students/

Dreher, H. M., Glasgow, M. E. S., & Schreiber, J. (2019). The use of 'high testing' in nursing education: Rhetoric or rigor? *Nursing Forum, 54*, 447–482. doi:10.1111/nuf.12363

Howard University Health Sciences Clinical Skills Center. (n.d.). *Standardized patients: History of standardize patients*. Retrieved from http://www.howard.edu/clinicalskills/cnt/standardized-patients/standardized -patients.html

Hunsicker, J., & Chitwood, T. (2017). High-stakes testing in nursing education: A review of the literature. *Nurse Educator, 43*(4), 183–186. doi:10.1097/NNE.0000000000000475

Jonathan Dorfman v. University of California, San Diego et al., Super. Ct. No. 37-2012-00101760-CU-WM -CTL (2015). Retrieved from http://www.courts.ca.gov/opinions/nonpub/D065865.PDF

Kim, J., Park, J., & Shin, J. (2016). Effectiveness of simulation-based nursing education depending on fidelity: A meta-analysis. *BMC Medical Education,16*, 152. doi:10.1186/s12909-016-0672-7

Morrison, S., Adamson, C., Nibert, A., & Hsia, S. (2005). HESI exams: An overview of reliability and validity. *Computers, Informatics, Nursing, 23*(3S), 39S–45S. doi:10.1097/00024665-200505001-00010

Park, Y. S., Hyderi, A., Heine, N., May, W., Nevins, A., Lee, M., … Yudkowsky, R. (2017). Validity evidence and scoring guidelines for standardized patient encounters and patient notes from a multisite study of clinical performance examinations in seven medical schools. *Academic Medicine, 92*(I–11S), S12–S20. doi:10.1097/ACM.0000000000001918

Preston, C. (2018, April 15). A prescription for poverty? A career in nursing. *NBC News*. Retrieved from https://www.nbcnews.com/news/us-news/prescription-poverty-career-nursing-n865236

Rezaei, R., & Mehrabian, G. (2014). A comparison of the scorings of real and standardized patients on physician communication skills. *Pakistan Journal of Medical Sciences, 30*(3), 664–666. doi:10.12669/ pjms.303.3255

Sideras, S., McKenzie, G., Noone, J., Markle, D., Frazier, M., & Sullivan, M. (2013). Making simulation come alive: Standardized patients in undergraduate nursing education. *Nursing Education Perspectives, 24*(6), 421–425. doi:10.5480/1536-5026-34.6.421

Sosa, M. E., & Sethares, K. A. (2015). An integrative review of the use and outcomes of HESI testing in baccalaureate nursing programs. *Nursing Education Perspectives, 36*(4), 237–243. doi:10.5480/14-1515

Vessey, W., & Brunnert, K. (2019). White Paper: RN HESI reliability scores (KR20s) for the 2017-2018 school year. *Elsevier*, pp. 1–2. Retrieved from https://pages.evolve.elsevier.com/rs/547-FPM-004/ images/2017-2018%20RN%20HESI%20Reliability%20Scores.pdf?aliId=eyJpIjoiZ0ZjR1o3NmpMQUMw MlRoUiIsInQiOiJFK0s0dDI5dTdqR3FkaDZ5M3BkXC9DZz09In0%253D

Warth, G. (2016, October, 26). Judge rules in favor of UCSD student accused of cheating, *sandiegotribune.com* Retrieved June 9, 2020 from https://www.sandiegouniontribune.com/news/education/sd-me-cheat-ucsd -20161003-story.html

Appendix

25.1

Rater Calibration and Rubric Guideline Development Protocol

I. You will receive the following materials for your case:

1. SP training materials (full case)
2. Gold-standard exemplar note highlighting key Hx and PE findings
3. Set of 10 patient notes written by students in previous years (this year if new case)
4. Scoring rubric and general scoring guidelines

II. Scoring team plenary meeting—1 hour
Goal: Develop a shared understanding of the note scoring rubric and how to use it
A. Before the meeting:

1. Review case training materials and exemplar note
2. Review the scoring rubric template and scoring guidelines

B. At the meeting:

1. Review the goals of the exam and pass/fail consequences
2. Review the note scoring rubric and general guidelines for use
3. Review an example of case-specific, level-specific guidelines
4. Review how to score notes online (if applicable)
5. Resolve any questions about the cases and exemplar notes

III. Case-specific calibration meetings—2 hours
Goal: Develop case-specific, level-specific scoring guidelines; calibrate raters
A. Before the meeting:

1. Review the case and exemplar note
2. Score the first three notes using the scoring rubric
3. Note any level-specific guidelines or scoring rules you start to develop
   a. Random example: Must list at least "fever × 2 days" and "productive cough" to get a Level-2 on Documentation section.
4. Bring the calibration notes and your scores for the first three notes to the calibration meeting.

B. At the meeting: Suggested timeline (2 hours total)

1. 10 minutes: Briefly review the exemplar note and key findings.
2. 40 minutes: Compare your scores for the first three notes. Discuss your reasoning and guidelines and come to an agreement on any discrepancies.

3. 20 minutes: Based on your discussions, draft level-specific guidelines for each domain. (What would it take to get a score of "3" for Documentation? etc.) Okay to leave some room for expert judgment and discretion regarding scoring.
4. 40 minutes: Score additional notes, one at a time, using the rubric and your preliminary guidelines. Compare scores, discuss, update guidelines.
5. Final 10 minutes: Make any final modifications to guidelines. Make a "clean copy" of final guidelines.
6. Give the clean copy and the scoring worksheets to your facilitator (if any).

C. After the meeting:
Score any of the 10 calibration notes that were not completed during the calibration meeting. Send scores and any comments to moderator.

Hx and PE, history and physical; SP, standardized patientaps/c.

Source: Reproduced with permission from Park, Y. S., Hyderi, A., Heine, N., May, W., Nevins, A., Lee, M., ... Yudkowsky, R. (2017). Validity evidence and scoring guidelines for standardized patient encounters and patient notes from a multisite study of clinical performance examinations in seven medical schools. *Academic Medicine, 92*(I–11S), S12–S20. doi:10.1097/ACM.0000000000001918

Changing the NCLEX-RN® to the Clinical Judgment Measurement Model: Educational, Legal, and Ethical Implications

INTRODUCTION

This chapter discusses the changes that are being made to the National Council Licensing Examination for Registered Nurses (NCLEX-RN®) licensing exam. Specifically, the authors discuss the clinical reasoning model in relation to cognitive information processing that will be needed to be successful. Related issues of cognitive load and overtaxed short-term store (STS) are included. A major change is the type of reasoning that will be required within the actual test items. We discuss Peirce's (1931–1958) abductive reasoning as a way to understand those changes. In addition to the changes in reasoning, the focus of probabilistic reasoning will also need to be understood by candidates. Finally, we provide a discussion about the changes that will need to occur in the classroom setting to prepare students for clinical reasoning on the test and to be clinically ready day one, as well as the legal and ethical implications. We first discuss the educational implications.

EDUCATIONAL IMPLICATIONS

The focus of this chapter is on the cognitive difficulty, or load, that will be inherent in the new NCLEX-RN exam (National Council of State Boards of Nursing [NCSBN], 2018). For those who have not seen the changes, we suggest examining the next generation NCLEX-RN material at www.ncsbn.org/next-generation-nclex.htm. Specifically, we will focus on five broad areas—the nursing clinical reasoning model (NCRM), information processing, cognitive load, abductive reasoning as part of the clinical reasoning model, and the downstream effects of potentially needed classroom changes. We will start with the NCRM because it is the central feature of the assessment changes.

CLINICAL REASONING MODEL

The NCRM has five major areas (Muntean et al., 2015). The five areas are Recognize Cues, Generate Hypotheses, Judge Hypotheses, Take Action, and Evaluate Outcomes (Figure 26.1).

While working with patients, nurses must recognize cues, pieces of information, or signs within the clinical problem space (Reed, 1972). Within the knowledge of that space, which is a domain-specific knowledge space, a nurse must keep all relevant information and discard irrelevant information. Here is where lack of knowledge or being cognitively overwhelmed by all the cues leads to poor decision-making in the next stage of hypothesis generation. For the purposes here, we are going to call hypotheses, diagnoses or scenarios, which will become critical later.

Owing to our cognitive architecture and functioning, we focus only on a subset of scenarios (Dougherty, Gettys, & Thomas, 1997). We can think of the cues as initially independent elements that need to be connected or integrated into the diagnosis so that an action can be taken. This cognitive work can create computational overload in working memory (Figure 26.2) while we are working through diagnoses (Johnson-Laird, 1999). When overload exists, incorrect hypothesis generations can occur based on differential cue focus. For example, overendorsed cues occur when a nurse overly weights or pays attention to a cue or set of cues that activates an incorrect hypothesis. Additionally, the focus can occur with an incomplete subset of relevant information that activates incorrect hypotheses, or a focus on all the correct cues and a rejection of incorrect cues, yet still activate a wrong hypothesis (Muntean et al., 2015).

At the point of hypothesis or hypotheses generation in the NCRM, nurses have to rank these developed scenarios with the criteria according to how well they explain the cues, or the probability, that is, likelihood that the diagnosis explains the cues (Tversky & Koehler, 1994). This is a focus on probabilistic thinking and not deterministic thinking (Cahan, Gilon, Manor, & Paltiel, 2003; Licata, 2007). The behaviors taken can be simple, such as there is one clear action, or complicated, where multiple actions could be possible. Once actions are taken, the effects of that decision can be evaluated (Johnson-Laird, 1999; Lewis, 1997). The timing of the decision and the effects vary from case to case, but once desired outcomes are observed, that part of the reasoning and action tasks end.

Building assessments based on this model is not simply information recognition, that is, traditional multiple-choice tests. This framework will provide an exceptionally different testing environment. The difference in magnitude will affect how students need to process information.

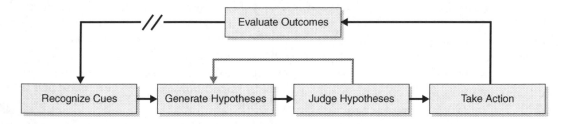

Figure 26.1 Nursing clinical reasoning model.

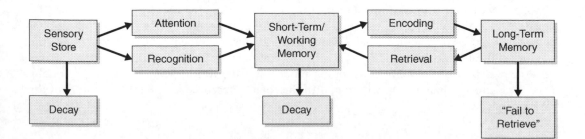

Figure 26.2 Main components of the information processing model.

COGNITION AND INFORMATION PROCESSING

What does all of this mean cognitively? The basic cognitive architecture we will use is the information processing model (IPM). In information processing, we simply discuss the three main components of sensory stores, working memory, aka, STS, and long-term memory (LTM) (Atkinson & Shiffrin, 1968; Baddeley, 2012; Miller, 1956). More complex and nuanced versions of the IPM exist but are outside the focus of this commentary (Figure 26.2).

Sensory stores are for each modality, such as visual or auditory, and decay quickly unless you pay attention to or recognize the information. For nurses, this is paying attention to patient and environmental cues. STS is of limited capacity in general, and if you do not work with the information in STS it will decay away. The information in STS can also be interfered with by other information. Try this yourself: Ask someone to remember eight numbers, and then keep talking to them about a topic. Quiz them at the end on both. This is hard to accomplish because the tasks are of different components. There are STS capacity limits with learning new information, and trying to listen at the same time creates interference (Bäuml & Kliegl, 2013; Wahlheim & Jacoby, 2011). This interference creates problems with encoding information into LTM. But, LTM is unlimited in capacity over long periods of time. Thus, the more information that is encoded and accessible from LTM, the easier it is to deal with new information in STS.

Think about all the cues that an expert nurse sees and easily processes using a massive and easily accessible knowledge and experience base from LTM that allows for a decision to be made. This is termed recognition primed decision (RPD) (Klein, 1993). RPD is why expert nurses were observed to be more proactive in collecting relevant cues and anticipating problems in order to identify patient problems (Hoffman, Aitken, & Duffield, 2009). Expert nurses recognize more cues and pay attention to them at the sensory stage, easily deal with them in limited STS based on a rich knowledge base efficiently accessible from LTM; they have recognition primed. And as the experience of the nurse increases, the nurse will be better able to reduce cues, information, to high-order schemata that "minimize the cognitive cost of maintaining elements in working memory" (Debue & Van De Leemput, 2014, p. 2). Schemata are organized knowledge structures and their interrelationships that allow us to work efficiently. The reduction to the schemata creates a computational advantage in STS, that is, STS is not overtaxed. Thus, the more information is encoded and easily retrievable, the less STS has to work. Education and experience help to build that massive computational advantage for experts. As a last example, when tracked eye movements of experienced doctors were examined, it was observed that they could fixate on cancer in a mammogram in less than 1.5 seconds (Kundel, Nodine, Conant, & Weinstein, 2007). This is the computational advantage and an indicator of primed recognition.

We can also examine this within a System 1 and System 2 model of cognition (Kahneman, 2011). System 1 is Automatized Knowledge (AK) and is running continuously—you have no normal control of this. As you look at these words, you are already interpreting them, and you cannot stop unless you are amazingly distracted by something like what is the square root of 2? At this moment you are stopping to think about the answer. When you have to stop and concentrate, you have just entered System 2, where you must concentrate for effortful mental activities. Effortful mental activities, information processing, can be discussed in relation to cognitive load.

COGNITIVE LOAD

Cognitive Load Theory (CLT) has a main assumption of a capacity-limited STS that can handle seven elements but operates on just two to four elements (Sweller, van Merriënboer, & Pass, 1998). Additionally, the information, those elements, must be dealt with (e.g., rehearsed) quickly, around 20 seconds, or all that information is lost, decays away. CLT focuses on the capacity and duration limitations related to novel information that is processed through the sensory store. But STS does not appear to have a limitation when processing old information retrieved from LTM (Ericsson & Kintsch, 1995; Sweller, 2003, 2004). For example, if someone starts signing, "I am just a bill, and I am only a bill..." Many people can finish the whole song because it is accessed as single schema from LTM.

STS load may be affected either by the intrinsic nature of the learning tasks themselves (intrinsic cognitive load) or by the manner in which the tasks are presented (extraneous cognitive load). Intrinsic is directly related to the learning material (or task) and defined by the number and interactivity of elements that have to be processed (Sweller, 1998).

The more novel or new cues to deal with, the higher the interactivity and, subsequently, the higher the load. An element is defined as "anything that needs to be or has been learned, such as concept or procedure" (Sweller, 2010, p. 24). Interactivity concerns the relationships among elements and the cognitive work, reasoning, that must be completed to determine an action. For example, a list of statistical symbols could be seen as low interactive material because these elements are not dependent, although learning to balance chemical equations represents high interactivity material (Sweller, 2010).

Extraneous cognitive load, in contrast, is load that is not necessary for learning and essentially acts as a distraction. A distraction or nonimportant cue that is attended to reduces STS capacity to deal with any important cues. Extraneous and intrinsic are additive in nature, and therefore the more complex the activity and distractions in the environment, the faster STS capacity is overwhelmed. This can lead to poor learning and poor decision-making.

Finally, germane load (GL) is defined as the mental resources that are devoted to acquiring and automating schemata in LTM (Sweller, 2010). For example, if intrinsic load is high and extraneous load is low, germane will be high because the student is devoting a massive amount of working memory resources to dealing with the materials.

REASONING

During the processing of information, that is, examining the cues from the patient or the health record in a test item, quite a bit of reasoning is occurring instantaneously. Most people have been introduced to inductive and deductive reasoning through their educational and work experiences. But focusing only on these will limit the development of clinical reasoning skills. We believe it is important to look at Peirce's tripartite model of reasoning, deductive, inductive, and, most importantly, abductive.

Peirce (1931–1958) stated,

> Deduction is the only necessary reasoning. It is the reasoning of mathematics. It starts from a hypothesis, the truth or falsity of which has nothing to do with the reasoning; and of course its conclusions are equally ideal. The ordinary use of the doctrine of chances is necessary reasoning, although it is reasoning concerning probabilities. Induction is the experimental testing of a theory. The justification of it is that, although the conclusion at any stage of the investigation may be more or less erroneous, yet the further application of the same method must correct the error. The only thing that induction accomplishes is to determine the value of a quantity. It sets out with a theory and measures the degree of concordance of that theory with fact. It can never originate any idea whatsoever. No more can deduction. All the ideas of science come to it by way of abduction. Abduction consists in studying facts and devising a theory to explain them. Its only justification is that if we are ever to understand things at all, it must be in that way. (CP5.145)

Unfortunately, we have relied almost solely on induction and deduction in nursing education programs and, in general, in the education field. To understand the pivotal role of abductive reasoning, it is important to situate it in an elaboration of Peirce's reasoning types (Shank & Cunningham, 1996). Peirce's (1931–1958) types of reasoning can be identified with six modes of abduction, three modes of induction, and one of deduction (Cunningham, 1998; Shank, 1994; Shank & Cunningham, 1996).

Briefly, the six modes of abduction are:
- Hunch (Open Iconic Tone)—possible evidence,
- Symptom (Open Iconic Token)—symptom of more general phenomenon,
- Metaphor/Analogy (Open Iconic Type)—Use of a Metaphor/Analogy to create potential rules or order,
- Clue (Open Indexical Token)—Sign of a past state of affairs, infer from a past state of affairs,
- Diagnosis/Scenario (Open Indexical Type)—Formation of rule based on available evidence, and
- Explanation (Open Symbolic Type)—Possible Formal Rule/General plausible explanation

As one reads the cues and evidence and uses that information to begin to build a diagnosis (hypothesis), abductive reasoning is occurring. We engage in abductive reasoning all day long. You can see this even in novels you have read or heard about. In *Pride and Prejudice*, Jane takes the cue (sign) of Mr. Bingley abruptly going away to London as an indication that he does not have affection for her (Scenario). Yet, Elizabeth takes this sign as a conspiracy in her scenario. These abductions can happen quickly, and we will miss them unless we try to pay attention.

During this abductive process, we are weighing evidence, building scenarios to potentially act on, and prioritizing those actions. Once we implement an action, we are testing our scenario (hypothesis in Nursing Clinical Judgement model). The results we obtain from testing let us make a conclusion or reengage in the abductive process because we did not obtain the results we were expecting. We enter into a state of doubt. When that doubt occurs, we reengage with the cues, abduction, and we have not been able to make a deductive-based statement at that point.

As the number of elements (intrinsic load) increases and interact, the abductive process is cognitively draining and absorbs STS capacity. As we engage in the process, we are trying to answer questions such as "What is happening? What should be prioritized? What actions are needed?" It is **not** a linear process; there are starts and stops and cognitive reorganization of information. Additionally, there is often a time demand.

Again, the reasoning is done quickly, so quickly you may not realize you are doing it (System 1). But you have education and years of clinical experience. Those in your classes at the associate or baccalaureate level do not. That difference of education and experience demands some serious changes to what we do in the classroom if they are going to be clinically ready day one. Now, as we build scenarios and work through what to prioritize, we are generally using a probabilistic system to make those decisions.

Probabilistic Reasoning-Subset to Abduction

Probabilistic reasoning for our illustrative purposes will be based on conditional probability. Others have argued for using fuzzy logic, but that is past the purpose of this commentary (Licata, 2007). Conditional probabilities are different than predicting a role of a fair die. With conditional probabilities, we have conditions that we are interested in using to decide on a probability. Such as, if Person H has symptoms X, Y, and Z, what is the probability that Q has the flu? This is traditionally written P (Flu | X, Y, Z) and read as the probability of having the flu, given conditions X, Y, and Z. This can also be viewed as if Person H shows the symptoms of X, Y, and Z, the probability that Q has the flu is P percent (Licata, 2007). Most importantly, there could be multiple diagnoses that are ranked by probabilities, such as flu, cold, and so on, in the form of differential diagnosis. This aligns with the ranking of hypotheses in the NCRM.

At this point, the abductive reasoning is on hold as a diagnosis is made. In the NCRM, the next step is taking action, and then evaluating that action, which again may lead back to abduction and new diagnosis development. But, owing to the probabilistic nature, there are decision thresholds that will exist in this process (Cahan et al., 2003). A threshold is a break point where one switches decisions, such as no treatment to running a test.

POTENTIAL CHANGES IN THE "CLASSROOM"

Based on the NCRM, the cognitive load and reasoning needed, there are some potential major changes for class designs. The first is that the life of lecturing on the chapter content using slides, PowerPoints, and so on, is going to be very limited when the exam and expectations are clinical reasoning in 24 to 48 months (i.e., depending on program length and design). The traditional class associated with remembering, understanding, and a bit of application of the knowledge that is activable from reading, studying, and listening to the lecture will not work as well. That information, to a certain extent, is inert information and needs to become active. There is a difference between asking what are the symptoms for PE or pneumonia and providing a scenario such as 43-year-old male, trouble breathing, nonsmoker, pulse normal, O_2 95%, low-grade fever, exhaustion, and not on any medications.

The role of the textbook will become information that must be consumed and understood before class and faculty will have to stop just lecturing on the text content. One of us has used this approach while teaching at high school and university levels and redeveloped "in-class" time for scenario, problem-solving, reasoning, and decision-making. We do not envision a full problem-based or project-based approach (Barrows, 1986; Barrows & Tamblyn, 1980). This is drastically different from a direct instruction approach (Beghetto, 2013; Beghetto & Schreiber, 2017).

Questioning Patterns

Behavioral modeling of the NCRM will be needed, forcing questioning patterns with students to change. Specifically, in courses faculty implement the IRE pattern, that is, Initiate, Respond, and Evaluate. It is a linear unconnected system. In this pervasive pedagogical mode, the faculty member asks a student a fact-based or even application question, the student responds, and the response is instantly evaluated by the faculty member (Beghetto, 2013; Beghetto & Schreiber, 2017; Mehan, 1979). Many faculty members do not realize they are engaging in this generic questioning pattern (Eagleman, 2011). This is killing ideas softly (Beghetto, 2013); for us it is killing clinical reasoning softly. After an IRE, everyone moves on to the next question. This is not pushing higher order thinking (Brookhart, 2010), but, simply, the live version of Skinner's teaching machine (Skinner, 1958), which kills any chance of students connecting material together for complex knowledge development.

Instead of asking what is a symptom for X, or a cluster of symptoms for Y, faculty will need to reset their questioning technique to the conditional probability focus: Given X, Y, and Z, what may be going on? Take 30 seconds and write down (a) What you think is going on? (b) What appears most important out of those cues? (c) How are they interrelated? (d) What is contradictory? (e) What do you think you know? (f) What would you ask? (g) Get ready to share.

The same material can be covered, but the cognitive demands are on the students, and they will need full engagement. Even in foundations courses, where there is core historical information, this can be accomplished. For example,

> "Why did the Institute of Medicine write *The Future of Nursing* report?"
> "What does 'highly educated' mean to you?"
> "What is the percentage of BSN-educated the IOM argues for, and why do you think they want that percentage?"
> "What does having that percentage of BSN-trained nurses do for the profession?"
> "Who benefits?"

These are much more cognitively engaging than asking:

> "What is the recommendation for the percentage of BSN-trained nurses?"

By changing the questions and focusing on higher order cognition, a major cognitive benefit is the natural occurrence of a juxtaposition of information (Shank, 2006). Juxtapositioning occurs when cues are put together and more open-formed questions are asked. This can aid in the development of abductive reasoning, prioritizing, using the NCRM, and learning differential diagnosis skills.

LEGAL CONSIDERATIONS

The proposed changes to the NCLEX-RN items currently under development are anticipated to go into effect tentatively on April 1, 2023. These proposed changes will make the exam more cognitively complex to respond to an increasingly complex practice setting. The technological advances in testing options have allowed test item writers the ability to create intricate cognitive models that can be transferred to assessment models to create these new items NCSBN (2018). Schools of Nursing should notify students in writing of these upcoming changes (once details are available) and revise their curriculum and exams to teach and test the Clinical Judgment Measurement Model, as well as provide additional support. In order for nursing programs to meet accreditation requirements, maintain their quality and reputation, and prepare the next generation of practitioners, faculty must adequately prepare their students for the revised NCLEX-RN exam and a more complex practice environment.

SUMMARY

To move students from entry level at a college or university to being prepared for the new NCLEX-RN and clinically ready day one is a daunting endeavor. Changes in delivery of content and behavioral expectations of students can go a long way in making this possible. You will also have to engage students differently, based on the IPM and reasoning process. Additionally, there will be a need to examine the types of cognitive load and reasoning in the items in faculty members' assessment. This also acknowledges that the load is very high early on and should decrease as they build their base and move to clinically ready. This is the trajectory each student should be on, with the overall goal of improving nursing clinical reasoning at entry.

ETHICAL CONSIDERATIONS

The need for a new exam structure was born of data suggesting that newly licensed nurses are required to make even higher complex decisions during the course of patient care. When a major change in a licensure exam and expectations occurs, faculty are ethically obligated to notify students of these changes and prepare the students and revise their respective curricula and evaluation methods accordingly. The American Association of University Professors (2002), in its founding document on academic freedom, identifies one of the "primary functions of universities as providing general instruction for students" (p. 182). Contextually, this function can be perceived more specifically within particular, especially professional and licensed, domains to prepare students as competent and knowledgeable within that domain. If the gatekeepers of the profession determine that a change in licensure exam is necessary for competent and knowledgeable professionals, then, absent reasoned and declared disagreement from educators in the profession, an obligation to prepare in the context of these changes is derived based on them. This seems like a no-brainer; however, the preparation of faculty to teach in a new way is complex. Many faculty do not have formal preparation in teaching and measurement. It is not likely that new nursing faculty educated in a clinical practice specialty, particularly those hired with limited or no teaching experience and limited or no education courses, can quickly establish the expertise to write strong, reliable, and valid complex test questions (using this new model) unless they have intensive faculty development and support over a certain period. Even some experienced faculty are challenged to write questions skillfully across the level of Bloom's Taxonomy (Dreher, Glasgow, & Schreiber, 2019). Ethical questions arise that are related to the time required to *educate the nurse educators* on this new type of model and develop reliable and valid exam questions so they can *effectively* educate students. There are also students who will be repeating the NCLEX-RN (because they failed their initial attempt or attempts) who have not been educated on the Clinical Judgment Measurement Model. Is it ethical to require them to take this new exam without any formal preparation on this new model? Will there be a transition period for these individuals repeating the NCLEX-RN? Implementing a new exam with immense changes requires a thoughtful transition plan involving a variety of stakeholders (including faculty and deans) and a very transparent communication plan.

 CRITICAL ELEMENTS TO CONSIDER

- Offer Faculty Development Sessions on the Clinical Judgment Measurement Model
- Consult experts in measurement and evaluation for assistance with test construction
- Offer workshops to students on the Clinical Judgment Measurement Model and advice on answering sample questions

- Offer individual faculty consultations in teaching the Clinical Judgment Measurement Model on their respective content and developing test items
- Notify students of this change in writing once more definitive information is available
- Use professionally developed tests that incorporate questions using the Clinical Judgment Measurement Model

References

Atkinson, R. C., & Shiffrin, R. M. (1968). Human memory: A proposed system and its control processes. In K. W.Spence & J. T. Spence (Eds.), Psychology of learning and motivation (Vol. 2, pp. 89–195). London, UK: Academic Press.

Baddeley, A. (2012). Working memory: Theories, models, and controversies. *Annual Review of Psychology*, *63*, 1–29. doi:10.1146/annurev-psych-120710-100422

Barrows, H. S. (1986). A taxonomy of problem-based learning methods. *Medical Education*, *20*(6), 481–486. doi:10.1111/j.1365-2923.1986.tb01386.x

Barrows, H. S., & Tamblyn, R. M. (1980). *Problem-based learning: An approach to medical education*. New York, NY: Springer Publishing Company.

Bäuml, K. H. T., & Kliegl, O. (2013). The critical role of retrieval processes in release from proactive interference. *Journal of Memory and Language*, *68*(1), 39–53. doi:10.1016/j.jml.2012.07.006

Beghetto, R., & Schreiber, J. B. (2017). Creativity and doubt (pp. 147–164). In B. Sriraman & R. Leikin (Eds.), *Creativity and giftedness: Interdisciplinary perspectives from mathematics and beyond*. Basel, Switzerland: Springer-Verlag.

Beghetto, R. A. (2013). *Killing ideas softly?: The promise and perils of creativity in the classroom*. Charlotte, NC: IAP.

Brookhart, S. M. (2010). *How to assess higher-order thinking skills in your classroom*. Alexandria, VA: Assessment and Curriculum Development.

Cahan, A., Gilon, D., Manor, O., & Paltiel, O. (2003). Probabilistic reasoning and clinical decision-making: Do doctors overestimate diagnostic probabilities? *QJM: An International Journal of Medicine*, *96*(10), 763–769. doi:10.1093/qjmed/hcg122

Cunningham, D. J. (1998). Cognition as semiosis: The role of inference. *Theory & Psychology*, *8*(6), 827–840. doi:10.1177/0959354398086006

Debue, N., & Van De Leemput, C. (2014). What does germane load mean? An empirical contribution to the cognitive load theory. *Frontiers in Psychology*, *5*, 1–12. doi:10.3389/fpsyg.2014.01099

Dougherty, M. R., Gettys, C. F., & Thomas, R. P. (1997). The role of mental simulation in judgments of likelihood. *Organizational Behavior and Human Decision Processes*, *70*(2), 135–148. doi:10.1006/obhd.1997.2700

Dreher, H. M., Smith Glasgow, M. E., & Schreiber, J. (2019). The use of 'high stakes testing' in nursing education: Rhetoric or rigor? *Nursing Forum*, *54*, 477–482. doi:10.1111/nuf.12363

Eagleman, D. (2011). *Incognito: The secret lives of the brain*. New York, NY: Pantheon.

Ericsson, K. A., & Kintsch, W. (1995). Long-term working memory. *Psychology Review*, *102*, 211–245. doi:10.1037/0033-295X.102.2.211

Hoffman, K. A., Aitken, L. M., & Duffield, C. (2009). A comparison of novice and expert nurses' cue collection during clinical decision-making: Verbal protocol analysis. *International Journal of Nursing Studies*, *46*(10), 1335–1344. doi:10.1016/j.ijnurstu.2009.04.001

Johnson-Laird, P. N. (1999). Deductive reasoning. *Annual Review of Psychology*, *50*(1), 109–135. doi:10.1146/annurev.psych.50.1.109

Kahneman, D., (2011). *Thinking, fast and slow*. New York, NY: Farrar, Straus and Giroux.

Klein, G. A. (1993). *A recognition-primed decision (RPD) model of rapid decision making* (pp. 138–147). New York, NY: Ablex Publishing Corporation.

Kundel, H. L., Nodine, C. F., Conant, E. F., & Weinstein, S. P. (2007). Holistic component of image perception in mammogram interpretation: Gaze-tracking study. *Radiology*, *242*(2), 396–402. doi:10.1148/radiol.2422051997

Lewis, M. (1997). Decision-making task complexity: Model development and initial testing. *The Journal of Nursing Education*, *36*, 114–120. doi:10.3928/0148-4834-19970301-06

Licata, G. (2007). Probabilistic and fuzzy logic in clinical diagnosis. *Internal and Emergency Medicine, 2*(2), 100–106. doi:10.1007/s11739-007-0051-9

Mehan, H. (1979). *Learning lessons*. Cambridge, MA: Harvard University Press.

Miller, G. A. (1956). The magical number seven, plus or minus two: Some limits on our capacity for processing information. *Psychological Review, 63*(2), 81. doi:10.1037/h0043158

Muntean, W. J., Lindsay, M., Betts, J., Woo, A., Kim, D., & Dickison, P. (2015). *Evaluating clinical judgment in licensure tests: Applications of decision theory*. Paper presented in the annual meeting of the American Educational Research Association in Chicago, IL.

National Council of State Boards of Nursing. (2018). *Next generation NCLEX project*. Retrieved from https://www.ncsbn.org/next-generation-nclex.htm

Peirce, C. S. (1931–1958). In C. Hartshorne, P. Weiss, & A. W. Burks (Eds.), *Collected papers of Charles Sanders Peirce*. Cambridge, MA: Harvard University Press.

Reed, S. K. (1972). Pattern recognition and categorization. *Cognitive Psychology, 3*, 382–407. doi:10.1016/0010-0285(72)90014-X

Shank, G. (1994). *Using semiotic reasoning in educational research: The legacy of Peirce's ten classes of signs*. Paper presented at the Annual Meeting of the Midwest Philosophy of Education Society, Chicago, IL.

Shank, G. (2006). Six alternatives to mixed methods in qualitative research. *Qualitative Research in Psychology, 3*(4), 346–356. doi:10.1177/1478088706070842

Shank, G., & Cunningham, D. J. (1996). Modeling the six modes of Peircean abduction for educational purposes. Paper presented at the annual meeting of the Midwest AI and Cognitive Science Conference, Bloomington, IN.

Skinner, B. F. (1958). Teaching machines. *Science, 128*(3330), 969–977. doi:10.1126/science.128.3330.969

Sweller, J. (1988). Cognitive load during problem solving: Effects on learning. *Cognitive Science, 12*, 257–285. doi:10.1207/s15516709cog1202_4

Sweller, J. (2003). Evolution of human cognitive architecture. In B. Ross (Ed.), *The psychology of learning and motivation* (Vol. 43, pp. 215–266). London, UK: Academic Press.

Sweller, J. (2004). Instructional design consequences of an analogy between evolution by natural selection and human cognitive architecture. *Instructional Science, 32*(1/2), 9–31. doi:10.1023/B:TRUC.0000021808.72598.4d

Sweller, J. (2010). Element interactivity and intrinsic, extraneous, and germane cognitive load. *Educational Psychology Review, 22*(2), 123–138. doi:10.1007/s10648-010-9128-5

Sweller, J., van Merriënboer, J. J. G., & Paas, F. (1998). Cognitive architecture and instructional design. *Educational Psychology Review, 10*, 251–296. doi:10.1023/A:1022193728205

Tversky, A., & Koehler, D. J. (1994). Support theory: A nonextensional representation of subjective probability. *Psychological Review, 101*, 547–567. doi:10.1037/0033-295X.101.4.547

Wahlheim, C. N., & Jacoby, L. L. (2011). Experience with proactive interference diminishes its effects: Mechanisms of change. *Memory & Cognition, 39*(2), 185–195. doi:10.3758/s13421-010-0017-4

27

Creating a Safe and Ethical Nursing Education Environment

Case Study 27.1
Creating a Safe and Ethical Environment

Your role: You are Professor Smith, the faculty member assigned to teach principles of nursing.

Michael Babaya is a 38-year-old international nursing student in the accelerated nursing program in his first clinical course, Principles of Nursing. Mr. Babaya has been on clinical warning for lack of clinical preparation and failure to meet clinical objectives related to basic skills. You initiated a learning contract with Mr. Babaya, and the laboratory faculty member has also worked extensively with him, but the results have been less than what is necessary to continue in the program. On the last clinical day, Mr. Babaya confronts you and demands to know if he passed the course. You respond by saying that his clinical performance is best addressed in your office, privately, rather than on the clinical unit, and offer to meet him later after clinical. Mr. Babaya raises his voice and begins to yell, "I demand to know *now*. Do you hear me!" He approaches you as he is making this statement, and for the first time, you are afraid for your safety and start backing away. As he continues to tell you how important it is for him to pass this course, concerned staff members call security, who come immediately and escort Mr. Babaya off the unit, telling him to calm down, get a grip, and go home. Security returns and records an official incident report of what happened.

The next evening, Mr. Babaya appears at your office at 7:30 p.m., where you are alone, working on end-of-term paperwork. Standing first in the doorway and then entering and sitting in a chair, he tries to convince you to pass him in the course. You are patient with him, and sympathetic, and you gently explain why you cannot change his grade. As the discussion ensues, he becomes increasingly angry. He stands up, leans over your desk, and in a rising voice exclaims, "You have to pass me! I quit my job and gave up everything for this program!" You are alarmed by his conduct, quite frightened, and hope that someone else is in the area and will respond.

Questions

- What are the immediate safety issues for the faculty member?
- How should the faculty member respond?
- Who should be notified with respect to the student's behavior?
- What safety precautions should the faculty member take given the recent circumstances?

BACKGROUND

As noted in other chapters, more and more students with behavioral health issues are arriving at universities. Higher education provides a totally different environment for these students than did high school: Not only does the student have more autonomy and less oversight, but also the duties owed to the student by the institution are far fewer. Moreover, core tenets of higher education are tolerance and respect for individuality and differences, meaning that "acting out" cannot be acceptable. The combination of these factors has the potential to cause uncomfortable, even threatening, situations not just in the classroom, but anywhere—on campus and off—and anytime.

A violent event requires the combination of a person with some (high or low) predisposing potential for violent behavior, a situation with elements that create some risk of violent events, and, usually, a triggering event (Reis & Ross, 1993). Under the law, people have the right to be free of the threat of violence, and this is protected by both the criminal law and the civil law of torts. A person commits an assault if he or she puts someone else in reasonable fear of being harmed and if the actor intended either to do the act that causes the fear or to cause the fear itself. Words alone are not enough to constitute assault, but they are if they are coupled with an act that suggests the ability to carry out the threat.

Virtually all student codes of conduct prohibit students from acts of violence or threats of violence, and the sanctions for violation are severe. But codes will never deter emotion. On Friday, February 12, 2010, University of Alabama Huntsville Professor Amy Bishop opened fire at a faculty meeting, killing three colleagues and wounding three others. Allegations emerged that a denial of tenure for Bishop played a role in the shootings (Bartlett & Wilson, 2010). The tragedies at Virginia Tech and Northern Illinois University have focused enormous attention on mental health issues and violence among college-aged students. In two separate attacks in 2007 in Blacksburg, Virginia, 32 Virginia Tech students and faculty were killed, before the gunman, who was a senior English major, killed himself. Less than a year later, in February 2008, on the campus of Northern Illinois University, a 27-year-old former graduate sociology student shot 22 victims and killed 6 (including himself) (Bohn, 2008). In 2002, a nursing student shot three nursing instructors to death at the University of Arizona and then killed himself ("Gunman in Arizona," 2002). As these tragic events indicate, faculty and administrators have good reason to be concerned for their safety. More recent college mass shootings include Umpqua Community College near Roseburg, Oregon, where in October 2019, a 26-year-old student enrolled at the college fatally shot an assistant professor and eight students in a classroom, before killing himself (Ford & Payne, 2015). The Virginia Tech University remained the largest massacre in U.S. history until the 2017 Las Vegas mass murder that killed 58 (Washington Post Staff, 2017).

The Clery Act, originally known as the Crime Awareness and Campus Security Act of 1990, the Jeanne Clery Disclosure of Campus Security Policy and Campus Crime Statistics Act (20 USC § 1092(f)) is the landmark federal law that requires colleges and universities across the United States to disclose information about crime on and around their campuses (U.S. Department of Education, Department of Postsecondary Education, 2016). The university must also report whether any of the crimes were motivated by race, gender, sexual orientation, religion, ethnicity, or disability, otherwise known as hate crimes. This will tell consumers (potential and current students, faculty, and staff) how safe the area is, but it is nothing more than historical fact. What is surmised is that many campus crime incidents, including theft, rape, and other sexual assaults, go unreported. In 2015, a national law firm used Clery Act open data to determine overall reports of crime and specific criminal acts for example sexual assault, motor vehicle theft, and other crimes using a roster of the Top 100 Colleges in the United States (Beltz, 2017). The top three schools for overall reports of crime were Stanford, UCLA, and the University of California Berkley. For motor vehicle theft, the top three schools were University of Maryland College Park, California State Polytechnic University, and Stanford. Because universities are often regarded as protected environments, incidents of violence are particularly shocking for the college campus and extended community. Another reason that college crime statistics may be underreported is a technical one—Where do a college's boundaries begin and end, and do areas of high student density off-campus housing count too? Today, students and their families must learn about campus crime statistics and ways to ensure their safety.

In response to acts and threats of violence, "user-friendly" harassment policies and complaint procedures are now common on university campuses. To minimize events of (and potential liability for) harassment, colleges and universities should make their antiharassment policies and procedures clear; publish and disseminate them as widely as possible; make sure there are hotlines in place to which reports can safely and effectively be made; and provide training to potential complaint handlers and faculty, staff, and students (Alger, 1998).

IDENTIFYING BEST PRACTICES IN NURSING EDUCATION

Faculty and administration need to be cognizant of triggering events that would cause a student with a propensity for violence to become violent. "A *triggering event* is a description of the immediate circumstances surrounding an act of violence and is not intended to convey a lack of agency or responsibility by perpetrators but rather to address conditions that may lead to violence" (Reiss & Roth, 1993). Increased vigilance and preventive measures during times of high stress—such as during midterm and final examinations—are recommended. For nursing faculty, the delivery of a clinical warning notice or grade of clinical failure could constitute a triggering event. During these times, faculty are cautioned to take preventive measures, such as alerting one's supervisor that a student will be receiving a failing grade. The faculty member should meet with the student during a high-traffic time when many faculty and staff members will be outside the conference room or office. The member should notify faculty and staff that they will be meeting with a student to deliver bad news. If the faculty member suspects that the student may become violent, they should notify security to be on standby as a precautionary measure. The university should also teach faculty how to identify behaviors that are consistent with harassment or potential violence, and it should also emphasize its zero tolerance for workplace harassment and violence (Equal Employment Opportunity Commission, 2010). There is also a growing literature on "how to deliver bad news," even to students. National Academic Advising Association is the national organization for academic advising, and they suggest the SPIKES acronym, which represents: Setting up an appointment, Perception, Invitation, Knowledge, Empathy, and Strategies and Summarize (Hammond, 2017). We have observed that nursing education can be a high-stress manor and suggest faculty and students should also be educated to report concerning behavior such as severe depression, anger outbursts, and fascination with weapons to university public safety officials. Equally important, complainants should be treated with respect and compassion, provided anonymity when possible, and given protection from retaliation or further harm.

One of the most serious present-day problems related to college safety is the peer harassment of a student or group of students. The harassment may be on grounds of race, national origin, ethnicity, gender, sexual orientation, religion, disability, or other factors such as fraternity hazing (Kaplin, Lee, Hutchens, & Rooksby, 2019). For example, as discussed in an earlier chapter, to hold a university liable for monetary damages for sexual peer harassment of one student by another student, the student would have to demonstrate: (a) a hostile environment exists in the school's program or activities, (b) the school knows or should have known about the harassment, and the school fails to take immediate and appropriate corrective action (62 Fed Reg. at 12039). After a university receives notice of the harassing conduct, it has a duty under Title IX to take some action to prevent the further harassment or harm of the student or students (Kaplin et al.,

2019). Student-to-student harassment is also the most common form of sexual harassment on campus. Eighty percent of the students who experienced sexual harassment on college campuses were harassed by a student or a former student (Silva & Hill, 2005), and these statistics are practically unchanged a decade later, where in a 2014 Department of Justice report, 80% of female student assaults were from someone they already knew (Sinozich & Langton, 2014). The American Association of University Women (AAUW; Silva & Hill, 2005) also showed that at colleges and universities "nearly one-third [of students] experience some form of physical harassment, such as being touched, grabbed, or forced to do something sexual" (p. 8).

College-wide prevention programs, and procedures by which there can be prompt and direct intervention, are critical in addressing and minimizing student–student harassment and violence. Harassment policies need to be widely publicized, as do the universities' methods for reporting and responding to incidents of harassment.

DISCUSSION OF CASE STUDY

In Case Study 27.1, it is important that the faculty member speak in a low tone, be empathetic to the student, and call him by his name. You can discuss how difficult the program is, how many students have difficulty in the first term, and how often students suffering from the anxiety and stress can be helped by seeking assistance from student health. You can promise to review his case again with the laboratory faculty member and speak again with him the following day.

Ideally, faculty members' offices should be so arranged that their chair is close to the door. This would help the faculty member exit the office quickly if necessary. Also, ideally, faculty members should avoid staying in their offices late at night or early in the morning, when the campus is isolated. If it is absolutely necessary to work late, then the faculty member should lock the office door and alert public safety or security that they are alone in the office.

Faculty should be particularly vigilant after giving students bad news. If possible, faculty office buildings should be locked during the evening hours. In this case, you should have declined to speak with the student about his situation, but scheduled a meeting with him first thing in the morning; if he refused that appointment, then you should have called security right then, before he had a chance to get upset. Now that this has occurred, you need to report him to the student conduct committee and the office of public safety for uncivil and threatening behavior. It was particularly concerning that Mr. Babaya appeared at the faculty member's office in the evening, when no one else was in the building, and could not control his anger on the clinical unit. It is difficult to predict if Mr. Babaya would resort to physical violence; however, his recent behavior is of great concern and warrants further investigation and action.

An emergency student protocol guide is also warranted in guiding the nursing faculty on the proper procedures in the event of a violent or potentially violent incident involving students or other personnel. These protocols serve as a resource in assisting faculty during interventions with students who may be in imminent danger to themselves or others. These protocols must be reviewed regularly by faculty. The easiest way to review these protocols is during a faculty meeting. We have also found an increase in the need for mental health counseling and intervention during exam week, and the Student Health Center is particularly aware of these trends. The need for management protocols for nursing students in crisis must be underscored.

In cases in which a student poses a significant safety risk, a university will convene a threat assessment task force with university officials made up of representatives of mental health counseling, public safety, student life, legal counsel, and, possibly, nursing academic administration (depending on the case) to evaluate the situation. They will consider whether the student is fit for educational responsibilities at this time and whether an involuntary leave or temporary suspension from specific educational activities is appropriate on the basis of an individualized assessment of the situation. Proper documentation that this assessment process was followed will help the institution defend itself in the event of legal challenge. In the event of a violent act, the police would be notified and take appropriate action. If the alleged perpetrator and victim are still on campus, as in *Kelly v. Yale University* (2003), the university is obligated to provide academic or residential accommodations to prevent possible future harassment or harm.

FINDINGS AND DISPOSITION

In Case Study 27.1, the faculty member informed Mr. Babaya that she could not make any decisions regarding his grade at that time and that she needed to review his clinical preparation sheets. She calmly told Mr. Babaya that she had to complete all the paperwork she was working on that night and that she would meet with him the next day and asked him to leave her office, and he complied with her request. The faculty member immediately closed and locked her door and called campus security. The security officer completed a report and escorted the faculty member to her car. The case was submitted to the student conduct committee and office of public safety. Based on the two incidents (clinical unit and office incidents) and clinical failure, the committee dismissed Mr. Babaya from the accelerated nursing program and included a "no readmit" notice in the file. The office of public safety sent Mr. Babaya written communication that he was no longer permitted on campus and to cease and desist from all communications with Professor Smith.

AN ETHICAL NURSING EDUCATION ENVIRONMENT

The first provision of the *American Nurses Association's Code of Ethics* (ANA, 2015) asserts a moral obligation to create "an ethical environment and culture of civility and kindness, treating colleagues, coworkers, employees, students, and others with dignity and respect" (p. 4). This imperative includes "an affirmative duty to act to prevent harm" (ANA, 2015, p. 4). What is particularly meaningful here is the invocation of an "affirmative duty." What this implies is that one's duty to foster an ethical environment is not limited to policing one's own behavior. That is, certainly one has a duty to refrain from engaging in unethical and unsafe behavior, but beyond that one needs to take active steps to ensure the work environment, whether a hospital, clinic, or educational institution, is safe and ethical. What this means in detail, in terms of specific acts, will require further examination.

Case Study 27.1 involves a student who displays threatening and potentially violent behaviors. Examples elsewhere in the chapter demonstrate that the risk of physical harm from both students and faculty is not unknown in the educational environment. But, of course, one has control over one's actions, but not over the actions of others. The mere assertion that such behavior is inappropriate and unethical does not take us very far. So given the fact that these types of risks are a reality, we must go further than this simplistic judgment. First, assuming it is true that we cannot control the actions of others, what we can control are our responses to others. And those reactions may either improve or aggravate and worsen a situation. This then transfers the burden of duty from the behavior of the threatening other to ourselves. Second, it may not be wholly true that we have no control over the actions of others. True, in the moment of the interaction and particularly with those of especially extreme and possibly pathological emotional states we likely have no control, but in terms of the "affirmative duty" to foster an ethical environment there are limited steps to take that may positively affect the behavior and disposition of others.

Both these considerations suggest an ethical outlook emphasizing the centrality of virtue. An ethics of principles and rules has a lot to offer, but it also has limits. In particular, as suggested previously, any coherent understanding of moral principle informs us that the actions in question, such as those of the student in Case Study 27.1, are clearly inappropriate and wrong. However, that judgment is so obvious as to be nearly trivial. And practically speaking, the best it can offer is to fulfill the "affirmative duty" to cultivate an ethical working environment through policy means such as indicated earlier in the chapter, implementing an emergency student protocol guide or convening a threat assessment task force. Such actions can surely be very effective and are necessary elements of cultivating an ethical working environment—especially given the past evidence of the likelihood of those types of events recurring. Virtue, as an understanding of ethical behavior, goes beyond a purely cognitive approach of rule following that seems characteristic of principle-based views on ethics.

Virtue theorists often describe a virtue approach operating at different levels of action and response. On the one hand, virtue ethics acknowledges that ethics is not just about what are sometimes called "hard cases," the types of dilemmas that courses in ethics typically focus on. These are cases that raise severe and unusual circumstances in which the morally correct decision is not easy to discern. Such education is certainly valuable for cultivating critical thinking and fostering a deeper understanding of theory and principle and possibly preparing students for those moments when they may face such situations. However, ethics is not just about these hard cases. It is also about the mundane activities and choices one makes in the course of one's life and profession (Fowers, 2005; MacIntyre, 2007; Tronto, 1993). Virtue ethics, through focus on a stable character, acknowledges the relevance of ethics for one's everyday life. A good character will carry one successfully and ethically through one's day and the mundane challenges one encounters. On the other hand, virtue ethicists also recognize the importance of the hard cases. Borrowing a metaphor from Aristotle, Veatch (1962) compares a virtuous character to a skilled pilot navigating stormy seas. Virtues help us navigate our own ethical and emotional storms. They enable "us to act intelligently ... in the face of our own feelings and impulses and emotions" (Veatch, 1962, p. 81). In other words, when we face difficult situations, virtues can help us navigate successfully. The difficulty of the situation can be due to the intemperate rhetoric and actions of a student or colleague but also due to the emotions that such behavior provokes in us. In such a threatening situation, the arising of such emotions may be involuntary, but our response to them is possibly something we can control or develop an ability to control.

Many principle-based theories of ethics—Kantian deontology, utilitarianism—emphasize impartiality, universality, and objective thought. In the pursuit of these formal standards, often they also deny any positive influence of emotion and perceive emotion as merely a hindrance to clear objective moral analysis and evaluation. Virtue ethics does not see emotion as necessarily a hindrance to either ethical analysis or to ethical action. In fact, distinct from these other approaches to ethics, the virtue approach does not acknowledge a clear division between reason and emotion (Carr & Steutel, 1999). Virtue ethics recognizes several positive means by which emotions function in ethical thought and conduct: (a) emotions aid us in attending to and testifying to what we care about; (b) emotions signal values to ourselves and others; (c) emotions are "modes of establishing values"; (d) emotions have intrinsic value themselves; and (e) emotions motivate action (Sherman, 1999, p. 42). In this way, virtues can be defined as "dispositions to feel and be moved by our various desires or emotions neither too weakly nor too strongly, but in a way that moves us to choose and act as reason would dictate..." (Curren, 1999, p. 67). In that tense situation in which an agitated, even threatening, other is confronting us, the various strong emotions that would likely arise could very well worsen the situation. A wise and virtuous person will be able to harness these emotions, not necessarily repress them, but direct them, in concert with a clear mind, to ease tension. Regarding the particular case for this chapter, the advice provided earlier in this chapter is to "speak in a low tone, be empathetic to the student, and call him by his name ... discuss how difficult the program is, how many students have difficulty in the first term, and how often students suffering from the anxiety and stress can be helped ... from student health." As with the navigation of stormy seas, this may not be a simple task, but it can be accomplished when appropriate virtues such as temperance, compassion, caring, prudence, modesty, and respect are in place.

Temperance refers to self-control, particularly in regard to desires and emotions. In the situation in question, this is likely the most important virtue. Whatever emotions arise in the heat of a moment like this—fear, anger, indignation, confusion, sympathy—these can either worsen the situation or guide us to a desirable outcome when properly managed. Compassion and caring are familiar virtues to nurses. In this case, when an agitated and threatening person is confronting us it can be difficult to respond with compassion and caring. But doing so can help in the encounter in understanding the suffering this person is undergoing—even if the response to that suffering is far out of proportion. Prudence, often interpreted as merely the ability to bring about the most useful outcome, in terms of virtue often refers to the ability to determine the proper moral outcome and do what is necessary to achieve that. The virtue of modesty refers to the proper perception of one's self, role, and ego. In a situation like this, emotions like indignation may tempt us to stand our ground and prove ourselves right in this situation. In the cold light of reason, you may well be right. But proving that may not be what is important at the moment. Modesty will keep your ego in check and help to focus on de-escalating the situation rather than proving yourself right. And respect, the recognition of the inherent value and dignity of another, like compassion and caring, can be difficult to access in a moment like this, in which the other is expressing no respect for you. But as with compassion and caring, respect as a virtue can alert us to the right of the other to their emotions—despite the disproportionate response to them. Thereby, instead of reflexively dismissing the concerns of the threatening person, we can take them properly into account.

Regarding an event such as the one in question, in the moment we cannot control the actions of another. However, part of the aforementioned affirmative duty to cultivate an ethical working environment and the broad duty to educationally prepare students is to prepare them in terms of ethics and character. A proper ethics education can and should take many forms. Students, especially in a professional program such as nursing, can be instructed through the employment of various theories, principles, case studies, and an examination of the professional code of ethics. Those are all valuable tools and strategies focusing on the important analytic and cognitive aspects of ethics education. Yet the virtue approach acknowledges more than the cognitive aspect of ethics and is arguably especially relevant for the ethics of nurses (Armstrong, 2006; Arries, 2005; Lützen & Barbarosa da Silva, 1996; Vanlaere & Gastmans, 2007). The duty to provide an ethics education is not exhausted by instruction in theory and principles. As important as that is, the development of character within the role of the nurse is also important to better ensure students become good and ethical nurses. Accordingly, Carr and Steutel (1999) assert that "positive moral and other human development is as much if not more, a matter of right affective nurture and good example and support … than of the disinterested mastery of rational principles of duty and obligation" (p. 252). Note the focus on affect from Carr and Steutel (1999). The ability to analyze a situation and objectively determine the moral path is truly valuable but less valuable when an agent lacks the proper affect or attitude, one which predisposes an agent to desire to act morally.

Discourse on moral education from the perspective of virtue ethics often presumes initial or primary education involving children (Carr & Steutel, 1999; Curren, 1999; Kupperman, 1999; Noddings, 2013; Slote, 1999; Spiecker, 1999). The complication of students at the tertiary level is that they are typically at least 18 years of age and thus come to a professional program with an established set of attitudes and dispositions. As Fowers (2005), for example, notes, some students may come to a professional program with good moral perception and others with less intact capacities for moral perception and other elements of character. Regardless of the good or bad, strong or weak character that a student brings to a professional program, it becomes the program's duty to help cultivate a character consistent with good nursing. Doing so includes techniques such as role modeling (Aristotle, 1941; Blum, 1994; Carr & Steutel, 1999; Fowers, 2005; Sherman, 1999). "The single most important way we teach ethics," Fowers (2005) stresses,

> is in the way that we convey to students and to one another, through all of our actions, what is important and what is trivial … through what we do or do not do, what we attend to or neglect, what we emphasize or marginalize…. We are constantly teaching ethics, sometimes explicitly, but much more of the time implicitly. (p. 196)

Other recommended teaching techniques include mirroring more conventional ethics education, utilization of the professional code of ethics (Fowers, 2005). Codes of ethics can communicate not only rules and principles but also deeper expectations in terms of attitude and disposition. Also, expanding the moral imagination through literary examples is often suggested as a means for cultivating character (Carr & Steutel, 1999; Fowers, 2005; Kupperman, 1999). The depth of emotion and meaningful narrative that literature often provides can reach students more deeply than simple study of theory. And case studies are often also cited as effective teaching tools (Fowers, 2005; Sherman, 1999). Through collective deliberation of case studies, students can become aware of their own fallibility and dependence on others, thereby forming virtues like modesty, humility, self-awareness, and openness to others. Kupperman (1999) even argues that any sufficiently challenging academic activity, even if not directly oriented toward ethics education, can help to build character. The quality and effectiveness of these techniques is not at all clear. As Carr and Steutel (1999) pointed out decades ago, more research is needed to identify "effective moral-educational strategies" (p. 252). And their observation still holds true.

One caveat must be kept in mind. The initial language characterizing the actions of the student involved in Case Study 27.1 is highly reflective of virtue ethics analysis: "some (high or low) predisposing potential for violent behavior," "impulsive acts." The investigation here, however, is focused on students whose problems are rooted in poorly formed character. Some of the other examples presented in the chapter are far more extreme and indicative of a pathological state of mind. It would be folly to assume a simple ethics education would be enough to resolve the issues affecting these students and faculty. Yet the line between these conditions may not be clear, particularly to the layman not prepared in psychological or psychiatric study. And this is why, as emphasized earlier, actions like providing emergency student protocol guides and outreach from campus health centers are so important.

Another type of undesirable behavior discussed in this chapter is peer harassment based on race, national origin, ethnicity, gender, sexual orientation, religion, disability, or other factors. This type of behavior also, perhaps even more so, is grounded in character. We can teach students that all persons are deserving of respect and that the ANA Code (2012) directs nurses to respect both colleagues and patients. In particular, the code prescribes "setting aside any bias or prejudice" in regard to providing nurses services (ANA, 2012, p. 1). And one could reasonably interpret that value of equality and respect to apply to one's peers and colleagues as well. These types of values and principles can and should be communicated to students. However, ethics includes more than just knowing, understanding, and even following commonly accepted rules and standards. Truly virtuous nurses will set aside bias and prejudice not simply to follow a predetermined rule but because they want to. They want to make others feel accepted and welcomed. They want to avoid excluding others. They want to acknowledge the value and dignity of others. They want to contribute to a harmonious working/ learning environment and even a better society. Virtuous nurses will have open, caring, and accepting dispositions and will not only conform to the values of the ANA Code of Ethics but will want to do so.

Once again, these are the types of virtues that need to be fostered in students, with the techniques outlined previously—but also with techniques in need of further study and development. For example, in regard to moral imagination, philosopher and ethicist Nussbaum (1995) details her application of Richard Wright's *Native Son* in teaching ethics to law students. She describes the University of Chicago, where she teaches, as an "island of privilege surrounded by poverty and urban decay, with a sharp boundary drawn between these areas" (Dahnke, 2007, p. 82). The themes of race, prejudice, and poverty in the novel are especially instructive to the largely privileged students in these environs and for those students who are likely to encounter many who are different from them in their future professional life. Referring to the privileged status of herself and her students, Nussbaum (1995) explains, "Almost all of us were in the position of Wright's Mary Dalton, when she says to Bigger Thomas that she has no idea how people live ten blocks away from her" (p. xiv). An expansion of moral imagination can affect someone more deeply than merely being instructed in commonly accepted principles.

In a similar vein, Fowers (2005) presents the case of a female second-year student in a doctoral program in applied psychology who

> was not completing assigned work in her graduate assistantship … had made offensive comments about gay men and lesbians and other individuals who did not share her conservative views … had several angry outbursts toward male coworkers … had been deceptive with several faculty members about her work, and that her attitude toward the faculty and her learning was dismissive and recalcitrant. (p. 199)

The student's academic work ranged from adequate to good. And the faculty acknowledged that the student had a right to her conservative beliefs but needed to learn to express them in a more mature and respectful manner. So, rather than expulsion from the program, the faculty "chose to focus on behaviors and outcomes that were central to their training program and ones that they could determine, observe, and evaluate themselves" (Fowers, 2005, p. 199). The student was placed on probation for a year and under close supervision of the director of training (DoT), who provided feedback regarding her disrespectful interpersonal behavior, offense caused to students and faculty, and loss of trust of students and faculty through deceptiveness. The DoT further advised the student that she had to improve her work performance in these respects to continue in the program. "This feedback," explains Fowers (2005), "was important in helping her to improve her performance in these areas, which was essential in her future work with people who might be alienated or harmed in similar ways" (p. 199). As with the experience of Nussbaum's law students reading *Native Son*, this feedback is meant not merely to provide simple rules to follow but to encourage engagement with and development of virtues like compassion in acknowledging and understanding the pain and experience of people who are different but nonetheless similar in terms of equality, dignity, and capacity to suffer. Further, the DoT counseled the student not only to refrain from similar behavior in the future but also to take steps to repair damaged relationships. Doing so would provide necessary forms of compensatory justice but also address her character more deeply through active atonement. And, finally, the DoT recommended, but did not require, personal therapy. The response of the faculty is geared toward instructing a student not merely to follow rules but to develop a character in line with the values and goals of the program. The results were that "following a brief period of defensiveness, this student took the feedback to heart and made clear and demonstrable improvements in all of these areas" (Fowers, 2005, p. 200). Fowers (2005), of course, emphasizes that such a positive outcome may not always occur. This is true, but such uncertainty does not itself abrogate the faculty obligation to provide the best ethics education possible.

SUMMARY

Unfortunately, there are not always red flags (e.g., harassment, anger management issues) to predict violent behavior; therefore, a comprehensive university approach that combines education, sound code of conduct policies, vigilance, and clear reporting mechanisms are in the best interest of the college community. Harassment and other violent behavior compromise the sense of community to which most universities aspire (Kaplin et al., 2019). Faculty, students, and staff all desire a safe campus environment. Individuals want to go about their daily lives without fear of physical, emotional, or psychological harm. Personal safety is a basic human need that must be upheld; therefore, violence prevention and safety promotion should be seen as a broader mission of all universities (Bickel & Lake, 1999; Roark, 1993).

 CRITICAL ELEMENTS TO CONSIDER

- Address attitudes and perceptions that contribute to violence through education, curriculum integration, and other efforts.
- Offer counseling to students at times of high stress, such as during midterm and final examinations.
- Deliver bad news to students during normal office hours in a private office located in a high-traffic area.
- Do not keep concerns related to student harassment to yourself. Alert your supervisor and public safety.
- Alert security ahead of time if you suspect that a student, faculty, or staff member may be violent when you deliver bad news.
- Alert security when you are working late, then lock your office and take necessary safety precautions.
- Educate faculty, students, and staff about the need to report behavior that threatens public safety.
- Educate and promote bystander intervention.
- Convey clear expectations for conduct among students, faculty, and staff.
- Create and disseminate comprehensive policies and procedures addressing behavior—strong enforcement of violent behavior sends a clear message about intolerance for violent behavior.
- Provide a range of support services for students, including mental health services, crisis management, and comprehensive services for victims.
- Offer campus safety classes in orientation and offer campus escort service.

- ▨ Establish comprehensive alcohol and other drug prevention programs.
- ▨ Do not keep your concerns related to aggressive, disturbing, or depressive behaviors to yourself. Notify your supervisor and the office of public safety with any questions/concerns.
- ▨ Determine whether a situation requires immediate intervention. (If the student appears to pose a danger to themselves or others, then contact security or public safety immediately.)
- ▨ If you feel uncomfortable or unsafe, trust your instincts.
- ▨ Faculty, students, and staff should register for the emergency notification system via text and email on cell phone.
- ▨ Publicize victim support services on campus.
- ▨ Convene a threat assessment task force.

Helpful Resources

- "Primary Prevention: Stopping Campus Violence Before It Starts." The Higher Education Center for Alcohol, Drug Abuse, and Violence Prevention: http://www.higheredcenter.org/files/prevention_updates/may2010.pdf
- American College Health Association: https://www.acha.org/
- Higher Education Center Resources: http://www.higheredcenter.org/pubs/violence.html
- The National Sexual Violence Resource Center (NSVRC): http://www.nsvrc.org
- Security on Campus: http://www.securityoncampus.org

References

Alger, J. R. (1998, September/October). Love, lust and the law: Sexual harassment in the academy. *Academe*, *84*, 34–39. Retrieved from https://eric.ed.gov/?id=EJ572067

American Nurses Association. (2015). *Code of ethics for nurses with interpretive statements*. Silver Spring, MD: Author.

Aristotle. (1941). *Nicomachean ethics*. In R. Mckeon (Trans Ed.), *The basic works of Aristotle*. New York, NY: Random House.

Armstrong, A. E. (2006). Towards a strong virtue ethics for nursing practice. *Nursing Philosophy*, *7*(3), 110–124. doi:10.1111/j.1466-769X.2006.00268.x

Arries, E. (2005). Virtue ethics: An approach to moral dilemmas in nursing. *Curationis*, *28*(3), 64–72. doi:10.4102/curationis.v28i3.990

Bartlett, T., & Wilson, R. (2010, June 17). Amy Bishop is indicted in 1986 shooting death of her brother. *The Chronicle of Higher Education*. Retrieved from http://chronicle.com/article/Amy-Bishop-Is-Indicted-in-1986/65970/

Beltz, B. (2017). Crime at the top 100 colleges in the U.S. *Huffing Post*. Retrieved from https://www.huffpost.com/entry/crime-at-the-top-100-colleges-in-the-us_b_6432864

Bickel, R. D., & Lake, P. F. (1999). *The rights and responsibilities of the modern university: Who assumes the risks of college life?* Durham, NC: Carolina Academic Press.

Blum, L. A. (1994). *Moral perception and particularity*. Cambridge, UK: Cambridge University Press.

Carr, D., & Steutel, J. (1999). The virtue approach to moral education. In D. Carr & J. Steutel (Eds.), *Virtue ethics and moral education* (pp. 241–255). New York, NY: Routledge.

Curren, A. (1999). Cultivating the intellectual and moral virtues. In D. Carr & J. Steutel (Eds.), *Virtue ethics and moral education* (pp. 67–81). New York, NY: Routledge.

Dahnke, M. D. (2007). *Film, art, and filmart: An introduction to aesthetic through film*. Lanham, MD: University Press of America.

Equal Employment Opportunity Commission. (2010). Harassment. *EEOC*. Retrieved from https://www.eeoc.gov/harassment

Ford, D., & Payne, E. (2015, October 2). Oregon shooting: Gunman dead after college rampage. *CNN*. Retrieved from https://www.cnn.com/2015/10/01/us/oregon-college-shooting/index.html

Fowers, B. J. (2005). *Virtue and psychology: Pursuing excellence in ordinary practices*. Washington, DC: American Psychological Association.

Gunman in Arizona wrote of plan to kill. (2002, October 22). *The New York Times*. Retrieved from https://www.nytimes.com/2002/10/31/us/gunman-in-arizona-wrote-of-plan-to-kill.html

Hammond, J. (2017). How to give bad news. *NACADA: Academic Advising Today*. Retrieved from https://nacada.ksu.edu/Resources/Academic-Advising-Today/View-Articles/How-to-Give-Bad-News.aspx

Kaplin, W. A., Lee, B. A., Hutchens, N. H., & Rooksby, J. H. (2019). *The law of higher education* (6th ed.). San Francisco, CA: John Wiley & Sons.

Kelly v. Yale University, WL 1563424, 2003 U.S. Dist. LEXIS 4543 (D. Conn. 2003).

Kupperman, J. J. (1999). Virtues, character, and moral dispositions. In D. Carr & J. Steutel (Eds.), *Virtue ethics and moral education* (pp. 199–209). New York, NY: Routledge.

Lützen, K., & Barbarosa da Silva, A. (1996). The role of virtue ethics in psychiatric nursing. *Nursing Ethics*, *3*(3), 202–211. doi:10.1177/096973309600300303

MacIntyre, A. (2007). *After virtue: A study in moral theory* (3rd ed.). Notre Dame, IN: Notre Dame University Press.

Noddings, N. (2013). *Caring: A relational approach to ethics and moral education* (2nd ed.) Berkeley: University of California Press.

Nussbaum, M. (1995). *Poetic justice: The literary imagination and public life*. Boston, MA: Beacon Press.

Reiss, A. J., Jr., & Roth, J. A. (1993). *Understanding and preventing violence: Vol. 1. Panel on the understanding and control of violent behavior*. Washington, DC: National Academy Press, National Research Council.

Roark, M. L. (1993). Conceptualizing campus violence: Definitions, underlying factors, and effects. *Journal of Student Psychotherapy*, *8*(1/2), 1–27. doi:10.1300/J035v08n01_01

Sherman, N. (1999). Character development and Aristotelian virtue. In D. Carr & J. Steutel (Eds.), *Virtue ethics and moral education* (pp. 35–48). New York, NY: Routledge.

Silva, C., & Hill, E. (2005). *Drawing the line on sexual harassment on campus*. Washington, DC: American Association of University Women Educational Foundation. Retrieved from https://www.aauw.org/files/2013/02/drawing-the-line-sexual-harassment-on-campus.pdf

Bohn, K. (2008, February 14). 6 shot dead, including gunman, at Northern Illinois University. *CNN*. Retrieved from http://www.cnn.com/2008/US/02/14/university.shooting/

Sherman, N. (1999). Character development and Aristotelian virtue. In D. Carr & J. Steutel (Eds.), *Virtue ethics and moral education* (pp. 35–48). New York, NY: Routledge.

Sinozich, S., & Langton, L. (2014). *Rape and sexual assault victimization among college-age females, 1995–2013*. Washington, DC: U.S. Department of Justice Office of Justice Programs Bureau of Justice Statistics. Retrieved from https://bjs.gov/content/pub/pdf/rsavcaf9513.pdf

Slote, M. (1999). Self-regarding and other-regarding virtues. In D. Carr & J. Steutel (Eds.), *Virtue ethics and moral education* (pp. 95–105). New York, NY: Routledge.

Spiecker, B. (1999). Habituation and training in early moral upbringing. In D. Carr & J. Steutel (Eds.), *Virtue ethics and moral education* (pp. 201–223). New York, NY: Routledge.

Tronto, J. C. (1993). *Moral boundaries: A political argument for an ethics of care*. New York, NY: Routledge.

U.S. Department of Education, Office for Civil Rights. (1997). *Sexual harassment guidance: Harassment of students by school employees, other students, or third parties*. Washington, DC: Author. Retrieved from https://www2.ed.gov/about/offices/list/ocr/docs/sexhar00.html

U.S. Department of Education, Department of Postsecondary Education. (2016). The handbook for campus safety and security reporting. Washington, DC: Author. Retrieved from https://www2.ed.gov/admins/lead/safety/handbook.pdf

Vanlaere, L., & Gastmans, C. (2007). Ethics in nursing education: Learning to reflect on care practices. *Nursing Ethics*, *14*(6), 758–766. doi:10.1177/0969733007082116

Veatch, H. B. (1962). *Rational man: A modern interpretation of Aristotelian ethics*. Bloomington: Indiana University Press.

Washington Post Staff. (2017, October 2). How the Las Vegas strip shooting evolved. *Washington Post*. Retrieved from https://www.washingtonpost.com/graphics/2017/national/las-vegas-shooting/

V

SPECIFIC ISSUES CONFRONTING ADJUNCT FACULTY IN THE CLINICAL AGENCY AND CLASSROOM

Confronting Adjunct Faculty Issues in the Classroom and Clinical Agency

TYPES OF ANECDOTAL ACTIONS BY ADJUNCT FACULTY IN THE CLASSROOM

We begin this chapter by making a very important point. Too often, not just in nursing, but in probably all departments in a college or university, the teaching by adjuncts is often characterized as somehow "less than" what is capable of the standing full-time faculty in the department. Writing for the American Association for the Advancement of Science, Benderly (2019) has written about a "systematic exploitation of adjunct and contingent faculty members."[1] These positions are usually low-paid, temporary appointments that do not include basic amenities, such as an office or even a desk; nor do they offer job security, health and retirement benefits, or professional advancement/recognition. Adjunct and contingent faculty provide over half of undergraduate teaching in the United States. Very often, adjunct faculty are not considered for a full-time position by a formal search committee, despite perhaps their proven teaching excellence. In addition, many of them have cumulated significant academic scholarly accomplishments and provide additional uncompensated support to the department, too. From our experience, with a persistent shortage of nursing faculty with a doctorate, nursing adjuncts may still have difficulty moving up the internal academic ranks. Commonly, if hired full-time, they are promoted only to a nontenure track rank, a clinical track. And at elite research-intensive schools/colleges of nursing, nursing search committees often follow the model of their fellow academic departments by not offering an interview to their own adjunct applicants. There is a large body of literature on the mistreatment of adjunct faculty in the "Academy,"[2] but it is beyond the scope of this chapter to address this issue (Childress, 2019; Jaschik, 2017). Our final point is this: Full-time faculty may be good or bad. Adjuncts can be good or bad. What is very different is the responsibilities that are required of the full-time faculty and adjunct faculty in their roles. However, expectations of performance in the classroom and clinical agency should be the

---

[1] Adjunct faculty are also referred to as contingent faculty. Some schools give them additional ranks, instead of simply "adjunct instructor," such as adjunct assistant, associate, or professor. Unfortunately, these additional ranks are more often not used, and we fully advocate that they should.
[2] The "Academy" is considered the full community of scholars involved in the educational enterprise. Although often considered tenure-track or tenured faculty and research faculty at colleges and universities, that is false, and it includes every individual contributing to education and knowledge generation in higher education.

same. Therefore, while our anecdotes have been observed by adjuncts, they could easily be likewise documented by others as having seen those anecdotes in full-time faculty as well.

Anecdotal Observations in the Classroom[3]

The professor:

- defaults to use of the traditional style of teacher-centered learning, where the teacher stands in front of the class and lectures to students. EAB Navigation has documented student attrition to classes where the faculty does not present information in an interesting or captive way, leading to less motivated students, course dropouts, failing grades, and ultimately probation and expulsion, or students who just withdraw from college (eab.com, 2019)
- overuses PowerPoint and reads the slides
- simply uses prepared textbook slides, indicating to students a lack of interest (or laziness) by the faculty in presenting their own slides
- underuses active learning or any alternative pedagogies in the classroom (even if the students are uninterested in them)
- has to adapt to students who don't have the required classroom text or may have an old edition (but fails to consider there are students who cannot afford either). What is the professor to do?
- tolerates persistence of late arrivals, which disrupts the teaching rhythm
- fails to take attendance, which is particularly detrimental to students who may not get the information again (students who only get the PowerPoints later lose the important context of the class presentation)
- refuses to use any technology in the classroom
- is afraid to call on students because the professor does not want to embarrass students
- calls on students to stimulate classroom discussion
- comes to class unprepared
- "wings" the class because the professor has taught the class for years
- has a syllabus that has been barely updated, even minimally, yearly
- is habitually late
- is unable to master the use of the "smart" classroom
- has low technology skills and prefers the way they were taught
- requires excess reading of a text that cannot reasonably be completely read by the student in one semester, instead of informing students the precise pages that must be read in preparation for the next class (has the faculty reread the content or read supplementary materials to enhance their preparation for the class?)
- has no blue print for the test or fails to follow a blue print (students can ask the faculty for a blue print on the first day of class and even examine their own test afterward to see if the faculty member adhered to the blue print—it can be done)
- commits the ultimate sin in nursing academia—uses no psychometrics to measure the reliability of the exam and then fails to make the necessary psychometric corrections[4]
- recycles the same questions semester after semester
- using electronic testing software, fails to adjust questions for the next exam when there are demonstrable problems with the question; an improved question for the next test would make the test more reliable
- is uncivil to students in the classroom

---

[3] We are purposefully not including the new teacher to online teaching. Although online courses are very prevalent in nursing education, these are not often given to a teacher teaching for the first time, but we admit this does occur. And it is not a wrong assumption that teaching an effective online course has a host of new pedagogies and technical skills to use.

[4] This is a damaging failure by a faculty or a department to ensure that the tests they administer are "fair." This may result in students failing a particular class or even being dismissed from the program—when perhaps in many (or all?) cases, their tests have not undergone this educational expectation, particularly in a clinical discipline. One of these authors took a deanship where the only review of a test was the number of students who got a particular item wrong, thus failing to examine the question's point biserial index.

- is not able to manage expected cultural issues in their presentation of the didactic content to students
- is unable to manage a classroom effectively
- is disorganized
- returns papers late
- fails to properly keep posted office hours
- fails *to attempt to align* the clinical faculty activities to the layout of the class content

This list is not comprehensive but is a good reminder to graduate students pursuing an academic career of some of the pitfalls and important reminders to create an ideal teaching/learning environment in the classroom.

There are two essential aspects to teaching a course that are essential: (a) presenting the course content in a way that students learn the content effectively and are able to apply that content in the rest of their nursing program and in professional practice; (b) effectively managing the classroom environment so that the effectiveness of teaching is sound or enhanced. Hall (2016) writes "… students dislike a disorganized class as much as we do! Students expect their instructors to have their 'stuff' together. Do you start your class on time or do you show up 'just in time?' Students watch you and make value judgments based on your actions" (p. 1). He also emphasizes that you set the tone for your course and class on the first day. From our experience, we caution new adjuncts faculty teaching in the classroom for the first time "not" to announce to the class that this your first-time teaching, unless you are asked by a student (which is unlikely). Openly disclosing this at the first class will only invite additionally scrutiny from your students. An analogy to this is when a newly practicing nurse is asked by the patient "Is this your first injection?" The student can respond honestly if indeed the student has had previous practice of the procedure in the lab and even more so if performed on a patient in clinical.

What is critical for the effectiveness of an adjunct, newly teaching a first class, is a proper orientation or assignment to a mentor. If the adjunct is teaching pediatrics, then it should often appropriately be a pediatric full-time faculty member (or even a highly experienced fellow adjunct faculty). It may be intimidating for a new teacher to teach a first class (all the authors of this text can recall this), but effective teaching is a long journey and not perfected in the first couple of years of teaching (or maybe never). Desaultes (2016) writes, "We meet our new students and begin to see novel behaviors, encounter unfamiliar and familiar words, and observe the mini-worlds that each student carries into our classrooms. We notice apathy, excitement, negativity, enthusiasm, and an array of cultures and belief systems" (p. 1). The question that the new teaching adjunct always faces is "where do I begin?"

Basic mentoring by an experienced teacher to a new adjunct faculty teaching in the classroom includes the following:

1. There is generally a syllabus already completed, whether it will be used in a traditional classroom or online. Often the syllabus cannot be changed, and the adjunct should inquire about this policy.
2. The adjunct will need the textbook(s) preordered so the adjunct can begin class preparation early. This may become very problematic if texts arrive late or if the adjunct is assigned the course at the last minute.
3. There is an orientation to the smart classroom or use of the technology that will be in the room.
4. Orientation to testing procedures. If testing software is used, a more extensive orientation to this procedure will be required.
5. If ebooks are used in the classroom, the adjunct will at minimum know how the students are using them and their functionality—we have often seen students using ebooks, whereas the faculty are unable to effectively use them in class.
6. The adjunct may need some general technology support or the college's online learning platform (LMS); even if a course is not taught online, there is a syllabus and gradebook shell embedded into every class (perhaps not always, but most institutions).

7. The adjunct will need a copy of any handbook that is focused on adjunct teaching, hopefully for teaching in the classroom, instead of just focusing on clinical teaching.

8. Policy and mechanics on grade submission and grade correction.

9. How to manage EAB or Starfish[5] (and perhaps other products) are student success platforms that aim for increased student retention and early alerts to both students and student support offices (advisement, tutoring, and even counseling—as long as FERPA[6] guidelines are ensured).

10. The adjunct faculty will need to be informed of all policies in the department, especially those that pertain to students and faculty responsibilities.

11. The adjunct faculty should have a peer evaluation of their classroom teaching early in the term, or at minimum by midterm, and understand the annual adjunct faculty evaluation and the reappointment process.

12. The adjunct should be fully aware of the program's emergency protocol for urgent student health or behaviors that require immediate attention.

Often a welcome letter from the dean is common to new adjuncts and returning adjuncts at the beginning of a semester. See Appendix 28.1 for a sample letter and sample contract information.

THE ROLE OF THE ADJUNCT FACULTY IN CLINICAL EDUCATION

There is a persistent shortage of nurses that is precipitated in part by a shortage in nursing faculty. This issue is further compromised by the unavailability of or limited clinical placements in healthcare facilities. The lack of clinical placements forces the nursing faculty to shift the skills-learning process from the healthcare environment to the clinical learning laboratory in nursing schools (Bloomfield, Fordham-Clarke, Pegram, & Cunningham, 2010; Bensfield, Olech, & Horsley, 2012). The shortage is magnified as budget constraints, an aging faculty, an increasing job competition with high compensation in the private nursing sector, and the inability of nursing schools to quickly produce larger numbers of nurse educators have all been cited as the reason for the nursing faculty shortage (Kring, Ramseur, & Parnell, 2013; Rosseter, 2019). There is an imminent vicious cycle existing among the shortage of nursing faculty, decreasing clinical placements, increased enrollment of nursing students with the exception of PhD students, and the graduation of skilled confident nurses to meet the nursing shortage in the healthcare environment. A solution to the nurse faculty shortage is one way in which nurse educators may arrest this cycle and increase the supply of skilled competent graduate nurses entering nursing practice.

The quality of care provided to patients in the hospital environment is strongly linked to the performance of clinical nursing skills by nurses, and the skills proficiency of the nursing staff is associated with healthcare outcomes (Aiken et al., 2012; Bloomfield et al., 2010). Hospitals demand nurses with experience and skills but are increasingly relying on inexperienced new nurses owing to the nursing shortage (Ball, Doyle, & Oocumma, 2015; Kring et al., 2013; Lubbe & Roets, 2014; Young, Acord, Schuler, & Hansen, 2014). The Institute of Medicine (IOM) stresses that new nurses should attain competence before entering practice and suggests that the education of nurses be directly linked to the quality of patient care (Cho & Choi, 2018; Hansen & Bratt, 2015). Nurse educators are therefore directly responsible for developing a curriculum that ensures newly prepared nurses are qualified and clinically equipped with the appropriate skill set (Ball et al., 2015; Felton & Royal, 2015; Wilson, Harwood, & Oudshoorn, 2015; Young et al., 2014).

The increasing shortage of nursing faculty coupled with limited clinical placement further challenges nurse educators to either locate or design teaching and learning opportunities for nursing students to attain clinical skills proficiency in the classroom, clinical learning laboratory, and healthcare facilities (Ball et al., 2015; Chicca & Shellenbarger, 2018; Wilson et al., 2015; Young et al., 2014). Increasing the supply of nurse faculty continues to be a challenge. The use of adjunct clinical instructors is a welcome addition to nursing education and may be a solution to the nursing faculty

---

[5] Starfish—www.starfishsolutions.com; EAB—https://eab.com/
[6] The Family Educational Rights and Privacy Act (FERPA; 20 U.S.C. § 1232g; 34 CFR Part 99) is a federal law that protects the privacy of student education records. The law applies to all schools that receive funds under an applicable program of the U.S. Department of Education.

shortage. However, there is difficulty in hiring experienced clinical instructors who practice and who are also equipped with the skills preparation for the role of adjunct clinical instructor. The American Association of Colleges of Nursing supports the use of adjunct faculty who are being provided with optimal orientation and ongoing faculty support, as one way to expand the supply of nursing faculty in both the clinical setting and in the classroom (Koharchik, 2014; Koharchik & Jakub, 2014; Rosseter, 2019). The use of adjunct nursing faculty may help narrow the nurse faculty shortage in clinical and classroom settings and assist nursing faculty to graduate skilled confident nurses who are ready for transition to nursing practice.

Adjunct faculty in clinical education nurtures novice student nurses and transforms them into confident graduate nurses with the basic knowledge, skills, and attitude necessary for transition to nursing practice. After weeks of practice on manikin/simulators (low, moderate, or high fidelity) in the clinical laboratory, the adjunct clinical faculty witnesses the students' first contact with the real-life patient in the healthcare environment or the clinical setting. The role of the clinical instructor is multifactorial. One important role of the adjunct clinical instructor is to assist students to connect what is learned in the classroom to clinical practice through mentoring, modeling, and molding. The instructor ensures that students meet the learning objectives and achieve the learning outcomes of the courses. Additionally, the adjunct clinical instructor assists the nursing faculty to carry out the mission and meet the goals of the nursing education department and the governing institution.

Meeting Departmental Goals

The adjunct faculty in clinical education assists the nursing faculty to achieve the goals of the nursing education unit. A comprehensive orientation session at the institution is provided before going into the healthcare environment. The orientation session enables new adjunct clinical faculty to meet seasoned adjunct and full-time faculty of the nursing education unit. Usually the chair of the nursing education unit or a designated faculty member conducts the orientation session. Human resources logistics related to compensation, hours of work, absences, holidays, and days off are covered. The facilitator reviews the mission and philosophy of the nursing department and the governing institution. The nursing curriculum, course syllabi, learning objectives, and student learning outcomes for the didactic, skills, and clinical component of the courses are reviewed. The adjunct clinical faculty is provided with ongoing guidance and direction on how to help students achieve the student learning outcomes for the courses.

Support for Nursing Faculty

The adjunct clinical instructor represents the nursing faculty in the clinical setting, provides support, and advocates for the nursing faculty. The instructor is responsible for ensuring that students achieve the clinical learning objectives of the course and, by extension, meet the outcomes of the program. The course syllabi with learning objectives of the lectures, skills lab, and clinical are reviewed in detail. The clinical instructor focuses on the weekly clinical objectives of the course and develops a plan for meeting each objective in the clinical setting with the students. The documents used in the healthcare environment are reviewed. Although there may be variations among institutions in the documents used, the student clinical evaluation tool, client assessment tool used for data collection, nursing care plans, concept maps, and skills checklists are basic documents used in the clinical setting. Both adjunct clinical nursing faculty and students are required to attend a mandatory orientation hosted at the healthcare agency. Faculty and students learn of the logistics such as fire and safety, security, and patient electronic health record-keeping systems for documentation and medication administration.

Important Aspects of Education in the Clinical Area by Adjunct Faculty

1. The clinical adjunct should have an orientation to all aspects of departmental technologies that the clinical adjunct might need, even if they are at a remote clinical agency.
2. The clinical adjunct must know the policies in the departmental adjunct handbook. It would be most unusual today for a nursing program not to have an adjunct handbook.

3. The clinical adjunct must have full knowledge of the clinical day: preconference, the clinical day, and postconference.

4. The clinical adjunct must be knowledgeable about agency policies that must be adhered to by all teaching faculty and students.

5. There are likely guidelines for the supervision of clinical adjuncts by the agency and guidelines that the adjunct clinical faculty must follow themselves with their clinical group.

6. The clinical adjunct must also be aware of student policies for participation in the clinical experience (lateness policy, absence policy, safety precautions, expected clinical preparation, evaluation, etc.).

7. The clinical adjunct must know and be prepared to deliver the proper feedback for remediation to expulsion from the clinical agency. These procedures vary from institution to institution, but it is common for a student to first be given an oral warning (for a minor infraction most likely). However, the clinical adjunct will document the oral warning. Sometimes, the student will be required to go for remediation, but often not if the infraction is easily corrected. Next is a written warning if the behavior is repeated or if a different infraction is committed. This almost always requires remediation and goals/outcomes that must be successfully remediated before the student is permitted to return to clinical. A subsequent infraction incurs a warning of clinical failure. This is really the last opportunity for the student to meet the clinical outcomes of the course. We suggest a very formal, tailored set of remediations that is developed by a clinical adjunct, course coordinator, and other designees. These are discussed with the student, who signs a document that he or she is signing the agreement and that in case of failure to successfully adhere to the remediations, the student will fail the clinical course. At any time for the degree of the infraction, the student can be immediately sent home from clinical, banned from the clinical agency, placed on immediate probation, or removed from clinical immediately and designated a failure in the course, expelled from the nursing department or even the college or university. The two nursing faculty of this text have seen all of these. It is also important that students are fully aware of their appeals process that they may file. This process should be in their student handbook and easy to access.

8. The clinical adjunct should collaborate with the course coordinator or teaching faculty concerned to best align clinical activities to the classroom content. This is not always a perfect alignment, but some degree of clinical activity can often be constructed.

9. The adjunct clinical faculty should fully establish their reporting lines back to the department for clinical issues.

10. Some of the classroom mentoring activities may be applied to the clinical adjunct, too.

One way to recruit additional clinical adjuncts on a yearly basis (it is suggested to do this once each spring, summer, and fall) is to have a faculty development recruitment session on: "How to Become a Clinical Nursing Adjunct." The second author of this text offered these sessions owing to an urgent need for more adjuncts on a semester basis with great success. The faculty joined him in his efforts to offer this half-day session to prospective adjuncts. Every event/session had very large attendance and a high rate of conversion of attendance to hire as an adjunct faculty member. Recruiting attendees occurred via website postings, emails to our current adjuncts to send the email/flyer to their friends who might be interested, and to the staff educator at many agencies. Attendees were asked to bring copies of their nursing license and résumé to the session so they could be screened for a possible clinical assignment. The faculty taught very short mini sessions on various topics such as the following:

- A quick review by the Dean of the School's mission and some highlights of the program. Many of the attendees were alumni of the school. Many of the attendees also came because they always wanted to be a clinical adjunct (often for supplementary pay) but did not know how to teach
- Spend 20 minutes on how to manage a 6-hour clinical day
- How to do a student clinical evaluation
- How to conduct a preconference

- How to conduct a postconference
- Ensuring safety in the clinical agency
- Some basic clinical teaching strategies (when to answer a student's question, when to ask the student to "think it through" instead, or when to ask the student to go find out the answer and perhaps discuss the issue for 5 minutes in the next clinical postconference, or other techniques/strategies)[7]
- Crucial conversations and other items

Teaching a clinical day or in the classroom is usually very rewarding to the adjunct. Sometimes, it leads adjuncts to greater interest in nursing education and the desire to obtain additional education/credentials (often a doctorate) to teach full-time. Some adjuncts continue to work for supplementary pay, and others serve as adjunct purely from the joy of knowing they are mentoring the next generation of nurses.

THE EVALUATION OF ADJUNCT FACULTY

In order to deliver effective teaching in the classroom or clinical agency, by any nursing faculty, whether full time, part time, or adjunct, requisite evaluation of that teaching or instruction must be performed if continuous improvement of the teaching mission is sought. This is, of course, required by our own departments, institutions, and regulators, including state boards of education, our nursing accrediting bodies, national accrediting bodies for colleges and universities (e.g., Middle States Commission on Higher Education),[8] and federal agencies such as the U.S. Department of Education.

The evaluation of adjuncts varies in programs, departments, and even in colleges or universities. Sometimes adjunct evaluation processes and procedures are standard across the college. Other times the adjunct evaluation is nursing program based, but in an otherwise superb adjunct nursing faculty clinical handbook, there is nothing on evaluation of the clinical faculty. Our view is that with so many adjunct faculty, particularly large nursing programs, we are concerned about the completeness of the adjunct clinical evaluation process. In another randomly selected nursing department, in their *Guidelines for the Clinical Experience: Manual and Forms Packet*, the evaluation of the adjunct faculty was stated as follows: "Clinical faculty may receive a written evaluation by the faculty of record or Undergraduate Chairperson as requested or needed."

Too often, the student evaluation of their clinical instructor (in form format) becomes the sole evaluation of the faculty. That does not seem fair, because it considers only the student perspective. Moreover, this document is heavily weighted in adjunct faculty reappointments. Generally, unless the student evaluation is completely disastrous, faculty who have less than average evaluations are given some mentoring or performance remediation warning. Repeated negative evaluations most often result in nonreappointment. Evaluation of clinical adjunct faculty is important to nursing accrediting agencies, but it is unclear to us whether this is a particular focus of the accreditors. Since nursing accreditations can last 10 years between review, from our own experiences, this has not been a focus. But accreditors usually do visit at least one agency during their review, and they speak to the clinical adjunct and students.

But we do see the immense challenge for course coordinators, program directors, clinical coordinators, or others in similar roles who have the responsibility for this activity. Moreover, the difficulties in regularly traveling to sometimes distant sites to evaluate large numbers of clinical faculty do impede the monitoring of new and more experienced adjuncts aside from student evaluations and sometimes a phone call to the nursing director of the unit. In one nursing program in a collective bargaining unit, after 10 consecutive semesters (5 years) of satisfactory teaching, the adjunct is given a 3-year contract. In other nursing programs there is an alternating period of evaluation, often performed in the earlier semesters of a new faculty teaching and longer for experienced adjunct faculty.

---

[7] One professor has used the "go find out" technique very useful. Students don't actually mind it and are usually asked to bring some kind of media (paper, poster, handout, etc.)—no PowerPoint (!), and usually everyone learns something new, even the clinical adjunct.

[8] Middle States serves Delaware, the District of Columbia, Maryland, New Jersey, New York, Pennsylvania, Puerto Rico, and the U.S. Virgin Islands, including distance education and correspondence education programs offered at those institutions.

We are not aware of any literature that examines a large cohort of nursing programs and their process for the role of evaluating clinical adjunct faculty. In a less contemporary time, it was very customary for someone from the program to visit the clinical site and speak with the adjunct clinical faculty member, talk to students, and perhaps to the administrator in charge. As mentioned previously, this is, unfortunately, less common, but there are unit directors who believe this is a minimal responsibility of the program, who we assume now recognize this is a practice of the past. There is a growing recognition that adjunct clinical faculty are now the backbone of any nursing program and, increasingly, full-time faculty do a lot less clinical teaching (Elder, Svoboda, Ryan, & Fitzgerald, 2016). We do not see this prevalence of adjunct clinical faculty decreasing in the future, but we do think the relationships between the adjunct clinical faculty and the department of nursing (particularly the course the adjunct is teaching in) need to improve and that the class and course content be better aligned. Hall and Chichester (2014) write, "It's important for nurse educators to continually work to remain effective in the clinical setting to provide an optimal learning environment for students and optimal working environment for staff" (p. 341). Finally, we believe there needs to be more support and recognition of these important partners in our educational enterprise of preparing the next generation of registered nurses.

CRITICAL ELEMENTS TO CONSIDER

- Review Faculty Handbook and adjunct faculty contracts with respect to adjunct faculty responsibilities.
- Consult the university attorney when experiencing personnel issues with adjunct faculty.
- Offer an adjunct faculty orientation and faculty development program.
- Assign a full-time faculty mentor or Director of Adjunct Faculty to mentor adjunct faculty.

ETHICAL CONSIDERATIONS

The prevalence of adjunct faculty has been increasing among all levels of colleges and universities and across all disciplinary fields, including nursing (Nica, 2017). The reasons for this are complex but are often related to financial concerns (Brennan & Magness, 2018b). Whatever the reasons, any use of adjunct faculty, especially the volume that currently exists, raises ethical concerns. A primary concern in the discourse of higher education is the treatment of adjunct faculty themselves. Adjunct faculty have been described as sweatshop workers, indentured servants, slaves, and exploited professors (Brennan & Magness, 2018a). There is currently a social, ethical, and financial debate occurring regarding higher education's use and treatment of adjunct faculty (Brennan & Magness, 2018a, 2018b; Shulman, 2019). Some adjunct faculty supplement their income from a profession related to their area of teaching. This is especially true of nursing adjuncts. However, some instead depend on adjunct course assignments, often from multiple institutions, as the primary, if not sole, source of their livelihood. The university receives competent teaching at a fraction of the cost of full-time, tenured, or tenure-track faculty. Adjunct faculty typically do not receive health insurance or any other benefits of full-time faculty and are paid what would not be considered a living wage (Brennan & Magness, 2018b; Shulman, 2019). The charge of exploitation is understandable. Of course, in the broader sociological and historical context of exploited workers, adjunct faculty may appear unusually privileged. Yet that does not resolve the question of exploitation *per se* or demonstrate that the common treatment of adjunct faculty is appropriately morally respectful. The low pay, lack of benefits, and lack of support often offered strongly imply some degree of use "as a means." Yet adjunct faculty are typically highly educated professionals able to read a contract and autonomously agree to its terms and often do so absent coercion. So while the debate regarding the systemic use and treatment of adjunct faculty continues, *we can at least ensure that our own adjunct faculty are treated as respectfully as possible and provided with all the support needed to teach and fulfill their own professional goals.*

Specifically, what does this entail? The beginning of this chapter noted the characterization of the instruction provided by adjunct faculty as "less than." Any hint of this attitude needs to be avoided, for no other reason than that several of the authors of this text can attest to the work ethics and the quality of the instruction provided by adjunct faculty—quality that often surpasses that of many full-time faculty. Support, including access to computers, copying services, and office space, should be available. Opportunities, including professional development, open to full-time faculty, should also be available to adjunct faculty. Provide and consider adjunct faculty for more permanent positions at the institution. Work toward better ensuring pay for adjunct faculty that is commensurate with the value they provide for the institution.

Much more could be and has been written on this question. The specifics of moral respect for adjunct faculty will vary depending on the nature of your adjunct faculty. Those supplementing the income of a preexisting professional life (such as nursing) may have different needs and expectations than those attempting to stitch together a livelihood through adjunct teaching. Earlier in this chapter, it was asserted that the expectations of adjunct faculty in terms of teaching quality and outcomes should be the same. Let us assume your adjunct faculty are providing quality education for your students. If they were not, they should not be adjunct or any other kind of faculty. Ensuring quality education is your primary duty as educators and as nurses in a faculty or administrative role. Thus, the fact that adjunct faculty have become, and, for the foreseeable future, will continue to be an integral part of achieving this goal, means that constant and proactive attention to ensuring respectful, nonexploitative treatment of your adjunct faculty needs to be a part of your overall ethical project.

SUMMARY

Adjunct faculty can be an asset in the classroom and clinical area as they bring a great deal of clinical and executive expertise. Adjunct faculty should be treated with respect and regard for the expertise they bring to the discipline. Adjunct faculty orientation, mentorship, and development programs are critical to adjunct engagement and success. If problems arise, direct communication, university counsel consultation, and additional mentoring are required to address any potential or actual issues.

References

Aiken, L. H., Sermeus, W., Heede, K. V., Sloane, D. M., Busse, R., McKee, M., ... Kutney-Lee, A. (2012). Patient safety, satisfaction, and quality of hospital care: Cross sectional surveys of nurses and patients in 12 countries in Europe and the United States. *British Medical Journal, 344*(7851), e1717. doi:10.1136/bmj.e1717

Ball, K., Doyle, D., & Oocumma, N. I. (2015). Nursing shortages in the OR: Solutions for new models of education. *Association of periOperative Registered Nurses Journal, 101*(1), 115–136. doi:0.1016/j.aorn.2014.03.015

Benderly, B. (2019). A warning from the academic underground of adjuncts and contingent faculty. Science. Retrieved from https://www.sciencemag.org/careers/2019/06/warning-academic-underground-adjuncts-and-contingent-faculty

Bensfield, L. A. M., Olech, M. J. M., & Horsley, T. L. M. (2012). Simulation for high-stakes evaluation in nursing. *Nurse Educator, 37*(2), 71–74. doi:10.1097/NNE.0b013e3182461b8c

Bloomfield, J., Fordham-Clarke, C., Pegram, A., & Cunningham, B. (2010). The development and evaluation of a computer-based resource to assist pre-registration nursing students with their preparation for objective structured clinical examinations (OSCEs). *Nurse Education Today, 30*(2), 113–117. doi:10.1016/j.nedt.2009.06.004

Brennan, J., & Magness, P. (2018a). Are adjunct faculty exploited: Some grounds for skepticism. *Journal of Business Ethics, 152*(1), 53–71. doi:10.1007/s10551-016-3322-4

Brennan, J., & Magness, P. (2019b). Estimating the cost of justice for adjuncts: A case study in university business ethics. *Journal of Business Ethics, 148*(1), 155–168. doi:10.1007/s10551-016-3013-1

Chicca, J., & Shellenbarger, T. (2018). Connecting with Generation Z: Approaches in nursing education. *Teaching and Learning in Nursing, 13*(3), 180–184. doi:10.1016/j.teln.2018.03.008

Childress, H. (2019). This is how you kill a profession: How did we decide that professors don't deserve job security or a decent salary? *Chronicle Review.* Retrieved https://www.chronicle.com/interactives/2019-03-27-childress

Cho, S. M., & Choi, J. (2018). Patient safety culture associated with patient safety competencies among registered nurses. *Journal of Nursing Scholarship, 50*(5), 549–557. doi:10.1111/jnu.12413

Desautels, L. (2016). Teachers, students, and the hero's journey. *The George Lucas Educational Foundation: Edutopia.* Retrieved from https://www.edutopia.org/blog/teachers-students-and-heros-journey

Elder, S, J., Svoboda, G., Ryan, L. A., & Fitzgerald, K. (2016). Work factors of importance to adjunct nursing faculty. *Journal of Nursing Education, 55*(5), 245–251. doi:10.3928/01484834-20160414-02

Felton, A,, & Royal, J. (2015). Skills for nursing practice: Development of clinical skills in pre-registration nurse education. *Nurse Education in Practice, 15*(1), 38–43. doi:10.1016/j.nepr.2014.11.009

Hall, C. J. (2016). College classroom management: The good, bad and ugly. *Dr. Christopher J. Hall. #Be Better.* Retrieved from https://chrisjhallsc.com/blog/2016/9/16/college-classroom-management-the-good-bad-and-ugly

Hall, N., & Chichester, M. (2014). How to succeed as an adjunct clinical nurse instructor. *Nursing & Women's Health, 18*(4), 341–344. doi:10.1111/1751-486X.12139

Hansen, J., & Bratt, M. (2015). Competence acquisition using simulated learning experiences: A concept analysis. *Nursing Education Perspectives, 36*(2), 102–107. doi:10.1111/1751-486X.12139

Jaschik, J. (2017). When colleges rely on adjuncts, where does the money go? *Inside Higher Ed.* Retrieved from https://www.insidehighered.com/news/2017/01/05/study-looks-impact-adjunct-hiring-college-spending-patterns

Koharchik, L. D. (2014). Delineating the role of the part-time clinical nurse instructor. *Journal of Nursing, 114*(5), 65–67. doi:10.1097/01.NAJ.0000446781.07147.3e

Koharchik, L. D., & Jakub, K. (2014). Starting a job as adjunct clinical instructor. *Journal of Nursing, 114*(8), 57–60. doi:10.1097/01.NAJ.0000453049.54489.d2

Kring, D. L., Ramseur, N., & Parnell, E. (2013). How effective are hospital adjunct clinical instructors? *Nursing Education Perspectives, 34*(1), 34–36. doi:10.5480/1536-5026-34.1.34

Lubbe, J. C., & Roets, L. (2014). Nurses' scope of practice and the implication for quality nursing care. *Journal of Nursing Scholarship, 46*(1), 58–64. doi:10.1111/jnu.12058

Nica, E. (2017). Has the shift to overworked and underpaid adjunct faculty helped education outcomes? *Educational Philosophy and Theory, 50*(3), 213–216. doi:10.1080/00131857.2017.1300026

Rosseter, R. (2019). *Fact sheet: Nursing faculty shortage.* Retrieved from https://www.aacnnursing.org/Portals/42/News/Factsheets/Faculty-Shortage-Factsheet.pdf

Shulman, S. (2019). The costs and benefits of adjunct justice: A critique of Brennan and Magness. *Journal of Business Ethics, 155*(1), 163–171. doi:10.1007/s10551-017-3498-2

Wilson, B., Harwood, L., & Oudshoorn, A. (2015). Understanding skill acquisition among registered nurses: The 'perpetual novice' phenomenon. *Journal of Clinical Nursing, 24*(23/24), 3564–3575. doi:10.1111/jocn.12978

Young, S., Acord, L., Schuler, S., & Hansen, J. M. (2014). Addressing the community/public health nursing shortage through a multifaceted regional approach. *Public Health Nursing, 31*(6), 566–573. doi:10.1111/phn.12110

Appendix

28.1

TO: ALL ADJUNCT FACULTY

FROM: XXX

                Dean and Professor, School of Nursing

RE: Summer 20XX Adjunct Contract

I want to welcome you to either your first or your returning semester and year to the School of Nursing at XXX. I am pleased that you are part of our teaching mission here. Adjunct nursing faculty have become an important backbone of most nursing programs in the United States, and I am glad you are teaching our students and helping us further the mission of XXX. Please feel free to contact me anytime, and do introduce yourself to me when you see me. We are really privileged at XXX to have such wonderful adjunct nursing faculty who contribute to the development of what is "The XXX Nurse!" The XXX nursing faculty are emphatic that ethics, civility, and professionalism be at the core of the kind of professional nurses that we all educate in our School of Nursing.

Computer user accounts/network IDs will be automatically created for all active adjunct faculty. The accounts also have an associated XXX email address that appears on your contract. It is essential that you activate your established XXX email account. Please review the enclosed Network Accounts for Adjunct Faculty information sheet, and visit the XXX virtual helpdesk at (http://www.XXX.edu/helpdesk) in order to do this. It is not acceptable to use outside email accounts (gmail/Yahoo, etc.) to communicate with students about official business of the School of Nursing or College.

Enclosed is your contract for the summer 20XX sessions. It is very important that you verify all information (both personal and academic) before signing this contract. Please also be sure your social security number, address, phone number, and course information are accurate before returning the signed contract.

<u>Contracts must be received by the School of Nursing at least 2 weeks prior to your start date in order to be processed in a timely fashion.</u> If not, your payments will be on a delayed pay date schedule, and the total stipend on your contract will be calculated/divided by the number of pay dates left in the Summer 20XX semester. The adjunct pay dates for summer 20XX are as follows:

6/03   6/17   7/15   7/29   8/12   8/26

Semester	From/To Dates	
SS I	06/01/XX–07/01/XX	(contract due in SON by 5/18/XX)
SS II	07/05/XX–08/06/XX	(contract due in SON by 6/21/XX)
Summer Inst 20XX	06/28/XX–07/30/XX	(contract due in SON by 6/14/XX)
Summer Module 1	06/30/XX–08/06/XX	(contract due in SON by 6/16/XX)
Summer Module 2	06/01/XX–08/06/XX	(contract due in SON by 5/18/XX)

If your contract is received in the School of Nursing by the due date, you should receive your first pay check approximately 1 to 2 weeks after the first day you worked and your last pay check approximately 1 to 2 weeks after the last day you worked.

All adjunct faculty, whether teaching in the classroom or clinical, are responsible to see that a course/teacher evaluation is completed by your students at the end of the semester. If there is no option to use an electronic evaluation and paper evaluations are used, the adjunct faculty member cannot in any way handle them once they are distributed. Completed evaluations must be collected by a student, placed in a confidential envelope, and returned to the Office of the Executive Assistant to the Dean. If you have any questions regarding any of these policies or any questions about the adjunct contract you received, please contact XXX, Undergraduate Clinical Placement Coordinator (for undergraduate courses) or XXX, Executive Assistant to the Dean @ (for graduate courses).

I am enclosing a copy of the School of Nursing Code of Conduct. The specifics of the code must be consistent in every classroom and clinical area in order to be able to enforce the penalties for violations. The elements that are critically important are the standards for use of cell phone and/or electronic devices and timeliness/attendance.

DO NOT ALLOW CELL PHONES OR ANY ELECTRONIC DEVICES WITHIN THE BUILDINGS OF THE CLINICAL AGENCIES. THERE IS NO EXCEPTION TO THIS POLICY. STUDENTS WHO HAVE THESE DEVICES OR ARE USING THESE DEVICES TO CALL, TEXT, OR TAKE PICTURES WILL FAIL CLINICAL IMMEDIATELY.

Students have failed clinical courses because they have been found to be using cell phones for personal business, except for urgent emergencies. These violations have major academic and financial repercussions for the students and risk our continued opportunities at the agencies. If you discover a student is in possession of or is using any electronic device for any purpose within the building, ask the student to leave the clinical area at once and notify the School of Nursing, Office of the Associate Dean, at XXX.

Students and faculty are expected to be on the clinical unit, designated area, or classroom ready to begin the preconference, the clinical experience, or a class. If students are late beyond the designated time or on a consistent basis, please ask the student to leave the class or clinical area, and notify the Office of the Associate Dean at XXX and the respective Clinical Course Coordinator. **Please be sure students have the contact number of the unit and/or an authorized person who is able to reach you as the faculty to give a message to the students.** Finally, the faculty are working on new clinical attendance, tardiness remediation, and clinical failure policies. If passed this term, these will be forwarded to you and included in the Adjunct Faculty Handbook.

If you have any questions regarding the policy, please contact me at any time.

Again, I am very grateful for your dedication to quality education and your willingness to share your talents and time with us. Please check our XXX/School of Nursing website for full-time employment opportunities now and in the future:

http://www.XXX.edu/employment-opportunities

All the best to you!

Attachments:

Adjunct Contract

Network Accounts Guidelines

ADP IPay Statement Instructions

Direct Deposit Authorization Form

Register to Receive Emergency Alerts/Weather-Related Announcements

School of Nursing Code of Conduct

29

Student–Faculty Professional Boundaries in the Academic and Clinical Environment

Case Study 29.1
Healthy Boundaries in the Classroom

Your role: You are Dr. Noah, a colleague of Dr. Jones, who is a statistics professor.

Dr. Jones has been teaching the introductory statistics course to graduate nursing students in the evening for several years. Over the years he has routinely gone with students of legal drinking age to the local pub for drinks after class. There has never been a complaint of excessive drinking or rowdy behavior, and Dr. Jones and the students who accompany him have generally developed relationships that could be perceived as being more friendly than professional. Not all the students join these after-class gatherings, and one student, in particular, has never attended. That student, Susan Wycliffe, files an email complaint with the Dean, complaining that she is being marginalized and being punished in class for "not attending these drinking binges with Dr. Jones like all the other students." The Dean sends the email to the statistics department chair, Dr. Zuvey, and tells him "to take care of it." Dr. Zuvey immediately notifies Dr. Jones by email that there has been a complaint about his going to the pub with students and to please meet with him. Dr. Jones is horrified by Dr. Zuvey's email and runs across the hall to you, his colleague, Dr. Noah, and asks you what he should do.

Questions
- What should you tell Dr. Jones?
- What should Dr. Zuvey tell Dr. Jones?
- Should Dr. Jones be disciplined for fraternizing with his graduate students?
- Should there be a university policy prohibiting fraternization between graduate faculty and graduate students?

Case Study 29.2
Healthy Boundaries in Clinical

Your role: You are Professor Fine and a close friend of Dr. Doyle.

Dr. Doyle comes to you one day and complains that she doesn't think the students in her psychiatric clinical group (junior-level BSN undergraduates) are sufficiently respectful of her or her authority and professional role as their teacher. You ask her to give you some examples. Dr. Doyle explains that sometimes when calling her Sarah, they speak to her as if she is their best friend. She states, "And when they say 'Hey Sarah!' I practically cringe." She goes on to say that she is having a hard time getting them to follow her instructions and confesses she sometimes feels as if they do not look upon her as their professor but as their friend. You ask Dr. Doyle why she does not require them to address her as Dr. Doyle or Professor Doyle instead of simply Sarah. Dr. Doyle replied that she always wanted to be more collegial with her undergraduate students and avoided the formal titles to promote a more egalitarian work environment. You ask, very bluntly, because you are a close friend and colleague of Dr. Doyle, "Well, do you think it's working?"

Questions

- What should you say next to Dr. Doyle?
- Do you think the casual manner of addressing faculty by their first name is problematic?
- Will the use of Dr. or Professor bring more civility to the clinical environment?
- Similarly, should faculty also address students by their first name if they are being addressed formally as "Dr." or "Professor"?
- Should there be a departmental policy on how students should address their professors, whether in the clinical or classroom setting?

HOW TO BEST ENFORCE STUDENT–FACULTY BOUNDARY AREAS IN THE ACADEMIC AND CLINICAL ENVIRONMENT: REVIEW OF THE LITERATURE

Setting professional boundaries between students and professors is no different from boundary setting in other professions, including the patient–therapist or the congregant–minister relationship. However, although therapists and ministers have an established code of ethical conduct, the student–teacher relationship has, for some reason, never been bound by a singular standard (Kitchener, 2000; Trull & Carter, 2004). Aultman, Williams-Johnson, and Schutz (2009) indicate that successful teaching and learning are integral to the student–teacher relationship, and in their study they reported that maintaining a balance between demonstrating care while maintaining a healthy, productive level of control in the classroom was the most recurring theme. Larkin and Mello (2010) highlight the medical student–physician teacher relationship in an issue of *Academic Medicine* and identify that the curricular content that addresses "the ethics of appropriate pedagogic and intimate relations between teaching staff and students, interns, residents, researchers, and other trainees" (p. 752) is rarely ever addressed. They go on to observe that "attraction and revulsion are normal aspects of the human psyche, but they must, as with all passions, be kept in check, lest one threaten the integrity of the academic environment" (p. 754).

Lack of proper student–teacher boundaries can lead to a variety of negative consequences, including sexual harassment, which is commonly cited as one of the most destructive outcomes of what Aultman et al. (2009) call "crossing the line." Students should be able to go to school free from experiencing sexual harassment or violence. That's the pledge that was made over 45 years ago by Title IX of the Education Amendments of 1972, which prohibited sex discrimination in any educational institution or program receiving federal funding. Research has found that women on college campuses and girls in junior high and high school continue to experience sexual harassment, sexual abuse or assault, and other crimes or behaviors that constitute sex discrimination under Title IX (American Association of University Women, 2018).

Henley (2009) and others also indicate that texting, emailing, and social networking sites are radically changing the historically traditional student–teacher relationship and placing new strains on the maintenance of healthy boundaries. Facebook, Twitter, blogs, and other cyber-based venues only add to the likelihood that student–teacher interaction will occur outside the classroom (Larkin & Mello, 2010). In the article "The Student–Teacher Relationship in a Texting World," Trotier (2008) indicates that beyond the frequency, the words used in texting, the topics shared, and the lack of discretion invite greater intimacy than in-person interactions. She recommends the following:

- Avoid engaging in inappropriate dialogue with students through the Internet.
- Avoid sending emails or text messages of a personal nature to students.
- Avoid being alone or in isolated situations with students, including social networking sites; this might be perceived as inappropriate in nature.
- Exercise extreme caution in connection with contact/Internet sites, including chat rooms, message boards, social networking, and news groups.

Faculty members are sometimes alone with students during office meetings or, in particular, during advisement. The important point to emphasize is that if there is any anxiety or concern about being alone with the student (e.g., the student has expressed greater than usual interest in you as the professor or has made comments or innuendos with sexual, intimate, or overly personal content), then the individual faculty member ought to meet with the student more publicly, with others around, or leave the office door open at all times. O'Connor (2005) notes that the current generation of students has a proclivity for using electronic media and gaming and recommends that educators try to find creative ways to use these educational media. She writes of her experience using instant messaging (IM) to improve writing skills. Although there is reason to be skeptical of this approach, especially in nursing education, Twitter, for instance, has been identified as being useful as a pedagogical approach to communicate real-time, health-related information (Dreher, 2009; Young, 2008).

There is an absence in the literature of how to properly address a college professor or teacher. The Internet is filled with anecdotal responses and advice. It is partly the culture of the university that often dictates the practice, and other times it really is the discipline. At Bryn Mawr College (a women's college in Pennsylvania), undergraduate and graduate students routinely call their professors by their first names; however, at South Carolina State University (a historically Black college in Orangeburg, South Carolina), students universally address their faculty as professor or doctor, creating a more formal campus culture.[1] Every possible form of address has been used in nursing schools between students and faculty, and without exception there are more faculty–student boundary issues when undergraduate students call the nursing professors by their first names. Pettigrew (2009) has a very engaging article, "What Do You Call a Professor? How to Play (and Win) the University Name Game," which gives practical advice to new college freshmen who face this issue. With master's students who are typically more mature, there are usually fewer boundary issues when professors request that students call them by their first name, although it is still common to see students use doctor or professor. With doctoral students who are being mentored as future colleagues, students are often requested to address faculty by first name, but many of them are uncomfortable doing so. The real question, particularly for undergraduate nursing faculty, is: What do you call your students? And the larger question remains, do you maintain a professional boundary between yourself and your students?

Observing professional boundaries in the clinical environment can be challenging in part because of the intense emotions evoked by some patient situations. Although sexual touching is always taboo,

---

[1] Academic dress is another example of university culture. For instance, business professors (particularly in MBA classes) tend to dress professionally for class (nursing administration faculty, too), but philosophy professors generally do not. Dress can establish boundaries, or the lack thereof, as can other forms of conduct.

it may be appropriate to use nonsexual touch to console a student, for example. Male nursing faculty generally exercise greater caution regarding physical distance and the use of nonsexual touch in the clinical environment (Lane & Corcoran, 2016; Zieber & Hagen, 2009). The faculty member should reflect on how to convey empathy and concern to students and avoid any misperceptions related to relationship boundaries.

DISCUSSION OF CASE STUDIES

Case Study 29.1

Recall the first question from Case Study 29.1, "What should you tell Dr. Jones?" After hearing of the accusation, Dr. Noah is also surprised because he does not believe that his friend and colleague Dr. Jones would ever treat any student in an arbitrary or unfair way. However, he always worried a bit about fraternizing with graduate students after class and was himself careful to do so only under special circumstances (e.g., after the last day or evening of class). Dr. Noah tells his friend that he should have been more cautious, stating, "You know, these days you have to be really careful around students. You can be accused of literally anything at anytime." He further advises, "You know, times have changed, I would probably cut out visiting pubs with these students, at least until this settles down." Dr. Jones is glad he shared these embarrassing details with his friend, but he is very weary of the process of being accused of something he clearly believes he did not do. As there is no special Ombudsman for the faculty, he feels more alone. He has heard about faculty being "thrown under the bus" even over an unproved accusation.

The second question is, what should Dr. Zuvey tell Dr. Jones? Dr. Jones met with the department chair, Dr. Zuvey, 2 days later, and Dr. Zuvey said, "Tell me about this incident. I have a disturbing email from a student of yours, but I certainly want to hear your side of this." Dr. Jones is clearly appreciative of this approach by his department chair because she is well known for doing diligent fact finding before acting on accusations or gossip. Dr. Jones explains that Ms. Wycliffe is perhaps the weakest student in the class and is often unprepared. He also states she does not interact well with her peers in class. To him it is obvious that she is using the "after-class activities" as an excuse for her poor performance and "getting her excuses and offense ready" if she gets a poor grade. Dr. Zuvey asks what classroom behaviors he would perceive as contributing to her alleged marginalization, and Dr. Jones says he does not know. He mentions that he perhaps calls on her less often, but that is because he does not want to embarrass her publicly by having her demonstrate she is not prepared. Dr. Zuvey informs Dr. Jones that she is not sure anything will come of this, but she does want him to "stop socializing after class." She tells him that although he may have only the best of intentions, drinking with students, even graduate students, is likely to contribute to a diminution in proper student–teacher boundaries. She further states that students who do not participate can imagine that you are secretly sharing information with those students who socialize with you that you are not providing in class. Dr. Jones agrees to cease the after-class pub activities.

Case Study 29.2

Recall the first question from Case Study 29.2: What should you say next to Dr. Doyle? Professor Fine had been in nursing education about 5 years longer than Dr. Doyle, and, having taught in both ADN and BSN programs, she had witnessed quite consistently that informality in both the classroom and clinical courses was usually an invitation to unprofessional student conduct. She told Dr. Doyle that she probably thought it was a bit late to try to have the students suddenly call her "Dr." midway through the semester, as that would draw unnecessary attention to it. She did, however, believe she could speak to her clinical group in preconference and voice her displeasure with some of informality of the clinical day. She told Dr. Doyle that her recommendation would be to remind them of the seriousness of their role as students in a clinical environment full of ill individuals and that from that day onward she wanted to see more professional attitudes for the duration of the semester, including less laughing and joking and a more proper professional demeanor befitting BSN students of the highest caliber. Dr. Doyle sighed and said, "I guess you're right."

FINDINGS AND DISPOSITION

Case Study 29.1

The third question is, should Dr. Jones be disciplined for fraternizing with his graduate students? In this case, he was not, as there really was no evidence of improper behavior with students off campus (e.g., intoxication or other breach of the code of conduct), and there was no institutional policy preventing (or even addressing) graduate faculty from socializing or fraternizing with graduate students; however, it is probably not wise from an optics perspective. The department chair could have probably forbidden Dr. Jones from socializing with graduate students after class permanently and put a faculty memo out. However, doing so might have raised a larger issue: one of precedent and establishing a "new policy" for her department that could be broadly applicable, and she wanted to avoid that based on one particular situation. In this case, Dr. Zuvey called the student in and inquired about her allegation of marginalization. Despite asking many different ways, she could not elicit from the student any instance of specific conduct (acts or omissions) either inside or outside the classroom. She told the student that she had not provided any evidence to support the charge, but she did indicate Dr. Jones had decided to stop going out with students after class for the rest of the term. The student seemed content with the response, and the complaint went no further. Dr. Zuvey informed the Dean that she had quashed the after-class pub activities and that she found no evidence to support the student's allegations about either binging or being treated differently in class. The Dean confirmed this is in a memo for the record.

The final question is, should there be a university policy prohibiting fraternization between graduate faculty and graduate students? In this case, Dr. Zuvey informed the Dean that there was no such policy at the university level except the university policy that addressed personal relationships and power differentials (e.g., when a supervisor wrongly engages in a relationship with a subordinate), but she reiterated that the university had affirmed that all individuals are entitled to freely choose their personal associations and relationships (Drexel University, 2013). She further stated that there was already a policy in both the undergraduate and graduate student nursing handbooks that specifically prohibited romantic or personal relationships between students and faculty who are actively teaching them and included prohibitions of such behaviors between students and any kind of preceptor or evaluator. Dr. Zuvey also arranged a faculty development program for the departmental faculty addressing legal issues concerning student–faculty fraternization. In the era of #MeToo trending, many different types of conversations about sexual harassment, faculty need to be aware of how their actions could be perceived and to protect themselves, the university, and students from potential issues.

Case Study 29.2

The second question is, do you think the casual manner of addressing faculty by their first names is problematic? Professor Fine was pretty adamant that it was problematic, and Dr. Doyle, although agreeing that she (Professor Fine) was probably correct, expressed some sadness that the lines between herself and her students needed to be drawn more rigidly. Philosophically, she would prefer to model collegiality to new and impressionable nursing undergraduates rather than to adhere to the traditional behaviors she had learned from her nursing education that had put the teacher on a pedestal. She also thought this traditional divide contributed to the rigidity of nursing practice in which students viewed nursing practice as black or white, with little room for higher-level critical thinking. Nevertheless, she decided that in the following semester she would try to use her "Dr." title to ascertain whether there really was a difference. For her, she needed more data before she would give up on her preferred teaching mode of professional address.

The third question is, will the use of "Doctor" or "Professor" bring more civility to the clinical environment? Dr. Doyle actually followed through with her experiment, and she found she created a more professional environment when the students addressed her as "Doctor." But Dr. Doyle did not simply change the way the students addressed her; she went one step further and resolved to stop addressing them by their first names also and began to address them as "Mr." and "Miss." For her, this satisfied her need for an egalitarian response in which each party (both student *and* professor) was more respectful of each other in their use of personal address.

In response to the fourth question, namely, whether faculty members should also address students by their first names if they are being addressed formally as "Doctor" or "Professor," it is suggested that Dr. Doyle's new practice actually be adopted. It certainly is not the most common practice in the clinical environment, but when faculty use it, it becomes a very powerful and actually equitable or democratic way to bring some formality and seriousness to the clinical environment. This does not mean, however, the clinical experience must be devoid of humor, but that humor should be used when appropriate and contribute to both a learning and healing environment.

The final question is, should there be a departmental policy on how students should address their professors whether in the clinical or classroom setting? A policy making forms of address mandatory should probably not be a requirement, but there should be a policy recommending forms of address for faculty in the student handbook.

RELEVANT LEGAL CASE

The Case of the Tenured Professor Moonlighting as a Phone-Sex Worker

In this case, reported by Schmidt in the *Chronicle of Higher Education* electronic edition (2010), a 48-year-old tenured associate professor of English, Dr. Lisa D. Chávez, was moonlighting as the phone-sex dominatrix "Mistress Jade" and posing in promotional and sexually suggestive pictures with one of her graduate students who was also working for the same phone-sex company, People Exchanging Power, in Albuquerque, New Mexico. Once it was discovered that Dr. Chávez was moonlighting in this job, she immediately quit and apologized for her serious lapse of judgment.

According to the *Chronicle* profile (Schmidt, 2010), graduate students in the creative writing program began working at People Exchanging Power because it paid well and in one case helped one of the students at the center of this case, 27-year-old Liz Derrington, gain more life experience to enhance her writing. At some point, Dr. Chávez needed extra income and also obtained part-time work there, too. Subsequently, Dr. Chávez encountered Ms. Derrington at the work site. This led to their becoming friendlier and ultimately posing for the company on its website. During this time, some of the graduate students in the program complained to other faculty about the sexually charged conversations occurring in Dr. Chávez's class. One professor took the allegations to the department chair, Dr. Jones, but no charges were filed. Later, photos of Dr. Chávez wound up on Dr. Jones's desk, with a note attached that read "appalled parents" (Schmidt, 2010, para. 15). Dr. Jones then asked another faculty member (and supervisor of Dr. Chávez), Dr. Warner, to investigate.

In late 2007, the provost and university administrators ruled that "Ms. Chávez had exercised bad judgment but did not find her guilty of allegations of maintaining a hostile learning environment, sexual harassment, or any other illegal activities or violations that suggested she was unfit for her job" (Schmidt, 2010, para. 24). Other tenured departmental members did not agree with the finding and continued to protest, vigorously accusing Ms. Chávez of "abuse of academic freedom and professional ethics that must govern the relationship between a professor and her student" (Schmidt, 2010, para. 26). Subsequently, one faculty resigned because she felt she could not protect her students, and three others have filed lawsuits against the university, including Dr. Chávez, who filed a lawsuit with the state claiming discrimination because she was Hispanic and bisexual. The creative writing program and English department continue to be in disarray; as the new department chair, Dr. Julie Shigekuni, states, "It becomes complicated, because I think that the lawsuits, and the kind of climate of antagonism and fear that is brought by the lawsuits, creates unpredictability. Students are uncertain about how the program is functioning and about the future of the program" (para 36). Dr. Chávez continues to teach in the department and creative writing program.

WHEN TO CONSULT THE UNIVERSITY COUNSEL

These situations are not likely to present issues for university counsel; they are most likely best handled within the department. If a student refuses to be appeased by the response to their complaint but continues to assert it (with greater force or to higher levels), then the Dean would be wise to consider seeking legal advice before any "last steps" are taken. This is particularly true if, as in her response, the student refuses to participate further in class.

SUMMARY

This chapter has explored the landscape of the boundaries between teachers and students. Gillespie (2002) has written about a transformation of the student–teacher relationship that incorporates a humanistic approach, which fosters the learning and growth of students and teachers—much like the philosophy that Dr. Doyle was struggling to implement in her own pedagogy. From both cases and the very messy real-life case of Dr. Chávez at the University of New Mexico, it is clear that the new social media technology makes the student–teacher relationship in some ways much more perilous. It is only going to get worse. Faculty now struggle with whether to give students a home phone number or a cell number, and the whole process of creating a relationship between students and faculty on social media is problematic. There is a lot to navigate these days to keep the student–teacher relationship focused on teaching and learning while maintaining the highest levels of professionalism. Whereas there are no hard rules about faculty and student forms of address, students (undergraduate and graduate) ought to use "Professor" and "Doctor" when appropriate (without obsessing over this) in academic settings and email.

ETHICAL CONSIDERATIONS

In general, the term "boundary" signifies "something that indicates a border or limit" ("Boundary," n.d.). Boundaries are conceptualized in relationships. In professional relationships, the term "boundaries" refers to rules that establish professional relationships as distinct from other relationships such as friendship, romantic, sexual, or familial (Austin, Bergum, Nuttgens, & Peternelj-Taylor, 2006; Owen & Zwahr-Castro, 2007). Nursing faculty are cautioned to remain in the "educator role" and provide educational support and avoid a student mental health counseling role or other forms of nonstudent–faculty relationships. Nursing faculty should also consult the National Council of State Board of Nursing's (2014) publication on boundaries. Recognition of when a boundary is becoming blurred or is being crossed is an important consideration for nursing faculty (Lane & Corcoran, 2016). Generally, when nursing faculty are clear about their professional boundaries and what constitutes a professional student–faculty relationship, the students are also clear. In the end, nursing faculty need to be cognizant of the principles that guide their ethical behaviors with students.

When professional boundaries are crossed and faculty engage in relationships beyond a student–faculty relationship, students and/or faculty are placed in ethically compromising situations. Boundaries in professional relationships help to clarify roles and identify proper and improper behavior. When boundary lines are blurred or crossed, a number of ethical problems may arise. A relationship with a student could itself become improper, drawing on a power differential between the parties that may exploit the less empowered student. Fair treatment of all students may be at risk. Once a boundary line is crossed, it can become difficult to ensure the favored student is not receiving different treatment, which may include favored treatment or even disfavored treatment, as in the case of a faculty member bending over backward not to appear unfair. One may even act in such a manner without realizing it. So it becomes especially important to maintain these boundaries to avoid both conscious and subconscious unfair treatment.

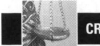

CRITICAL ELEMENTS TO CONSIDER

- The best way to clear up any confusion about your preference for a mode of personal address is to simply tell the students your requirements on the first day of class. That usually clears up the problem immediately, assuming you act thereafter in conformity with your declaration.
- Visit the university website and human resources website to see if there are any institutional policies regarding faculty fraternizing with students. Appreciate the fact that the question presented in these relationships is not just "fact" but "appearance." What is perceived, accurate or not, is the reality.
- Fraternization with undergraduate students, especially in the presence of alcohol (even with undergraduates of legal age), is highly discouraged. Students are predictably enamored with professors: their knowledge, experiences, and confidence. Faculty must be on guard to detect "more" than this attitude. Signs that a student is overly attracted to, attentive to, or preoccupied with you warrant exceptional faculty measures that discourage the continuation of such behaviors. If you have not experienced the situation before, seek the advice of a colleague promptly.
- Fraternization with graduate students is more acceptable, but, again, it can be complicated, so we caution faculty to use good judgment.
- Be very wary of participating in social media interactions with any students (especially, but not limited to, whom you are teaching) in your class via social media sites (e.g., Facebook, Twitter). This does not mean there are no pedagogically appropriate uses of them, but these must be devised and monitored very carefully by the faculty member.
    - Use the university email system when communicating with students and avoid personal email addresses, texting, and so forth, that can be misinterpreted by students.
    - Avoid friending students on Facebook and other social media forums.
    - Refer to the National Council of State Boards of Nursing, *A Guide to Professional Boundaries* at https://www.ncsbn.org/ProfessionalBoundaries_Complete.pdf

Helpful Resources

- Academic Coach: Earnest exhortations and random tidbits for dissertating graduate students, postdoctoral job hunters, and tenure-track faculty. (2005, October 26). *Doctor, professor, hey you* [Web log post]. Retrieved from http://successfulacademic.typepad.com/successful_academic_tips/2005/10/doctor _professo.html
- The Gradcafe: Where something is always brewing. (2010, February 18). *Re: How do you address a professor?* [Web log comment]. Retrieved from http://forum.thegradcafe.com/topic/9610-how-do-you -address-a-professor/

References

American Association of University Women. (2018). *Schools are still underreporting sexual harassment and assault.* Retrieved from https://www.aauw.org/article/schools-still-underreporting-sexual-harassment-and-assault/

Aultman, L. P., Williams-Johnson, M. R., & Schutz, P. A. (2009). Boundary dilemmas in teacher-student relationships: Struggling with "the line." *Teaching and Teacher Education, 25*(5), 636–646. doi:10.1016/j.tate.2008.10.002

Austin, W., Bergum, V., Nuttgens, S., & Peternelj-Taylor, C. (2006). A re-visioning of boundaries in professional helping relationships: Exploring other metaphors. *Ethics & Behavior, 16*, 77–94. doi:10.1207/s15327019eb1602_1

Brooks, D. (2011). *The social animal: The hidden sources of love, character and. achievement.* New York, NY: Random House.

Boundary. (n.d.). In *The Free Dictionary's online dictionary*. Retrieved from http://www.thefreedictionary.com/boundaries

Dreher, H. M. (2009). Twittering about anything, everything and even health. *Holistic Nursing Practice*, *23*(4), 217–221. doi:10.1097/HNP.0b013e3181aece81

Drexel University. (2013). *Human resource policy: Nepotism, employment of relatives and consensual amorous relationships policy*. Retrieved from https://drexel.edu/hr/resources/policies/dupolicies/hr46/

Gillespie, M. (2002). Student-teacher connection in clinical nursing education. *Journal of Advanced Nursing*, *37*(6), 566–576. doi:10.1046/j.1365-2648.2002.02131.x

Henley, J. (2009, September 23). Blurred boundaries for teachers. *Guardian*. Retrieved from http://www.guardian.co.uk/education/2009/sep/23/teacher-pupil-sexual-relationship

Larkin, G. L., & Mello, M. J. (2010). Commentary. Doctors without boundaries: The ethics of teacher-student relationships in academic medicine. *Academic Medicine*, *85*(5), 752–755. doi:10.1097/ACM.0b013e3181d7e016

Kitchener, K. S. (2000). *Foundations of ethical practice, research, and teaching in psychology*. Mahwah, NJ: Lawrence Erlbaum.

Lane, A. M., & Corcoran, L. (2016). Educator or counselor? Navigating uncertain boundaries in the clinical environment. *Journal of Nursing Education*, *55*(4), 189–195. doi:10.3928/01484834-20160316-02

National Council of State Boards of Nursing. (2014). *A nurse's guide to professional boundaries*. Retrieved from https://www.ncsbn.org/ProfessionalBoundaries_Complete.pdf

O' Connor, A. (2010, May 5). Instant Messaging: Friend or Foe of Student Writing?." *New Horizons*. n. pag. Web.

Owen, P. R., & Zwahr-Castro, J. (2007). Boundary issues in academia: Student perceptions of faculty–student boundary crossings. *Ethics & Behavior*, *17*, 117–129. doi:10.1080/10508420701378065

Pettigrew, T. (2009). What do you call a professor? How to play (and win) the university name game. *On Campus: Mcleans*. Retrieved from http://oncampus.macleans.ca/education/2009/08/30/what-do-you-call-a-professor/

Schmidt, P. (2010, September 12). In professor-dominatrix scandal, U. of New Mexico feels the pain. *Chronicle of Higher Education*. Retrieved from http://chronicle.com/article/In-Professor-Dominatrix/124369/

Trotier, G. (2008, December). The student-teacher relationship in a texting world. *School Law Solutions*. Retrieved from https://www.dkattorneys.com/publications/student-teacher-relationship-texting-world/

Trull, J. E., & Carter, J. E. (2004). *Ministerial ethics: Moral formation for church leaders* (2nd ed.). Grand Rapids, MI: Baker Academic.

Young, J. R. (2008, February 29). Forget Email: New Messaging Service Has Students and Professors ATwitter. *Chronicle of Higher Education*, *54*(25), A15.

Zieber, M. P., & Hagen, B. (2009). Interpersonal boundaries in clinical nursing education: An exploratory Canadian qualitative study. *Nurse Education in Practice*, *9*, 356–360. doi:10.1016/j.nepr.2008.10.008

30

Addressing Students With Mental Health Issues or Psychiatric Disabilities

Case Study 30.1
Mental Health

Your role: You are the Chair of the nursing department, Dr. Barrett.

Laura Helms is a 23-year old BSN Second Degree Nursing student, enrolled in the 12-month accelerated program, with a previous degree in Social Work from your university. She is in her first semester of the Second Degree Program and enrolled in Fundamentals of Nursing Practice and Health Assessment. Faculty report that Laura cannot stay focused in the nursing skills lab. She is easily distracted and does not fully listen to instructions or complete tasks. She also frequently goes to the bathroom to wash her hands. Faculty note that her hands are dry and red which appears to be a result of frequent handwashing. She has not yet passed the skills competency assessment for Fundamentals of Nursing Practice to enter the clinical portion of the program. Her clinical faculty member has doubts that Laura will be able to pass the core basic clinical skills for clinical readiness given her current performance. Laura's mother has called your office requesting to meet with you, stating that Laura is being held back from clinical and "targeted" because she has a mental health history. She is afraid that being held back from clinical will destroy Laura.

Questions
- What information do you need to consult?
- Would you, as Chair, meet with Mrs. Helms, Laura's mother?
- Would you permit Laura to attend clinical?

LEGAL PRINCIPLES AND REVIEW OF THE LITERATURE

Nursing programs are seeing higher numbers of students with mental health and related disabilities as the number of college students with psychiatric disabilities in general has increased. College counseling centers across the United States are reporting increased frequency and greater severity of students' mental health concerns, such as depression, suicidal thoughts, sexual assaults, and personality disorders (Kucirka, 2017) and the prevalence of anxiety and mood disorders has grown (American College Health Association, 2015; Kaplan & Reed, 2004). Factors such as public awareness of mental health disorders, improved assessment and diagnosis, earlier intervention, improved treatments, and decreased stigma related to mental illness account for some of these changes (Kaplan & Reed, 2004; Silverman, 2004). Interventions, including medications, diminish symptoms and enable students with mental health disorders to be more productive and academically successful (Cleary, Horsfall, Baines, & Happell, 2012; Souma, Rickerson, & Burgstahler, 2002). In addition, greater numbers of students have been diagnosed and treated effectively in high school, leading to a higher likelihood that these students are able to enter college (Brockelman & Scheyett, 2015; Osberg, 2004).

The transition from high school to college marks the start of young adulthood, which is also the age of onset for many mental health illnesses (Eisenberg, Hunt, & Speer, 2013). Psychiatric illnesses are often diagnosed in young adulthood and may very well be triggered by stressful situations germane to college life. Some of the stressors that contribute to the development of mental health problems in college students include living in a new environment, sharing a confined place such as a dormitory room, peer pressure, greater academic demands, and less structure (Cleary et al., 2012; Cook, 2007). New students are faced with these multiple changes during their transitions to college life, and they may be further magnified by the physical absence of parents, family members, and structural supports available through home life and high school. Current, emerging, or previously diagnosed mental health disabilities may or may not be disclosed to those in the university.

Nursing majors have additional pressures associated with clinical education during this stressful time. The nursing major is unique in the college or university setting in that program requirements overlap both academic and clinical healthcare settings; students are required to adjust to both the university's academic requirements and conduct policies and the clinical agency's policies related to practice and professional conduct. This chapter explores the challenging decisions that must be made when nursing students have mental health or related disabilities. Although awareness of the needs of this group of students and sensitivity to potential biases by the various stakeholders involved in their education are required, faculty and administrators must also consider their relationships with, responsibilities to, and obligations to, both the educational and healthcare institutions. As stated by Marks (2007) and that which still holds true today, "Educators in nursing schools continue to ask whether people with disabilities have a place in the nursing profession, while the more salient question is, 'When will people with disabilities have a place in the nursing profession?'" (p. 70). Marks's comment reflects an evolving understanding of diversity and disability in the profession, as well as the need to reconceptualize some of the assumptions and standards associated with nursing education and practice.

Nursing faculty should anticipate that the increased number of students with mental health issues may translate into increases in the number of nursing majors who experience some type of mental health problem while in the program. Nursing faculty should also anticipate that there is a higher expectation that all faculty members be prepared to identify psychologically distressed students and provide appropriate support and mental health referrals. It will be necessary for nursing faculty members to understand their roles and responsibilities as a faculty member and allow mental healthcare to be provided by a mental health practitioner or appropriate healthcare provider. Professional boundary issues are important from a legal perspective, so nursing faculty are not considered healthcare providers responsible for the student's health. Faculty must adhere to their responsibilities in the faculty role and own institutional policies. Nursing faculty should not provide psychological counseling or treatment but refer the student to the appropriate healthcare provider (Lane & Corcoran, 2016).

DISCUSSION OF CASE STUDY

Dr. Barrett consults with the clinical faculty member to obtain more details about Laura's performance in the nursing skills laboratory. She also consults Laura's file. She notes that Laura had a 1-year medical leave in her first undergraduate degree. Laura also has an academic accommodation for decreased distraction during testing, preferably a quiet, individual testing room. Dr. Barrett tells Mrs. Helms that she cannot speak or meet with her unless she has Laura's permission by completing a signed FERPA (Family Educational Rights and Privacy Act) release. Dr. Barrett also states that Laura is an adult second-degree student and needs to be present at the meeting to discuss her own academic performance. Laura appears rather nervous during the meeting and is constantly looking at her phone or out the window. Laura does not appear to have insight into her clinical performance in the skills laboratory when the matter is discussed. She notes that Laura's hands are indeed very red and dry. During the meeting, Mrs. Helms discloses that Laura had a depressive episode during her first undergraduate degree. Dr. Barrett asked Laura if she had any recent thoughts about wanting to harm herself and Laura stated she did not. You inform Mrs. Helms and Laura that you will investigate the matter and be back in contact with Laura as you want to consult with the Dean and Legal Counsel.

Developmental Psychiatric Disabilities

An emerging challenge for universities in general and for nursing programs, faculty, and administrators specifically, is the increasing number of students on campus with neurodevelopmental disabilities such as Asperger syndrome (Marsh & Wilcoxon; 2015; VanBergeijk, Klin, & Volkmar, 2008). A large cohort of children diagnosed with a neurodevelopmental disability have reached college age; an increasing number of children explicitly diagnosed with autism spectrum disorder are also being admitted to colleges based on their academic skills (May, 2014; VanBergeijk et al., 2008). Many of these are students who previously would have been categorized as having Asperger syndrome, which is no longer specifically included as a diagnostic category. These students often have received extensive support in high school via the Individuals with Disabilities Education Act, and may require a variety of accommodations for success in the university setting. Individuals on the autism spectrum often have comorbid psychiatric conditions, particularly anxiety and depression, which add complexity to the challenges they may face in the social, academic, and clinical realms (May, 2014; VanBergeijk et al., 2008). There is minimal literature documenting the academic success or career choices of college students with neurodevelopmental disorders in general, and none has been found for nursing education specifically. However, based on these students' increased prevalence in the population (Kirsch, Doerfler, & Truong, 2015), it is likely that nursing programs and faculty will encounter students with complex issues and needs related to these conditions and will need to make decisions regarding their academic and/or clinical progress.

Faculty Perspective

In 1973, section 504 of the Rehabilitation Act introduced the first piece of disability-specific legislation to protect students with disabilities from discrimination. Nearly 20 years later, in 1990, the Americans with Disabilities Act (ADA) went into effect and clarified that people with disabilities are not only to be protected from discrimination but are also eligible for reasonable accommodations in order to fully and equally enjoy the goods, services, facilities, privileges, advantages, or accommodations of an entity. In order to be eligible for accommodations at the university level, it is the student's responsibility to register with the Office of Disabilities and (depending on the procedure at the given institution) ensure that an accommodation notice is provided to each professor in a reasonable amount of time before the accommodation is to be used. It is the responsibility of the university to ensure that all reasonable accommodations are provided for students with disabilities (Meloy & Gambescia, 2014).

Unlike primary and secondary teacher preparation programs, few, if any, faculty preparation programs include content on teaching college students with mental health disabilities. Faculty may have significant knowledge deficits regarding this population of students (Ashcroft et al., 2008; Meloy & Gambescia, 2014). Increased knowledge and understanding of the legal and educational issues involved and consideration of the unique factors related to clinical nursing education can guide faculty members to be supportive of students who are managing their disabilities effectively, to recognize students at risk, and to refer them appropriately. However, faculty must also be cognizant of the fact that students at universities are not required to disclose mental health or related disabilities, unless they are seeking disability accommodations. Nursing faculty need to be able to identify students who may have issues emerging from mental health or similar disabilities to support student learning and concurrently minimize safety risks in both students and patients (Maheady, 1999; Matt, Maheady, & Fleming, 2015). It is recommended that faculty refer a student to the office of disability services (ODS) when faculty suspects a disability and anticipates the clinical practice implications of an accommodation if granted (Meloy & Gambescia, 2014).

There is a distinct and critical difference between classroom accommodations and clinical accommodations. The ODS personnel and clinical faculty members must be knowledgeable about the influence of a clinical accommodation and its impact, if any, on patient care and patient safety. For example, although it may be quite reasonable for the ODS to establish an accommodation of extended time for completing a classroom examination, an accommodation of this nature would have serious safety implications in the clinical area if provided during medication administration and testing. There is a need for collaborative dialogue and planning between the ODS and the nursing program when nursing students are eligible for accommodations that extend to the clinical area. When a person with a mental health disability is experiencing illness symptoms that could endanger the safety or well-being of a patient in a clinical setting, there must be an emergent process to address this situation to ensure that patient safety remains a priority, as well as the safety of the student. Management of these types of situations involves clear communication and full understanding of clinical practice responsibilities as well as clinical and academic policies and federal regulations. Furthermore, it is essential to ensure that university administrators address both the rights of the student with a disability, and the obligation to ensure the safety of others, especially patients.

MAJOR STAKEHOLDERS

The faculty member responsible for the clinical education of nursing majors is typically an employee or agent of the university who serves as a bridge between the university and clinical institutions. Whereas the relationship between a faculty member in the classroom and the student is quite delineated, the role of the clinical faculty member in undergraduate programs is more complex. Clinical faculty can assist the student in obtaining accommodations to fulfill their educational requirements by directing them to ODS (Helms, Jorgensen, & Anderson, 2006; Lane & Corcoran, 2016). The ODS will also seek information from the faculty or program leader to confirm the requirements of the course or program. The ODS can determine that the condition does not amount to a disability and can deny the request, at which time the best practice is for the rejection letter to request the submission of any additional information that the student believes might make the ODS change its decision. Once the ODS determines that a disability is involved and the person is eligible for an accommodation (known as a qualified individual), the ODS engages in an interactive discussion to devise a plan that is acceptable to the ODS, the university, and the student. The ADA stipulates that the individual needing services is responsible for the cost associated with the diagnosis and assessment of the disability (Drexel University College of Nursing and Health Professions, 2019).

An accommodation verification letter (AVL), issued by the ODS following the interactive discussion, is used as the communication tool to inform faculty and staff of the reasonable accommodations that have been approved for the particular student. The AVL is specific and precise and ensures the student of nothing other than what is specifically stated in the letter, so it eliminates any guesswork or discretion by the faculty or staff (which could then readily be perceived as unfair by students not receiving those benefits; Figure 30.1). Once an AVL is issued to a student by the ODS, it is the student's responsibility to share that AVL with faculty or administrators if the student wants to receive the approved accommodations. If the student never shares the AVL with any professors,

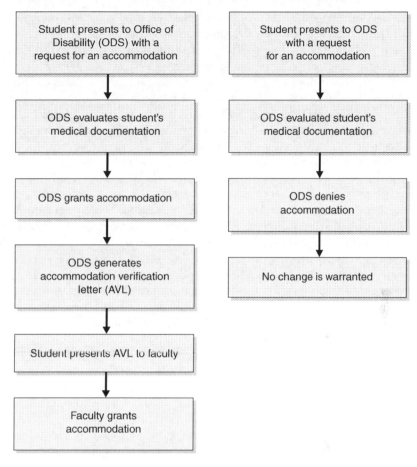

Figure 30.1 Disability accommodation process.

then neither the university nor any of the professors assigned to teach the student will be expected or required to provide any accommodations. In fact without an AVL, faculty should never provide students with disability accommodations of any kind.

It must be noted that faculty and staff who receive the AVL, which lists the approved accommodations, are not provided with information on the underlying disability. Under FERPA, the ODS is not permitted to share the details of a student's disability with anyone at the university unless there is a legitimate education interest. Beyond FERPA, most ODS offices consider disability information confidential and often require a student's consent before the ODS will share the details of the student's disability with anyone other than the student. An academic administrator of the nursing program will also have no knowledge of the student's underlying disability.

UNIVERSITY-DIRECTED ACCOMMODATIONS DECISIONS

Although many students with a disability will register with the ODS, others choose not to disclose a disability; this may be the case for students with mental health disabilities who are concerned about stigma and believe that they will not be treated fairly. When nursing students with undisclosed conditions experience mental health symptoms and exhibit distress in the classroom and/or the clinical area, a different type of problem-solving is required involving a more complex set of stakeholder considerations. For example, faculty may not be clear about how to manage an emergency situation for a student who is experiencing a psychiatric crisis. It is a best practice for a university to have an emergency student protocol in place to assist faculty in supporting the student who is an imminent danger to themselves. It is important that faculty members be aware of distress signals, methods of immediate intervention, and sources of help for students. Few programs appear to have such protocols (Cook, 2007), but these are necessary to protect the safety and integrity of students with emerging mental health problems. Protocols should offer clear guidance to faculty in recognizing student distress and directing students to an appropriate intervention.

A student may not recognize that they are not well enough to participate in a clinical rotation providing care for sick, vulnerable patients and could refuse to take a temporary leave from the clinical experience. At the same time, university officials may be reticent to remove the student from their clinical rotation, as officials may be fearful that they are violating the student's rights or unnecessarily harming their educational progress. Clinical faculty teaching students with emerging mental health problems have other, competing obligations including addressing needs of other students, maintaining patient safety, and maintaining collaborative relationships with nursing leadership and staff at clinical agencies. In managing such at-risk student situations, faculty, nursing administrators, and institutional officials will want to act in a manner that does not violate the legal rights of the individual student and give rise to potential legal liability. To accomplish this, the institution can conduct a direct threat review prior to initiation of any involuntary leave or suspension. The objective of this review is to assess whether the student poses a direct threat to themselves or to others, and whether the institution could or could not provide a reasonable accommodation that would reduce or eliminate that threat. As part of this assessment, the institution determines whether there is a high probability of substantial harm and not just a slightly increased, speculative, or remote risk. The institution will need to conduct an individualized and objective assessment about whether the student can continue to participate in the institution's programs safely, based on a reasonable medical judgment relying on the most current medical knowledge or the best objective evidence. The assessment should determine the nature, duration, and severity of the risk, the probability that the potential threatening injury will actually occur, and whether reasonable modifications of policies, practices, or procedures will sufficiently mitigate the risk (Lee & Abbey, 2008; May, 2014).

In the event that the student refuses to take a temporary leave from the clinical experience while having a mental health crisis, a university can convene a threat assessment task force with university officials made up of representatives of mental health counseling, public safety, student life, legal counsel, and nursing academic administration to evaluate the situation and the student's fitness for clinical educational responsibilities at this time and to consider whether an involuntary leave or temporary suspension from specific educational activities is appropriate based on an individualized assessment of the situation. Proper documentation that this assessment process was followed will help the institution defend itself in the event of legal challenge.

In an effort to manage students in crisis effectively, universities have developed protocols on substance abuse and emergency student situations to guide faculty when students are in such a situation. These protocols serve as a resource in assisting faculty during interventions with students who may be in imminent danger to themselves or others. The need for management protocols for nursing students in crisis, particularly those with suspected mental health disabilities, cannot be underestimated. Academic nursing programs need to be cognizant of the safety of the student and the patient, as well as the student's ADA rights as they pertain to this situation, especially nursing students with mental health problems who have responsibilities in the clinical area.

FINDINGS AND DISPOSITION

Dr. Barrett consults with the Dean who arranges a meeting with Legal Counsel. During the meeting, you review the Nursing Program's Technical Standards and Laura's observed behaviors. After the meeting, it is decided that the chair will meet with Laura and request a medical clearance from her psychiatrist stating that she can meet the nursing program's technical standards in order to remain in a clinical course at this time. Remember, Laura has yet to meet the basic clinical skills competency to enter the clinical phase of the program. The Chair and Dean did not want to put Laura under undue stress in the nursing skills laboratory when it is apparent that she is not well and had concerns about her ability to meet the program's technical standards. Dr. Barrett also agrees to speak to Laura's psychiatrist, Dr. Morgan (if Laura agrees) to give him additional information about the competencies required for an academic nursing program and faculty's observations about Laura's behaviors. After seeing Laura and consulting the nursing program's technical standards, Dr. Morgan (Laura's psychiatrist) informs Laura that he cannot medically clear her at this time. Laura takes a medical leave of absence, providing documentation from her psychiatrist. Laura returned to the nursing program after a medical leave. Her academic program plan was revised to allow her to complete the program in 2 years rather than the original 1-year time frame.

Nursing Faculty Decisions

Nursing faculty members need to be comfortable addressing the technical standards or essential job competencies required for nursing students to perform patient care safely in the clinical area. Having an open, supportive dialogue about the ODS and the management of students who have a mental health disability may encourage students to seek an AVL and assist them with managing their learning process with support. In addition, nursing faculty need to learn how to have the kinds of conversations with students that employers have with employees related to essential functions of their job. Nursing students must be able to independently, with or without reasonable accommodation, meet technical standards related to (a) observation; (b) communication; (c) motor skills; (d) intellectual, conceptual, and quantitative abilities; (e) essential behavioral and social attributes; and (f) ability to manage stressful situations. For example, the student must be able to adapt to and function effectively in stressful situations in both the classroom and clinical settings, including emergency situations. Students will encounter multiple stressors while in their nursing programs. Rather than focus on the specific disabling conditions, medications, or treatment, faculty can manage a situation best by focusing on the student's behavior or function. Furthermore, when faculty encounter problems in the clinical setting when a student engages in problematic behavior or is in crisis, it is important for the faculty member to be proactive and engage the student about counseling and the ODS and its services. It is also a best practice for schools of nursing to specify these behavioral standards that they view as essential for a student to participate in a program.

Without a thorough working knowledge of disability law, nursing faculty members may devolve to their clinical nursing roles and attempt to diagnose or clinically intervene with a student. However, as noted elsewhere in this book, the legal case law clearly cautions faculty that doing so could well be held to create a special relationship that then imposes special responsibilities and liabilities. Rather than helping, faculty may be unintentionally hurting the student or at least increasing the likelihood of harm occurring to the student or others. For example, in one case, a clinical faculty member spoke to a particular student on the phone almost daily in an effort to help the student address her anxiety related to clinical performance. When the faculty member in question placed the student on clinical warning, the student felt betrayed and became depressed; the student had perceived the faculty member as a close friend and confidant. In this situation, it would have been best for the clinical faculty member to have referred the student to the student counseling center, rather than have attempted to counsel the student, as this could be considered a special relationship. It is best for faculty to refer students to the university counseling center, as would be expected from faculty members from other academic disciplines. Psychiatric/mental health nursing faculty members are especially cautioned not to establish a special relationship with students. In the academic setting, the faculty member is a teacher not a therapist (Cook, 2007).

Nursing faculty members also have an ethical duty to protect the public. The majority of clinical experiences are outside the college and in hospitals, and other clinical settings. As such, nursing programs, students, and faculty are subject to the procedures and policies of that institution. Today, distance learning adds yet another dimension to addressing anyone with mental health issues and the environment where student learning is taking place. In particular, the nursing student with mental health problems may be at a clinical site that is quite a distance from the student's respective college in today's distance learning environment. In this scenario, clinical supervision presents a new set of challenges for students with mental health issues, as well as for the faculty member attempting to supervise the student from a distance. The faculty member is not on site and is therefore unable to recognize the student who may be exhibiting mental health problems. The faculty member may make site visits only a few times a semester or may rely on a preceptor's observations. In this situation, the student is not being supervised as closely as they would be supervised in a usual clinical educational setting. Therefore, it would be important for the faculty member to orient the preceptor to contact the faculty member and document any signs that might indicate student mental health distress. Furthermore, the faculty member should be sure to share the university's emergency protocol guide and related policies with the preceptor and/or clinical faculty member, as well as other relevant policies in orientation.

In addition, faculty should understand that disability accommodations should not be provided to any student, unless a current, signed AVL has first been produced. It is also important for faculty to appreciate what is required to be kept confidential, and what is not, under both FERPA and the Health Insurance Portability and Accountability Act (HIPAA). The ability to share information is complicated if the disclosure is to be made outside of the institution (e.g., hospital to academic institution) or academic program (e.g., nursing faculty to university administrator). Many faculty incorrectly believe that FERPA and HIPAA absolutely prohibit such disclosures, and for that reason fail to make timely and critically important reports of behaviors of concern to institutional administrators. In fact, it is permissible to disclose information in connection with an emergency if knowledge of information is necessary to protect the health or safety of the student or other individuals. A failure to share such information within the university results in lost opportunities for early intervention, may complicate effective management of these situations, and may result in both harm (to student or others) and liability (to faculty or university).

Problem-Solving Strategies

Situational accommodation decisions would definitely benefit from the development of clear policies for both faculty and students. It would also be useful to develop comprehensive education about (a) the role of the administrator in facilitating the integration of students into the educational community; (b) the different types of accommodations that can address people's disabling conditions, helping them to be successful in completing educational requirements; (c) the best approaches to management of communication and emergency challenges; and (d) what types of campus resources are available to students with a disability. In addition, a comprehensive disabilities education program needs to be developed for nursing academic administrators, faculty members, and students to interpret clearly their legal obligations, rights, and remedies (Hirshfield & Woolf, 2005; Meloy & Gambescia, 2014).

Universities can support their faculty members, more specifically their nursing faculty members, by making sure that they have clear policies and procedures to manage the types of emergency situations that involve the rights of the person with a disability, the care and safety of patients, the care and safety of the student at risk, and the safety of other students involved. For example, faculty development sessions can be offered to new faculty members to acquaint them with behaviors that warrant concern as well as the appropriate action to take in these situations, with periodic reinforcement of this information to ensure awareness and accessibility of these possibilities (Box 30.1).

FERPA was designed to establish the rights of students, inspect and review their education records, prevent the release of educational records to third parties without permission of the student, and provide guidelines for the correction of inaccurate or misleading data through formal and informal hearings. Students also have the right to file complaints with the FERPA office concerning alleged failures by the university to comply with FERPA. The university's interpretation of FERPA and its emergency exceptions should be emphasized in the university's polices and faculty development sessions (Baker, 2005).

Case law has clearly noted that a student's psychiatric disability does not exempt them from academic policies and technical standards. All students with or without disabilities or related accommodations must demonstrate that they are "otherwise qualified" to meet all programmatic requirements or are subject to denial of continued academic progression and even dismissal (*Betts v. Rector and Visitors of the University of Virginia*, 2005; *Hash v. University of Kentucky*, 2004; Meloy & Gambescia, 2014).

Box 30.1
Faculty Recommendations on Managing a Student With Mental Health Issues

1. Recognize signs of psychological/behavioral distress and/or substance abuse.
2. Talk with the student privately about your concerns arising from the student's recent behavior or conduct. Share your observations and make an assessment of the urgency of the situation. *During this discussion the faculty member should focus on describing the behavior or conduct that is causing concern, rather than the suspected causes of that behavior or conduct (i.e., psychiatric illness). Even where strongly indicated, the faculty member should avoid diagnosis of psychological illness until the student mentions it.*
3. Determine if the situation requires immediate intervention. *The most basic criteria are whether the student is an immediate danger to themselves others. If this is the case, the faculty member needs to contact security or public safety representatives immediately. It is imperative that the student receive appropriate evaluation and subsequent treatment.*
4. Do not isolate yourself when dealing with a student with a serious mental health issue. Consult with academic nursing administrators and staff at the university's counseling center, legal department, public safety/police and disability services to access their special expertise for managing these difficult situations.

Source: Adapted from Ashcroft, T., Chernomas, W., Davis, P., Dean, R., Seguire, M., Shapiro, C., & Swiderski, L. M. (2008). Nursing students with disabilities: One faculty's journey. International Journal of Nursing Education Scholarship, 5(1), 1–26. doi:10.2202/1548-923X.1424

RELEVANT LEGAL CASES

Schieszler v. Ferrum College, No. 7:02CV00131 (W.D. Va. 2002)

Shin v. Massachusetts Institute of Technology, No. 020403, 2005 WL 1869101 (Mass. Super. Ct. June 27, 2005)

Nguyen v. Massachusetts Institute of Technology, 96 N.E.3d 128 (Mass. 2018)

Nursing faculty are cautioned from forming "special relationships" and counseling students with mental health issues based on the case law described in the following. The law clearly shapes university policies that are related to students with mental illness. The recent increase in the number of suicides on campus (and the attendant reporting of them by the media) has fueled litigation that challenges the traditional approach to suicide (holding the victim accountable). Universities are usually challenged on one of the following legal theories: duty to protect, duty to prevent, and permitting or allowing the cause (Smith & Fleming, 2007).

In more publicized cases, *Schieszler v. Ferrum College* (2002) and *Shin v. Massachusetts Institute of Technology* (*MIT*; 2005), the parents of students who committed suicide argued that universities have a special relationship with their students that impose a duty on the school to protect the students even from themselves. In *Schieszler v. Ferrum College* (2002), the student, Michael Frentzel, hung himself with a belt. Distraught after a fight with his girlfriend, Mr. Frentzel was seen banging his head against a wall and heard talking about killing himself. This was reported by other students in his dormitory to college officials, but the officials did not do what a jury later decided was required of them. The court held that the college was liable for his death based on the foreseeability of the suicide and the special relationship it had with him because college employees knew that the student had threatened to kill himself, had self-inflicted injuries, and had a history of emotional problems (Cohen, 2007).

Elizabeth Shin was a student at MIT who killed herself by setting herself on fire. While a freshman, she had required a week-long hospitalization for suicidal behavior based on an overdose of Tylenol with codeine. Following hospitalization, Ms. Shin gave permission for her parents to be notified. Ms. Shin, her parents, and the MIT medical team decided that the student should receive care from the medical team at MIT. In her sophomore year, Ms. Shin again required hospitalization for mental health issues and recovered at home. Upon her return from spring break, Ms. Shin told her friends that she intended to kill herself—and her friends immediately called the university, who alerted the medical team. The team scheduled an appointment to discuss her case the next day, but Ms. Shin committed suicide that same night. The parents filed a wrongful death suit against the university, the medical team, and others. MIT was granted summary judgment, but the medical team was not. The court based its finding on the duty of care that the medical team owed Ms. Shin and on its conclusion that a special relationship existed between them and Ms. Shin because they had a specific knowledge that she was at high risk for suicide and it was likely that she would hurt herself without proper supervision (Pavela, 2006). The lawsuit was settled out of court for an undisclosed amount (Cohen, 2007).

In a later case against MIT, *Nguyen v. Massachusetts Institute of Technology* (2018), the court held that a university has a special relationship with a student and a corresponding duty to take reasonable measures to prevent student suicide where the university has actual knowledge of a student's suicide attempt that occurred while enrolled at the university or recently before matriculation, or a student's stated plans or intentions to commit suicide. The court went on to explain that the duty is not triggered merely by the university's knowledge of a student's suicidal ideation without any stated plans or intention to act on such thoughts. In the *Nguyen* case, the court ultimately ruled that no special relationship was created and there was no duty established because the student did not tell any MIT staff of any plans or intentions to commit suicide or of previous suicide attempts prior to enrollment and had not told any of his mental health providers he was considering suicide. The court also considered that non-clinicians are not expected to be able to diagnosis suicidal intent.

Stress, anxiety, and depression—either alone or combined with other psychiatric disorders—can lead students to act out in a variety of unfortunate ways, including considering suicide. It will be impossible for faculty or administrators to know whether the student is serious; they must not place themselves in the position of making that kind of judgment. Both of these cases illustrate the need for faculty members to find help *immediately* for a student who has verbally or textually voiced the intention (or the idea) to commit suicide; they should not attempt to help suicidal students themselves because doing so would qualify them as having a special relationship with the student. Nor is it enough just to diagnose the situation properly: Immediate action is required. Scheduling an appointment for the student with a specialist for "the next day" is too risky, as shown in *Shin v. Massachusetts Institute of Technology* (2005). Instead, if university faculty members directly or indirectly hear of suicidal intent, then they should immediately report the incident and do whatever they can to get the student help—for example, taking the student to the ED—as soon as possible. If the student commits suicide and the courts rule that the university did not act on their knowledge to protect the student, then the university and the faculty personally may be held liable.

SUMMARY

It is imperative that nursing faculty bring attention to this very significant issue of educating nursing students who are living with a mental health or related disability. Although many of these students will manage their disabilities with no need for accommodations, there will continue to be a need to manage emergent problem situations related to mental health status of nursing students, particularly as these situations influence clinical practice. It is clear that faculty would benefit from both education opportunities and protocols related to the management of accommodations for nursing students with mental health or related disabilities to support the decisional procedures for both academic and clinical healthcare settings.

ETHICAL CONSIDERATIONS

Nursing faculty members should anticipate that their students may experience psychological distress at times as a result of academic, transitional, or familial/relationship stressors. These stressors may trigger or exacerbate underlying mental health issues that commonly occur in young adulthood. Other students may have an existing psychiatric disability. Nursing education occurs in an academically rigorous, high-stakes learning environment. Nursing students have also been found to have more anxiety and depression than the general population due to demanding curriculum, stress associated with caring for acutely ill patients, balancing classroom and clinical education work, and the high volume of testing (Chernomas & Shapiro, 2013). Students with existing mental health issues or psychiatric disabilities are at greater risk for exacerbation of their illness during times of stress. Proactive faculty development opportunities related to "recognizing and handling psychologically distressed students" are required, so faculty are prepared to identify students in distress, support them, and refer appropriately (Cleary et al., 2012). Nearly one third of newly admitted college students report a history of mental illness (Marsh & Wilcoxon, 2015), so faculty preparation is an ethical consideration. Faculty and the Office of Disability can collaboratively create programs to help students build self-awareness and coping skills and mobilize support systems for students to assist with coping skills related to stress (Aradilla-Herrero, Tomas-Sabado, & Gomez-Benito, 2014). As nursing faculty, we have competing obligations, the student and patient. Faculty also need to be cognizant of their own biases with respect to mental illness when making decisions related to a student's fitness for clinical rotations.

As stated, nursing faculty has competing obligations, the student and patient. The potential conflict of these obligations is especially emphasized regarding the issue of nursing students' mental health. On the one hand, faculty have a duty to recognize and provide resources for students suffering from mental health problems. On the other hand, faculty have a duty to protect patients and future patients who may be at risk of impaired practice. Both parties are worthy of care and respect. Providing care for the students will also provide protection for patients, but care for the students must be recognized as care for their own sake, not simply as a means to protect patients.

Nursing faculty members should anticipate that their students may experience psychological distress at times as a result of academic, transitional, or familial/relationship stressors. These stressors may trigger or exacerbate underlying mental health issues that commonly occur in young adulthood. Nursing education occurs in an academically rigorous, high-stakes learning environment. Nursing students have also been found to have more anxiety and depression than the general population due to demanding curriculum, stress associated with caring for acutely ill patients, balancing classroom and clinical education work, and the high volume of testing (Chernomas & Shapiro, 2013). Other students may have an existing psychiatric disability. Students with existing mental health issues or psychiatric disabilities are at greater risk for exacerbation of their illness during times of stress.

Proactive faculty development opportunities related to "recognizing and handling psychologically distressed students" are required, so faculty are prepared to identify students in distress, support them, and refer appropriately (Cleary et al., 2012). Nearly one third of newly admitted college students report a history of mental illness (Marsh & Wilcoxon, 2015), so faculty preparation is an ethical consideration. Faculty and the Office of Disability can collaboratively create programs to help students build self-awareness and coping skills and mobilize support systems for students to assist with coping skills related to stress.

Nursing faculty also need to consider the student's mental health and the student's ability to meet patient care obligations. In our current culture, university faculty are concerned about a student's personal academic goals, but they also need to consider the capacity of students to meet patient care obligations in the face of challenges involving mental health. And finally, faculty also need to be cognizant of their own biases with respect to mental illness when making decisions related to a student's fitness for clinical rotations.

CRITICAL ELEMENTS TO CONSIDER

- Consult the university attorney. *(Note:* University administrators and legal counsel are not clinicians and may not fully appreciate the specific safety implications of an accommodation respective to the clinical arena.)
- Consult the ODS.
- Consult with the student counseling office.

- Know university policies and procedures as well as the appropriate state laws. The university's interpretation of FERPA and its emergency exceptions should be emphasized.
- Initiate an emergency protocol for any reference to harm self or others or extreme emotional distress.
- Focus on the academic performance and conduct of the student only, and do not diagnose the student.
- Contact the director or dean or department chair regarding the distressed student.
- Refer the student to the student counseling center.
- Do not provide an accommodation without official accommodation from the office of disability.
- Be familiar with the nursing program's technical standards.
- Implement preventive strategies such as emails related to student counseling services during times of high stress such as midterms and finals.
- Offer faculty development sessions to faculty related to best practices in addressing students with mental health issues and psychiatric disabilities, particularly warning signs that warrant attention.

References

American College Health Association. (2015). *American College Health Association National College Health Assessment II: Spring 2015 Reference Group Executive Summary*. Linthicum, MD: ACHA.

Aradillo-Herrero, A., Tomas-Sabado, J., & Gomez-Benito, J. (2014). Associations between emotional intelligence, depression and suicide risks in nursing students. *Nurse Education Today*, 34, 520–525. doi:10.1016/j.nedt.2013.07.001

Ashcroft, T., Chernomas, W., Davis, P., Dean, R. A., Seguire, M., Shapiro, C. R., & Swiderski, L. M. (2008). Nursing students with disabilities: One faculty's journey. *International Journal of Nursing Education Scholarship*, 5(1), 1–26. doi:10.2202/1548-923X.1424

Baker, T. R. (2005). Notifying parents following a college student suicide attempt: A review of case law and FERPA, and recommendations for practice. *National Association of Student Personnel Administrators Journal*, 42, 513–533. doi:10.2202/1949-6605.1538

Betts v. Rector and Visitors of the University of Virginia, 145 Fed. Appx. 7 (4th Cir. 2005).

Brockelman, K. F., & Scheyett, A. M. (2015). Faculty perceptions of accommodations, strategies, and psychiatric advance directives for university students with mental illnesses. *Psychiatric Rehabilitation Journal*, 38(4), 342–348. doi:10.1037/prj0000143

Chernomas, W. M., & Shapiro, C. (2013). Stress, depressions, and anxiety among undergraduate nursing students. *International Journal of Nursing Education Scholarship*, 10(1), 255–266. doi:10.1515/ijnes-2012-0032

Cleary, M., Horsfall, J., Baines, J., & Happell, B. (2012). Mental health behaviours among undergraduate nursing students: Issues for consideration. *Nurse Education Today*, 32, 951–955. doi:10.1016/j.nedt.2011.11.016

Cohen, V. K. (2007). Keeping students alive: Mandating on-campus counseling saves suicidal college students' lives and limits liability. *Fordham Law Review*, 75, 3081.

Cook, L. J. (2007). Striving to help college students with mental health issues. *Journal of Psychosocial Nursing*, 45(4), 40–44. doi:10.3928/02793695-20070401-09

Drexel University College of Nursing and Health Professions. (2017). Bachelor of Science Program Co-operative Education Program Student Handbook. Retrieved from http://www.pages.drexel.edu/~cnhp/pdf/Co-op-Student-Handbook.pdf

Eisenberg, D., Hunt, J., & Speer, N. (2013). Mental health in American colleges and universities: Variation across student subgroups and across campuses. *Journal of Nervous and Mental Disease*, 201, 60–67. doi:10.1097/NMD.0b013e31827ab077

Hash v. Univ. of Kentucky, 138 S.W.3d 123 (Ky. Ct. App. 2004).

Helms, L., Jorgensen, J., & Anderson, M. A. (2006). Disability law and nursing education: An update. *Journal of Professional Nursing*, 22(30), 190–196. doi:10.1016/j.profnurs.2006.03.005

Hirshfield, S. J., & Woolf, S. R. (2005). Sex, religion, and politics: New challenges in discrimination law. *The Chronicle of Higher Education, 51*(38), B10.

Kaplan, B., & Reed, M. (2004, March). College student mental health: Plan designs, utilization, trends and costs. *Student Health Spectrum.* p. 31–33.

Kirsch, D. J., Doerfler, L. A., & Truong, D. (2015). Mental health issues among college students: Who gets referred for psychopharmacology evaluation? *Journal of American College Health, 63,* 50–56. doi:10.1080/07448481.2014.960423

Kucirka, B. G. (2017). Navigating the faculty–student relationship: Interacting with nursing students with mental health issues, *Journal of the American Psychiatric Nurses Association, 23*(6), 393–403. doi:10.1177/1078390317705451

Lane, A. M., & Corcoran, L. (2016). Educator or counselor? Navigating uncertain boundaries in the clinical environment. *Journal of Nursing Education, 55*(4), 189–195. doi:10.3928/01484834-20160316-02

Lee, B. A., & Abbey, G. E. (2008). College and university students with mental disabilities: Legal and policy issues. *The Journal of College and University Law, 34*(2), 349–391.

Maheady, D. (1999). Jumping through hoops, walking on egg shells: The experiences of nursing students with disabilities. *Journal of Nursing Education, 38*(4), 162–170. doi:10.3928/0148-4834-20000501-05

Marks, B. (2007). Cultural competence revisited: Nursing students with disabilities. *Journal of Nursing Education, 46*(2), 70–74. doi:10.3928/01484834-20070201-06

Marsh, C. N. & Wilcoxon, S. A. (2015). Underutilization of mental health services among college students: An examination of system related barriers. *Journal of College Student Psychotherapy, 29,* 227–243. doi:10.1080/87568225.2015.1045783

Matt, S. B., Maheady, D., & Fleming, S. E. (2015). Educating nursing students with disabilities: Replacing essential functions with technical standards for program entry criteria. *Journal of Post-secondary Education and Disability, 28*(4), 461–468.

May, K. A. (2014). Nursing faculty knowledge of the Americans with Disabilities Act. *Nurse Educator, 19*(5), 241–245. doi:10.1097/NNE.0000000000000058

Meloy, F., & Gambescia, S. F. (2014, May/June). Guidelines for response to student requests for academic considerations: Support vs. enabling. *Nurse Educator, 39*(3), 138–142. doi:10.1097/NNE.0000000000000037

Nguyen v. Massachusetts Institute of Technology, 96 N.E.3d 128 (Mass. 2018).

Osberg, T. M. (2004). A business case for increasing college mental health services. *Behavioral Health Management, 24*(5), 33–36.

Pavela, G. (2006). Should colleges withdraw students who threaten or attempt suicide? *Journal of American College Health, 54*(6), 367–370. doi:10.3200/JACH.54.6.367-371

Schieszler v. Ferrum College, No. 7:02CV00131 (W.D. Va. 2002).

Section 504 of the 1973 Rehabilitation Act (29 U.S.C. § 794) (1978) and Title II and III of the 1990 Americans With Disabilities Act (42 U.S.C. § 12132).

Shin v. Massachusetts Institute of Technology, No. 020403, 2005 WL 1869101 (Mass. Super. Ct., June 27, 2005).

Silverman, M. M. (2004). College student suicide prevention: Background and blueprint for action. *Student Health Spectrum,* 13–20.

Smith, R.B., & Fleming, D. L. Student Suicide and Colleges' Liability. *Chronicle of Higher Education, 53*(33), B24.

Souma, A., Rickerson, N., & Burgstahler, S. (2002). Academic accommodations for students with psychiatric disabilities. *DO-IT, University of Washington,* 1–4.

VanBergeijk, E., Klin, A., & Volkmar, F. (2008). Supporting more able students on the autism spectrum: College and beyond. *Journal of Autism and Developmental Disorders, 38,* 1359–1370. doi:10.1007/s10803 -007-0524-8. Retrieved from https://mijn.bsl.nl/supporting-more-able-students-on-the-autism-spectrum -college-and/547540

31

A Bad Action: Is It Ethical, Illegal, or Both?

INTRODUCTION

It is all too easy to confuse law and morality. What they most fundamentally have in common is that they are normative systems, which means that they provide rules and values meant to direct human action. They are not the only normative systems that weigh upon us. Etiquette, fashion, institutional policy, and social convention are also normative systems. However, arguably, law and morality weigh upon us as normative systems more than any others. This weight can also understandably lead to conflicts. Their imperatives can be quite strong, and when they conflict, it can be difficult to decide which path to follow. In the general course of life, however, they likely coincide. Many acts are both moral and legal. Some are both immoral and illegal. But some are moral while illegal and others immoral while legal. Most actions people perform in their daily lives likely qualify as both legal and moral. And some acts like theft, murder, and assault are largely considered both illegal and immoral. But an act such as lying is legal but might be considered immoral.[1] And rushing someone in emergent medical need to the hospital, while breaking the speed limit, is illegal but might be judged moral. All of this points to a complex and nuanced relationship between these two normative systems. And given their weight and the potential for conflict, it becomes important to understand each of them deeply in order to examine those situations when they may conflict.

LAW VERSUS MORALITY

The first contrast to make between law and morality is that laws are primarily aimed at regulating external actions or actions in the public realm in order to protect the interests of individuals and promote the public good. Morality, though, focuses on actions within one's private life and even one's private thoughts. This is particularly true within a liberal democratic society. In a theocratic society, in which morality is perceived and enforced within an accepted (or imposed) religious point of view, the distinction between law and morality can break down. Whereas in liberal democratic societies, we recognize the existence of a private sphere in which individuals have a high degree of sovereignty without legal or other type of government interference. The public sphere, in which we commingle with our fellow citizens in politics, commerce, and other areas of public life, is far more regulated by law. This is because one of the primary functions of law is to maintain civil order. Thus, those acts which could cause harm (physical harm, harm to property, violation of legal rights) are

---

[1] Lying, of course, in some circumstances, such as testifying under oath, can have civil and criminal repercussions. However, lying in general, in the course of one's private life, is not illegal.

those primarily regulated by law. Respect of the private sphere by law and government translates to respect to persons as individuals able to choose their own good, make their own personal decisions, build their own lives, and follow their own conceptions of morality. This view of legal regulation is sometimes conceptualized in terms of moral and political philosopher John Stuart Mill's (1910) harm principle: "The only purpose for which power can be rightfully exercised over any member of a civilized community, against his will, is to prevent harm to others" (p. 73). Essentially, this means that each individual should be legally free to do anything they wish so long as someone else is not harmed. This idea is also sometimes expressed in the cliché, "Your right to swing your arm ends where my nose begins." This principle also implies that self-harming acts ought not to be regulated. The assumption is that a rational, competent person who is performing an action with the potential for self-harm (heavy alcohol use, use of illicit drugs, cigarette smoking) has the ability to understand the consequences of their actions and choose to perform those actions nonetheless. It is not the state's place to protect someone against themselves.

As attractive as this principle might sound, a couple of caveats must be noted. First, although most liberal democratic states likely operate under some explicit or implicit version of this principle, it is unlikely that any political state follows it with absolute stringency. Second, due to the uncertain nature of some underlying concepts, it may not even be possible for any state to follow this principle with absolute stringency in a clear and uniform sense. As to the first caveat, in our own society we arguably violate the harm principle with laws against recreational drug use, prostitution, and limitations on the selling of alcohol. The reason, one might say, particularly for these examples, is a lingering pre-Enlightenment religion-based legal moralism. Even Mill in one case argued for a limitation of what might appear to be a merely self-regarding act, maintaining that one should not be allowed to voluntarily become a slave to another. Certainly, this would seem a rare and unlikely choice, but it would appear to be allowed according to a strict interpretation of the harm principle. Mill (1910), however, found it contradictory for one to use his liberty "to abdicate his liberty" (p. 158). In addition, the rather stringent standard that prevents a state from protecting citizens from themselves may be too context independent to be tenable. Are there cases in which it would be good to protect people from their own desperation, such as with usury laws? Can we always be confident in the full autonomy of persons when they act in potentially self-harmful manners? Should we protect people from themselves when they are scammed and misinformed by those who would exploit their naïveté and credulousness? Should we recognize the legitimacy of gratuitous contracts?

As to the second caveat, there is uncertainty regarding what might count as harm regarding the division between the private and public spheres. Mill (1910) conceptualized harm in terms of limitation or violation of individual interests or rights. This conceptualization is rather broad and not limited to physical harm but likely does not include emotional harm. Thus, one may have a right to insult or even emotionally abuse another. However, if "harm" were to include emotional harm, that restriction would likely infringe too far on other rights like the right to free expression. But more importantly, if one follows the effects of a presumably self-regarding act far enough, one is likely to find some harm done to another. For example, rock climbing might on its face seem like a choice that only places oneself at potential risk. However, if a rock climber is in need of rescue, now rescuers may be at risk. If a rock climber is injured and in need of extensive medical treatment, payment for that treatment may weigh upon others. If payment is public through government programs, that effect upon others is clear. But even payment through private insurance might be said to become a burden upon uninvolved others in drawing upon the premiums of other insured persons and potentially raising those payments in the future. Or, if in a system of rationing, care or resources provided for this injured rock climber is drawn away from care or resources needed by others, this too would seem to demonstrate an effect (harm) of the rock climber's actions upon others. However, there comes a point at which following this line of causation becomes ridiculous. For this reason, Mill (1910) attempted to limit far flung, fanciful claims of harm. The understanding of harm to others (in terms of which acts should be regulated or prohibited by the government) should be those harms caused "directly, and in the first instance" by one's actions (Mill, 1910, p. 75). In other words, "indirect" harms or harms caused indirectly by one's actions should not be reasons to legally prohibit or regulate an act or practice. This restriction does not fully resolve the problem, however, as the line between direct effect and indirect effect is not always clear. For this reason we get debates in our society regarding issues like tobacco smoking in public spaces, wearing seatbelts in motor vehicles, and motorcyclists wearing helmets. These issues have all been defended as merely self-regarding acts, and thus beyond the control of legal regulation. Certainly, tobacco use, not wearing seatbelts, and not wearing motorcycle helmets all present dangers to the individuals involved, but do they also pose harms to others that are direct enough to justify legal regulation? Are the potential harms to others (secondhand smoke, the physical force of one's own untethered body in the confined space of an automobile, and the costs of severe head trauma) direct enough to warrant regulation of these behaviors? Regarding these particular examples, we have mostly answered yes.[2] But when these questions were being contested, there was much disagreement about where to draw that line. And that line continues to be uncertain and negotiable.

Relatedly, the line between the private sphere and the public sphere is also not always clear enough to function as a distinct criterion for applying the law. Though theoretically distinct areas of life, according to German philosopher Jürgen Habermas (2000), they are equiprimordial, meaning that they are equally fundamental and also rely on one another's realization to be fully realized. Having a fully realized private life depends upon the proper and full realization of the public sphere and vice versa. Due to this co-dependence, the line between the public and private may not always be clear. The interpretation of the public and the private in relation to spheres of experience is by no means wholly objective or absolute. It may be clear that an action like brandishing and discharging a firearm in a common, populated area is a public act that should be regulated, and engaging in consensual sexual activity in one's home is private and should not be regulated. However, it was not long ago that domestic violence was considered by many as merely a private matter between a married couple, with which the government should not interfere (Solic, 2015). Also, currently, one of the primary points of contention regarding the moral/legal issue of abortion is whether the act is one of the private or public sphere. The common discourse from the pro-choice perspective is that abortion is a private act between a woman and her physician and thus should be free of government interference. According to the pro-life perspective, abortion is not merely a self-regarding act but one that harms others (fetuses) who should be viewed as having legal rights worthy of protection by the government. This does not mean that the public/private division in determining where the law applies is a useless standard, but it can't operate as a specific, purely objective, and absolute standard. It is one that is continuously undergoing negotiation and adjustment.

While the common distinction is that law addresses external or public activities and morality private ones, morality does still address public life. The areas of social ethics and professional ethics address our actions in the public sphere. Common social issues like abortion, the death penalty, and genetic engineering, while legal issues, are also issues of public ethical discourse. And of course professional ethics—the ethics of physicians, nurses, lawyers, educators, and so on—address and regulate the actions of professionals as they practice and provide services among the public.

The idea that morality addresses the private sphere may even include the realm of thought. Beliefs and opinions are often judged moral or immoral. Racist, sexist, or homophobic beliefs may be considered morally improper. It is not just the acts that these beliefs inspire that are immoral, some may say, but the thoughts themselves. One of the most famous philosophical investigations into the morality of thought and belief is Clifford's (1999) essay "The Ethics of Belief." In this essay, originally published in 1877, Clifford argues that one has not only an intellectual obligation but indeed a *moral* obligation not to believe a claim until sufficient evidence is presented. Being credulous, that is, believing before sufficient evidence is presented, is not only intellectually dishonest and possibly imprudent, but also morally dishonest and even socially and personally harmful, according to Clifford. The law, as stated, focuses on external actions or actions in the public realm. However, there are even times when law takes internal mental states into account. *Mens rea* is a legal concept that from Latin literally means "guilty mind." The principle of *mens rea* is that for one to be legally liable for a criminal act one must have a "guilty mind" and be aware of one's actions; that is, one must have criminal intent. Prosecutors, judges, and juries do not of course have direct access to defendants'

---

[2] All but three states have motorcycle helmet laws (Insurance Institute for Highway Safety, 2019). New Hampshire is the only state without a seatbelt law, except one for drivers and passengers under 18 (Government Highway Safety Association, 2019). Only seven states have no laws restricting smoking at private worksites, restaurants, or bars (Centers for Disease Control and Prevention, 2011).

minds, but certain external acts can be used to infer a guilty intent or *mens rea*. Similarly, federal laws and state laws include different degrees of murder, some of which are identified by mental states like premeditation and malice aforethought. And once again, authorities cannot directly perceive these in the accused but can infer them from actions.

Another distinction between law and morality relates to enforcement. Law has the force of the government behind it to enforce laws through the coercion of punishment. The enforcement of morality is comprised primarily of public disapprobation or tainted reputation. Outside of theocratic regimes with institutionalized "morality police," there are generally no bodies with the power to enforce morality and ensure that all citizens follow moral rules.[3] Social and professional ethics are the areas in which overlap with the law occurs the most. Our moral views on issues like abortion and the death penalty feed into the laws governments pass regarding them, despite the ideal that in a liberal democratic society no one vision of the good should be imposed upon all. And the laws we have on these issues likely also have an influence on individuals' moral views regarding them (Mentovich & Zeev-wolf, 2018). Similarly, professional ethics often overlap with legal issues. Such overlap occurs every semester of a healthcare ethics or nursing ethics course when a student responds to a case involving questions of confidentiality with a simple invocation of HIPAA. Yes, the Health Insurance Portability and Accountability Act (HIPAA) of 1996 provides legal protections for patient confidentiality and outlines punishments for breaches of confidentiality. However, it is a mistake to assume outside of or prior to HIPAA, there is no acknowledgment of the importance of confidentiality in patient care. Confidentiality is one of the moral principles emphasized in the Hippocratic Oath, while respect for autonomy (considered by many currently as the most important of moral principles in healthcare ethics) is completely ignored. In 1996, the U.S. Congress wanted to send the message that confidentiality in healthcare is so important that it should have the force of law and coercion of potential punishment behind it in order to provide even more protection than mere moral disapprobation. Along these lines, it is also worth noting that in the study and education of social ethics and professional ethics, the analysis and evaluation of landmark legal cases is often central. To teach about abortion, cases like *Roe v. Wade* (1973) and *Planned Parenthood v. Casey* (1992) are indispensable. To teach end-of-life ethics, the Quinlan case (*In re Quinlan*, 1976) and Cruzan case (*Cruzan v. Director, Missouri Department of Health*, 1990), along with *In re Helga Wanglie* (1991) and *Washington v. Glucksberg* (1997) provide rich context for discussion and exploration of central ethical issues. Whereas ethics in general only has the enforcement of reputation and social disapprobation behind it, as noted in Chapter 5, Basic Primer on Applied Ethics, professional ethics often include mechanisms of coercive enforcement such as loss or suspension of license to practice. And for officers and employees of the federal government, statutes outline specific penalties for ethics violations. This last especially may unnecessarily conflate law and morality. In this case, an ethics violation is in fact a legal violation. To refer to these violations as ethics violations seems almost superfluous. Perhaps doing so invokes a standard of excellence and a perspective that surpasses mere rule following, which, though in practice, requires only rule following.

One simple distinction between law and morality is that laws are created and modified by legislative bodies. This imputes intentional and procedural qualities of laws. They can be merely created, modified, and annulled by a recognized body of authority. Ethical rules and principles do not work this way but develop or evolve organically within a community of valuers. They do undergo change, but an authoritative body cannot merely change moral rules with the wave of a hand—or an official, procedural wave of hand. Ethics, in general, is not procedural. However, as noted in Chapter 5, Basic Primer on Applied Ethics, professional ethics can often take on a procedural quality as a means of more strictly and uniformly regulating conduct among members of the profession. Change in ethical rules typically occurs slowly, usually due to changes in society, environment, or moral perception. This last reason for moral rule change points to a deeper question. Moral rules do change within a society; however, that may not be the same as ethics or morality itself changing. To assert that ethics itself changes implies a view of moral relativism. An objective view of ethics would affirm that ethics

---

[3] The governor of Alabama has recently signed a law allowing a megachurch to install its own police force with powers similar to those of the state police. This body may not be quite the same as the "morality police" found within some theocratic countries, but it seems on its face uncomfortably similar (Gonzalez, 2019).

itself stays the same (at least generally), but society's perception of ethics changes—hopefully for the better. In our society, various forms of gender and racial oppression have been viewed as morally acceptable, or even obligatory, in the past. As we have evolved in acknowledging the rights and proper respect of various minorities, we have to either accept that treatment of these minorities in the past was morally good *then* but not *now*, or that such treatment was always wrong (objectively) but we did not recognize the wrongness at the time. Also, due to the procedural nature of law, the law only requires that one meet the specific inscribed requirements. Ethics often demands more than simply refraining from breaking rules, but going beyond that to good and benevolent action. This is particularly true from a perspective of virtue ethics in which moral education and self-improvement and an ideal of moral excellence (not mere rule following) is to be pursued.

Finally, for the purpose of clear and just enforcement, law needs a degree of certainty, while morals have a greater degree of flexibility and variability. The law depends upon clear and distinct definitions, which may not always hold up outside the law. A simple example is the age of majority. In this society we recognize the age of majority as 18. This means that there are certain rights, privileges, and responsibilities afforded 18-year-olds but not 17-year-olds, such as the right to vote and make one's own medical decisions. However, there is nothing magical that happens to one's mentality upon one's 18th birthday. And it is very possible to find 17-year-olds with greater maturity and decision-making abilities than some persons much older. Yet for the purpose of applying legal rights and responsibilities, a legal expediency is necessary. It would be inefficient and inconvenient to have to apply some form of individual psychological test for the many mundane rights and responsibilities of adult citizens and residents for each individual. There are some exceptions regarding minors' rights built into the law like the mature minor doctrine in the context of medical decisions, the process of emancipation, and legal exceptions in relation to reproductive choices. But these are procedural exceptions that cannot of course locate and empower every minor capable of making mature decisions. This mechanism toward expediency does have its downsides, however. The cliché, "the law is an ass," appeals to one of these. Because of these dictated legal standards and rules applying universally but perhaps ill-fitting certain specific situations, the law receives a reputation for being stubborn and incompatible with common sense.

Because moral rules (outside of procedural professional ethics) are not distinctly delineated and dictated, some degree of flexibility and variability is inevitable and perhaps necessary. Moral principles often conflict and thus are in need of deliberation through the application of practical judgment in order to resolve conflicts. There is also the problem that moral judgments and systems vary even within a society and even more so among different societies. In order to reach consensus or have any fruitful moral discourse, some degree of flexibility will be needed.

IS THERE A MORAL OBLIGATION TO FOLLOW THE LAW?

Laws include coercive penalties to help ensure obedience and civil order. People of course try to avoid unpleasant repercussions, and so it is expected that they will generally follow laws. However, even absent penalties, is there warrant for respecting and following the law? Are there deeper *moral* reasons one should avoid breaking laws? Of course, in the case of some laws a legal violation qualifies as a moral violation as well. Acts like theft, murder, and rape are typically judged immoral as well as illegal. However, there are many laws, the violation of which would not be patently immoral. Would there be a similar moral imperative to respect and follow these laws?

There are two major theories regarding the foundation of law. The first, natural law theory,[4] maintains, according to the overlap thesis, that laws are founded in a preexisting understanding of morality (Bix, 2010). That is, a law (or a proper law) needs to be derived from a moral principle or value. One of two important implications of the overlap thesis (depending on which version of the theory you appeal to) follows from this: If a law is not moral in itself, it is either not a law at all (Augustine, 1973; Blackstone, 2016), or it does not meet the ideal of what a law *should be* (Finnis,

---

[4] It is important not to confuse this theory of natural law with the natural law theory of morality discussed in the previous chapter. It is easy to confuse them because they have the same name and share some basic principles and intuitions. However, one addresses the essence of morality and the other the essence of law and the law's relationship to morality.

2011). On the one hand, according to the view of theorists like Blackstone and Augustine, immoral or unjust laws are not laws at all. As expressed by St. Augustine: *lex injustia non est lex*, "an unjust law is not a law."[5] Under this interpretation, an unjust law is a law in name only. It has no legitimate authority, and one should feel free to reject and disobey it and should not be punished for doing so. On the other hand, the view of theorists like John Finnis is that an unjust law is in fact a legitimate law, but not a good one. Such laws should be removed or amended to meet basic standards of morality. This view is more famously expressed in Martin Luther King's (2018) "Letter from a Birmingham Jail": "There are two types of laws: there are *just* and there are *unjust* laws.... A just law is a man-made code that squares with the moral law or the law of God" (p. 503). King (2018) maintained that a law can be unjust in four different ways: (a) the law is generally inconsistent with the moral law; (b) the law degrades human personality; (c) the law is inflicted upon a minority by a majority who is itself not subject to the law; or (d) the law is inflicted upon a minority who had no say in creating it. King of course famously advocated, and practiced himself, a civil disobedience of transgressing unjust laws in order to fight to change or remove them. Because King (2018) affirmed this second interpretation of natural law, he maintained that one should accept the punishment for breaking even an unjust law. For, even though an unjust law is unjust, it is still a law: "One who breaks an unjust law must do it *openly, lovingly* ... and with a willingness to accept the penalty" (King, 2018, p. 504).

The competing theory of law and morality, legal positivism, conceives laws as an expression of conventionalism and created by an authoritative body possibly out of whole cloth. Legal positivism rejects the overlap thesis and instead affirms the separation thesis: There is no conceptual overlap between law and morality; they are conceptually and completely distinct and different normative systems and areas of life (Coleman & Leiter, 2010). For a law to be a legitimate law it need not meet some test for morality. Whereas, according to legal positivism and the separation thesis, there is no conceptual overlap between law and morality, there still may be content overlap, meaning that many immoral actions may also be illegal or many moral actions may also be legal. However, according to legal positivism, these instances of consistency are merely incidental and adventitious. The authority and legitimacy of the law rests wholly in the authority and power of the perceived lawmakers, not in some perceived moral foundation. Although there is no moral basis for law, it may not be the case that laws are created in a purely arbitrary or self-serving manner. Law, even absent an essential relation to morality, can have the objective of maintaining social order or protecting and promoting the well-being of the populace. But at the same time, there is nothing, according to legal positivism, that would guarantee law functioning in this manner. For any unjust law would be functionally and authoritatively equivalent to any just law. Thus, under a natural law theory interpretation, one who breaks the law is also violating morality, regardless of whether the act is patently immoral in itself. But under the theory of legal positivism, breaking the law does not logically entail a moral violation.

Because of the contributions of thinkers like St. Augustine and St. Thomas and because of the common conflation and confusion of the natural law theory of morality and the natural law theory of the law, natural law theory is often assumed to include an essential religious element or religious presuppositions. It is true that natural law theory is often developed in terms of law's connection to a sense of religious morality. However, it is possible to conceive natural law theory in a secular manner as well. King (2018) suggests this duality in the quote given previously when he defines a just law as one that "squares with the moral law or the law of God" (p. 503). Here, "moral law" is left open to possible secular interpretation. This moral law could be one of nonreligious origin and basis. It is indeed true that King conceived of morality from within a faith tradition, but he still leaves room in his comment on natural law for those who do not. Indeed, the roots of natural law theory in the West can be found in pre-Christian Greek philosophy, in the thinking of Aristotle, Plato, and Socrates (Bix, 2002). While the relationship among law, morality, and religion for these three thinkers is rather complex and not one of complete separation, the connections are not what we typically

---

[5] This quote is commonly attributed to Augustine, but I have not encountered this specific quote in my reading of Augustine. It is likely a more succinct paraphrase of a statement from his book *On Free Will*.

conceive from our modern perspective.[6] For these three, justice in morality and law is to be determined through rational contemplation and deliberation. The Middle Ages saw a rise in acknowledging an essential relation between religion and morality (and by extension through natural law theory, to the law). The Renaissance and Enlightenment saw a move away from a religious interpretation of natural law with, first, a return to Classical texts and ideas (Renaissance) and, second, the concomitant rise of secular moral and political theories (Enlightenment): utilitarianism, Kantian ethics, liberal democracy. Contemporary approaches to secular natural law theory may focus on elaborating the meaning of rights and responsibilities in relation to facts of human nature while attempting to resolve the is–ought distinction (Weinreb, 2004).

As noted, if natural law theory is true, then one has a moral duty (not just a duty of prudence or self-interest) to follow the law. But could we say the same if legal positivism were the correct theory? Without providing an ultimate answer to this long-standing debate in legal theory, we can further explore the question of a possible moral obligation to follow the law even with the assumptions of legal positivism. Most persons, it seems, are generally law-abiding. This is not to say that most persons have not broken some laws, even with impunity. Most persons likely have broken what they consider to be minor laws: speeding infractions, rolling stops, jaywalking. This could be seen as pointing to an underlying view of legal positivism: These minor laws, while generally effective for maintaining social order, serve no inherent moral purpose and can be overridden by one's personal, practical needs or interests. "I am running late for work. A speed limit is largely an arbitrary line. Exceeding the speed limit by a small amount will serve my interests in getting to work on time without significantly endangering myself or anyone else." However, consider a person who intentionally violates what many would consider more serious laws: theft, armed robbery, murder, rape. Your typical (generally) law-abiding citizen will have negative feelings regarding such a person. These negative feelings are likely inspired by the moral quality of the lawbreaker's actions. These more serious infractions are often (as in the examples provided) perceived as both illegal and immoral. However, these negative feelings may be associated with something more than the purely moral nature of the actions. There may be a concern with the actual legal violations involved. But why? What is the source of this scorn for lawbreakers as *lawbreakers*, not just as moral transgressors?

One possible answer to this question is that when one breaks a law, one disrespects the state and political apparatus that creates the law. Under this interpretation we, as citizens (or possibly merely as residents), have not only a legal but a moral obligation to the state in which we live. This type of obligation is first (probably) and most famously developed in Plato's dialogue *The Crito*. In this dialogue Socrates sits in prison awaiting his execution. His friends suggest the possibility of escape in order to avoid what they deem to be an unjust punishment. Socrates disagrees and argues that it is his obligation to remain and accept the punishment deemed appropriate and just by the state. To do otherwise, argues Socrates, would destroy the state, defy his implicit consent to the law, neglect a supposed natural duty to the state, and disregard the gratitude one owes to the state. These have all turned out to be infamously problematic arguments. First, it is patently not true that any specific instance of defying the law (like Socrates avoiding execution) will destroy the state. The only way to make sense of such a dramatic claim is from an absolutist, quasi-Kantian perspective that immorality is a form of logical incoherence, thereby destroying the coherence of the system itself. But practically speaking, it simply is not true that Socrates's escape would destroy Athens. Second, the claim that one, simply by continuing to live in a society, implicitly consents to any rule of the state is highly dubious. The argument assumes that leaving a state is similar to leaving a club in which one loses interest. But it is not a simple matter to uproot oneself from a political state when one does not agree with it. In fact, doing so can be so difficult that rather than implicit consent to obey, the situation might be better described as a form of coercion. Third, Socrates assumes that citizens have a parent–child relationship with the state and thus a natural duty to obey like a child's natural duty to obey the parent. The analogy itself is dubious, but is especially problematic in considering the possibility of an abusive parent. And to assume that a citizen owes whatever a state demands due to gratitude for what

---

[6] What I mean by this is far more complex that can be developed in this context. However, as just a hint of what I mean, I can point to Aristotle's conception of God not as a personal being but as an attractive and good force toward which everything is leading. In this way, God for Aristotle is essentially associated with everything good but not as a creative or judgmental presence as is typically conceived today.

the state provides (protection, resources, etc.) perverts the nature of gratitude, as the creditor cannot demand any and everything of the debtor.[7] It seems that a coherent moral obligation to the state to obey the laws is difficult to defend. In addition to these specific responses to Socrates, one could also point out the difficulty of conceptualizing a moral duty to a "state." It seems natural to understand a moral duty to an individual, a person. However, a political state is a different type of thing. A state is a conceptual fiction, not a moral agent.

If one does not clearly have a moral obligation to the state to obey laws, there may instead be actual persons (moral agents) to whom we could say that we morally owe a duty to obey the law. A common argument in support of this view is known as the "fair play argument," which is a species of social contract thinking (Hart, 1958; Luban, 1988; Rawls, 2001). Returning to the lawbreaker and the average citizen's scorn for the lawbreaker, one means of conceiving the lawbreaker and their actions is in terms of being a "free rider." A free rider is one who reaps the benefits of a system without contributing to that system. For example, some years ago, following a severe snowstorm which left much of the city buried under several feet of snow and the city's resources stretched to their limit, my neighbors and I found ourselves immobilized with the street clogged with snow and cars buried. Without an explicit collective decision, the neighborhood all came out to shovel the snow, clear the street, and uncover automobiles. This phenomenon provided a unique and unusual sense of community in which all contributed to a shared good of a clear street and the individual goods of disinterred cars. Now, imagine someone who watches all this occur from a window, from the warmth and security of home. When the neighbors finish clearing the street, this bystander calmly leaves their apartment, walks to their car, and drives off as the exhausted neighbors stare in amazement. Clearly, bad feelings would arise among the neighbors regarding this individual due to free-riding, the use or exploiting of the efforts of others absent any personal contributions. There appears something inherently unfair in this. The lawbreaker might be seen in a similar light by the average law-abiding citizen. The non-shoveling individual places themselves above or beyond others in the neighborhood, benefiting from that to which they refused to contribute. The lawbreaker also places themselves above others, as someone not beholden to the rules (laws) of society but benefiting from the goods of society nonetheless.[8] Such actions also suggest moral failings such as arrogance, disregard for the needs of others, and selfishness. Without assuming an inherent morality in the law, the fair play argument identifies a moral duty owed to one's fellow citizens to follow the law nonetheless. This, however, assumes that the law is itself of value to citizens. Otherwise, there would be no interest for individuals to follow the law at all. Thus, the fair play argument assumes that laws must be generally beneficial (Luban, 1988). Just as the act of clearing snow in the neighborhood is beneficial and one benefiting from it imposes a duty to participate equally, the benefit one individually gains from the law imposes a duty, out of fairness, to comply with the law.

But is it always morally wrong to break the law? Consider the non-shoveling neighbor again. Perhaps this neighbor did not participate in the collective shoveling because of a heart condition, or a need to care for a sick relative. In such instances, the free-rider might be excused. Their free-riding is not borne of moral failings like selfishness but extenuating circumstances that make it difficult or impossible to contribute the same as the rest of the community. By analogy, could there be circumstances that might justify a failure to comply with a law, or even a blatant defiance of a law? If, as in the extended snow shoveling example, there are extenuating circumstances that make an individual unable to follow a law, then it seems reasonable to excuse that individual from that law. However, there may also be conditions regarding a law itself in which a violation could appear morally justified. The fair play argument holds that a law should be generally beneficial in order for an individual to be obligated to follow it (Luban, 1988). To say that a law is generally beneficial is to say that it secures, promotes, or encourages some good for society. Absent some beneficence, it would be difficult to assert that any individual should comply with any law, absent absolute coercion. Further, to say that a law should be *generally* beneficial means that the law should not "confer benefits on one group

---

[7] These counterarguments to Socrates's position adapted from Luban (1988).

[8] This example is a combination of an actual personal experience and an adaptation of a case presented by Luban (1988).

at the expense of others" (Luban, 1988, p. 43). In other words, a law should not be discriminatory and unfair. This criterion is itself expressed in the Fourteenth Amendment of the Constitution: "No state shall … deny any person within its jurisdiction the equal protection of the laws." Thus, as noted earlier, social and legal reformers like Martin Luther King (2018) identify discriminatory laws as laws that are degrading, that are inflicted upon a minority by a majority while excepting the majority from the restriction or penalty, or that are inflicted upon a minority who has no say in their creation. To break a law for one's individual benefit and assumed exceptionalism bespeaks of moral failings, of "unilaterally exempting oneself from the shared conditions of the community" (Luban, 1988, p. 42). However, to break a law as an act of resistance against a law that does not meet basic standards of fairness can itself be seen as a courageous, moral act—an act aimed at seeking justice overall. Breaking laws for one's personal benefit demonstrates an arrogance and selfishness, a contempt for others which denies or neglects the personhood and equal interests of others in one's community. Whereas, breaking an unjust law holds no such implications: "The fact that a law is wrong or is overwhelmingly stupid means that noncompliance with it exhibits no disrespect for one's fellows, and thus that there is no obligation to obey it in the first place" (Luban, 1988, p. 45).

One last point: I earlier affirmed that most law-abiding citizens likely were not completely law-abiding, that everyone or nearly everyone has broken some (presumably) minor laws. Yet, these law-abiding citizens feel a lack of fairness from the lawbreaker, as with the neighbor who blithely drove off after refusing to help clear the street of snow. Does that make these law-abiding citizens hypocrites? Perhaps. From my experience, people who violate minor laws likely do not see themselves as immoral or evil. They are wrong for the (minor) laws they violate merely for their own benefit or convenience. However, they tend to employ forms of rationalization to absolve themselves (at least to themselves) of these sins: "Everyone does it" or "It's not a big deal." The former excuse smacks of a "two wrongs" fallacy morally speaking. But in terms of the law, it may not be so simple. One further condition of the fair play argument is that a law that legitimately commands obedience must be one that most people comply with (Luban, 1988). In terms of fairness, if most people contravene a law with impunity, the moral imperative for any individual to comply with the law weakens in recognition of the lack of fairness of most benefiting from flouting from the law with impunity. The latter excuse, "It's not a big deal," while mostly a rationalization, may have some weight. If one were to adopt a strict Kantian moral position, outside of proportional punishment, the severity of a crime would be irrelevant. Wrong is wrong. A murderer and a jaywalker are both equally lawbreakers. However, such strict Kantianism is likely difficult to defend. Rather, it seems more reasonable that the severity of a crime roughly reflects the character of the lawbreaker. Yes, the jaywalker is wrong for jaywalking, but clearly the crimes jaywalking and murder are not comparable. Kant at least acknowledges this in terms of retribution but still takes a simple and dogmatic approach to one's status as a rule breaker. The consequences of one's actions are not wholly dispositive of the moral quality of those actions or one's character. However, those consequences are not irrelevant either. The law-abiding citizen who may have broken some minor laws in the past may be a bit hypocritical. But there clearly can be a reasoned, commonsensical distinction between such a person and one who explicitly violates the law with an assumption of exceptionalism and contempt for one's fellow persons.

NORMATIVE DOMINANCE: WHICH IS MORE IMPORTANT? LAW OR MORALITY?

Answering this question may depend on what we mean by "more important"? If one judges merely avoiding punishment as more important, then clearly following the law has greater weight. However, it is not clear that merely avoiding punishment is what matters most in life. As humans we have values that provide meaning for our lives and sometimes preserving those values may be worth risking punitive consequences.

As noted at the beginning of this chapter, law and morality comprise distinct normative systems, among many other normative systems. And among these many normative systems, law and morality seem especially weighty. But also noted at the beginning of the chapter, sometimes law and morality may conflict. Many acts are both moral and legal. Many are both immoral and illegal. However, there are also acts that are moral but illegal and some that are immoral but legal. When we face such situations, which should we choose to follow: the law or morality? The question here falls under the concept of normative dominance. When different types of normative systems conflict, which should be acknowledged as dominant? For example, fashion is another normative system indicated at the beginning of the chapter. Fashion norms dictate or suggest the way people should dress. There may not be one particular type of fashion norm. There may be different normative sets for different socioeconomic classes or different ethnicities or different genders. It can be a very complex and dynamic normative system. However, it generally is not viewed as having a high degree of normative dominance.[9] Consider the wearing of animal fur. There are people who find the cultivation, creation, and wearing of animal fur as highly immoral. Perhaps if we lived in a pre-industrial society in which wearing animal fur was the only means of surviving very cold weather, the morality of the practice might be judged differently. But that is not the situation in which we find ourselves. We have many alternatives for warm clothing that do not pose the same level of harm to animals. And so, the cultivation and killing of animals to wear seems unnecessary, an unnecessary infliction of harm upon sentient creatures. Making such a sartorial choice in our milieu appears to have value only in terms of aesthetics and status. One wearing a fur who is confronted with these moral problems associated with the cultivation and wearing of fur might respond with a statement such as, "But it looks good." Many people, understandably, even those who do not consider themselves animal rights advocates, would find that response crass and insensitive; that is, morally bankrupt. For most people of any moral sensitivity, even those with refined fashion sense, morality is perceived as normatively dominant to fashion. But when addressing the question of normative dominance as it relates to law and morality, is the answer equally as clear?

We recognize the state as having power over us, even though in a representative democracy "we the people" are theoretically the government, or at least those who endorse and endow the formal government with power. The enforcement of law is part of that power. If we want to live prosperously and peacefully in society, then presumably it benefits us to obey the law. Living contrary to the law opens us up to civil litigation and criminal penalty. Of course, those consequences can befall even the most law-abiding citizens, but following legal strictures seems the best bet to avoid them. Thus, the motivation for obeying the law does not follow simply from a desire not to be punished. It also comes from a desire to live a good life within a particular social structure. Motivation for obeying the law may also be a matter of simple character. Some people merely may not have it in them to be a thief or to sell dangerous and illicit products in order to make money. Here, we begin to loop back to the theme of the previous section. If laws (or at least proper and legitimate laws) are founded in morality, then there are not merely prudential, self-serving reasons for obeying the law but moral ones as well.

This progression also begins to point to an answer on normative dominance. Identifying the question of character in relation to law and the possible moral foundation of law suggests a greater normative dominance in morality. If morality indeed provides a foundation for law or a collective moral reason for obeying the law, as in the fair play argument, it does appear more fundamental and presumably more dominant. What this means is that in a conflict between law and morality, *typically* one should choose to follow morality. It may not be prudent to establish that principle in any more strict or absolutist sense than this. In any particular case one may have to consider the degree of moral and legal wrong involved and the moral and legal consequences involved. That is, it might be justifiable to commit a minor moral wrong in order to follow a more serious legal requirement. It may not be possible to foresee all such situations and thus not prudent to establish a stricter principle.

But what does it mean to say that a conflict may exist between law and morality? If natural law theory is correct, then laws are themselves moral. That is not exactly true. Natural law theory is more normative than descriptive. Laws *should* be moral. They may not always be moral in nature. According to natural law theory, as indicated earlier, immoral laws are either not laws at all (despite what the state might say) or they do not meet the ideal of what a law should be. If a law is not really a law or not a legitimate law, then one no longer has a moral obligation to obey it. Even if an immoral law merely

---

[9] I will make one exception regarding this statement in terms of gender fashion norms, in which for much of our cultural history, policing the proper clothes for the proper genders has been perceived as highly important. But two points about this exception: First, this norm appears to be currently undergoing change and opening up in recognition of the complexity of gender and greater respect for those who are transgender and transsexual; second, this particular fashion norm has been closely allied with perceived ethical norms regarding the proper behavior and separation of the genders and sexes. Thus, the importance of this fashion norm is more truly found within the ethical side of it.

does not meet the ideal of what a law should be, then we at least have a moral duty to reform and repair the law. Even under legal positivism and the fair play argument, if there is a moral obligation under a sort of social contract to obey the law, that obligation breaks down when the law in question does not provide a general benefit to society or apply to people equally. In contemporary society, of course, the quintessential example of this type of situation is the American Civil Rights Movement of the 20th century, particularly the activism and thought of Martin Luther King, Jr.

Earlier in this chapter I quoted King defining a moral law as one "that squares with the moral law or the law of God" (2018, p. 503). King was a man of faith, a Christian; thus, much of his thought and activism were inspired and driven by religious principle. More specifically, he had a moral religious interpretation of Christian doctrine which the discriminatory laws and social structures in the United States at the time (and possibly currently as well to some extent) violated. King was a Baptist minister, so that of course makes sense. At the same time, he was open-minded and strategic enough to realize that he could not communicate to all merely within a narrow moral/religious point of view which not all whom he may wish to contend with might share. So, in the preceding quote, he disjunctively refers also to the "moral law." This is a complex term with much background, both religious and secular. In terms of secular background, the most well-known use of this particular term comes from the work of Kant. Kant too was a highly religious, Christian man. However, in his work on ethics, he attempted to develop his analysis and theory as secularly as possible. One does not have to be a Christian or theist at all to evaluate or even adopt the moral views of Kant's philosophy. The moral law from this perspective is founded in reason. Reason, which exists independently of human desire or bias, provides a stable reality to what morality is; that is, it can give the status of "law." If an objective morality exists (in the form of moral law), then we can easily test law against it and know which laws we should have, which laws we should morally violate, which laws we should change. However, even if objective morality does exist, the situation is not that simple.

Objective morality may exist, but our confidence in being able to access it and know what comprises it is not absolute. The employment of King as an example in this discussion is possibly a bit facile. From our current historical perspective, it is easy to look back upon King, his thoughts, and his activism and say he was right to challenge the law. He was right that the law was unjust and discriminatory. However, it is important to remember that many people at the time did not agree and saw him as a mere scofflaw or worse. Consider a similar activist today engaging in civil disobedience. Many could see that person as a troublemaker or mere provocateur. But in decades to come, that person could become a great hero. Knowing whether such a person is a troublemaker or a hero today is more of a challenge. Consider Timothy Quill. In 1991, palliative physician Dr. Timothy Quill (1991) "stunned the medical community" (Connolly, 1998, p. 201) when he announced in the pages of *The New England Journal of Medicine* that he had aided, at her request, a terminally ill patient in ending her life by prescribing barbiturates. In 1991, physician-assisted suicide was legal nowhere in the United States. Thus, in the act itself, and especially in the public nature of this announcement, he was placing himself at legal risk. He explains his moral view as inclusive of an advocacy for control and dignity in patients' deaths. Yet, previous to this event, that was limited to legally sanctioned instances of withdrawal of life-sustaining treatment. But in crossing the line to *actively* contributing to the ending of a patient's life in this case, he refers to the value of his patient's independence, her fear of a lingering death, and his fear of the family dealing with a violent death. "I also felt strongly," wrote Quill (1991), "that I was setting her free to get the most out of the time she had left, and to maintain dignity and control on her own terms until her death" (p. 693). Yet, at the same time, he also expressed some uncertainty when he writes of her request "stretching" him profoundly and of an uneasy feeling from exploring boundaries. This uncertainty and emotional disturbance is to be expected and is likely a sign of a thoughtful, conscientious person in the midst of a novel and difficult decision. Thus, in his mind at least, he was acting morally yet contravening widely accepted medical ethics at the time as well as the law. Public opinion, the majority of the medical establishment, and the law would condemn his actions, yet he believed he was morally justified. As a result of this publication, he was investigated by authorities in Monroe County, New York. His case went before a grand jury, but the grand jury declined to indict. Today, physician-assisted suicide is legal in several states—though still not in the state of New York where Quill aided his patient. Quill (along with other physicians) was later involved in a suit against the state of New York claiming that the state's law prohibiting physician-assisted suicide violated the equal protection clause of the Fourteenth Amendment (*Vacco v. Quill*, 1997). The U.S. Supreme Court ruled against Quill in a unanimous decision.

Given the state of our moral discourse on physician-assisted suicide, it may still be reasonable to be unsure whether Quill was responding morally to a law that may be immoral in itself. That is a matter we are still working through in terms of our social ethics. But is a moral dissenter of law themselves thinking their act is moral enough? That, I believe, is not a question to which a general answer can be given. We have to consider the act in question and the thinking behind the act. What about when *you* face a situation like this? It is possible, though not likely, that the whole world is wrong while you are right. It is possible that you and a minority of others are right, while the majority is wrong. But it will ultimately come down to you, your reasoning, and your conscience. In class, I tell my students that I cannot, from the safety of a classroom, counsel them to break the law if they believe the law is immoral. That can only be their decision. You have to consider the values involved, the repercussions (legal and moral), and your own integrity and conscience. What is doing the (morally) right thing worth to you in this particular instance? Only you can answer that question.

FOSTERING INTERPERSONAL VIRTUES

"It is as natural to seek virtue and to avoid vice as to seek health and avoid disease."

—Dickinson (1909, p. 1626)

As noted previously, where law and morality most obviously intersect is in the context of actions that have a public effect, that involve others, their needs and interests. Educationally speaking, these concerns can in part be addressed through instruction in ethical theories based in principle: Kantian deontology, utilitarianism, and so forth. But arguably, that is not enough (Carr & Steutel, 1999; Curren, 1999; Fowers, 2005; Kupperman, 1999; Vanlaere & Gastmans, 2007). Ethics transcends mere rule following or even intellectual apprehension of right and wrong. Particularly, in relation to good nursing care, one needs as well "a moral inner attitude" of "depth of interest and the empathy [a] nurse has for patients" (Vanlaere & Gastmans, 2007, p. 760). Ethical character then requires a particular affect or attitude disposing one to do the right thing. One needs the correct motivation in order to inspire one to act, to follow what the intellect tells one is right, and also to act properly in mundane or emergency situations without in-depth analysis. As expressed rather dramatically by Carr and Steutel (1999), "In the absence of properly ordered affect, any explicit formal or informal teaching of moral rules or principles could only be so much wasted toil" (p. 250). Thus, a proper moral education should address not just the intellectual apprehension of right and wrong but the underlying character of the developing nurse as well. In terms of "fostering interpersonal virtues," there are three elements we must consider as indicated by the three terms in that titular concept.

Virtue theorists sometimes divide virtues into the categories of self-regarding virtues and other-regarding (interpersonal) virtues (Slote, 1999). Self-regarding virtues, such as prudence, resourcefulness, and temperance (especially in regard to personal affairs), are those that primarily involve one's actions as they affect oneself, toward advancing one's own well-being. Sometimes such attitudes or dispositions are perceived as selfish, that ethics should primarily or only be about our actions toward others. But this need not be the case. Indeed, Provision 5 of the *American Nurses Association's Code of Ethics* focuses squarely on virtues such as these. Most of the principle-based theories focus on other-regarding acts, but even they note the distinction and acknowledge some limited importance of ethical action toward oneself. The second version of Kant's categorical imperative, for example, asserts an obligation to treat everyone, even oneself, always as an end, never as a means only (Kant, 2012). And the principle of utility is typically interpreted as including one's own happiness in any hedonic calculation equal to all others (Bentham, 1988; Mill, 1910). Though, these are quite limited appeals to self-regarding ethics. Virtue ethics more emphatically weighs the value of both self-regarding and other-regarding ethics and also coheres more closely with our natural relations with others. Common principle-based theories like Kantian deontology and utilitarianism include an emphasis on impartiality in moral judgment and action. For much of public action, impartiality can be an important and desirable value, cultivating justice and equality and restraining unfairness and bias. However, much of our lives occur at the intersection of the public and the personal where cold impartiality is intuitively problematic. Impartiality, strictly interpreted, would have us treat our friends, family, coworkers, and so forth the same as any stranger. And there may be instances in which we should do that. For example, in a time of rationing it may be proper not to be partial regarding personal relationships. However, for most of our daily lives and activities, it not only makes sense to treat others in regard to their relationships with us, but it would be socially disastrous to do otherwise. Virtue ethics provides a clearer foundation for understanding the morality of doing so.

Virtues are character dispositions, meaning that they are elements of who we are as persons, expressed through affect and attitude influencing behavior, inclinations, and temperament. A person of good character will want to do what is moral, enjoy doing what is moral, and will know how to determine the moral choice in a difficult situation. Aristotle defines four types of character. The highest form is the virtuous. A virtuous person typically does what is moral without need to appeal to complex argument or principle but can do so when needed. The virtuous person has inclinations to do what is right and happily follows those inclinations. The second type, the continent person, also often does the right thing but does not have as many virtues as the virtuous person. Thus, they are often tempted to act improperly or immorally, but will usually resist temptation. The incontinent person, the third type, experiences immoral temptations, like the continent person, but unlike the continent, the incontinent will often give in to temptation. And lastly, the vicious person lacks many, if not all, virtues. Their character is instead comprised mostly of vices. Thus, the vicious person is drawn toward the immoral through personal inclinations. The vicious person will typically be inclined to and make the immoral choice. In moral education, the virtuous character is typically seen as the ideal to achieve. We want people who not only choose to do the right thing but are inclined to and want to do the right thing because it is right. This grounding of character in good motivation better ensures moral action than merely instruction in moral rules or even cognitive understanding of right and wrong. But even a continent character is desirable. A moral person is sometimes tempted by improper urges, but it is also seen as a strength of character to resist this temptation. In the moral education of nursing students, in addition to theoretical and cognitive understanding of ethics, these states of character should also be aimed for.

What virtues need to be taught? Which character traits qualify as virtues is a long-standing debate in the study of virtue ethics. Two types of answers are typically provided in response. First, virtue theorists often identify virtues as character traits manifested by a virtuous person (Lachman, 2009). For this reason, moral role models or moral exemplars are often utilized as examples to emulate. Critics will sometimes point out the circularity of this approach in that virtues are defined as the qualities of a virtuous person and a virtuous person is described as virtuous due to the virtues they possess. So, second, virtue is also tied to some teleological goal. Aristotle related virtues in terms of achieving what he considered the goal of human life: *Eudaimonia*. This term is often translated as happiness, but many scholars instead prefer to translate it as "flourishing," as that concept seems more consistent with Aristotle's broader theoretical view of human life. What this means, then, is that one's goal in life is to flourish or achieve one's full potential as a human being. Virtues, then, are those character traits that aid one in flourishing in one's life. Aristotle's approach here is arguably highly abstract and debatable in terms of a theory of human nature. Thus, virtues since have been defined in various different manners, resulting in many contrasting lists of what traits count as virtues.

One recent and promising attempt to resolve these conflicts is from ethicist Alasdair MacIntyre (2007). MacIntyre, instead of being mired in contentious theories of human nature, narrowed and particularized the grounding of virtues in relation to what he calls "practice." By practice he means a socially established, self-regulated cooperative activity aimed toward achieving particular goods. Virtues, then, can be more clearly, specifically, and objectively defined as those traits that help one achieve the goods of a specific practice. Thus, if nursing can be understood as a practice, and I think it can, then in identifying the specific goods of nursing one can then clearly identify the virtues needed to achieve those goods. Given the interpersonal essence of nursing practice, interpersonal virtues such as generosity, conscientiousness, and veracity are essential. In this way, now we can identify the meaning and purpose of virtue and also objectively identify and justify what traits qualify as virtues.

It is thus necessary to foster these interpersonal virtues in students being prepared for the important and sensitive work of nursing. Unfortunately, little is known about the effectiveness of pedagogical techniques for character development and virtue education and more research in this area is needed if we are going to confidently recommend effective techniques (Carr & Steutel, 1999; Kristjánsson, 2013). Although there have been some valuable studies toward these ends, more still needs to be done (Arthur & Carr, 2013). Nevertheless virtue theorists and moral educators have identified several techniques with the potential to transmit and instill the virtues needed for good citizenship, good humanity, or, potentially, good nursing.

First, drawing on ancient insights from Aristotle, a commonly recommended teaching technique is the use of role models in the form of moral exemplars (Blum, 1994; Carr & Steutel, 1999; Fowers, 2005; Lachman, 2009; Sherman, 1999; Vanlaere & Gastmans, 2007). Role models can be well-known virtuous contemporary or historical figures such as Albert Schweitzer, Oskar Schindler, or Florence Nightingale (Blum, 1994; Lachman, 2009). And thus study of such historical figures can have value not just for historical knowledge but to help develop characters through emulating these persons. The technique of role models provides in-depth instruction "through the narratives, stories, and drama of someone who has been there, faced the music and made choices" (Sherman, 1999, p. 37). Role models can also be those with whom students have daily interaction like faculty. As Fowers (2005) contends, the most important form of moral education is from the behavior of faculty themselves, expressing what is important and what is of value through their very actions. Whether the role model put forth is a famous contemporary personality, an historical figure, or someone familiar to the student, what is pedagogically important is that the role model be someone "concrete and meaningful to the individual" (Sherman, 1999, p. 36). A role model who is abstract and alien from the experience and lifeworld of the student will likely not have a meaningful effect. Although it is possible that exposure to a somewhat alien role model could expand the student's world and even deepen their moral outlook.

Vanlaere and Gastmans (2007) advocate a particular form of role modeling in nursing ethics education that they refer to as critical companionship. More fully developed by Titchen (2000), critical companionship is a form of mentorship "guiding student nurses to the completion of their clinical internship" (Vanlaere & Gastmans, 2007, p. 763). The student's mentor or critical companion guides her in evolving critical reflection on practice. Ultimately, critical companionship encourages nurses to develop as person-centered, evidence-based practitioners by combining "the expressive and intuitive processes of relationships and creativity with rational processes of analysis, critique and evaluation of practice and its knowledge" (Vanlaere & Gastmans, 2007, p. 764). A review of this technique in practice demonstrated that nurses developed a self-reflective, person-centered approach (Wright & Titchen, 2003).

Some nursing programs offer a course or courses dedicated to instruction in ethics, while others teach ethics absent a dedicated course but instead claim to "thread" ethics education throughout the curriculum (Grady et al., 2008). There is some debate as to which is the better method, but I would contend that both are necessary. Employing a threaded approach exclusively risks debasing the study of ethics and corroding the expertise of ethicists by assuming that any professional with sufficient experience qualifies as an expert in ethics. Employing a dedicated course approach exclusively neglects the importance of faculty role models that Fowers (2005) identifies.

A second commonly cited technique for teaching virtue and improving character is the use of various forms of fiction and literature (Carr & Steutel, 1999; Kupperman, 1999; Nussbaum, 1995). Fictional characters can also function as role models. In addition, novels and other forms of fiction and literature can "strengthen the moral imagination" and explore the morality of character in challenging situations (Kupperman, 1999, p. 207). Nussbaum (1995) advocates especially for the use of novels as the depth of detail of the novel form allows for extensive development of character and analysis of response to difficult events. However, other forms of fictional, narrative expression, such as film, have the potential to provide a fruitful exploration of character and provide as well of possible role model. For example, the 1997 HBO film *Miss Evers' Boys* provides an intriguing character study in the context of a relatively powerless person attempting to maintain moral integrity in the face of powerful institutional constraints. The central character of Miss Evers (Alfre Woodard), a nurse involved in the infamous Tuskegee Syphilis Study from its beginning until its end, displays at first quite praiseworthy virtues for a nurse. However, she is challenged to maintain her own moral integrity in the face of various forces. First is the moral orientation of obedience to physicians in which she was trained. It became clear to her that despite being taught to always follow doctors' orders, those orders were not always morally acceptable. Second are the institutional constraints placed upon her in working within the federal government. Her character manifests conflicts between self-regarding virtues such as moral integrity and other-regarding (interpersonal) virtues displayed in scenes in which she struggles to get along with her superiors and fulfill requests of theirs that she finds morally troubling. She may or may not qualify as a true moral exemplar, but her struggles and difficulties as a person and a nurse can provoke important introspection on the potential conflicts one could face in the context of institutional constraints.

A third commonly cited technique for teaching virtues is the use of case studies (Fowers, 2005; Sherman, 1999). The use of case studies may more typically be perceived as a tool for teaching ethics from a more cognitive, theoretic, or principle-based perspective. A case study presents a real or fictional situation in which a difficult moral issue arises. The goal then is, through discussion, application of theory and principle, possibly appeal to precedent and applicable codes of ethics, to reach the most morally justifiable resolution. However, in the collective practice of investigating a case study, both self-regarding and interpersonal virtues can be cultivated. Working with others, taking into account the thoughts and perspectives of others, the realization of relevant perspectives and opinions different from one's own, and reaching a reasonable conclusion through dialectical reasoning can help instill and foster interpersonal virtues like open-mindedness, tolerance, patience, courtesy, docility, gratitude, flexibility, and veracity. The cognitive aspect of case study pedagogy is also relevant to the teaching of virtue. In Aristotle's structure of virtue ethics, one unique and uniquely important virtue is practical wisdom. The virtues mentioned so far in this section fall under the category of moral virtues. Moral virtues are distinctive as being learned through habit and repetition. In the words of Aristotle, "states of character arise out of like activities" (Aristotle, 1941, p. 953/1103b 21–22). In other words, we become honest by doing honest acts; we become courteous by doing courteous acts. Repetition works from the outside in, as the acts develop into dispositions. Practical wisdom is a different kind of virtue, an intellectual virtue. And according to Aristotle, as an intellectual virtue, practical wisdom is learned not through habit and repetition but with a more cognitive approach through intellectual study. Practical wisdom refers to the ability to apply reason to moral problems. The proper, moral attitude or affect, as already noted, is needed for virtuous character. But in order to consistently act morally, more than the intention or inclination to act morally is needed. The ability to take complex situations into account and reach a reasonable conclusion consistent with moral character is also necessary, "a reasoned and true state or capacity to act with regard to human goods" (Aristotle, 1941, p. 1027/1140b 20–22). Aristotle uses the metaphor of an archer in which the right choice is the bull's-eye. Moral virtue provides the inclination to hit the bull's-eye, but practical wisdom provides the aim. Without practical wisdom, moral virtues, no matter how well intended, can miss the mark.

SUMMARY

Many acts are both moral and legal. Some are both immoral and illegal. But some are moral while illegal and others immoral while legal. Most actions people perform in their daily lives likely qualify as both legal and moral. As discussed, some acts like theft, murder, and assault are largely considered both illegal and immoral. As noted earlier, more research is needed to increase our knowledge as to the best techniques for ethics education. The techniques outlined here are commonly used and seem commonsensical. Indeed, they may even be seen as trivial because they appear so simple and "no more than glorified common sense" (Carr & Steutel, 1999, p. 253). However, that itself may reflect a strength of the virtue approach. The pedagogical techniques appear to be common sense because the virtue approach so clearly reflects the reality of our moral situation and the nature of moral development. Nursing faculty need to reflect on how to best incorporate applied nursing ethics education in their respective curricula as it is indeed needed.

CRITICAL ELEMENTS TO CONSIDER

- Law and morality are both weighty normative systems.
- According to one theory of the law, natural law theory, laws must be moral themselves either to be laws at all or to be proper or legitimate laws.
- According to another theory of the law, legal positivism, laws do not have to be moral themselves to be legitimate laws. Law and morality are completely distinct and separate normative systems.
- Even under the theory of legal positivism, a general moral obligation to follow the law can be conceived according to the fair play argument.
- Even accepting the fair play argument, not all laws are equally legitimate. One can (and perhaps should) defy and/or work to change a law which is unfair or discriminatory.
- Generally speaking, morality has moral dominance over the law. That is, morality is more foundational and fundamental and should be followed when the two conflict.
- Although morality has normative dominance, there may be cases, when considering real-world situations and consequences, in which following the law instead of morality might be justified. It is up to the moral agent to determine in that case what is most important and what is worth risking.

Helpful Resources

- A brief video discussing the distinction between law and morality: https://www.youtube.com/watch?v=T94agavDVUw
- A video explaining Jürgen Habermas' concept of the public sphere and applying those ideas to the contemporary context of the internet: https://www.youtube.com/watch?v=R1K46oK3xTU
- A discussion/debate on natural law theory vs. legal positivism between University of Chicago Law School philosopher of law Brian Leiter and Yale Law School professor Scott Shapiro: https://www.youtube.com/watch?v=V51588_U5nw

References

Aristotle. (1941). Nicomachean ethics (R. Mckeon, Trans.). In R. Mckeon (Ed.), *The basic works of Aristotle.* New York, NY: Random House.

Arthur, J., & Carr, D. (2013). Character in learning for life: A virtue-ethical rationale for recent research on moral and values education. *Journal of Beliefs & Values, 34*(1), 26–35. doi:10.1080/13617672.2013.759343

Augustine. (1973). On free will. In A. Hyman & J. J. Walsh (Eds.), *Philosophy in the middle ages: The Christian, Islamic, and Jewish traditions* (pp. 33–64). Indianapolis, IN: Hackett Publishing Company.

Bentham, J. (1988). *The principles of morals and legislation.* Amherst, NY: Prometheus Books.

Bix, B. (2002). Natural law theory: The modern tradition. In J. L. Coleman & S. Shapiro (Eds.), *Oxford handbook of jurisprudence and philosophy of law* (pp. 61–103). Oxford, UK: Oxford University Press.

Bix, B. (2010). Natural law theory. In D. Patterson (Ed.), *A companion to philosophy of law and legal theory* (pp. 211–227). Oxford, UK: Blackwell Publishing.

Blackstone, W. (2016). *The Oxford edition of Blackstone's: Commentaries on the laws of England: Book I: Of the rights of persons.* Oxford, UK: Oxford University Press.

Blum, L. A. (1994). *Moral perception and particularity.* Cambridge, UK: Cambridge University Press.

Carr, D., & Steutel, J. (1999). The virtue approach to moral education. In D. Carr & J. Steutel (Eds.), *Virtue ethics and moral education* (pp. 241–255). New York, NY: Routledge.

Centers for Disease Control and Prevention. (2011, April 22). *State smoke-free laws for worksites, restaurant, and bars: United States, 2000-2010.* Retrieved from https://www.cdc.gov/mmwr/preview/mmwrhtml/mm6015a2.htm

Clifford, W. K. (1999). The ethics of belief. In T. Madigan (Ed.), *The ethics of belief and other essays* (pp. 70–96). Amherst, MA: Prometheus.

Coleman, J. L., & Leiter, B. (2010). Legal positivism. In D. Patterson (Ed.), *A companion to philosophy of law and legal theory* (pp. 228–248). Oxford, UK: Blackwell Publishing.

Connelly, R. J. (1998). Death with dignity: Fifty years of soul-searching. *Journal of Religion and Health, 37*(3), 195–213. doi:10.1023/A:1022981721537

Cruzan v. Director, MDH, 497 U.S. 261 (1990).

Curren, R. (1999). Cultivating the intellectual and moral virtues. In D. Carr & J. Steutel (Eds.), *Virtue ethics and moral education* (pp. 67–81). New York, NY: Routledge.

Dickinson, G. L. (1909). *The Greek view of life* [Kindle DX version]. Staten Island, NY: Project Gutenberg/College of Staten Island Library.

Finnis, J. (2011). *Natural law and natural rights.* Oxford, UK: Oxford University Press.

Fowers, B. J. (2005). *Virtue and psychology: Pursuing excellence in ordinary practices.* Washington, DC: American Psychological Association.

Gonzalez, R. (2019, June 20). *New Alabama law permits church to hire its own police force.* Retrieved from https://www.npr.org/2019/06/20/734591147/new-alabama-law-permits-church-to-hire-its-own-police-force

Government Highway Safety Association. (2019). *Seat belts.* Retrieved from https://www.ghsa.org/state-laws/issues/Seat-Belts

Grady, C., Danis, M., Soeken, K. L., O'Donnell, P., Taylor, C., Farrar, A., & Ulrich, C. M. (2008). Does ethics education influence the moral action of practicing nurses and social workers? *American Journal of Bioethics, 8*(4), 4–11. doi:10.1080/15265160802166017

Habermas, J. (2000). *The inclusion of the other: Studies in political theory.* Cambridge, MA: MIT Press.

Hart, H. L. A. (1958). Legal and moral obligation. In A. I. Melden (Ed.), *Essays in moral philosophy* (pp. 82–107). Seattle, WA: University of Washington Press.

In re Quinlan, 355 A.2d 647 (N.J. Super. Ct. 1976).

In Re the conservatorship of Helga M. Wanglie, No. PX-91-283, 4th Judicial District (Dist. Ct., Probate Ct. Div., Hennepin County, Minn. 1991).

Insurance Institute for Highway Safety. (2019, May). *Motorcycles.* Retrieved from https://www.iihs.org/topics/motorcycles#helmet-laws?topicName=Motorcycles

Kant, I. (2012). In M. Gregor & J. Timmerman (Trans. Ed.), *Groundwork of the metaphysics of morals.* Cambridge, UK: Cambridge University Press.

King, M. L., Jr. (2018s). Letter from a Birmingham jail. In S. M. Cahn (Ed.), *Exploring philosophy: An introductory anthology* (pp. 499–511). New York, NY: Oxford University Press.

Kristjánsson, K. (2013). Ten myths about character, virtue and virtue education: Plus three well-founded misgivings. *British Journal of Education Studies, 61*(3), 269–287. doi:10.1080/00071005.2013.778386

Kupperman, J. J. (1999). Virtues, characters, and moral dispositions. In D. Carr & J. Steutel (Eds.), *Virtue ethics and moral education* (pp. 199–209). New York, NY: Routledge.

Lachman, V. D. (2009). *Ethical challenges in health care: Developing your moral compass.* New York, NY: Springer Publishing Company.

Luban, D. (1988). *Lawyers and justice: An ethical study.* Princeton, NJ: Princeton University Press.

MacIntyre, A. (2007). *After virtue: A study in moral theory* (3rd ed.). Notre Dame, IN: Notre Dame University Press.

Mentovich, A., & Zeev-wolf, M. (2018). Law and moral order: The influence of legal outcomes on moral judgment. *Psychology, Public Policy, and Law, 24*(4), 489–502. doi:10.1037/law0000175

Mill, J. S. (1910). *Utilitarianism, liberty, and representative government.* New York, NY: E. P. Dutton.

Nussbaum, M. (1995). *Poetic justice: The literary imagination and public life.* Boston, MA: Beacon Press.

Planned Parenthood v. Casey, 505 U.S. 833 (1992).

Quill, T. (1991). Death and dignity: A case of individualized decision making. *New England Journal of Medicine, 324*, 691–694. doi:10.1056/NEJM199103073241010

Rawls, J. (2001). Legal obligation and the duty of fair play. In S. Freeman (Ed.), *John Rawls: Collected papers* (pp. 117–129). Cambridge, MA: Harvard University Press.

Roe v. Wade, 410 U.S. 113 (1973).

Sherman, N. (1999). Character development and Aristotelian virtue. In D. Carr & J. Steutel (Eds.), *Virtue ethics and moral education* (pp. 35–48). New York, NY: Routledge.

Slote, M. (1999). Self-regarding and other-regarding virtues. In D. Carr & J. Steutel (Eds.), *Virtue ethics and moral education* (pp. 95–105). New York, NY: Routledge.

Solic, P. (2015). Private matter or public crisis? Defining and responding to domestic violence. *Origins: Current Events in Historical Perspective, 8*(10). Retrieved from http://origins.osu.edu/article/private-matter-or -public-crisis-defining-and-responding-domestic-violence

Titchen, A. (2000). Professional craft knowledge in patient-centred nursing and facilitation of its development (Doctoral dissertation). Oxford, UK: University of Oxford.

Vacco v. Quill, 521 U.S. 793 (1997).

Vanlaere, L., & Gastmans, C. (2007). Ethics in nursing education: Learning to reflect on care practices. *Nursing Ethics, 14*(6), 758–766. doi:10.1177/0969733007082116

Washington v. Glucksberg, 521 U.S. 702 (1997).

Weinreb, L. L. (2004). A secular theory of natural law. *Fordham Law Review, 72*(6), 2287–2300. Retrieved from http://web.b.ebscohost.com.proxy.library.csi.cuny.edu/ehost/pdfviewer/ pdfviewer?vid=2&sid=6ad32dbd-68de-4d5a-97a8-b5712d8a0bab%40pdc-v-sessmgr01

Wright, J., & Titchen, A. (2003). Critical companionship: Part 2: using the framework. *Nursing Standard, 18*(10), 33–38. doi:10.7748/ns2003.11.18.10.33.c3506

Index

Printed in the United States
by Baker & Taylor Publisher Services